Reemergence of Established Pathogens in the 21st Century

Emerging Infectious Diseases of the 21st Century

Series Editor: I. W. Fong

Professor of Medicine, University of Toronto
Head of Infectious Diseases, St. Michael's Hospital

Recent volumes in this series

INFECTIONS AND THE CARDIOVASCULAR SYSTEM: New Perspectives
Edited by I. W. Fong

REEMERGENCE OF ESTABLISHED PATHOGENS IN THE 21ST CENTURY
Edited by I. W. Fong and Karl Drlica

A Continuation Order Plan is available for this series. A continuation order will bring delivery of each new volume immediately upon publication. Volumes are billed only upon actual shipment. For further information, please contact the publisher.

Reemergence of Established Pathogens in the 21st Century

Edited by

I. W. Fong

University of Toronto, St. Michael's Hospital
Toronto, Ontario, Canada

and

Karl Drlica

The Public Health Research Institute
Newark, New Jersey

Kluwer Academic / Plenum Publishers
New York, Boston, Dordrecht, London, Moscow

Library of Congress Cataloging-in-Publication Data

Reemergence of established pathogens in the 21st century / Ignatius W. Fong and Karl Drlica.
p. cm.—(Emerging infectious diseases of the 21st century)
Includes bibliographical references and index.
ISBN 0-306-47500-6
1. Drug resistance in microorganisms. 2. Communicable diseases—Epidemiology. I.
Fong, I. W. (Ignatius W.) II. Drlica, Karl. III. Series.
[DNLM: 1. Communicable Diseases, Emerging—etiology. 2. Communicable Diseases,
Emerging—drug therapy. WA 110 R327 2003]
QR177 .R446 2003
616.9–dc21

2002040669

ISBN: 0-306-47500-6

© 2003 Kluwer Academic/Plenum Publishers
233 Spring Street, New York, NY 10013

http://www.wkap.nl/

10   9   8   7   6   5   4   3   2   1

Permissions for books published in Europe: *permissions@wkap.nl*
Permissions for books published in the United States of America: *permissions@wkap.com*

Printed in the United States of America

Contributors

Rafael Cantón Servicio de Microbiología, Hospital Ramón y Cajal, Madrid, Spain

Karl Drlica Public Health Research Institute, 225 Warren St., Newark, NJ 07103

Ignatius W. Fong Chief of Infectious Disease, St. Michael's Hospital, University of Toronto, Toronto, Ontario, Canada, M5B 1W8

Nina E. Glass Centers for Disease Control and Prevention, Atlanta, GA

Gilbert Greub Unité des Rickettsies, CNRS UMR 6020, IFR48 Faculté de Médecine, Université de la Méditerranée 27, Boulevard Jean Moulin 13385 Marseille, France

Kevin C. Kain Center for Travel and Tropical Medicine, University Health Network, Toronto General Hospital, Toronto, Ontario, Canada

Maria Kolia Research Fellow in Infectious Disease, St. Michael's Hospital, University of Toronto, Canada

Malak Kotb Department of Surgery and Microbiology and Immunology, University of TN, Memphis, TN 38163, and Veterans Affairs Medical Center, Research Service, Memphis TN 38104

Mona Loufty Fellow in Infectious Diseases, Department of Medicine, University of Toronto, Ontario, Canada

Donald E. Low Department of Microbiology, Mount Sinai Hospital, Toronto, Ontario, Canada, M5G 1X5

José L. Martínez Departaments de Biotecnología Microbiana, Centro Nacional de Biotecnología (CSIC), Madrid, Spain

Allison McGeer Department of Microbiology, Mount Sinai Hospital and the University of Toronto, Toronto, Ontario, Canada, M5G 1X5

Maria Morosini Servicio de Microbiología, Hospital Ramón y Cajal, Madrid, Spain

Barbara E. Murray Center for the Study of Emerging and Re-Emerging Pathogens, Division of Infectious Diseases, Department of Internal Medicine, and Department of Microbiology and Molecular Genetics, The University of Texas Medical School, Houston, Texas

Esteban C. Nannini Center for the Study of Emerging and Re-Emerging Pathogens, Division of Infectious Diseases, Department of Internal Medicine, University of Texas Medical School, Houston, Texas

Anna Norrby-Teglund Center for Infectious Medicine, Department of Medicine, Karlinska Institutet, Huddinge University Hospital, Stockholm, Sweden

Didier Raoult Unité des Rickettsies, CNRS UMR 6020 IFR48 Faculté de Médecine, Université de la Méditerranée 27, Boulevard Jean Moulin 13385 Marseille, France

Renee Ridzon Chief of Outbreak Investigations Section, Division of Tuberculosis Elimination, Center's for Disease Control and Prevention, Atlanta, Georgia

Philip Spradling Medical Epidemiologist, Varicella Activity, Child Vaccine-Preventable Diseases Branch, Centers for Disease Control and Prevention, Atlanta, Georgia

Cynthia Whitney Respiratory Diseases Branch, Division of Bacterial and Mycotic Diseases, National Center for Infectious Diseases, Centers for Disease Control and Prevention, Atlanta, Georgia

Xilin Zhao Public Health Research Institute, 225 Warren St., Newark, NJ 07103

Preface

In the closing decade of the last century, we saw warnings that infectious diseases will require much more attention from patients and physicians in the 21st century. Recently discovered diseases such as AIDS pose a major threat to the population at large, and to that threat has been added the re-emergence of established pathogens, microbes that were readily treatable in the past. Since infectious diseases already play a major role in the burden of illness and mortality, health care providers and planners are worried.

A large proportion of the problem is man-made, arising mainly from the unnecessary overuse of antimicrobials in hospital and community settings and from the agricultural misuse of the agents in animal feed. A consequence has been a dramatic increase in resistant strains of bacteria that were considered conquerable several decades ago. Community infections caused by multi-resistant pneumococci serve as an example. These organisms were readily treated with penicillin, but now the spread of penicillin-resistant *Streptococcus pneumoniae* from continent to continent is becoming a worldwide problem. This is a major concern because pneumococcal infections are common in the community, being the leading cause of pneumonia, sinusitis, and meningitis. Resistant bacteria in hospitals are also becoming more prevalent. We have become accustomed to hearing about methicillin-resistant *Staphylococcus aureus* (MRSA) and vancomycin-resistant enterococci (VRE), but now we have to be concerned about multidrug-resistant coliform bacteria and pseudomonads. The potential impact is enormous, as it involves expensive infection control measures, longer hospital stays, increased overall health care costs, increased morbidity, and potentially greater mortality. It also involves expensive and potentially toxic new agents, if we are lucky enough to find some (bringing new compounds to market is increasingly difficult and expensive). Parasites and fungal infections will give us the same problems. For example, chloroquine-resistant *Plasmodium falciparum* is now present in most countries where malaria is endemic.

Re-emergence of established pathogens can also be driven by increases in virulence. An example is the resurgence of severe invasive group A streptococcal infections that result in a dreaded *fasciitis* ("flesh-eating disease" as labeled by the lay press), toxic shock syndrome, and septicemia. Another is trench fever, a disease associated with the great world wars. It is now making a reappearance (or being recognized) among the inner city homeless population.

   With this book we have tried to provide the specialist and trainee in microbiology, infectious disease, infection control, and epidemiology with an up-to-date and authoritative review of problematic infections that we are facing in the new century. We hope that the work fosters a better understanding of the issues and new ideas for preventing and controlling infectious diseases.

I. W. FONG AND K. DRLICA

Contents

Section II

Resistant Bacteria and Resurgence

Chapter 3

**Antibiotic-Resistant *Streptococcus pneumoniae*: Implications
for Management in the 21st Century**
Cynthia G. Whitney and Nina E. Glass

Chapter 4

MRSA in the 21st Century: Emerging Challenges
Ignatius W. Fong and Maria Kolia

Chapter 5

Vancomycin-Resistant Enterococci
Esteban C. Nannini and Barbara E. Murray

Chapter 6

Multi-Resistant *Enterobacteriaceae* in Hospital Practice
Maria I. Morosini, Rafael Cantón, and José L. Martínez

              5.2.1. Antibiotic Policies 224
     6. New Agents on the Horizon 231
     References.. 232

Chapter 7

Multidrug-Resistant Tuberculosis
Philip Spradling and Renee Ridzon

     1. Overview 245
        1.1. History 245
        1.2. Definition 246
        1.3. Public Health Importance 247
     2. Epidemiology 248
        2.1. Domestic 248
        2.2. International 250
     3. Production and Perpetuation of MDRTB 256
        3.1. Mechanisms of Resistance 256
        3.2. Clinical Errors 256
        3.3. Host Factors 257
        3.4. Transmission and Outbreaks 258
        3.5. Programmatic and Institutional Factors 259
        3.6. Substandard Antituberculosis Drugs 261
     4. Diagnosis 261
        4.1. Risk Factors for MDRTB 261
        4.2. Drug Susceptibility Tests 262
        4.3. New Methodologies for Rapid Detection of Drug Resistance 263
     5. Treatment 264
        5.1. General Principles 264
        5.2. Second-Line Antituberculosis Drugs, Toxicity, and
             Cross-Resistance 265
        5.3. Surgical Intervention 270
        5.4. Novel Therapies 271
        5.5. Treatment Outcomes 272
     6. HIV Infection and MDRTB 272
        6.1. Impact of HIV on the Epidemiology of MDRTB 272
        6.2. Impact on Diagnosis and Treatment 275
        6.3. Impact on Treatment Outcomes 277
     7. Prevention 277
        7.1. Provider-Based 277
        7.2. Institutional and Program-Based 278
        7.3. Treatment of Persons Exposed to MDRTB 279
        7.4. BCG and Vaccines 280
     8. Summary 281
     References.. 282

Chapter 8

**Controlling Antibiotic Resistance: Strategies Based on the
Mutant Selection Window**
Karl Drlica and Xilin Zhao

Section III

Resistant Parasitic Infections

Chapter 9

Drug-Resistant Malaria
Mona R. Loutfy and Kevin C. Kain

Section I

The Changing Spectrum of Bacterial Infections

1

Severe Invasive Group A Streptococcal Infections

Anna Norrby-Teglund, Allison McGeer,
Malak Kotb, and Donald E. Low

1. INTRODUCTION

Emerging infections can be defined as those diseases that have newly appeared in the population, or have existed but are rapidly increasing in incidence or geographic range. Reasons for disease emergence may include changes in the pathogen, the host, or the environment. The dynamics may be sufficiently complex that the occurrence appears inexplicable. The reemergence of severe group A streptococcal (GAS) infections is an excellent example of an emerging, or more correctly reemerging, infectious disease.

Severe GAS infections have long been recognized and the history of GAS disease has been characterized by periodic changes in severity of disease. Streptococcal infections were recognized by Greek physicians in the 5th century. Sydenham described the disease as "febris scarlatina" as early as 1664 (Katz & Morens, 1992). This description clearly differentiated this disease from measles and other rashes, which allowed outbreaks of scarlet fever to be documented throughout the world. The most severe forms of streptococcal disease were well known long before the discovery of the bacterium. Hippocrates recorded epidemic erysipelas and clinical descriptions of a disease that we would clinically refer to today as necrotizing fasciitis (NF) (Descamps et al., 1994).

In the United States during the mid part of the last century there was a dramatic decline in the occurrence and mortality of scarlet fever (Quinn, 1982). This occurred without an associated decrease in pharyngitis due to GAS and with continuing severe infections and their sequelae in developing countries (Kaplan, 1993). This decline in severity began in the 1930s, before the advent of antibiotics for the treatment of streptococcal disease, and continued up to and including the 1970s (Kaplan, 1996). The mortality declined from 72% in the pre-antibiotic era to 7–27% (Duma et al., 1969; Hable et al., 1973; Keefer et al., 1937). However in the early 1980s reports began to appear that described not only

Reemergence of Established Pathogens in the 21st Century
Edited by Fong and Drlica, Kluwer Academic/Plenum Publishers, New York, 2003

an increased mortality due to GAS bacteremia (35–48%), but also anecdotal reports emphasizing a rapidly fatal outcome in bacteremic patients presenting with shock (Goepel et al., 1980). This syndrome has been designated as the streptococcal toxic shock syndrome (STSS), and is commonly associated with specific M types (Gaworzewska & Colman, 1988; Hoge et al., 1993a; Martin & Hoiby, 1990; Schwartz et al., 1990; Stromberg et al., 1991).

In addition to the increase in STSS during the 1980s, there were increased reports of NF (Chelsom et al., 1994; Cone et al., 1987; Demers et al., 1993; Kaul et al., 1997; Stevens et al., 1989). The hallmark of NF is infection of the subcutaneous tissue and fascia that often results in necrosis with relative sparing of the underlying muscle. The diagnosis can be made if histopathology demonstrates both necrosis of superficial fascia and polymorphonuclear infiltrate and edema of the reticular dermis, subcutaneous fat, and superficial fascia. From 1992 to 1995, the annual incidence of NF increased 4-fold in Ontario, Canada from 0.85 per million population to 3.5 per million ($p < 0.001$) (Kaul et al., 1997).

2. MICROBIOLOGY

Streptococci are Gram-positive, catalase-negative facultatively anaerobic bacteria forming spherical or ovoid cells less than 2 μm in diameter. Streptococci are nutritionally fastidious, with variable nutritional requirements, and growth on complex media is enhanced by the addition of blood or serum. Glucose and other carbohydrates are metabolized fermentatively, and lactic acid is produced as the major metabolic end product. Gas is not produced as the result of glucose metabolism. Isolates of streptococci produce the enzyme leucine aminopeptidase, but production of pyrrolidonly arylamidase (PYR) is rare among streptococci, occurring only in isolates of group A streptococci (*Streptococcus pyogenes*) and some strains of *Streptococcus pneumoniae* (Ruoff, 1995). β-Hemolytic, bacitracin-susceptible, PYR-positive, large-colony-forming streptococci with Lancefield's group A antigen are included in the species *S. pyogenes*. The manifestations of GAS infections in humans are diverse in both clinical presentation and morbidity. Pharyngitis and impetigo are common childhood illnesses with few complications. Infrequently, GAS causes invasive disease, of which the most serious presentation is necrotizing soft-tissue infection with associated shock and multisystem organ failure.

3. PATHOGENESIS

GAS express numerous virulence factors, both surface-associated and secreted, which interact with immune cells and other factors of the host to promote colonization, growth, dissemination, and survival of the organism.

The surface-attached virulence factors, including among others hyaluronic acid capsule, M- and M-like proteins, Protein F1, C5a-peptidase, and α_2-macroglobulin binding protein, are pivotal in the primary stages of infection involving bacterial adherence, colonization, and evasion of phagocytosis (Boyle, 1995; Fischetti, 1989; Rasmussen et al.,

1999). Surface-associated streptococcal virulence factors interact with a variety of human proteins, such as immunoglobulins, fibronectin, fibrinogen, albumin, plasminogen, kininogen, complement factor C5a, and regulators of the complement system, thereby promoting attachment of the bacteria to host cells and tissue, as well as evasion of phagocytosis (Table 1.1).

The systemic effects seen in patients with severe invasive GAS infections, such as STSS and NF, are largely triggered by inflammatory mediators induced in response to microbial factors (Figure 1.1). The pro-inflammatory activity is mediated by both strepto-coccal cell wall components as well as secreted factors (Table 1.2). Peptidoglycan and

Table 1.1

Surface-Associated Virulence Factors of Group A Streptococci and their Major Human Ligands

Name	Human ligand(s)	Reference(s)
Hyaluronic acid capsule	CD44	Ashbaugh et al. (1998), Cywes et al. (2000), Dale et al. (1996), Husmann et al. (1997), Moses et al. (1997), Schrager et al. (1998), Wessels and Bronze (1994)
M-protein family:	Albumin,	Boyle (1995), Fischetti (1989), Navarre and
M/Emm	Fibrinogen	Schneewind (1999)
Mrp/FcrA	IgG, IgA	
Enn	Kininogen	
	Fibronectin	
	Factor H	
	Plasminogen	
	C4BP	
	CD46 (MCP)	
	N-CAM	
Protein F1/SfbI	Fibronectin	Boyle (1995), Cunningham (2000),
	Fibrinogen	Fischetti (1989), Navarre and Schneewind (1999)
Lipoteichoic acid	Fibronectin	Hasty et al. (1992), Simpson and Beachey (1983)
Fibronectin-binding protein FBP54	Fibronectin	Courtney et al. (1994, 1996)
Glyceraldehyde-3-phosphate dehydrogenase	Fibronectin Plasmin	Pancholi & Fischetti (1992) Winram & Lottenberg (1996)
Protein F2	Fibronectin	Jaffe et al. (1996)
Serum opacity factor/SfbII	Fibronectin	Courtney et al. (1999), Kreikemeyer et al. (1995), Rakonjac et al. (1995)
α-enolase	Plasminogen	Pancholi and Fischetti (1998)
C5a peptidase	Anaphylatoxin C5a	Ji et al. (1997), Wexler et al. (1985)
R28	Not defined	Stalhammar-Carlemalm et al. (1999)
Streptococcal protective antigen (Spa)	Not defined	Dale et al. (1999), McLellan et al. (2001)
Collagen-like protein (Scl) A and B	Not defined	Lukomski et al. (2000), Rasmussen and Bjorck (2001), Rasmussen et al. (2000)
α_2-macroglobulin-binding protein (GRAB)	α_2-macroglobulin	Rasmussen et al. (1999)
Streptococcal cystein protease/SpeB	Laminin Intergrins	Hytonen et al. (2001), Stockbauer et al. (1999)

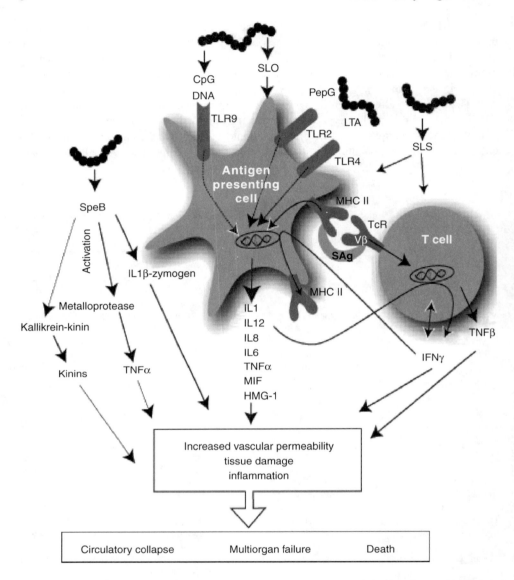

Figure 1.1. Induction of pro-inflammatory responses by group A streptococcal virulence factors. Lipoteichoic acid (LTA), peptidoglycan (PepG), and unmethylated CpG DNA activate antigen presenting cells through Toll-like receptors (TLR), to induce various cytokines, among others IL12 which promoted IFNγ production by T cells. Superantigens (SAg) interact with MHC class II molecules (MHC II) and the T cell receptor (TcR) to activate both cell types resulting in high production of cytokines. The cysteine protease, streptococcal pyrogenic exotoxin (SpeB), also promotes a pro-inflammatory response. Streptolysin O and S (SLO, SLS) are cytotoxic and pro-inflammatory.

lipoteichoic acid in the Gram-positive cell wall have been shown to activate leukocytes and trigger production of pro-inflammatory cytokines, including interleukin (IL)1β, IL6, IL8, IL12, tumour necrosis factor (TNF)α, and chemokines, as well as other inflammatory mediators, such as inducible nitric oxide synthetase (Bhakdi et al., 1991; Card et al., 1994;

Table 1.2
Streptococcal Virulence Factors with Pro-Inflammatory Activity

Name	Location	Proposed host receptor(s)	Reference(s)
Peptidoglycan	Cellbound	TLR2	Medzihtov and Janeway (2000), Sriskandan and Cohen (1999)
Lipoteichoic acid	Cellbound	TLR2, TLR4	Medzihtov and Janeway (2000), Sriskandan and Cohen (1999)
Superantigens	Secreted	TcR and MHC class II	Kotb (1995), McCormick et al. (2001)
Streptolysin O	Secreted	Not defined	Hackett and Stevens (1992), Shanley et al. (1996)
Unmethylated CpG DNA	Secreted	TLR9	Chatellier and Kotb (2000), Hemmi et al. (2000)
Cysteine Protease/SpeB	Secreted/cell bound	Cytokine-precursors and metalloproteases	Burns et al. (1996) Kapur et al. (1993a, 1993b)

Note: The table includes only receptors or substrates involved in the pro-inflammatory response.

Heumann et al., 1994; Keller et al., 1992; Mattsson et al., 1993; Morath et al., 2001; Riesenfeld-Orn et al., 1989; Standiford et al., 1994; Stylianos et al., 1991; Timmerman et al., 1993; Wang et al., 2000a, 2000b). Activation of innate immunity occurs via the Toll signalling pathway, in particular, Toll-like receptors (TLR) 2 and 4 (Figure 1.1 and Table 1.2) (Medzihtov & Janeway, 2000). Engagement of these TLRs triggers several intra-cellular signal transduction pathways, resulting in activation of the transcription nuclear factor (NF)-$\kappa\beta$, and subsequent induction of expression of pro-inflammatory genes (Medzihtov & Janeway, 2000).

The ability of purified peptidoglycan and lipoteichoic acid to trigger pathologic inflammatory conditions has been demonstrated in various animal models including exper-imental meningitis and septic shock (De Kimpe et al., 1995a, 1995b; Kengatharan et al., 1996; Spika et al., 1982; Tuomanen et al., 1985). In a rat model of septic shock, it was shown that although administration of lipoteichoic acid resulted in moderate hypotension, it did not trigger multiorgan failure and death (De Kimpe et al., 1995a, 1995b). However, when lipoteichoic acid was administered together with peptidoglycan a synergistic effect was achieved and the anaesthetized rats experienced shock and multiorgan failure (De Kimpe et al., 1995a, 1995b; Kengatharan et al., 1996).

Superantigens are by far the most potent streptococcal factors in induction of pro-inflammatory responses, and have therefore been implicated as crucial players in the pathogenesis of STSS and NF (Kotb, 1995; McCormick et al., 2001). There are several dif-ferent superantigens produced by GAS including streptococcal pyrogenic exotoxins (Spe) A, B, C, F, G, H, J (Kotb, 1995; Proft et al., 1999), streptococcal superantigen (SSA) (Mollick et al., 1993), and the streptococcal mitogenic exotoxin Z and Z-2 (Kamezawa et al., 1997; Proft et al., 1999). Most GAS strains express several different superantigens, although the repertoire of genes encoding superantigens varies between GAS strains (McCormick et al., 2001). It seems likely that several different superantigens can trigger invasive GAS diseases and that more than one superantigen are produced by the bacteria during the infection.

The "super" activity of superantigens is achieved by their ability to circumvent the normal rules for antigen processing and presentation, which results in excessive activation and release of inflammatory mediators. Superantigens interact, without prior cellular processing and outside the conventional antigen-binding cleft, with the relatively invariable Vβ-regions of the T cell receptor and MHC class II molecules on antigen presenting cells (APC) (Figure 1.1) (Marrack & Kappler, 1990). Each superantigen has a characteristic Vβ-specificity, and activates preferentially T cells expressing certain Vβ-elements, which may account for 5–20% of the naive T cell population. Interaction with MHC class II molecules differ between superantigens and preferential binding to certain alleles occur (reviewed in [Kotb, 1995; McCormick et al., 2001]). Interestingly, although there is significant difference in the primary sequence of the superantigens, they all share a common three-dimensional structure, which includes a folding of the superantigen into different domains, one amino-terminal hydrophobic β-barrel domain and a carboxy-terminal β-grasp domain (reviewed in Kotb, 1998). This common tertiary structure has been targeted in the development of superantigen antagonist (Arad et al., 2000; Visvanathan et al., 2001). The potential use of these antagonists as a novel therapeutic strategy is discussed in more detail below.

Another mediator of pro-inflammation is unmethylated oligonucleotides containing cytidine–phosphate–guanosine (CpG) motifs (Chatellier & Kotb, 2000; Klinman et al., 1996; Krieg, 1995). Unmethylated CpG DNA is exclusively found in prokaryotes, and has been shown to activate macrophages, dendritic cells, and B-cells, thereby triggering production of IL1, IL6, TNFα, IL12, IL10, and Th1 type of cytokines (reviewed by Heeg et al., 1998). Activation of cellular responses by CpG DNA was recently reported to be mediated by TLR9 (Figure 1.1 and Table 1.2) (Hemmi et al., 2000). Although streptococcal DNA generally have a low GC-content, certain important virulence genes, such as the genes encoding M-proteins, have been reported to have relatively high frequencies of immunostimulatory CpG motifs (Chatellier & Kotb, 2000).

The streptococcal cysteine protease, also called SpeB, is an important virulence factor with multiple activities, including superantigenic as well as proteolytic activity. By virtue of its proteolytic activity, SpeB modulates several host defense systems including the cytokine, kallikrein-kinin, coagulation, and complement system, and has therefore been suggested to contribute to tissue destruction and the systemic effects seen in fulminant GAS infections (Figure 1.1). Numerous physiologically important host proteins, including IL1β-precursor (Kapur et al., 1993a), metalloproteases (Burns et al., 1996), the extracellular matrix proteins vitronectin and fibronectin (Kapur et al., 1993b), and kininogens (Herwald et al., 1996), are substrates for SpeB. Cleavage of human IL1β-precursor and activation of metalloproteases that cleaves the precursor form of TNFα, result in generation of bioactive pro-inflammatory IL1β and TNFα (Burns et al., 1996). The pro-inflammatory response can be further augmented by SpeB-cleavage of kininogen resulting in release of pro-inflammatory kinins and consequently increased vascular permeability and inflammation (Herwald et al., 1996). SpeB is not only active as a secreted factor, but also in a cell-bound form with ability to function as an adhesin interacting with laminin and glycoproteins (Hytonen et al., 2001).

Several studies have supported a critical role of SpeB in the pathogenesis of GAS infections, including among others analyses of humoral immunity in patients with invasive GAS infections, where a lack of acute-phase antibodies were associated with invasive disease (Basma et al., 1999; Norrby-Teglund et al., 1994). Reduced morbidity and mortality of invasive GAS disease could be demonstrated in mice following immunization against SpeB (Kapur et al., 1994), administration of a protease inhibiting synthetic peptide (Bjorck et al., 1989), or genetic inactivation of the gene encoding SpeB (Hoe et al., 1999; Kuo et al., 1998; Lukomski et al., 1997; Svensson et al., 2000a). SpeB was also found to exacerbate the pro-inflammatory cytokine response and lung injury induced in rats by streptolysin O (SLO) and streptococcal cell wall fragments (Shanley et al., 1996). However, there are also several conflicting reports demonstrating either no effect of SpeB or even an association between SpeB expression and decreased virulence of the bacteria (Ashbaugh et al., 1998; Kansal et al., 2000; Raeder et al., 2000). One potential explanation for this could be that several important cell-associated virulence factors of GAS, including M-protein, protein H, and C5a peptidase, can be cleaved by SpeB resulting in either loss of, or altered properties of, essential virulence factors for the bacteria (Berge & Bjorck, 1995; Raeder et al., 1998). Thus, the role of SpeB in GAS pathogenesis is highly complex and remains to be defined.

Pro-inflammatory responses are also induced by SLO, which acts in synergy with both the superantigen SpeA (Hackett & Stevens, 1992) and as already mentioned above with SpeB (Shanley et al., 1996). In an experimental murine skin model, SLO-deficient strains were found to be attenuated in virulence, and although the bacteria disseminated in the animals, they were less likely to cause lethal infection than wild type strains (Limbago et al., 2000).

4. CLINICAL ENTITIES AND EPIDEMIOLOGY

The resurgence of severe disease was recognized not only by the increase in occurrence of STSS and NF, but also by an increase in severity and incidence of other clinical entities including GAS pneumonia and soft tissue infection (Low et al., 1997; Sharkawy et al., 2002).

4.1. STSS

STSS was defined by criteria established by The Working Group on Severe Streptococcal Infections (The Working Group on Severe Streptococcal Infections, 1993). Patients were considered to have STSS if they had hypotension in combination with two or more of the following: acute renal failure, coagulation abnormalities, liver abnormalities, acute respiratory distress syndrome, generalized rash and NF. Epidemiological studies revealed that the majority of these outbreaks, although reported from different countries and on different continents, were caused predominantly by GAS strains of M1 and M3 serotypes (Cockerill et al., 1997; Eriksson et al., 1999; Holm et al., 1992; Kaul et al., 1999; Kiska et al., 1997; Martin & Hoiby, 1990; Nakashima et al., 1997; Stromberg et al., 1991; Svensson et al., 2000b; Upton et al., 1996). However, while serotypes M1 and M3 accounted for the vast majority of strains isolated from cases of STSS and NF during the recent outbreaks, many other M types, including some non-typable strains, are known to cause these disease (Cunningham, 2000; Stevens, 1992).

Davies et al. (1996) characterized 323 cases of invasive GAS disease from the Ontario streptococcal study group (OSSG), a prospective, population-based surveillance study of all invasive GAS infections in Ontario, Canada. Out of the 13% of the cases that were classified as having STSS (annual rate, 0.2 per 100,000 population), 31 fulfilled the consensus definition of the syndrome, 4 were dead on arrival to the hospital, and 7 died shortly after admission without having sufficient information available for classification. The patients who had the STSS were older than the other patients (median age, 61, as compared with 38; $p < 0.001$) and more likely to have an underlying chronic illness (71%, as compared with 51%; $p = 0.03$). The overall mortality rate was 81% among patients with the STSS (65% among those whose illness met the consensus definition), as compared with 5% among those without the syndrome ($p < 0.001$). The distribution of sites of infection were soft tissue (30%), bacteremia without focus (15%), arthritis (15%), upper respiratory tract (10%), adenitis (8%), NF (6%), pneumonia (5%), peritonitis (4%), and meningitis (2%). Laupland et al. (2000) described the incidence and clinical features of invasive GAS disease in children from the OSSG. There were 1.9 cases of invasive GAS disease per 100,000 children per year. STSS occurred in 7% of cases: six with bacteremia without focus, three with NF, two with pneumonia (one with cellulitis and one with peritonitis), two with cellulitis, and one each with pharyngitis and an infected iliac vein thrombus. Children under 10 years of age were less likely to be diagnosed with STSS than children 10 years of age and older ($p = 0.002$). They found that chickenpox infection was associated with a 58-fold increased risk of acquiring invasive GAS disease.

4.2. Necrotizing Fasciitis

In addition to the increase in STSS during the 1980s, there were increased reports of NF (Chelsom et al., 1994; Demers et al., 1993; Kaul et al., 1997; Stevens et al., 1989). The hallmark of NF is infection of the subcutaneous tissue and fascia that often results in necrosis with relative sparing of the underlying muscle. The diagnosis can be made if histopathology demonstrates both necrosis of superficial fascia and polymorphonuclear infiltrate and edema of the reticular dermis, subcutaneous fat, and superficial fascia. In the absence of examined specimens, the diagnosis requires the presence of gross fascial edema and necrosis detected at surgery (Kaul et al., 1997). Kaul et al. (1997) reported on 77 cases of streptococcal NF gleaned from the OSSG. From 1992 to 1995, the annual incidence of NF increased 4-fold from 0.85 per million population to 3.5 per million ($p < 0.001$). The majority (71%) of adult cases occurred in persons with at least one chronic underlying illness. Nine (12%) infections occurred in a chronically ischemic limb in patients with diabetes and/or peripheral vascular disease. None of the children affected had underlying chronic medical conditions. However, in four of eight cases occurring in children (and in four of five cases in children less than 10 years of age), NF occurred as a complication of chickenpox. Use of nonsteroidal anti-inflammatory drugs (NSAIDs) prior to admission was reported by 26% of the cases where information was available. Eight patients had been taking NSAIDs chronically, and three had taken them because of pain associated with the acute illness.

The most common primary site of infection was the lower extremity (53%), followed by the upper extremity (29%), trunk (9%), groin/perineum (8%), and face (1%). Forty-nine percent of patients had significant hypotension. Forty-six percent of cases (35 of 75 from whom blood cultures were obtained) were bacteremic. The majority of patients (73%) had an elevated white blood cell count; however in 20% of patients white cell counts were within the normal range, and in 7% they were low. Acute renal failure was present in 35% of patients, coagulopathy in 29%, and 28% of patients had liver function test abnormalities. Overall, 49% of cases met the case definition for STSS.

In Laupland's study (Laupland et al., 2000) 10 children (4%) had NF, 3 of whom had STSS. In contrast to cellulitis, which was distributed across all body sites, 8 of 10 cases of NF occurred in the lower limb ($p = 0.001$), and 5 of 8 of these initially involved the thigh and/or groin. One patient (10%) with NF died at presentation to the emergency department. No other patients with NF alone or in combination with STSS died. In univariate analysis, only the presence of antecedent chickenpox was associated with the diagnosis of NF ($p = 0.007$). In multivariable analysis, both in all cases and in the subset with soft-tissue infections, only chickenpox was associated with the diagnosis of NF.

Haywood et al. (1998) reviewed 20 consecutive patients identified from the OSSG, that had been cared for in Toronto. The average age of all patients was 58 years (ranging from 33 to 89 years, with a median age of 55.5 years). A physician had seen seven (35%) patients in the 48 hr prior to admission. Their signs and symptoms were such that they were diagnosed with a condition other than NF. Fifty-five percent of patients had an underlying chronic illness. The body distribution of NF involved upper extremity (35%), lower extremity (30%), and trunk (35%). One patient developed a postoperative surgical wound infection that resulted in necrotizing fasciitis, which was found to be secondary to an asymptomatically colonized healthcare worker who was present during surgery. Clinical presentation of patients within the first 48 hr included hypotension (85%), use of vasopressors (55%), renal impairment (45%), coagulopathy (55%), liver involvement (25%), acute respiratory distress syndrome, ARDS (15%), and a rash (35%). Forty percent of all patients met the criteria of STSS.

Clinically it appears that STSS is a separate entity from NF. The studies from Britain and Sweden, which reported an increase in severe GAS infection, did not report the concomitant presence of NF (Colman et al., 1993; Gaworzewska & Colman, 1988; Stromberg et al., 1991). Martin and Hoiby (1990) in their report of an increase in incidence and severity of GAS disease in Norway, due primarily to M1 strains, reported only a small number of cases of necrotizing fasciitis. Hoge et al. (1993b) carried out a retrospective survey of the medical records from all 10 hospitals in Pima County, Arizona, to identify sterile site isolates of GAS between 1985 and 1990. They found significant changes in the clinical spectrum of invasive infections with an increase in patients with clinical features of STSS during the last three years of the study. Necrotizing fasciitis was not associated with shock or any of the other clinical features of STSS, suggesting that fasciitis was not a component of the syndrome. Kaul et al. (1997) found only 36 of 77 cases of GAS necrotizing fasciitis associated with STSS. McGeer et al. (1998) reviewed all M3 disease identified in the OSSG data base between 1992 and 1998. There were 1,335 cases of invasive GAS disease (2/100,000 population) of which M3 serotypes represented 7.1% of isolates. Non-M3 isolates were more likely to be associated with soft-tissue infection without fasciitis ($p = 0.001$), whereas M3 isolates were more likely to be associated with necrotizing fasciitis ($p = 0.001$). M3 was also associated with increased severity of systemic disease, including STSS.

4.3. Soft-Tissue Infections

Soft-tissue infections are common diseases, which are rarely life threatening and can usually be managed without hospital admission. They are most commonly due to GAS. In order to better characterize patients with soft-tissue infections due to GAS in this era of emerging prevalence and severity of GAS infections, Sharkawy et al. (2002) characterized 474 cases of invasive GAS soft-tissue infections from the OSSG data base. The incidence of invasive disease with a soft tissue focus varied from 0.62 per 100,000 population per year in 1992 to 1.29 per 100,000 population per year in 1995; $p < 0.001$. Most of this variability was in the rate of NF, which ranged from 0.08 per 100,000 per year in 1992 to 0.49 per 100,000 per year in 1995. The incidence of all invasive soft-tissue disease including NF was highest in the elderly. Fifty percent of cases occurred in patients with at least one chronic underlying illness, of which diabetes mellitus and alcoholism were the most common. The overall case fatality rate was 13%. In multivariate analysis of factors identifiable at presentation hypotension, increased age, and underlying chronic illness were significantly associated with an increased case-fatality rate. None of 198 patients (including 92 who were bacteremic) without hypotension or chronic underlying illness died. Of the 158 patients with chronic underlying illness but no hypotension for whom age was known, 1 of 96 aged younger than 65 years died, compared to 9 of 62 aged 65 years or older ($p = 0.001$). Patients with positive blood cultures were more likely to die (61/315, 19%, vs. 7/205, 3.4%, $p < 0.001$) and to have severe systemic disease (37/301, 12%, vs. 10/203, 4.9%, $p = 0.008$). Patients with infection due to M1 and M3 strains were more likely to have NF than other patients. Patients infected with M3 strains were also more likely to die: 11/40 (28%) patients infected with M3 strains died, compared to 11/105 (10%) of those infected with M1 strains, and 36/293 (12%) of those infected with strains of other serotypes. Sharkaway's data, while limited to disease due to GAS, support the contention that cellulitis is seldom life threatening and can usually be managed in an outpatient setting. All patients in this series were admitted to hospitals, and had positive sterile site cultures, and 60% were bacteremic. Despite this, no patients without chronic underlying illness or hypotension died, and the case fatality rate in patients under the age of 65 with underlying illness was 1%.

4.4. Pneumonia

In the pre-antibiotic era GAS pneumonia was a common clinical entity accounting for 3–5% of community acquired pneumonia (CAP) (Keefer et al., 1941). Most cases occurred following outbreaks of viral illness, commonly influenza or measles (Keefer et al., 1941; MacCallum, 1919; Parker, 1979). Cases also occurred following GAS pharyngitis or tonsillitis (Keefer et al., 1941). Underlying chronic lung disease was a predisposing factor. Typical clinical features included the sudden onset of high fever and pleuritic chest pain and the frequent development of pleural effusions and empyema (Basiliere et al., 1968; Keefer et al., 1941; MacCallum, 1919; Parker, 1979). Fatal outcomes were common and may have occurred in up to 50% of cases (MacCallum, 1919).

The incidence of GAS pneumonia declined significantly over the first half of the 20th century (Basiliere et al., 1968). Despite this, several large outbreaks of GAS pneumonia were described in military personnel in the 1960's (Basiliere et al., 1968; Welch et al., 1961). Unlike previously described outbreaks, these were not linked to preceding viral illnesses. Despite this the clinical presentation and the frequent occurrence of empyema were identical to previous descriptions of the disease.

Since the 1960s the incidence of GAS pneumonia has dramatically declined. Numerous case series examining the etiologic agents of CAP have failed to detect any contribution from the GAS (Bates et al., 1992; Fang et al., 1990; Lieberman et al., 1996; Lim et al., 1989). No further large outbreaks have been reported and only a handful of case reports exist describing the modern presentation of GAS pneumonia.

As noted previously, over the last 15 years the incidence of severe GAS infections has been rising. Whether these changes have lead to resurgence of GAS pneumonia or to a change in the clinical or epidemiological features of this illness has not been directly addressed.

Muller et al. (2000) described the clinical and epidemiological features of 222 patients with invasive GAS pneumonia identified through the OSSG between 1992 and 1999. The yearly incidence of GAS pneumonia rose from 0.16 per 100,000 per year in 1992 to 0.35 per 100,000 in 1999 paralleling an increase in the incidence of all invasive GAS infections in the same cohort. GAS pneumonia occurred predominantly during the winter months, with a striking nadir in infections in August/September of each year. The median age was 56 years and ranged from 1 day to 100 years. A significant chronic illness was identified in 61% patients. The majority of cases were community acquired (179, 81%). Four of these cases were subsequent to other nonpharyngeal, culture-confirmed GAS infections in household contacts. One patient's spouse had been admitted three days previously with GAS bacteremia, another patient's spouse had been admitted the previous day with epiglottitis due to GAS, a third patient's child had been treated for GAS vulvitis 1 week prior to his presentation, and one 3-week old child's mother had had GAS endometritis.

Blood cultures were positive in 178 patients (78%); five of these patients also had GAS isolated from cultures of pleural fluid. Of the 44 patients with negative blood cultures or where blood cultures had not been done, GAS was isolated from pleural fluid in 37, and cultures of autopsy lung tissue in 7. The predominant M-types were M1 (38%) followed by M3 (11%), M12 (8%), and M6 (5%).

The case fatality rate was 38% compared with 12% for remainder of the cohort of invasive GAS infection ($p < 0.001$) and 26% (58 of 221) of patients with NF ($p = 0.008$). The progression of fatal cases was rapid with a median time to death of 2 days. In multivariate analysis, only the presence of STSS and increasing age were associated with a higher case fatality rate. Although the case fatality rate increased significantly with age, significant mortality occurred in young adults. The case fatality rate in previously healthy patients aged 1–65 years was 18% (9 of 49). The incidence of invasive GAS pneumonia during the period of our study ranged from 0.16 to 0.35 per 100,000 population with a trend toward increasing frequency. Data from the Centers for Disease Control and Prevention's (CDC) Active Bacterial Core (ABC) surveillance reports for 1997 and 1999 suggest that similar frequencies of invasive GAS disease and GAS pneumonia occur in the United States (Schuchat et al., 2001). Their data show an incidence of invasive GAS of 3.5 per 100,000 population with 11% representing pneumonia. Although the overall incidence of GAS pneumonia is low compared with common causes of community acquired pneumonia such as *S. pneumoniae*, it occurs with a frequency similar to that of other less common but well recognized causes of severe CAP such as *Staphylococcus aureus*. In a population based study by Marston et al. (1997) 0.3% cases in which a definite etiologic agent was identified were due to GAS compared with 0.4% due to *S. aureus*. The most striking findings of this study are the case fatality rate associated with GAS pneumonia, the high incidence of STSS, and the rapid progression to death that occurred in fatal cases. The overall case fatality rate of 38% is consistent with the 30–60% mortality found in bacteremic GAS pneumonia in other studies (Barnham & Anderson, 1997; Davies et al., 1996; Demers et al., 1993; Martin & Hoiby, 1990), and considerably higher than the case fatality rate of NF in our cohort of invasive GAS infection. The case fatality rate for GAS pneumonia is also higher than that reported for community acquired bacteremic pneumococcal pneumonia, estimated at 12–20% in recent studies (Metlay et al., 2000).

5. TREATMENT MODALITIES

5.1. Antimicrobials

Conventional therapy of invasive GAS infections has consisted of antimicrobials and, when necessary in severe invasive disease, support of vital functions for those patients with STSS and surgery for those patients with NF. Penicillin and cephalosporins are the antimicrobials most frequently used for treating GAS pharyngitis, cellulites, and impetigo. However, concern has been raised that in more severe infections the organism is less likely to respond to β-lactam antibiotics. Stevens et al. (1988) were able to show that penicillin was ineffective in a mouse model of myositis due to GAS if treatment was delayed ≥2 hr after initiation of treatment. The targets for the β-lactams are the penicillin binding proteins (PBPs), enzymes responsible for the formation of the peptidoglycan in the cell wall of the bacteria. The PBPs are expressed during the log-phase of growth, but in large inocula infections they are not expressed during the stationary phase of growth. Stevens et al. (1993) found that in addition to decreased binding of radiolabeled penicillin by all PBPs in stationary cells, PBPs 1 and 4 were undetectable at 36 hr. They speculated that the loss of certain PBPs during stationary-phase growth in vitro might account for the failure of penicillin in both experimental and human cases of severe streptococcal infection.

Stevens et al. (1988) found that antimicrobials that inhibit protein synthesis were able to improve survival over penicillin in a mouse model of myositis. Survival of erythromycin-treated mice was greater than that of penicillin-treated mice and untreated controls, but only if treatment was begun within 24 hr. Mice receiving clindamycin had survival rates of 100%, 100%, 80%, and 70%, even if the treatment was delayed 0, 2, 6, and 16.5 hr, respectively (Stevens et al., 1988). There are several possible explanations for the greater efficacy of clindamycin in the treatment of severe GAS infections (Stevens, 1999). In vitro and in vivo data support the concept that clindamycin efficacy is not affected by inoculum size or stage of growth and in fact may suppress the synthesis of PBPs (Stevens et al., 1993; Yan et al., 1993, 1994). Other mechanistic actions of clindamycin in invasive GAS disease include enhanced opsonization of streptococci through suppression of bacterial M protein expression (Gemmell et al., 1981), reduced capsular expression, and suppression of bacterial toxin synthesis, including superantigens (Mascini et al., 2001; Sriskandan et al., 1997). Finally there is evidence that clindamycin can function as an immune modulator by suppressing synthesis of TNF-α from monocytes.

Although GAS have remained exquisitely sensitive to penicillin, resistance to the macrolides and clindamycin have emerged worldwide. Resistance to macrolides in GAS arises by two distinct mechanisms: (i) ribosomal modification resulting from the presence of an Erm methylase; and (ii) drug efflux conferred by a membrane protein encoded by the *mefA* gene. Presence of an Erm methylase confers cross-resistance to erythromycin, clindamycin, and streptogramin B-type compounds (MLS$_B$ phenotype). MLS resistance in GAS is encoded by two types of methylase gene: the *erm* (AM) [*erm* (B)] and the recently described *erm* (TR). The latter has also been associated with inducible resistance to clindamycin when using a double disc diffusion test. Resistance resulting from efflux is encoded by the *mefA* gene. This resistance is specific for 14- and 15-member macrolides (erythromycin, azithromycin, and clarithromycin); 16-member macrolides (e.g., josamycin) are not affected and neither are clindamycin or streptogramin B-type compounds (M-phenotype). Therefore depending on the prevalence of resistance and the mechanism of resistance either erythromycin or clindamycin or both may not be active against the infecting GAS. Therefore, an approach for severe invasive GAS infection has been to utilize a combination of penicillin and clindamycin, since the penicillin provides coverage against 100% of GAS strains.

5.2. Novel Therapeutic Strategies

The conventional wisdom is that patients with severe GAS infections require antimicrobials, supportive therapy to manage their hypotension and multiorgan failure, and surgery for the removal of devitalized tissue. However, as with severe invasive *Streptococcus pneumoniae* disease, there has been a failure to influence mortality (Davies et al., 1996; Hook et al., 1983). Often patients succumb to their infection before antimicrobials can have any beneficial effect, despite supportive care of the intensive care unit and extensive debridement, emphasizing the importance of research in immune modulation therapy.

The finding that low levels of protective antibodies against the M-protein and superantigens correlated with invasive GAS disease highlighted the importance of antibodies in protection against these infections, and suggested that immunoglobulins might be a potential adjunctive therapy (Basma et al., 1999; Eriksson et al., 1999; Holm et al., 1992;

Mascini et al., 2000; Norrby-Teglund et al., 1994). In order for an immunoglobulin therapy to be efficacious, broad antibody specificity would be required to cover all the different serotypes of GAS and the whole spectrum of superantigens as well as other important virulence factors. Intravenous immunoglobulin (IVIG) exhibits high polyspecificity generated by antibodies pooled from several thousands of donors, and IVIG is commonly used as therapy in various autoimmune and immunodeficiency diseases, as well as in Kawasaki disease.

Several different modes of actions that contribute to the beneficial effect in autoimmune and systemic inflammatory diseases have been described for IVIG. These include blockade of Fc-receptors on reticuloendothelial cell system and phagocytic cells, modulation of Fc receptor expression, interference with activated complement, modulation of cytokine responses, modulation of immune cell functions, interaction with idiotype–antiidiotypic network, antigen-neutralization, and selection of immune repertoires (Ballow, 1997; Mouthon et al., 1996). A crucial pathway by which IVIG exerts its anti-inflammatory activity was recently identified in a murine model of immune thrombocytopenia and involved increased expression of the Fc inhibitory receptor for IgG, FcγRIIB, and consequently abrogated platelet destruction by macrophage phagocytosis (Samuelsson et al., 2001). Mechanistic actions directly related to the pathogenesis of invasive GAS infections, such as antigen neutralization, bacterial opsonization, as well as cytokine modulation, are discussed further below.

Opsonizing antibodies that promote phagocytosis and bacterial clearance of several pathogenic microorganisms, including GAS, have been demonstrated in IVIG preparations (Basma, 1998; Weisman et al., 1994; Yang et al., 1989). These opsonizing anti-M1 antibodies were found to be conferred on the patients upon IVIG therapy, since elevated opsonizing titers were demonstrated in post-therapy plasma (Basma, 1998). Thus, increased bacterial clearance through opsonizing antibodies against GAS might be a potential mechanistic action of IVIG contributing to clinical efficacy. However, an experimental murine model of necrotizing fasciitis that compared the efficacy of clindamycin, penicillin, and IVIG, alone or in combination, failed to support this hypothesis (Patel et al., 2000). Efficacy of the various treatment regimens was assessed based on quantitative bacterial clearance, and IVIG did not enhance killing of the M3 strain used. Thus, further studies are warranted to define the exact role of IVIG conferred opsonic antibodies in the efficacy of IVIG therapy in severe invasive GAS infections.

IVIG also contains neutralizing antibodies against several different GAS superantigens. These antibodies potently inhibit the proliferative and cytokine-inducing capacity of GAS superantigens in vitro at physiological concentrations of IVIG (Norrby-Teglund et al., 1996a, 1996b; Skansen-Saphir et al., 1994). IVIG has been shown to inhibit several SSAs, including SpeA, SpeB, and SpeC (Norrby-Teglund et al., 1996a, 1996b). In addition, culture supernatants prepared from GAS strains of different serotypes including M1, M3, M4, M6, and M28, were used as crude preparations of secreted virulence factors, and all tested supernatants were completely inhibited by IVIG (Norrby-Teglund et al., 1998). Thus, IVIG exhibits an extraordinary broad specificity against GAS virulence factors, which is transferred to the patients upon administration of IVIG with subsequent increased superantigen-neutralizing activity in patients' plasma (Norrby-Teglund et al., 1996a, 1996b). This inhibitory activity of IVIG is not exclusive for GAS superantigens, also superantigens produced by *S. aureus* are potently inhibited by IVIG (Darville et al., 1997;

Takei et al., 1993). Furthermore, antibodies against other important streptococcal virulence factors including DNaseB and SLO have also been found in IVIG preparations
(Lissner et al., 1999; Stegmayr et al., 1992).

Analyses of different IVIG preparations containing varying concentrations of IgG,
IgA, and/or IgM revealed that they varied in opsonizing and toxin-neutralizing capacity,
and variation in inhibitory activity was even observed between lots of the same preparation (Hiemstra et al., 1994; Norrby-Teglund et al., 1998, 2000). IgA and IgM were found
to be potent inhibitors of GAS superantigens, and in the case of SpeA the most efficient
neutralization was achieved by a preparation containing a mixture of IgG, IgA, and IgM
(Norrby-Teglund et al., 2000). These findings suggest that optimization of IVIG therapy
may be achieved by changing the type or lot of IVIG preparation; however, this remains to
be proven in a clinical setting.

IVIG is a powerful modulator of cytokine production, not only via direct antigen-
neutralizing, but also through immunomodulatory activities that are mediated by pathways
not yet completely understood. These pathways are believed to include Fc-interactions,
soluble immune components, and induction of regulatory cytokines. A strong induction of
IL1ra have been shown in human monocytes following culture on adherent IgG (Arend
et al., 1991) or coculture with IVIG (Andersson et al., 1996; Poutsiaka et al., 1991). Also
IL8 production is induced in human monocytes following coculture with IVIG (Andersson
et al., 1996; Ruiz de Souza et al., 1995). IL1ra is well known to exert anti-inflammatory
activity due to its interaction with IL1 signaling; however, the effect of IL8 as an anti-
inflammatory agent is not as clearly defined but has been suggested to inhibit the accumulation of neutrophils at the sites of inflammation when induced systemically (Asano &
Ogawa, 2000).

IVIG was shown in vitro to be a strong inhibitor of superantigen-induced lymphokine
production, with the strongest suppression seen for the Th1 cytokines IFNχ and TNFβ, as
their production was almost completely abolished (Andersson et al., 1996; Norrby-
Teglund et al., 1996b, 2000; Skansen-Saphir et al., 1994). This inhibitory effect was seen,
although to a lesser extent, even when addition of IVIG was delayed 24 hr poststimulation
with superantigen. These findings suggest that additional mechanisms of IVIG, aside from
antigen-neutralization, contribute to the inhibitory effect (Andersson et al., 1996; Skansen-
Saphir et al., 1994). A differential effect of IVIG was noted on superantigen-induced
monokine production with upregulated IL8 and decreased IL6 production (Andersson
et al., 1994). Studies on the effect of IVIG on superantigen induced IL1 production have
reported conflicting results, as one study demonstrated no effect on IL1 production
(Skansen-Saphir et al., 1994), whereas the other reported a significant reduction of IL1
(Norrby-Teglund et al., 2000). Thus, superantigen-induced lymphokine production is
potently suppressed by IVIG, and the monokine production may also be modulated by
IVIG, but further studies are required to define the effect of IVIG on superantigen induced
monokines. However, since the Th1 type of cytokines are the hallmark of a superantigen
response, the powerful inhibition of these cytokines by IVIG most likely represents a major
mechanistic action of IVIG contributing to clinical efficacy.

Cytokine modulation by IVIG have also been shown in vivo in several diseases,
including among others severe invasive GAS infections where patients showed decreased
levels of TNFα and IL6 (Kaul et al., 1999; Nadal et al., 1993); Guillain-Barré syndrome
patients who showed a selective down-regulation of pro-inflammatory cytokines (Sharief

et al., 1999), and Kawasaki patients who demonstrated elevated IL1ra and IL8, as well as decreased pro-inflammatory cytokines following IVIG therapy (Leung et al., 1989).

Several case reports have demonstrated clinical improvement after IVIG therapy of patients with severe invasive GAS infections including STSS, NF, and necrotizing myositis (Barry et al., 1992; Cawley et al., 1999; Chiu et al., 1997; Lamothe et al., 1995; Mahieu et al., 1995; Nadal et al., 1993; Perez et al., 1997; Stegmayr et al., 1992; Yong, 1994).

There have been three studies conducted of IVIG therapy in patients with NF (Haywood et al., 1998; Kaul et al., 1997; Muller et al., 2001). In the study by Kaul et al. (1997), a reduction in mortality rate (10% compared to 37%) was noted between IVIG-treated patients as compared to the nontreated controls. However, only age, hypotension, and bacteremia were independently associated with mortality of streptococcal necrotizing fasciitis. Muller et al. (2001) described six patients with severe GAS disease and soft tissue involvement that were managed conservatively. Treatment in all cases included clindamycin, a β-lactam, and high-dose IVIG. All patients were hypotensive and three patients developed STSS. One patient had limited exploratory surgery without debridement. One patient had repeated bedside drainage of her olecranon bursa. No other patient had surgery. All patients survived.

An observational cohort study designed to evaluate the efficacy of IVIG therapy in patients with STSS was conducted in Canada (Kaul et al., 1999). The study included 21 cases that were treated with IVIG during 1994–1995, and 32 nontreated controls identified through OSSG's active surveillance during 1992–1995. Multivariate analysis revealed that IVIG therapy and a lower acute physiology and chronic health evaluation II (APACHE) score was significantly associated with survival. One confounding factor in the material was that IVIG-treated cases were more likely to have received clindamycin therapy than the controls. Therefore, a secondary multivariate analysis considering only cases and controls that had received clindamycin was performed, and APACHE II score and IVIG therapy remained the two variables associated with survival. Further support for the use of IVIG was provided by in vitro studies of blood samples collected pre- and post-IVIG therapy (Kaul et al., 1999). Neutralizing activity against culture supernatant prepared from the patient's own infecting isolate increased significantly post-therapy, and the majority of patient's plasma caused 80–100% inhibition of the bacterial supernatants. Since the material included patients infected with GAS strains of varying serotype, this supports the in vitro findings that IVIG have a very broad spectrum of superantigen-neutralizing antibodies. IVIG therapy also resulted in a significantly reduced TNFα and IL6 production in peripheral blood mononuclear cells in four patients tested (Kaul et al., 1999). Thus, together these data suggest that the clinical improvement achieved by IVIG therapy is partly attributed to inhibition of the superantigens produced by the clinical isolates, and a reduction in the pro-inflammatory response.

The treatment of necrotizing fasciitis has emphasized the importance of early surgical intervention for diagnosis or surgical debridement and/or hyperbaric oxygen (Bisno & Stevens, 1996). Early aggressive surgery has been advocated in order to reduce the systemic inflammatory response and the spread of local infection (Stevens, 1999). Hyperbaric oxygen is recommended in order to administer oxygen at greater than normal pressure so as to lead to better wound healing. Unfortunately, both procedures usually occur at a time when the patient is most unstable and therefore interferes with monitoring and treatment. In addition, there is no evidence to support the use of hyperbaric oxygen and there is new

Table 1.3

Recommendations for the Treatment of Streptococcal Toxic Shock Syndrome

Penicillin 4 MU iv q6h
Plus
Clindamycin 900 mg iv q6h (discontinue at 72–96 hr, as long as the patient is hemodynamically stable and local disease is no longer progressing).
Plus
Intravenous immunoglobulin 2 g/kg iv for 1 dose (consider second dose of 1 g/kg at 72 hr only if patient remains hemodynamically unstable or local disease continues to progress).

information we may allow surgery to be delayed until the patient is stable and the degree of surgery required is better defined, thereby reducing unnecessary tissue debridement and/or amputation (Brown et al., 1994; Muller et al., 2001). IVIG has resulted in a reduction in the mortality associated with STSS and possibly a reduction in morbidity and mortality in patients with necrotizing fasciitis (Haywood et al., 1998; Kaul et al., 1997).

Antibiotic and IVIG treatment regimens are presented in Table 1.3.

6. PREVENTION

Prevention of streptococcal infections occurs naturally by acquisition of immunity to one or several streptococcal virulence factors. Considering that severe invasive GAS infections are such rare occurrences among the population despite widespread exposure to virulent GAS strains in communities, natural immunity most likely plays a very important role. However, the complexity of GAS pathogenesis involving several serotypes and toxins/superantigens, makes the development of a vaccine highly challenging. There are several strategies of vaccine development currently being pursued (Table 1.4).

The main target for a streptococcal vaccine has been the anti-phagocytic M-protein, since it is a major protective antigen of GAS. In 1962, Lancefield and colleagues (Lancefield, 1962) demonstrated that type-specific anti-M protein antibodies protected against infection in a murine model, and that recovery from infection in humans was related to the presence of type-specific anti-M antibodies. However, the protection was type-specific, and the individuals remained susceptible to infection by other serotypes. Considering that there exist over 100 different M-serotypes, type-specificity poses a major challenge in the design of M-protein vaccines. Another important issue with M-protein vaccines is that certain areas of the M-proteins have been shown to contain epitopes that evoke antibodies to human tissue including myocardium (Dale & Beachey, 1985), renal glomeruli (Kraus & Beachey, 1988), cartilage (Baird et al., 1991), and brain (Bronze & Dale, 1993). Hence, it is essential that these regions be avoided in a vaccine construct, and that the selected region only contains protective epitopes. One approach to overcome the problem of type-specificity and to increase the spectrum of protection has been to develop multivalent vaccines (Beachey et al., 1988; Dale, 1999a). Multivalent vaccines containing N-terminal fragments of several different M-proteins linked in tandem has been developed and demonstrated to be immunogenic. A recent study by Dale (1999b) reported a hexavalent M-protein vaccine, which was shown to be immunogenic and to evoke protective

Table 1.4
Vaccine Candidates in Group A Streptococcal Infections

Streptococal factor	Targeted region	Reference(s)
M-protein	N-terminal N- and C-terminal C-terminal	Bessen and Fischetti (1990), Brandt et al. (2000), Dale (1999a), Medaglini et al. (1995), Pruksakorn et al. (1994)
C5a peptidase	scpA gene with deleted signal sequence and cell wall anchor	Ji et al. (1997)
Cysteine protease/SpeB	The whole molecule	Kapur et al. (1994)
Group A carbohydrate	The whole molecule	Salvadori et al. (1995)
Streptococcal Protective Antigen (Spa)	N-terminal	Dale et al. (1999), McLellan et al. (2001)
Fibronectin-binding protein SfbI	Fibronectin-binding	Guzman et al. (1999), Schulze et al. (2001)
Fibronectin-binding protein FBP54	The whole molecule	Kawabata et al. (2001)

antibodies against all serotypes included in the construct. Brandt et al. (Brandt et al., 2000) recently reported a novel multi-epitope vaccine strategy, in which the construct included a minimum non-cross-reactive peptide from the conserved C-terminal half of the M-protein that was linked to seven serotypic peptides from the N-terminal region. The construct demonstrated good immunogenicity and protection in mice.

There are also other non-M-protein derived vaccine candidates, including C5a-peptidase, streptococcal cysteine protease (SpeB), streptococcal protective antigen (SPA), group A carbohydrate, and fibronectin-binding proteins (Table 1.4). One advantage with these candidates is that they provoke serotype-independent immunity, and can provide protection against heterologous GAS strains. With the recent advancements in multi-epitope vaccines, it seems plausible that future streptococcal vaccines may combine multiple streptococal antigens, thereby providing broad-spectrum immunity.

The occurrence of outbreaks of GAS in communities, especially clusters of STSS and/or NF, has raised concern about the transmissibility of the organism and the need for prophylaxis. DiPersio et al. (1996) described two clusters of GAS disease that occurred within separate family units. Davies et al. (1996) in their prospective study were able to estimate the incidence of invasive disease among contacts of persons with invasive GAS. They found that the risk to family members of patients' households was 2.9 per 1,000, almost 200 times the risk in the general population, supporting the use of chemoprophylaxis in patients' close contacts. The use of prophylaxis when severe disease occurs in such a setting is supported by the observation that subsequent cases are often also severe (Couper, 1997).

Numerous hospital-based case series have been reported on the clinical spectrum of pediatric invasive GAS disease and have identified that varicella-zoster virus (VZV) infection commonly precedes these infections, especially in cases of NF (Brogan et al., 1995; Davies et al., 1994; Doctor et al., 1995; Peterson et al., 1996a, 1996b; Vugia et al., 1996; Wheeler et al., 1991; Wilson et al., 1995).

Laupland et al. (2000) describe the incidence and clinical features of invasive GAS disease in children from the OSSG to better quantify the risk of this disease following chickenpox infection. There were 1.9 cases of invasive GAS disease per 100,000 children per year. Fifteen percent of children identified had preceding chickenpox infection, which significantly increased the risk for acquisition of invasive GAS disease (Relative Risk, RR: 58; 95% Confidence Interval, CI: 40–85). Children with invasive GAS and recent chickenpox were more likely to have NF (RR: 6.3; 95% CI: 1.8–22.3). The most striking finding of this study is the observation that VZV infection is associated with a 58-fold increased risk of acquiring invasive GAS disease in children. It is not clear why chickenpox infection increases the risk for GAS infection so dramatically.

Although the attack rate for invasive GAS disease following chickenpox is relatively low at 5.2 per 100,000, it is important that 15% of all pediatric invasive GAS infection in Laupland's study, including 50% of NF cases, followed VZV infection. Because there is an effective, safe vaccine for chickenpox available, many cases of invasive GAS disease, including NF, may potentially be preventable by chickenpox vaccination of young children. Laupland et al. (2000) estimated the impact of universal chickenpox vaccination effectiveness in preventing invasive GAS infection using the following assumptions: (1) vaccine coverage would be 80%; (2) vaccine efficacy for preventing chickenpox manifested by any skin lesions would be 85%; (3) vaccine would be administered at 1 year of age; and (4) the risk of invasive GAS infection would be equal in vaccinated and nonvaccinated children with skin lesions following wild type VZV infection. Based on their data and these assumptions, they estimated that universal vaccination of 1-year-old children would prevent at least 10% of all invasive GAS infections. Given that their estimates of vaccine efficacy (85%) and coverage (80%) are conservative, the effect of vaccination is likely greater than 10%. These data lend further support to the arguments in favor of introducing VZV vaccination into the routine childhood regimen.

7. FUTURE DIRECTIONS

At present the conventional therapy of severe invasive GAS infections includes clindamycin in combination with penicillin, supportive therapy to manage their hypotension and multiorgan failure, and surgery when indicated. However, the persistently high mortality rates demonstrate the need for adjunctive therapy in these diseases. The most promising therapies today seem to be agents that target several different streptococcal factors and/or host systems involved in sepsis. One such therapy is IVIG that has been shown to interact with GAS pathogenesis at several different stages (reviewed in Norrby-Teglund & Stevens, 1998), and in vitro data together with a case-control study strongly supports a clinical efficacy of IVIG as adjunctive therapy for STSS patients (Kaul et al., 1999).

By virtue of their pivotal role in the pathogenesis of the severe invasive GAS infections, superantigens are obvious targets for intervention. However, there are several different GAS superantigens with the potential for causing disease, hence, the intervention would need to be polyspecific. Despite significant difference in the primary sequence of the superantigens, they all share a common three-dimensional structure. Using this common tertiary structure, researchers have managed to produce peptides that inhibited the induction of cytokines and protected against lethal shock in experimental models of superantigen-induced toxic shock (Arad et al., 2000; Visvanathan et al., 2001). Similarly, using site-directed mutagenesis of the conserved receptor-binding regions in superantigens, vaccines were generated that protected against lethal shock (Ulrich et al., 1998).

References

Andersson, J., Skansen-Saphir, U., Sparrelid, E., & Andersson, U. (1996). Intravenous immune globulin affects cytokine production in T lymphocytes and monocytes/macrophages. *Clin Exp Immunol, 104* (Suppl 1), 10–20.

Andersson, U., Bjork, L., Skansen-Saphir, U., & Andersson, J. (1994). Pooled human IgG modulates cytokine production in lymphocytes and monocytes. *Immunol Rev, 139*, 21–42.

Arad, G., Levy, R., Hillman, D., & Kaempfer, R. (2000). Superantigen antagonist protects against lethal shock and defines a new domain for T-cell activation. *Nat Med, 6*, 414–421.

Arend, W. P., Smith, M. F., Jr., Janson, R. W., & Joslin, F. G. (1991). IL-1 receptor antagonist and IL-1 beta production in human monocytes are regulated differently. *J Immunol, 147*, 1530–1536.

Asano, T., & Ogawa, S. (2000). Expression of IL-8 in Kawasaki disease. *Clin Exp Immunol, 122*, 514–519.

Ashbaugh, C. D., Warren, H. B., Carey, V. J., & Wessels, M. R. (1998). Molecular analysis of the role of the group A streptococcal cysteine protease, hyaluronic acid capsule, and M protein in a murine model of human invasive soft-tissue infection. *J Clin Invest, 102*, 550–560.

Baird, R. W., Bronze, M. S., Kraus, W., Hill, H. R., Veasey, L. G., & Dale, J. B. (1991). Epitopes of group A streptococcal M protein shared with antigens of articular cartilage and synovium. *J Immunol, 146*, 3132–3137.

Ballow, M. (1997). Mechanisms of action of intravenous immune serum globulin in autoimmune and inflammatory diseases. *J Allergy Clin Immunol, 100*, 151–157.

Barnham, M., & Anderson, A. W. (1997). Non-steroidal anti-inflammatory drugs: A predisposing factor for streptococcal bacteremia. In Horaud (Ed.), *Streptococci and the host*. New York: Plenum Press.

Barry, W., Hudgins, L., Donta, S. T., & Pesanti, E. L. (1992). Intravenous immunoglobulin therapy for toxic shock syndrome. *JAMA, 267*, 3315–3316.

Basiliere, J. L., Bistrong, H. W., & Spence, W. F. (1968). Streptococcal pneumonia. Recent outbreaks in military recruit populations. *Am J Med, 44*, 580–589.

Basma, H. (1998). Opsonic antibodies to the surface M protein of group A streptococci in pooled normal immunoglobulins (IVIG): Potential impact on the clinical efficacy of IVIG therapy for severe invasive group A streptococcal infections. *Infect Immun, 66*, 2279–2283.

Basma, H., Norrby-Teglund, A., Guedez, Y., McGeer, A., Low, D. E., El-Ahmedy, O., Schwartz, B., & Kotb, M. (1999). Risk factors in the pathogenesis of invasive group A streptococcal infections: Role of protective humoral immunity. *Infect Immun, 67*, 1871–1877.

Bates, J. H., Campbell, G. D., Barron, A. L., McCracken, G. A., Morgan, P. N., Moses, E. B., & Davis, C. M. (1992). Microbial etiology of acute pneumonia in hospitalized patients. *Chest, 101*, 1005–1012.

Beachey, E. H., Bronze, M., Dale, J. B., Kraus, W., Poirier, T., & Sargent, S. (1988). Protective and autoimmune epitopes of streptococcal M proteins. *Vaccine, 6*, 192–196.

Berge, A., & Bjorck, L. (1995). Streptococcal cysteine proteinase releases biologically active fragments of streptococcal surface proteins. *J Biol Chem, 270*, 9862–9867.

Bessen, D. E., & Fischetti, V. A. (1990). Differentiation between two biologically distinct classes of group A streptococci by limited substitutions of amino acids within the shared region of M protein-like molecules. *J Exp Med, 172*, 1757–1764.

Bhakdi, S., Klonisch, T., Nuber, P., & Fischer, W. (1991). Stimulation of monokine production by lipoteichoic acids. *Infect Immun, 59*, 4614–4620.

Bisno, A. L., & Stevens, D. L. (1996). Streptococcal infections of skin and soft tissues. *N Eng J Med, 334*, 240–245.

Bjorck, L., Akesson, P., Bohus, M., Trojnar, J., Abrahamson, M., Olafsson, I., & Grubb, A. (1989). Bacterial growth blocked by a synthetic peptide based on the structure of a human proteinase inhibitor. *Nature, 337*, 385–386.

Boyle, M. D. (1995). Variation of multifunctional surface binding proteins—a virulence strategy for group A streptococci? *J Theor Biol, 173*, 415–426.

Brandt, E. R., Sriprakash, K. S., Hobb, R. I., Hayman, W. A., Zeng, W., Batzloff, M. R., Jackson, D. C., & Good, M. F. (2000). New multi-determinant strategy for a group A streptococcal vaccine designed for the Australian Aboriginal population. *Nat Med, 6*, 455–459.

Brogan, T. V., Nizet, V., Waldhausen, J. H., Rubens, C. E., & Clarke, W. R. (1995). Group A streptococcal necrotizing fasciitis complicating primary varicella: A series of fourteen patients. *Pediatr Infect Dis J, 14*, 588–594.

Bronze, M. S., & Dale, J. B. (1993). Epitopes of streptococcal M proteins that evoke antibodies that cross-react with human brain. *J Immunol, 151*, 2820–2828.

Brown, D. R., Davis, N. L., Lepawsky, M., Cunningham, J., & Kortbeek, J. (1994). A multicenter review of the treatment of major truncal necrotizing infections with and without hyperbaric oxygen therapy. *Am J Surg, 167*, 485–489.

Burns, E. H., Jr., Marciel, A. M., & Musser, J. M. (1996). Activation of a 66-kilodalton human endothelial cell matrix metalloprotease by *Streptococcus pyogenes* extracellular cysteine protease. *Infect Immun, 64*, 4744–4750.

Card, G. L., Jasuja, R. R., & Gustafson, G. L. (1994). Activation of arachidonic acid metabolism in mouse macrophages by bacterial amphiphiles. *J Leukoc Biol, 56*, 723–728.

Cawley, M. J., Briggs, M., Haith, L. R., Jr., Reilly, K. J., Guilday, R. E., Braxton, G. R., & Patton, M. L. (1999). Intravenous immunoglobulin as adjunctive treatment for streptococcal toxic shock syndrome associated with necrotizing fasciitis: Case report and review. *Pharmacotherapy, 19*, 1094–1098.

Chatellier, S., & Kotb, M. (2000). Preferential stimulation of human lymphocytes by oligodeoxynucleotides that copy DNA CpG motifs present in virulent genes of group A streptococci. *Eur J Immunol, 30*, 993–1001.

Chelsom, J., Halstensen, A., Haga, T., & Hoiby, E. A. (1994). Necrotising fasciitis due to group A streptococci in western Norway: Incidence and clinical features. *Lancet, 344*, 1111–1115.

Chiu, C. H., Ou, J. T., Chang, K. S., & Lin, T. Y. (1997). Successful treatment of severe streptococcal toxic shock syndrome with a combination of intravenous immunoglobulin, dexamethasone and antibiotics. *Infection, 25*, 47–48.

Cockerill, F. R. I., MacDonald, K. L., Thompson, R. L., Roberson, F., Kohner, P. C., Besser-Wiek, J., Manahan, J. M., Musser, J. M., Schlievert, P. M., Talbot, J., Frankfort, B., Steckelberg, J. M., Wilson, W. R., Osterholm, M. T., & The Investigation Team. (1997). An outbreak of invasive group A streptococcal disease associated with high carriage rates of the invasive clone among school-aged children. *JAMA, 277*, 38–43.

Colman, G., Tanna, A., Efstratiou, A., & Gaworzewska, E. (1993). The serotypes of *Streptococcus pyogenes* present in Britain during 1980–1990 and their association with disease. *J Med Microbiol, 39*, 165–178.

Cone, L. A., Woodward, D. R., Schlievert, P. M., & Tomory, G. S. (1987). Clinical and bacteriologic observations of a toxic shock-like syndrome due to *Streptococcus pyogenes. N Engl J Med, 317*, 146–149.

Couper, R. (1997). Invasive group A streptococcal infections. *N Engl J Med, 336*, 513.

Courtney, H. S., Dale, J. B., & Hasty, D. L. (1996). Differential effects of the streptococcal fibronectin-binding protein, FBP54, on adhesion of group A streptococci to human buccal cells and HEp-2 tissue culture cells. *Infect Immun, 64*, 2415–2419.

Courtney, H. S., Hasty, D. L., Li, Y., Chiang, H. C., Thacker, J. L., & Dale, J. B. (1999). Serum opacity factor is a major fibronectin-binding protein and a virulence determinant of M type 2 *Streptococcus pyogenes*. *Mol Microbiol, 32*, 89–98.

Courtney, H. S., Li, Y., Dale, J. B., & Hasty, D. L. (1994). Cloning, sequencing, and expression of a fibronectin/fibrinogen-binding protein from group A streptococci. *Infect Immun, 62*, 3937–3946.

Cunningham, M. W. (2000). Pathogenesis of group A streptococcal infections. *Clin Microbiol Rev, 13*, 470–511.

Cywes, C., Stamenkovic, I., & Wessels, M. R. (2000). CD44 as a receptor for colonization of the pharynx by group A Streptococcus. *J Clin Invest, 106*, 995–1002.

Dale, J. B. (1999a). Group A streptococcal vaccines. *Infect Dis Clin North Am, 13*, 227–243, viii.

Dale, J. B. (1999b). Multivalent group A streptococcal vaccine designed to optimize the immunogenicity of six tandem M protein fragments. *Vaccine, 17*, 193–200.

Dale, J. B., & Beachey, E. H. (1985). Epitopes of streptococcal M proteins shared with cardiac myosin. *J Exp Med, 162*, 583–591.

Dale, J. B., Chiang, E. Y., Liu, S., Courtney, H. S., & Hasty, D. L. (1999). New protective antigen of group A streptococci. *J Clin Invest, 103*, 1261–1268.

Dale, J. B., Washburn, R. G., Marques, M. B., & Wessels, M. R. (1996). Hyaluronate capsule and surface M protein in resistance to opsonization of group A streptococci. *Infect Immun, 64*, 1495–1501.

Darville, T., Milligan, L. B., & Laffoon, K. K. (1997). Intravenous immunoglobulin inhibits staphylococcal toxin-induced human mononuclear phagocyte tumor necrosis factor alpha production. *Infect Immun, 65*, 366–372.

Davies, H. D., Matlow, A., Carroll, K., & Curley, F. J. (1994). Apparent lower rates of streptococcal toxic shock syndrome and lower mortality in children with invasive group A streptococcal infections compared with adults. *Pediatr Infect Dis J, 13*, 49–56.

Davies, H. D., McGeer, A., Schwartz, B., Green, K., Cann, D., Simor, A. E., Low, D. E., & The Ontario Group A Streptococcal Study Group. (1996). Invasive group A streptococcal infections in Ontario, Canada. *N Eng J Med, 335*, 547–554.

De Kimpe, S. J., Hunter, M. L., Bryant, C. E., Thiemermann, C., & Vane, J. R. (1995a). Delayed circulatory failure due to the induction of nitric oxide synthase by lipoteichoic acid from *Staphylococcus aureus* in anaesthetized rats. *Br J Pharmacol, 114*, 1317–1323.

De Kimpe, S. J., Kengatharan, M., Thiemermann, C., & Vane, J. R. (1995b). The cell wall components peptidoglycan and lipoteichoic acid from *Staphylococcus aureus* act in synergy to cause shock and multiple organ failure. *Proc Natl Acad Sci USA, 92*, 10359–10363.

Demers, B., Simor, A. E., Vellend, H., Schlievert, P. M., Byrne, S., Jamieson, F. B., Walmsley, S., & Low, D. E. (1993). Severe invasive group A streptococcal infections in Ontario, Canada: 1987–1991. *Clin Inf Dis, 16*, 792–800.

Descamps, V., Aitken, J., & Lee, M. G. (1994). Hippocrates on necrotising fasciitis. *Lancet, 344*, 556.

DiPersio, J. R., File, T. M., Jr., Stevens, D. L., Gardner, W. G., Petropoulos, G., & Dinsa, K. (1996). Spread of serious disease-producing M3 clones of group A streptococcus among family members and health care workers. *Clin Inf Dis, 22*, 490–495.

Doctor, A., Harper, M. B., & Fleisher, G. R. (1995). Group A beta-hemolytic streptococcal bacteremia: Historical overview, changing incidence, and recent association with varicella. *Pediatrics, 96*, 428–433.

Duma, R. J., Weinberg, A. N., Medrek, T. F., & Kunz, L. J. (1969). Streptococcal infections: A bacteriologic and clinical study of streptococcal bacteremia. *Medicine, 48*, 87–127.

Eriksson, B. K., Andersson, J., Holm, S. E., & Norgren, M. (1999). Invasive group A streptococcal infections: T1M1 isolates expressing pyrogenic exotoxins A and B in combination with selective lack of toxin-neutralizing antibodies are associated with increased risk of streptococcal toxic shock syndrome. *J Infect Dis, 180*, 410–418.

Fang, G. D., Fine, M., Orloff, J., Arisumi, D., Yu, V. L., Kapoor, W., Grayston, J. T., Wang, S. P., Kohler, R., & Muder, R. R. (1990). New and emerging etiologies for community-acquired pneumonia with implications for therapy. A prospective multicenter study of 359 cases. *Medicine (Baltimore), 69*, 307–316.

Fischetti, V. A. (1989). Streptococcal M protein: Design and biological behavior. *Clin Microbiol Rev, 2*, 285–314.

Gaworzewska, E., & Colman, G. (1988). Changes in the pattern of infection caused by *Streptococcus pyogenes. Epidem Inf, 100*, 257–269.

Gemmell, C. G., Peterson, P. K., Schmeling, D., Kim, Y., Mathews, J., Wannamaker, L., & Quie, P. G. (1981). Potentiation of opsonization and phagocytosis of *Streptococcus pyogenes* following growth in the presence of clindamycin. *J Clin Invest, 67*, 1249–1256.

Goepel, J. R., Richards, D. G., Harris, D. M., & Henry, L. (1980). Fulminant *Streptococcus pyogenes* infection. *Brit Med J, 281*, 1412.

Guzman, C. A., Talay, S. R., Molinari, G., Medina, E., & Chhatwal, G. S. (1999). Protective immune response against *Streptococcus pyogenes* in mice after intranasal vaccination with the fibronectin-binding protein SfbI. *J Infect Dis, 179*, 901–906.

Hable, K. A., Horstmeirer, C., Wold, A. D., & Washington, J. A. (1973). Group A β-hemolytic streptococcemia: Bacteriologic and clinical study of 44 cases. *Mayo Clin Proc, 48*, 336–339.

Hackett, S. P., & Stevens, D. L. (1992). Streptococcal toxic shock syndrome: Synthesis of tumor necrosis factor and interleukin-1 by monocytes stimulated with pyrogenic exotoxin A and streptolysin O. *J Infect Dis, 165*, 879–885.

Hasty, D. L., Ofek, I., Courtney, H. S., & Doyle, R. J. (1992). Multiple adhesins of streptococci. *Infect Immun, 60*, 2147–2152.

Haywood, C. T., McGeer, A., & Low, D. E. (1998). Clinical experience with 20 cases of group A streptococcus necrotizing fasciitis and myonecrosis: 1995–1997. *Abstract of Canadian Society for Plastic Surgeons Annual Meeting*. Ref Type: Abstract.

Heeg, K., Sparwasser, T., Lipford, G. B., Hacker, H., Zimmermann, S., & Wagner, H. (1998). Bacterial DNA as an evolutionary conserved ligand signalling danger of infection to immune cells. *Eur J Clin Microbiol Infect Dis, 17*, 464–469.

Hemmi, H., Takeuchi, O., Kawai, T., Kaisho, T., Sato, S., Sanjo, H., Matsumoto, M., Hoshino, K., Wagner, H., Takeda, K., & Akira, S. (2000). A Toll-like receptor recognizes bacterial DNA. *Nature, 408*, 740–745.

Herwald, H., Collin, M., Muller-Esterl, W., & Bjorck, L. (1996). Streptococcal cysteine proteinase releases kinins: A novel virulence mechanism. *J Exp Med, 184*, 665–673.

Heumann, D., Barras, C., Severin, A., Glauser, M. P., & Tomasz, A. (1994). Gram-positive cell walls stimulate synthesis of tumor necrosis factor alpha and interleukin-6 by human monocytes. *Infect Immun, 62*, 2715–2721.

Hiemstra, P. S., Brands-Tajouiti, J., & van Furth, R. (1994). Comparison of antibody activity against various microorganisms in intravenous immunoglobulin preparations determined by ELISA and opsonic assay. *J Lab Clin Med, 123*, 241–246.

Hoe, N. P., Nakashima, K., Lukomski, S., Grigsby, D., Liu, M., Kordari, P., Dou, S. J., Pan, X., Vuopio-Varkila, J., Salmelinna, S., McGeer, A., Low, D. E., Schwartz, B., Schuchat, A., Naidich, S., De Lorenzo, D., Fu, Y. X., & Musser, J. M. (1999). Rapid selection of complement-inhibiting protein variants in group A Streptococcus epidemic waves. *Nat Med, 5*, 924–929.

Hoge, C. W., Schwartz, B., Talkington, D. F., Breiman, R. F., MacNeill, E. M., & Englender, S. J. (1993a). The changing epidemiology of invasive group A streptococcal infections and the emergence of streptococcal toxic shock-like syndrome. *JAMA, 269*, 585–589.

Hoge, C. W., Schwartz, B., Talkington, D. F., Breiman, R. F., MacNeill, E. M., & Englender, S. J. (1993b). The changing epidemiology of invasive group A streptococcal infections and the emergence of streptococcal toxic shock-like syndrome. A retrospective population-based study [published erratum appears in *JAMA*, 1993, Apr 7, *269(13)*, 1638] [see comments]. *JAMA, 269*, 384–389.

Holm, S. E., Norrby, A., Bergholm, A. M., & Norgren, M. (1992). Aspects of pathogenesis of serious group A streptococcal infections in Sweden. *J Infect Dis, 166*, 31–37.

Hook, E. W., Horton, C. A., & Schaberg, D. R. (1983). Failure of intensive care unit support to influence mortality from pneumococcal bacteremia. *JAMA, 249*, 1055–1057.

Husmann, L. K., Yung, D.-L., Hollingshead, S. K., & Scott, J. R. (1997). Role of putative virulence factors of *Streptococcus pyogenes* in mouse models of long-term throat colonization and pneumonia. *Infect Immun, 65*, 1422–1430.

Hytonen, J., Haataja, S., Gerlach, D., Podbielski, A., & Finne, J. (2001). The SpeB virulence factor of *Streptococcus pyogenes*, a multifunctional secreted and cell surface molecule with strepadhesin, laminin-binding and cysteine protease activity. *Mol Microbiol, 39*, 512–519.

Jaffe, J., Natanson-Yaron, S., Caparon, M. G., & Hanski, E. (1996). Protein F2, a novel fibronectin-binding protein from *Streptococcus pyogenes*, possesses two binding domains. *Mol Microbiol, 21*, 373–384.

Ji, Y., Carlson, B., Kondagunta, A., & Cleary, P. P. (1997). Intranasal immunization with C5a peptidase prevents nasopharyngeal colonization of mice by the group A Streptococcus. *Infect Immun, 65*, 2080–2087.

Kamezawa, Y., Nakahara, T., Nakano, S., Abe, Y., Nozaki-Renard, J., & Isono, T. (1997). Streptococcal mitogenic exotoxin Z, a novel acidic superantigenic toxin produced by a T1 strain of *Streptococcus pyogenes*. *Infect Immun, 65*, 3828–3833.

Kansal, R. G., McGeer, A., Low, D. E., Norrby-Teglund, A., & Kotb, M. (2000). Inverse relation between disease severity and expression of the streptococcal cysteine protease, SpeB, among clonal M1T1 isolates recovered from invasive group A streptococcal infection cases. *Infect Immun, 68*, 6362–6369.

Kaplan, E. (1993). Global assessment of rheumatic fever and rheumatic heart disease at the close of the century. The influences and dynamics of population and pathogens: A failure to realize prevention? (The T. Duckettt Jones Memorial Lecture.) *Circulation, 88*, 1964–1972.

Kaplan, E. L. (1996). Recent epidemiology of group A streptococcal infections in North America and abroad: An overview. *Paediatrics, 97*, 945–948.

Kapur, V., Maffei, J. T., Greer, R. S., Li, L. L., Adams, G. J., & Musser, J. M. (1994). Vaccination with streptococcal extracellular cysteine protease (interleuki-1β convertase) protects mice against challenge with heterologous group A streptococci. *Microb Pathog, 16*, 443–450.

Kapur, V., Majesky, M. W., Li, L. L., Black, R. A., & Musser, J. M. (1993a). Cleavage of interleukin 1 beta (IL-1 beta) precursor to produce active IL-1 beta by a conserved extracellular cysteine protease from *Streptococcus pyogenes*. *Proc Natl Acad Sci USA, 90*, 7676–7680.

Kapur, V., Topouzis, S., Majesky, M. W., Li, L. L., Hamrick, M. R., Hamill, R. J., Patti, J. M., & Musser, J. M. (1993b). A conserved *Streptococcus pyogenes* extracellular cysteine protease cleaves human fibronectin and degrades vitronectin. *Microb Pathog, 15*, 327–346.

Katz, A. R., & Morens, D. M. (1992). Severe streptococcal infections in historical perspective. *Clin Infect Dis, 14*, 298–307.

Kaul, R., McGeer, A., Low, D. E., Green, K., Schwartz, B., Ontario Group A Streptococcal Study, & Simor, A. E. (1997). Population-based surveillance for group A streptococcal necrotizing fasciitis: Clinical features, prognostic indicators and microbiologic analysis of 77 cases. *Am J Med, 103*, 18–24.

Kaul, R., McGeer, A., Norrby-Teglund, A., Kotb, M., Schwartz, B., O'Rourke, K., Talbot, J., The Canadian Streptococcal Study Group, & Low, D. E. (1999). Intravenous immunoglobulin therapy in streptococcal toxic shock syndrome—A comparative observational study. *Clin Inf Dis, 28*, 800–807.

Kawabata, S., Kunitomo, E., Terao, Y., Nakagawa, I., Kikuchi, K., Totsuka, K., & Hamada, S. (2001). Systemic and mucosal immunizations with fibronectin-binding protein FBP54 induce protective immune responses against *Streptococcus pyogenes* challenge in mice. *Infect Immun, 69*, 924–930.

Keefer, C. S., Inglefinger, F. J., & Spink, W. W. (1937). Significance of hemolytic streptococci bacteraemia: A study of two hundred and forty six patients. *Arch Intern Med, 60*, 1084–1097.

Keefer, C. S., Rantz, L. A., & Rammelkamp, C. H. (1941). Hemolytic streptococcal pneumonia and empyema: A study of 55 cases with special reference to treatment. *Ann Intern Med, 14*, 1533–1550.

Keller, R., Fischer, W., Keist, R., & Bassetti, S. (1992). Macrophage response to bacteria: Induction of marked secretory and cellular activities by lipoteichoic acids. *Infect Immun, 60*, 3664–3672.

Kengatharan, K. M., De Kimpe, S. J., & Thiemermann, C. (1996). Role of nitric oxide in the circulatory failure and organ injury in a rodent model of Gram-positive shock. *Br J Pharmacol, 119*, 1411–1421.

Kiska, D. L., Thiede, B., Caracciolo, J., Jordan, M., Johnson, D., Kaplan, E. L., Gruninger, R. P., Lohr, J. A., Gilligan, P. H., & Denny, F. W., Jr. (1997). Invasive group A streptococcal infections in North Carolina: Epidemiology, clinical features, and genetic and serotype analysis of causative organisms. *J Infect Dis, 176*, 992–1000.

Klinman, D. M., Yi, A. K., Beaucage, S. L., Conover, J., & Krieg, A. M. (1996). CpG motifs present in bacteria DNA rapidly induce lymphocytes to secrete interleukin 6, interleukin 12, and interferon gamma. *Proc Natl Acad Sci USA, 93*, 2879–2883.

Kotb, M. (1995). Bacterial pyrogenic exotoxins as superantigens. *Clin Microbiol Rev, 8*, 411–426.

Kotb, M. (1998). Superantigens of Gram-positive bacteria: Structure–function analyses and their implications for biological activity. *Curr Opin Microbiol, 1*, 56–65.

Kraus, W., & Beachey, E. H. (1988). Renal autoimmune epitope of group A streptococci specified by M protein tetrapeptide Ile–Arg–Leu–Arg. *Proc Natl Acad Sci USA, 85*, 4516–4520.

Kreikemeyer, B., Talay, S. R., & Chhatwal, G. S. (1995). Characterization of a novel fibronectin-binding surface protein in group A streptococci. *Microb Pathog, 19*, 299–315.

Krieg, A. M. (1995). CpG DNA: A pathogenic factor in systemic lupus erythematosus? *J Clin Immunol, 15*, 284–292.

Kuo, C. F., Wu, J. J., Lin, K. Y., Tsai, P. J., Lee, S. C., Jin, Y. T., Lei, H. Y., & Lin, Y. S. (1998). Role of streptococcal pyrogenic exotoxin B in the mouse model of group A streptococcal infection. *Infect Immun, 66*, 3931–3935.

Lamothe, F., D'Amico, P., Ghosn, P., Tremblay, C., Braidy, J., & Patenaude, J. V. (1995). Clinical usefulness of intravenous human immunoglobulins in invasive group A streptococcal infections: Case report and review. *Clin Inf Dis, 21*, 1469–1470.

Lancefield, R. C. (1962). Current knowledge of the type specific M antigens of group A streptococci. *J Immunol, 89*, 307–313.

Laupland, K. B., Davies, H. D., Low, D. E., Schwartz, B., Green, K., & McGeer, A. (2000). Invasive group A streptococcal disease in children and association with varicella-zoster virus infection. Ontario Group A Streptococcal Study Group. *Pediatrics, 105*, E60.

Leung, D. Y., Cotran, R. S., Kurt-Jones, E., Burns, J. C., Newburger, J. W., & Pober, J. S. (1989). Endothelial cell activation and high interleukin-1 secretion in the pathogenesis of acute Kawasaki disease. *Lancet, 2*, 1298–1302.

Lieberman, D., Schlaeffer, F., Boldur, I., Lieberman, D., Horowitz, S., Friedman, M. G., Leiononen, M., Horovitz, O., Manor, E., & Porath, A. (1996). Multiple pathogens in adult patients admitted with community-acquired pneumonia: A one year prospective study of 346 consecutive patients. *Thorax, 51*, 179–184.

Lim, I., Shaw, D. R., Stanley, D. P., Lumb, R., & McLennan, G. (1989). A prospective hospital study of the aetiology of community-acquired pneumonia. *Med J Aust, 151*, 87–91.

Limbago, B., Penumalli, V., Weinrick, B., & Scott, J. R. (2000). Role of streptolysin O in a mouse model of invasive group A streptococcal disease. *Infect Immun, 68*, 6384–6390.

Lissner, R., Struff, W. G., Autenrieth, I. B., Woodcock, B. G., & Karch, H. (1999). Efficacy and potential clinical applications of Pentaglobin, an IgM-enriched immunoglobulin concentrate suitable for intravenous infusion. *Eur J Surg Suppl, 584*, 17–25.

Low, D. E., Schwartz, B., & McGeer, A. (1997). The reemergence of severe group A streptococcal disease: An evolutionary perspective. In W. M. Scheld, D. Armstrong, & J. M. Hughes (Eds.), *Emerging infections 1* (pp. 93–123). Washington, DC: ASM Press.

Lukomski, S., Nakashima, K., Abdi, I., Cipriano, V. J., Ireland, R. M., Reid, S. D., Adams, G. G., & Musser, J. M. (2000). Identification and characterization of the scl gene encoding a group A Streptococcus extracellular protein virulence factor with similarity to human collagen. *Infect Immun, 68*, 6542–6553.

Lukomski, S., Sreevatsan, S., Amberg, C., Reichardt, W., Woischnik, M., Podbielski, A., & Musser, J. M. (1997). Inactivation of *Streptococcus pyogenes* extracellular cysteine protease significantly decreases mouse lethality of serotype M3 and M49 strains. *J Clin Invest, 99*, 2574–2580.

MacCallum, W. G. (1919). *The pathology of the pneumonia in the United States army camps during the winter of 1917–1918* (Monograph No. 10). New York: Rockefeller Institute for Medical Research.

Mahieu, L. M., Holm, S. E., Goossens, H. J., & Van Acker, K. J. (1995). Congenital streptococcal toxic shock syndrome with absence of antibodies against streptococcal pyrogenic exotoxins. *J Pediatr, 127*, 987–989.

Marrack, P., & Kappler, J. (1990). The staphylococcal enterotoxins and their relatives. *Science, 248*, 705–711.

Marston, B. J., Plouffe, J. F., File, T. M., Jr., Hackman, B. A., Salstrom, S. J., Lipman, H. B., Kolczak, M. S., & Breiman, R. F. (1997). Incidence of community-acquired pneumonia requiring hospitalization. Results of a population-based active surveillance study in Ohio. The Community-Based Pneumonia Incidence Study Group. *Arch Intern Med, 157*, 1709–1718.

Martin, P. R., & Hoiby, E. A. (1990). Streptococcal serogroup A epidemic in Norway 1987–1988. *Scand J Infect Dis, 22*, 421–429.

Mascini, E. M., Jansze, M., Schellekens, J. F., Musser, J. M., Faber, J. A., Verhoef-Verhage, L. A., Schouls, L., van Leeuwen, W. J., Verhoef, J., & van Dijk, H. (2000). Invasive group A streptococcal disease in the Netherlands: Evidence for a protective role of anti-exotoxin A antibodies. *J Infect Dis, 181*, 631–638.

Mascini, E. M., Jansze, M., Schouls, L. M., Verhoef, J., & van Dijk, H. (2001). Penicillin and clindamycin differentially inhibit the production of pyrogenic exotoxins A and B by group A streptococci. *Int J Antimicrob Agents, 18*, 395–398.

Mattsson, E., Verhage, L., Rollof, J., Fleer, A., Verhoef, J., & van Dijk, H. (1993). Peptidoglycan and teichoic acid from *Staphylococcus epidermidis* stimulate human monocytes to release tumour necrosis factor-alpha, interleukin-1 beta and interleukin-6. *FEMS Immunol Med Microbiol, 7*, 281–287.

McCormick, J. K., Yarwood, J. M., & Schlievert, P. M. (2001). Toxic shock syndrome and bacterial superantigens: An update. *Annu Rev Microbiol, 55*, 77–104.

McGeer, A., Willey, B., Schwartz, B., Green, K., Bernston, A., Trpeski, L., Talbot, J., Group A Streptococcal Study, & Low, D. E. (1998). Epidemiology of invasive GAS disease due to M3 serotypes in Ontario, Canada. *38th Interscience Conference on Antimicrobial Agents and Chemotherapy*, Abstract no. 577. Abstract.

McLellan, D. G., Chiang, E. Y., Courtney, H. S., Hasty, D. L., Wei, S. C., Hu, M. C., Walls, M. A., Bloom, J. J., & Dale, J. B. (2001). Spa contributes to the virulence of type 18 group A streptococci. *Infect Immun, 69*, 2943–2949.

Medaglini, D., Pozzi, G., King, T. P., & Fischetti, V. A. (1995). Mucosal and systemic immune responses to a recombinant protein expressed on the surface of the oral commensal bacterium *Streptococcus gordonii* after oral colonization. *Proc Natl Acad Sci USA, 92*, 6868–6872.

Medzihtov, R., & Janeway, C. J., Jr. (2000). Innate immunity. *N Engl J Med, 5*, 338–344.

Metlay, J. P., Hofmann, J., Cetron, M. S., Fine, M. J., Farley, M. M., Whitney, C., & Breiman, R. F. (2000). Impact of penicillin susceptibility on medical outcomes for adult patients with bacteremic pneumococcal pneumonia. *Clin Infect Dis, 30*, 520–528.

Mollick, J. A., Miller, G. G., Musser, J. M., Cook, R. G., Grossman, D., & Rich, R. R. (1993). A novel superantigen isolated from pathogenic strains of *Streptococcus pyogenes* with aminoterminal homology to staphylococcal enterotoxins B and C. *J Clin Invest, 92*, 710–719.

Morath, S., Geyer, A., & Hartung, T. (2001). Structure–function relationship of cytokine induction by lipoteichoic acid from *Staphylococcus aureus*. *J Exp Med, 193*, 393–397.

Moses, A. E., Wessels, M. R., Zalcman, K., Alberti, S., Natanson-Yaron, S., Menes, T., & Hanski, E. (1997). Relative contributions of hyaluronic acid capsule and M protein to virulence in a mucoid strain of the group A Streptococcus. *Infect Immun, 65*, 64–71.

Mouthon, L., Kaveri, S. V., Spalter, S. H., Lacroix-Desmazes, S., Lefranc, C., Desai, R., & Kazatchkine, M. D. (1996). Mechanisms of action of intravenous immune globulin in immune-mediated diseases. *Clin Exp Immunol, 104*(Suppl. 1), 3–9.

Muller, M. P., McGeer, A., Low, D. E., & Ontario Group A Streptococcal Study. (2001). Successful outcomes in six patients treated conservatively for suspected necrotizing fasciitis (NF) due to group A streptococcus (GAS). *41st Interscience Conference on Antimicrobial Agents and Chemotherapy*. Ref Type: Abstract.

Muller, M. P., McGeer, A. J., Low, D. E., & the Ontario Group A Streptococcal Study Group. (2000). Clinical and epidemiological features of group A streptococcal pneumonia in Ontario, Canada: 1992 to 1996. *40th Interscience Conference on Antimicrobial Agents and Chemotherapy*. Ref Type: Abstract.

Nadal, D., Lauener, R. P., & Braegger, C. P. (1993). T cell activation and cytokine release in streptococcal toxic shock-like syndrome. *J Pediatr, 122*, 727–729.

Nakashima, K., Ichiyama, S., Iinuma, Y., Hasegawa, Y., Ohta, M., Ooe, K., Shimizu, Y., Igarashi, H., Murai, T., & Shimokata, K. (1997). A clinical and bacteriologic investigation of invasive streptococcal infections in Japan on the basis of serotypes, toxin production, and genomic DNA fingerprints. *Clin Infect Dis, 25*, 260–266.

Navarre, W. W., & Schneewind, O. (1999). Surface proteins of Gram-positive bacteria and mechanisms of their targeting to the cell wall envelope. *Microbiol Mol Biol Rev, 63*, 174–229.

Norrby-Teglund, A., Basma, H., Andersson, J., McGeer, A., Low, D. E., & Kotb, M. (1998). Varying titers of neutralizing antibodies to streptococcal superantigens in different preparations of normal polyspecific immunoglobulin G: Implications for therapeutic efficacy [see comments]. *Clin Infect Dis, 26*, 631–638.

Norrby-Teglund, A., Ihendyane, N., Kansal, R., Basma, H., Kotb, M., Andersson, J., & Hammarstrom, L. (2000). Relative neutralizing activity in polyspecific IgM, IgA, and IgG preparations against group A streptococcal superantigens. *Clin Infect Dis, 31*, 1175–1182.

Norrby-Teglund, A., Kaul, R., Low, D. E., McGeer, A., Andersson, J., Andersson, U., & Kotb, M. (1996a). Evidence for the presence of streptococcal superantigen neutralizing antibodies in normal polyspecific IgG (IVIG). *Infect Immun, 64*, 5395–5398.

Norrby-Teglund, A., Kaul, R., Low, D. E., McGeer, A., Newton, D. W., Andersson, J., Andersson, U., & Kotb, M. (1996b). Plasma from patients with severe group A streptococcal infections treated with normal polyspecific IgG (IVIG) inhibits streptococcal superantigen-induced T cell proliferation and cytokine production. *J Immunol, 156*, 3057–3064.

Norrby-Teglund, A., Pauksens, K., Holm, S. E., & Norgren, M. (1994). Relation between low capacity of human sera to inhibit streptococcal mitogens and serious manifestations of disease. *J Inf Dis, 170*, 585–591.

Norrby-Teglund, A., & Stevens, D. L. (1998). Novel therapies in streptococcal toxic shock syndrome: Attenuation of virulence factor expression and modulation of the host response. *Curr Opin Infect Dis, 11*, 285–291.

Pancholi, V., & Fischetti, V. A. (1992). A major surface protein on group A streptococci is a glyceraldehyde-3-phosphate-dehydrogenase with multiple binding activity. *J Exp Med, 176*, 415–426.

Pancholi, V., & Fischetti, V. A. (1998). Alpha-enolase, a novel strong plasmin(ogen) binding protein on the surface of pathogenic streptococci. *J Biol Chem, 273*, 14503–14515.

Parker, M. T. (1979). Necropsy studies of the bacterial complications of influenzae. *J Infect, 1*(Suppl 2), 9–16.

Patel, R., Rouse, M. S., Florez, M. V., Piper, K. E., Cockerill, F. R., Wilson, W. R., & Steckelberg, J. M. (2000). Lack of benefit of intravenous immune globulin in a murine model of group A streptococcal necrotizing fasciitis. *J Infect Dis, 181*, 230–234.

Perez, C. M., Kubak, B. M., Cryer, H. G., Salehmugodam, S., Vespa, P., & Farmer, D. (1997). Adjunctive treatment of streptococcal toxic shock syndrome using intravenous immunoglobulin: Case report and review. *Am J Med, 102*, 111–112.

Peterson, C. L., Mascola, L., Chao, S. M., Lieberman, J. M., Arcinue, E. L., Blumberg, D. A., Kim, K. S., Kovacs, A., Wong, V. K., & Brunell, P. A. (1996a). Children hospitalized for varicella: A prevaccine review. *J Pediatr, 129*, 529–536.

Peterson, C. L., Vugia, D. J., Meyers, H. B., Chao, S. M., Vogt, J., Lanson, J., Brunell, P. A., Kim, K. S., & Mascola, L. (1996b). Risk factors for invasive group A streptococcal infections in children with varicella: A case–control study. *Pediatr Infect Dis J, 15*, 151–156.

Poutsiaka, D. D., Clark, B. D., Vannier, E., & Dinarello, C. A. (1991). Production of interleukin-1 receptor antagonist and interleukin-1 beta by peripheral blood mononuclear cells is differentially regulated. *Blood, 78*, 1275–1281.

Proft, T., Moffatt, S. L., Berkahn, C. J., & Fraser, J. D. (1999). Identification and characterization of novel superantigens from *Streptococcus pyogenes*. *J Exp Med, 189*, 89–102.

Pruksakorn, S., Currie, B., Brandt, E., Martin, D., Galbraith, A., Phornphutkul, C., Hunsakunachai, S., Manmontri, A., & Good, M. F. (1994). Towards a vaccine for rheumatic fever: Identification of a conserved target epitope on M protein of group A streptococci. *Lancet, 344*, 639–642.

Quinn, R. W. (1982). Epidemiology of group A streptococcal infections—their changing frequency and severity. *Yale J Biol Med, 55*, 265–270.

Raeder, R., Harokopakis, E., Hollingshead, S., & Boyle, M. D. (2000). Absence of SpeB production in virulent large capsular forms of group A streptococcal strain 64. *Infect Immun, 68*, 744–751.

Raeder, R., Woischnik, M., Podbielski, A., & Boyle, M. D. (1998). A secreted streptococcal cysteine protease can cleave a surface-expressed M1 protein and alter the immunoglobulin binding properties. *Res Microbiol, 149*, 539–548.

Rakonjac, J. V., Robbins, J. C., & Fischetti, V. A. (1995). DNA sequence of the serum opacity factor of group A streptococci: Identification of a fibronectin-binding repeat domain. *Infect Immun, 63*, 622–631.

Rasmussen, M., & Bjorck, L. (2001). Unique regulation of SclB—a novel collagen-like surface protein of *Streptococcus pyogenes*. *Mol Microbiol, 40*, 1427–1438.

Rasmussen, M., Eden, A., & Bjorck, L. (2000). SclA, a novel collagen-like surface protein of *Streptococcus pyogenes*. *Infect Immun, 68*, 6370–6377.

Rasmussen, M., Muller, H. P., & Bjorck, L. (1999). Protein GRAB of *Streptococcus pyogenes* regulates proteolysis at the bacterial surface by binding alpha2-macroglobulin. *J Biol Chem, 274*, 15336–15344.

Riesenfeld-Orn, I., Wolpe, S., Garcia-Bustos, J. F., Hoffmann, M. K., & Tuomanen, E. (1989). Production of interleukin-1 but not tumor necrosis factor by human monocytes stimulated with pneumococcal cell surface components. *Infect Immun, 57*, 1890–1893.

Ruiz de Souza, V., Carreno, M. P., Kaveri, S. V., Ledur, A., Sadeghi, H., Cavaillon, J. M., Kazatchkine, M. D., & Haeffner-Cavaillon, N. (1995). Selective induction of interleukin-1 receptor antagonist and interleukin-8 in human monocytes by normal polyspecific IgG (intravenous immunoglobulin). *Eur J Immunol, 25*, 1267–1273.

Ruoff, K. L. (1995). Streptococcus. In P. R. Murray, E. J. Baron, M. A. Pfaller, F. C. Tenover, & R. H. Yolken (Eds.), *Manual of clinical microbiology*. (pp. 299–307). Washington: ASM Press.

Salvadori, L. G., Blake, M. S., McCarty, M., Tai, J. Y., & Zabriskie, J. B. (1995). Group A streptococcus-liposome ELISA antibody titers to group A polysaccharide and opsonophagocytic capabilities of the antibodies. *J Infect Dis, 171*, 593–600.

Samuelsson, A., Towers, T. L., & Ravetch, J. V. (2001). Anti-inflammatory activity of IVIG mediated through the inhibitory Fc receptor. *Science, 291*, 484–486.

Schrager, H. M., Alberti, S., Cywes, C., Dougherty, G. J., & Wessels, M. R. (1998). Hyaluronic acid capsule modulates M protein-mediated adherence and acts as a ligand for attachment of group A Streptococcus to CD44 on human keratinocytes. *J Clin Invest, 101*, 1708–1716.

Schuchat, A., Hilger, T., Zell, E., Farley, M. M., Reingold, A., Harrison, L., Lefkowitz, L., Danila, R., Stefonek, K., Barrett, N., Morse, D., & Pinner, R. (2001). Active bacterial core surveillance of the emerging infections program network. *Emerg Infect Dis, 7*, 92–99.

Schulze, K., Medina, E., Talay, S. R., Towers, R. J., Chhatwal, G. S., & Guzman, C. A. (2001). Characterization of the domain of fibronectin-binding protein I of *Streptococcus pyogenes* responsible for elicitation of a protective immune response. *Infect Immun, 69*, 622–625.

Schwartz, B., Facklam, R. R., & Breiman, R. F. (1990). Changing epidemiology of group A streptococcal infection in the USA. *Lancet, 336*, 1167–1171.

Shanley, T. P., Schrier, D., Kapur, V., Kehoe, M., Musser, J. M., & Ward, P. A. (1996). Streptococcal cysteine protease augments lung injury induced by products of group A streptococci. *Infect Immun, 64*, 870–877.

Sharief, M. K., Ingram, D. A., Swash, M., & Thompson, E. J. (1999). I.v. immunoglobulin reduces circulating proinflammatory cytokines in Guillain–Barre syndrome. *Neurology, 52*, 1833–1838.

Sharkawy, A., Low, D. E., Saginur, R., Gregson, D., Schwartz, B., Jessamine, P., Green, K., & McGeer, A. (2002). Severe group A streptococcal soft-tissue infections in Ontario: 1992–1996. *Clin Infect Dis, 34*, 454–460.

Simpson, W. A., & Beachey, E. H. (1983). Adherence of group A streptococci to fibronectin on oral epithelial cells. *Infect Immun, 39*, 275–279.

Skansen-Saphir, U., Andersson, J., Bjorck, L., & Andersson, U. (1994). Lymphokine production induced by streptococcal pyrogenic exotoxin-A is selectively down-regulated by pooled human IgG. *Eur J Immunol, 24*, 916–922.

Spika, J. S., Peterson, P. K., Wilkinson, B. J., Hammerschmidt, D. E., Verbrugh, H. A., Verhoef, J., & Quie, P. G. (1982). Role of peptidoglycan from *Staphylococcus aureus* in leukopenia, thrombocytopenia, and complement activation associated with bacteremia. *J Infect Dis, 146*, 227–234.

Sriskandan, S., & Cohen, J. (1999). Gram-positive sepsis. Mechanisms and differences from Gram-negative sepsis. *Infect Dis Clin North Am, 13*, 397–412.

Sriskandan, S., McKee, A., Hall, L., & Cohen, J. (1997). Comparative effects of clindamycin and ampicillin on superantigenic activity of *Streptococcus pyogenes*. *J Antimicrob Chemother, 40*, 275–277.

Stalhammar-Carlemalm, M., Areschoug, T., Larsson, C., & Lindahl, G. (1999). The R28 protein of *Streptococcus pyogenes* is related to several group B streptococcal surface proteins, confers protective immunity and promotes binding to human epithelial cells. *Mol Microbiol, 33*, 208–219.

Standiford, T. J., Arenberg, D. A., Danforth, J. M., Kunkel, S. L., VanOtteren, G. M., & Strieter, R. M. (1994). Lipoteichoic acid induces secretion of interleukin-8 from human blood monocytes: A cellular and molecular analysis. *Infect Immun, 62*, 119–125.

Stegmayr, B., Bjorck, S., Holm, S., Nisell, J., Rydvall, A., & Settergren, B. (1992). Septic shock induced by group A streptococcal infection: Clinical and therapeutic aspects. *Scand J Infect Dis, 24*, 589–597.

Stevens, D. L. (1992). Invasive group A streptococcus infections. *Clin Infect Dis, 14*, 2–11.

Stevens, D. L. (1999). The flesh-eating bacterium: What's next? *J Infect Dis, 179*(Suppl. 2), S366–S374.

Stevens, D. L., Gibbons, A. E., Bergstrom, R., & Winn, V. (1988). The Eagle effect revisited: Efficacy of clindamycin, erythromycin and penicillin in the treatment of streptococcal myositis. *J Infect Dis, 158*, 23–28.

Stevens, D. L., Tanner, M. H., Winship, J., Swarts, R., Ries, K. M., Schlievert, P. M., & Kaplan, E. (1989). Severe group A streptococcal infections associated with a toxic shock-like syndrome and scarlet fever toxin A. *N Eng J Med, 321*, 1–7.

Stevens, D. L., Yan, S., & Bryant, A. E. (1993). Penicillin-binding protein expression at different growth stages determines penicillin efficacy in vitro and in vivo: An explanation for the inoculum effect. *J Infect Dis, 167*, 1401–1405.

Stockbauer, K. E., Magoun, L., Liu, M., Burns, E. H., Jr., Gubba, S., Renish, S., Pan, X., Bodary, S. C., Baker, E., Coburn, J., Leong, J. M., & Musser, J. M. (1999). A natural variant of the cysteine protease virulence factor of group A Streptococcus with an arginine–glycine–aspartic acid (RGD) motif preferentially binds human integrins alphavbeta3 and alphaIIbbeta3. *Proc Natl Acad Sci USA, 96*, 242–247.

Stromberg, A., Romanus, V., & Burman, L. G. (1991). Outbreaks of group A streptococcal bacteremia in Sweden: An epidemiologic and clinical study. *J Infect Dis, 164*, 595–598.

Stylianos, S., Wakabayashi, G., Gelfand, J. A., & Harris, B. H. (1991). Experimental hemorrhage and blunt trauma do not increase circulating tumor necrosis factor. *J Trauma, 31*, 1063–1067.

Svensson, M. D., Scaramuzzino, D. A., Sjobring, U., Olsen, A., Frank, C., & Bessen, D. E. (2000a). Role for a secreted cysteine proteinase in the establishment of host tissue tropism by group A streptococci. *Mol Microbiol, 38*, 242–253.

Svensson, N., Oberg, S., Henriques, B., Holm, S., Kallenius, G., Romanus, V., & Giesecke, J. (2000b). Invasive group A streptococcal infections in Sweden in 1994 and 1995: Epidemiology and clinical spectrum. *Scand J Infect Dis, 32*, 609–614.

Takei, S., Arora, Y. K., & Walker, S. M. (1993). Intravenous immunoglobulin contains antibodies inhibitory to activation of T-cells by staphylococcal superantigens. *J Clin Invest, 91*, 602–607.

The Working Group on Severe Streptococcal Infections. (1993). Defining the group A streptococcal toxic shock syndrome. Rationale and consensus definition. *JAMA, 269*, 384, 390–391.

Timmerman, C. P., Mattsson, E., Martinez-Martinez, L., De Graaf, L., Van Strijp, J. A., Verbrugh, H. A., Verhoef, J., & Fleer, A. (1993). Induction of release of tumor necrosis factor from human monocytes by staphylococci and staphylococcal peptidoglycans. *Infect Immun, 61*, 4167–4172.

Tuomanen, E., Liu, H., Hengstler, B., Zak, O., & Tomasz, A. (1985). The induction of meningeal inflammation by components of the pneumococcal cell wall. *J Infect Dis, 151*, 859–868.

Ulrich, R. G., Olson, M. A., & Bavari, S. (1998). Development of engineered vaccines effective against structurally related bacterial superantigens. *Vaccine, 16*, 1857–1864.

Upton, M., Carter, P. E., Orange, G., & Pennington, T. H. (1996). Genetic heterogeneity of M type 3 group A streptococci causing severe infections in Tayside, Scotland. *J Clin Microbiol, 34*, 196–198.

Visvanathan, K., Charles, A., Bannan, J., Pugach, P., Kashfi, K., & Zabriskie, J. B. (2001). Inhibition of bacterial superantigens by peptides and antibodies. *Infect Immun, 69*, 875–884.

Vugia, D. J., Peterson, C. L., Meyers, H. B., Kim, K. S., Arrieta, A., Schlievert, P. M., Kaplan, E. L., & Werner, S. B. (1996). Invasive group A streptococcal infections in children with varicella in Southern California. *Pediatr Infect Dis J, 15*, 146–150.

Wang, F. D., Liu, I. M., & Liu, C. Y. (2000a). In vitro activity of quinupristin/dalfopristin and other antibiotics against ampicillin-resistant enterococcus faecium. *Chung Hua I Hsueh Tsa Chih (Taipei.), 63*, 119–123.

Wang, J. E., Jorgensen, P. F., Almlof, M., Thiemermann, C., Foster, S. J., Aasen, A. O., & Solberg, R. (2000b). Peptidoglycan and lipoteichoic acid from *Staphylococcus aureus* induce tumor necrosis factor alpha, interleukin 6 (IL-6), and IL-10 production in both T cells and monocytes in a human whole blood model. *Infect Immun, 68*, 3965–3970.

Weisman, L. E., Cruess, D. F., & Fischer, G. W. (1994). Opsonic activity of commercially available standard intravenous immunoglobulin preparations. *Pediatr Infect Dis J, 13*, 1122–1125.

Welch, C. C., Tombridge, T. L., Baker, W. J., & Kinney, R. J. (1961). Beta-hemolytic streptococcal pneumonia. Report of an outbreak in a military population. *Am J Med Sci, 242*, 157–167.

Wessels, M. R., & Bronze, M. S. (1994). Critical role of the group A streptococcal capsule in pharyngeal colonization and infection in mice. *Proc Natl Acad Sci USA, 91*, 12238–12242.

Wexler, D. E., Chenoweth, D. E., & Cleary, P. P. (1985). Mechanism of action of the group A streptococcal C5a inactivator. *Proc Natl Acad Sci USA, 82*, 8144–8148.

Wheeler, M. C., Roe, M. H., Kaplan, E. L., Schlievert, P. M., & Todd, J. K. (1991). Outbreak of group A streptococcus septicemia in children. Clinical, epidemiologic, and microbiological correlates [see comments]. *JAMA, 266*, 533–537.

Wilson, G. J., Talkington, D. F., Gruber, W., Edwards, K., & Dermody, T. S. (1995). Group A streptococcal necrotizing fasciitis following varicella in children: Case reports and review. *Clin Infect Dis, 20*, 1333–1338.

Winram, S. B., & Lottenberg, R. (1996). The plasmin-binding protein Plr of group A streptococci is identified as glyceraldehyde-3-phosphate dehydrogenase. *Microbiology, 142*(Pt. 8), 2311–2320.

Yan, S., Bohach, G. A., & Stevens, D. L. (1994). Persistent acylation of high-molecular-weight penicillin-binding proteins by penicillin induces the postantibiotic effect in *Streptococcus pyogenes*. *J Infect Dis, 170*, 609–614.

Yan, S., Mendelman, P. M., & Stevens, D. L. (1993). The in vitro antibacterial activity of ceftriaxone against *Streptococcus pyogenes* is unrelated to penicillin-binding protein 4. *FEMS Microbiol Lett, 110*, 313–317.

Yang, K. D., Bathras, J. M., Shigeoka, A. O., James, J., Pincus, S. H., & Hill, H. R. (1989). Mechanisms of bacterial opsonization by immune globulin intravenous: Correlation of complement consumption with opsonic activity and protective efficacy. *J Infect Dis, 159*, 701–707.

Yong, J. M. (1994). Necrotising fasciitis. *Lancet, 343*, 1427.

2

Bartonella Infections Resurgence in the New Century

Gilbert Greub and Didier Raoult

1. INTRODUCTION

Until recently, there were only two known human diseases due to *Bartonella* species. The first one, trench fever, due to *Bartonella quintana*, transmitted by the human body louse (*Pediculus humanus*), affected over 1 million troops during World War I (Kostrzewski, 1949). It presented an epidemic character during 1939–1945 and became rare after World War II. The second one, Carrion's disease, due to *Bartonella bacilliformis*, thought to be transmitted by sand flies of the genus *Lutzomyia*, is limited to certain regions of the Andes (Alexander, 1995).

In 2001, as many as seven *Bartonella* sp. have been recognized as causative agents of several human diseases, including bacillary angiomatosis, cat-scratch disease, chronic bacteremia, chronic lymphadenopathy, meningoencephalitis, stellar retinitis, myelitis, granulomatous hepatitis, endocarditis, osteomyelitis, and peliosis hepatitis (Jacomo & Raoult, 2002; Tables 2.1 and 2.2). This increased knowledge on human *Bartonella* pathogenesis, was mainly afforded by the availability of modern clinical microbiology diagnostic tools, the development of which was triggered by the recognition of the emerging role of *Bartonella* in AIDS-related diseases.

In view of the biodiversity of *Bartonella* sp., their wide pattern of human diseases, their numerous vectors, and the ongoing description of new species of *Bartonella*, the present review will probably be outdated within the next decade. However, it intends to present the current knowledge on *Bartonella* microbiology, taxonomy, epidemiology, clinical features, diagnostic approaches, and treatments.

2. MICROBIOLOGY

2.1. Description of the Genus

The current genus *Bartonella* was deeply extended by reclassifying in it the genus *Rochalimea* (Brenner et al., 1993) and the genus *Grahamella* (Birtles et al., 1995). Thus,

Reemergence of Established Pathogens in the 21st Century
Edited by Fong and Drlica, Kluwer Academic/Plenum Publishers, New York, 2003

Table 2.1

Bartonella Sp., Reservoir Host, and Human Pathogenicity

Species	Reservoir	Vector	Human pathogenicity	Reference
B. alsatica	Rabbits	Fleas or ticks		Heller et al. (1999)
B. bacilliformis	Humans	Phlebotomines	Carrion's disease (Oroya fever and verruga peruana)	Maguina (1998)
B. birtlesii	Rats			
B. clarridgeiae	Cats	Fleas	Cat scratch disease?	
B. doshiae	Rats			Birtles et al. (1995)
B. elizabethae	Rats	Fleas	Endocarditis, neuroretinitis	
B. grahamii	Rats		Uveitis	Birtles et al. (1995)
B. henselae	Cats	Fleas (Ticks?)	Cat-scratch disease, peliosis hepatis, bacillary angiomatosis, endocarditis, bacteremia, neuroretinitis.	
B. koehlerae	Cats	Fleas		Droz et al. (1999)
B. peromysci	Mice			Birtles et al. (1995)
B. quintana	Humans	Human body lice	Bacillary angiomatosis, trench fever, endocarditis, chronic bacteremia	Vinson and Fuller (1961)
B. schoenbuchii	Deer			Dehio (2001b)
B. talpae	Moles			Birtles et al. (1995)
B. taylori	Rats			Birtles et al. (1995)
B. tribocorum	Rats			Heller et al. (1998)
B. vinsonii subsp. arupinensis	Cattle		Endocarditis (to be confirmed)	Welch et al. (1999)
B. vinsonii subsp. berkhoffii	Dogs	Fleas and ticks	Endocarditis	Breitschwerdt et al. (1999)
B. vinsonii subsp. vinsonii	Voles			Kordick et al. (1996)
B. weissii	Deers, cattle, elks			Chang et al. (2000)

it comprises only one species in 1993 (*B. bacilliformis*) and now includes 17 species and proposed species and three subspecies (Table 2.1). The genus was defined as containing Gram-negative, oxidase-negative, fastidious aerobic rods, which grow better at 25°C (*B. bacilliformis*) or 37°C (other species) on media containing 5% or more rabbit, sheep, or horse blood in the presence of 5% CO_2 (Birtles et al., 1995). Their G + C contents were found to range from 38.5% to 41% (Birtles et al., 1995).

2.2. Phylogeny

Genotypic studies based on the analysis of the sequences relatedness of 16s rRNA established the phylogenic position of the genus *Bartonella*, demonstrating its relatedness to other alpha-2 *Proteobacteria* including *Brucella* sp., *Afipia* sp., *Bradyrhizobium* sp., and

Table 2.2
Some Clinical Entities Associated with *Bartonella* Infections in Humans

	First clinical description	Risk factors	Clinical presentation	Diagnostic approach	Species involved
Carrion' disease					
Oroya fever	1869	Nonnative°	Acute febrile, hemolytic anemia, or mild fever with body pain, nausea, and headache	Blood smear, Blood culture	*B. bacilliformis*
Verruaga peruana	1571		Exophytic or miliary skin eruption	Histology + culture of skin biopsy	*B. bacilliformis*
Trench fever	1914	Lice infestation, poor hygiene	Relapsing fever, headache, and body pain	Blood culture, serology	*B. quintana*
Bacillary angiomatosis	1983	Immunosuppresion (mainly HIV), cat, homelessness	Red and papular cutaneous lesions (± lymphadenopathy, osteolysis, fever, weight loss, etc.)	Histology, culture, and PCR of biopsy	*B. quintana*, *B. henselae*
Bacillary peliosis	1990	Immunosuppression (mainly HIV)	Abdominal pain, fever, hepatosplenomegaly	Histology, culture, and PCR of biopsy	*B. henselae*
Cat-scratch disease	1950	Cat (dog) scratch or bite	Lymphadenopathy (± mild fever, body pain, and headache)	PCR or culture of lymph node, serology	*B. henselae*, *B. clarridgeiae*
Ocular involvement	1889		Conjunctival ulceration, stellar retinitis, neuroretinitis		*B. henselae*, *B. grahamii*§
Chronic bacteremia	1995	Homelessness, lice, alcoholism	Fever, headache, leg pain, and thrombocytopenia	Blood culture (± serology)	*B. quintana*
Endocarditis	1993	Lice, homelessness, Alcoholism, cats	Fever, dyspnea on exertion, bibasal lung rales, cardiac murmur, embolic phenomena, and vegetations*	Serology, blood culture	*B. quintana*, *B. henselae*, *B. vinsonii*,§ *B. elizabethae*§

° Of endemic areas (Peru, Ecuador, Colombia, Bolivia, Chili, Guatemala); *insidious course with severity of signs reported to date probably reflecting diagnostic delay; §only one reported case.

Bosea sp. (Figure 2.1a) (Birtles et al., 1995; Brenner et al., 1993). However, it failed defining the intragenus phylogeny, as their 16s rRNA sequence similarity ranged from 97.5 to 99.9
between *Bartonella* sp. (Droz et al., 1999; Heller et al., 1998, 1999; Kordick et al., 1997).

The 16s–23s rRNA intergenic spacer region (ITS) has been recently shown to be
useful for inferring *Bartonella* phylogeny (Houpikian & Raoult, 2001a). Thus, five well-
supported lineages were identified within the genus and the proposed phylogenetic
organization was consistent with that resulting from protein-encoding gene sequence comparisons. Further, partial ITS amplification and sequencing offers a sensitive means of
intraspecies differentiation of *Bartonella henselae, Bartonella clarridgeiae*, and *B. bacilliformis* isolates, as each strain had a specific sequence. Contrary to previous hypothetical
controversies on the reliability of such highly variable sequences as indicator of evolution
(Birtles et al., 2000; Roux & Raoult, 1995), the ITS-derived phylogeny appears to be a useful tool for investigating the evolutionary relationships of *Bartonella* sp. and to identify
Bartonella sp.

Intraspecies phylogeny was also assessed by sequence comparisons of partial
sequence of the citrate synthase (*gltA*) (Birtles & Raoult, 1996; Joblet et al., 1995) and the
60 kDa heat-shock protein (*groEL*) (Marston et al., 1999; Zeaiter et al., 2002a) encoding
genes. The *groEL*-based phylogeny (Figure 2.1b) allowed distinction of four subgroups,
including: (1) *B. henselae* and *Bartonella quintana*; (2) *Bartonella elizabethae, Bartonella
tribocorum, Bartonella grahamii*, and *Bartonella taylorii*; (3) the *Bartonella vinsonii* subspecies; and (4) *Bartonella birtlesii* and *Bartonella weissi* (Zeaiter et al., 2002a). However,
the high bootstrap values of the *gltA* trees obtained when using neighbor-joining or maximum likelihood (Birtles & Raoult, 1996) highlighted the usefulness of that gene in
Bartonella phylogeny. Thus, the assessment of the precise intragenus phylogeny of
Bartonellaceae should be cautious and ideally based on the comparisons of multiple
sequences genes. An attempt to precise this intragenus phylogeny while using all 4 above-
mentioned genes identified 6 evolutionary clusters (Houpikian & Raoult, 2001b). *B. bacilliformis* and *B. clarridgeiae* appeared to be divergent species both being the unique
flagellated species; *B. henselae, Bartonella koehlerae*, and *B. quintana* clustered together,
as well as *B. vinsonii* subsp. *vinsonii* and *B. vinsonii* subsp. *berkhoffii*; the fifth group
included *Bartonella* sp. isolated from various rodents; and the sixth *B. tribocorum, B. elizabethae, B. grahamii*, and several strains isolated from rodents.

In conclusion, the phylogeny of Bartonellaceae remains confused and the use of
sequences of other genes such as those coding for the riboflavin synthetase (*ribC*)
(Bereswill et al., 1999), the RNA polymerase β subunit (*rpoB*) (Renesto et al., 2001a,
2001b) and the cell division protein (*ftsZ*) (Kelly et al., 1998), till now hampered by the
lack of some *Bartonella* sequences, may help in the future precising it.

2.3. Diagnostic Methods

Apart from histology, which gave a suggestive pattern and could reveal the presence
of bacteria, culture, serology, and molecular-based techniques are the main diagnostic laboratory approaches of *Bartonella*-related infectious diseases. Their respective diagnosis
efficiency, limitations, and pitfalls are highly dependent on the clinical syndrome, species

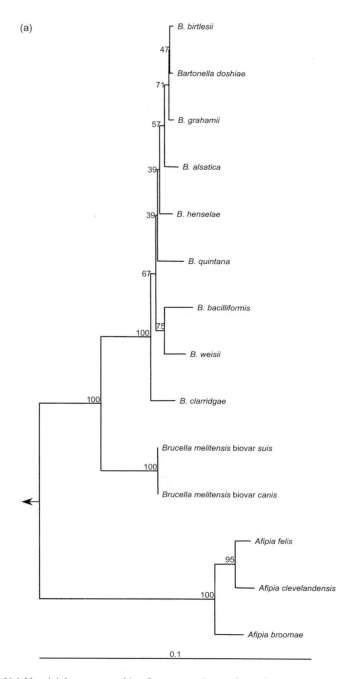

Figure 2.1 Neighbor-joining trees resulting from comparisons of complete sequences of (a) 16s rRNA- and (b) groEL-encoding genes of (a) different *Proteobacteria* and (b) all *Bartonella* sp. identified to date, respectively. The values at each node represent the percentage of times each branch was found in 100 bootstrap replicates.

(b)

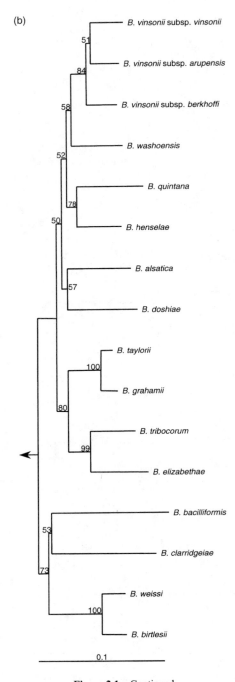

Figure 2.1 Continued

involved, sample analyzed, and expertise of the laboratory. The increasing sensitivities and specificities of microbiology diagnostic techniques were determinant in defining novel clinical entities and in establishing the role of some *Bartonella* sp. in these emerging or reemerging diseases.

2.3.1. Histology

Chronic inflammatory infiltrates (histiocytic), perivascular inflammation, endothelial cell proliferation, and swelling are the main histologic features found on skin biopsies taken from subjects suffering from *Carrion's disease* (Amano et al., 1997; Kosek et al., 2000). Skin biopsies will often show the presence of silver-stained organisms (Amano et al., 1997).

Histologic examination of skin biopsy is an effective approach for diagnosing *bacillary angiomatosis*, at least helpful in differentiating the cutaneous involvement from Kaposi sarcoma lesions. Hematoxylin–eosin stained sections reveal lobular proliferation of blood vessels in the dermis (Leboit, 1995; Wong et al., 1997). The proliferating epithelioid endothelial cells typically lined the vascular channels, sometimes even protruding in the vascular lumen (Figure 2.2a). Aggregates of bacteria, can be seen especially with Warthin–Starry silver stain, acridine orange, or immunofluorescence. The elicited inflammation explains the presence of edema in early lesions and fibrosis in later stages (Borczuk et al., 1998).

Though bacteria could also be seen with appropriate stains of liver sections taken from subjects with *peliosis hepatitis*, its histological characteristics are mainly the presence of dilated vessels and blood-filled spaces dispersed all over the hepatic parenchyma (Figure 2.2b) (Perkocha et al., 1990; Walter & Mockel, 1997).

In lymph nodes removed from patients presenting with *cat-scratch disease*, the histology will depend on the stage of disease: lymphoid and reticulum hyperplasia precede the formation of a micro-abscess surrounded by granulomatous reaction (Figure 2.2c), in which bacteria can only be seen using adequate stains.

Histology of valves taken from persons suffering from a *Bartonella endocarditis* also demonstrated the presence of bacteria organized in clusters of variable size, mainly in the valvular vegetations (Figure 2.2d) (Lepidi et al., 2000). Mononuclear cell infiltrates, fibrosis, and calcifications were more frequently seen than histiocytic infiltrates and focal granulomatous inflammation (Lepidi et al., 2000).

2.3.2. Culture

Though being fastidious organisms, *Bartonella* sp. can be isolated from biopsies or blood by inoculation on various blood agar or into tissue culture. Cultures on human endothelial cells (ECV 304) using the shell-vial centrifugation technique was shown to be about 10 times more sensitive than plating on agar for the recovery of *Bartonella* from valvular samples of patients presenting with *Bartonella* endocarditis ($p < 0.0005$) (La Scola & Raoult, 1999). Increased recovery rate of *Bartonella* sp. from blood was also observed by using shell-vial instead of axenic culture ($p = 0.045$) (La Scola & Raoult, 1999). However, cell-based culture being not widely available, agar plating remains an attractive alternative for nonreference centers. Numerous media have been shown to allow recovery

(a)

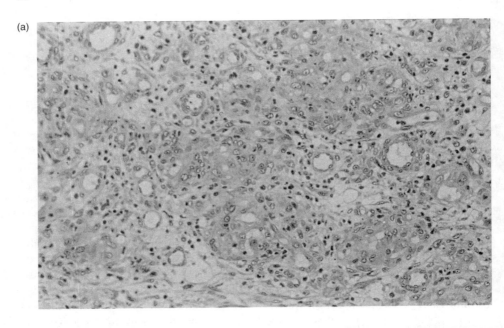

(b)

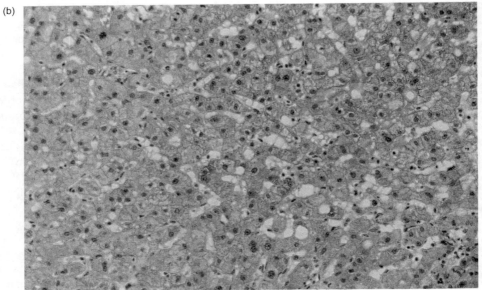

Figure 2.2. (a) Cutaneous bacillary angiomatosis. Lobular proliferation of endothelial cells, vascular channels lined with protuberant endothelial cells, and inflammatory infiltrate with numerous neutrophils scattered throughout the lesion (Hematoxylin–phloxine–saffron stain, original magnification 250×). Courtesy of H. Lepidi, Marseille. (b) Hepatis peliosis. Peliotic spaces filled with erythrocytes are surrounded by cords of hepatocytes (Hematoxylin–phloxine–saffron stain, original magnification 250×). Courtesy of H. Lepidi, Marseille.

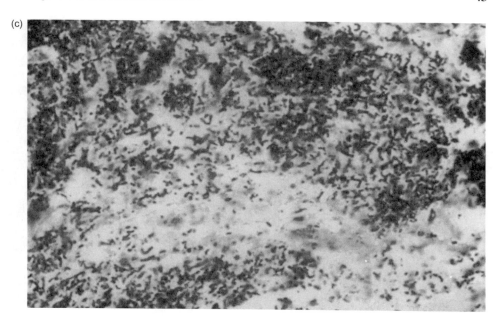

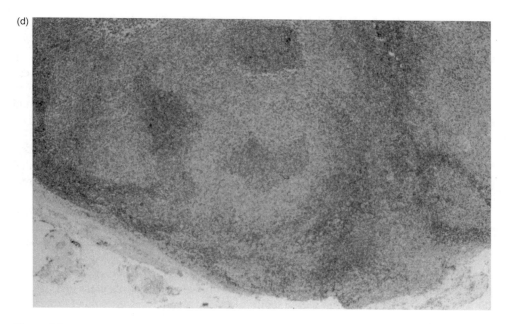

Figure 2.2. (c) *Bartonella* endocarditis. Resected valve with *B. henselae* infection showing darkly stained bacilli organized in numerous clusters of argyrophilic bacteria present in the valvular vegetation (Warthin–Starry silver stain, original magnification). Courtesy of H. Lepidi, Marseille. (d–e) Cat-scratch disease lymphadenitis. Lymph node specimen showing (d) a cortical abscess surrounded by granulomatous inflammation near the subcapsular sinus (Hematoxylin–eosin, original magnification 40×) and showing.

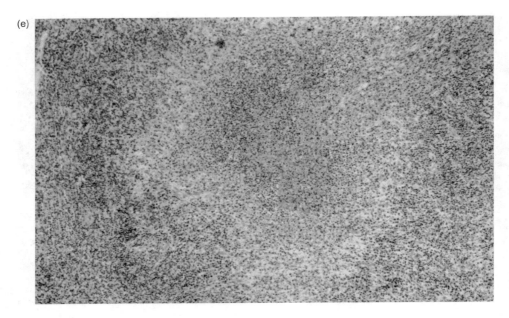

Figure 2.2.   Cat-scratch disease lymphadenitis. Lymph node specimen showing (e) a granuloma with central suppuration (Hematoxylin–eosin, original magnification 40×). Courtesy of H. Lepidi, Marseille.

of *Bartonella* sp. including chocolate agar (Dolan et al., 1993; Koehler et al., 1992; Slater et al., 1990), sheep blood (Clarridge et al., 1995; Regnery et al., 1992; Schmidt et al., 1996), rabbit blood (Regnery et al., 1992), CDC anaerobic blood agar (Dolan et al., 1993), peptone horse serum yeast extract broth (Cockerell et al., 1991; Wong et al., 1995), horse serum (Cockerell et al., 1991; Wong et al., 1995), and trypticase soy fildes horse serum broth (Cockerell et al., 1991; Wong, et al., 1995). Blood cultures have been shown to be especially valuable in disseminated infections such as bacillary angiomatosis, endocarditis, and chronic bacteremia in homeless people (La Scola & Raoult, 1999). *Bartonella* sp. have been isolated from blood by direct plating or by prolonged incubation in automated systems such as the BacT/Alert (La Scola & Raoult, 1999; Tierno et al., 1995). Direct whole blood plating was, however, shown to be considerably less effective than plating 7 day's blood culture broth (La Scola & Raoult, 1999). Despite a significant growth in blood culture broth, the small amount of CO_2 produced often prevents detection by the automated system (Tierno et al., 1995). Consequently, Gimenez or acridine orange staining and subculture on blood or chocolate agar could increase *Bartonella* recovery (Larson et al., 1994; La Scola & Raoult, 1999; Raoult et al., 1996; Spach et al., 1995). Use of isolator blood-lysis tubes that contain sodium polyanetholsulfonate (an anticoagulant that inhibits the bactericidal effect of blood) and saponin (a substance that lyses erythrocytes and leucocytes and liberates, if any, intracellular organisms) was shown to increase *Bartonella* recovery from blood (Brenner et al., 1997). Brenner et al. (1997) also demonstrated that freezing EDTA blood samples increased *Bartonella* isolation rate. This is currently the preferred technique. As prolonged incubation time is required, moist atmosphere will help prevent desiccation of the media.

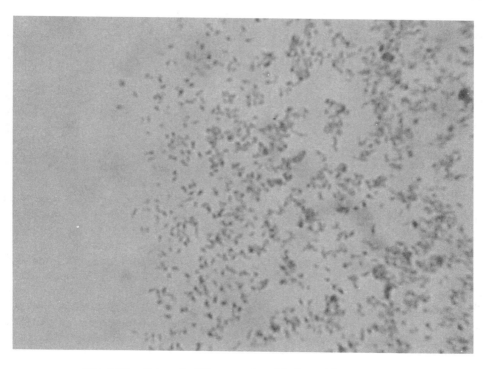

Figure 2.3. *B. henselae* (Gimenez stain, original magnification 1000×).

Isolation from agar plate or shell-vial of a nonmotile, oxidase-negative, catalase-negative (Drancourt & Raoult, 1993), Gimenez-positive (Figure 2.3), Gram-negative, pleomorphic curved rod (Birtles et al., 1995), should prompt suspicion towards the possibility of being a *Bartonella* sp. Initially reported to be inert biochemically to conventional bacteriological tests, the Bartonellaceae were found to exhibit some positive reactions when adding 100 mg/ml hemin to the medium used in commercial identification tests (Drancourt & Raoult, 1993). However, further identification is mainly based on sequencing genes, such as 16s rRNA, citrate synthase, or ITS coding-gene (La Scola & Raoult, 1999).

2.3.3. Molecular Tools

To overcome the poor sensitivity of culture-based methods, polymerase chain reaction (PCR) amplification and sequencing of 16s rRNA has been developed and was shown efficient in detecting *Bartonella* sp. in biopsy samples, taken from patients suffering from bacillary angiomatosis (Dauga et al., 1996; Matar et al., 1999), cat-scratch diseases (Bergmans et al., 1997; Dauga et al., 1996; Sander et al., 1999), endocarditis (Raoult et al., 1996; Wilck et al., 2001), and Carrion's disease (Amano et al., 1997). The molecular approach could also potentially help in describing novel entities associated with *Bartonella* sp. infections, such as the recognition of the association between *B. henselae* and bacillary angiomatosis by 16s rRNA amplification and sequencing (Relman et al., 1990). The main pitfall of the broad-range PCR approach is the risk of contamination, which may not be completely eluded even with careful reagent preparations and isolation procedures. Thus, amplification of other target genes such as *rpoB* (Renesto et al., 2001b) or *htrA* (Sander et al., 1999), which will have less conserved sequence, will reduce the risk of contamination. To increase the sensitivity of the PCR and to improve species differentiation, use of species-specific oligonucleotide probes, which hybridize in the amplified region, could be useful (Sander & Penno, 1999). To preclude the need for sequencing, which in past years was associated with a huge work burden, the use of PCR–restriction fragment length polymorphism was proposed (Matar et al., 1999). Nowadays, with the simplification of sequencing technique and with the availability of more specific primers, designed to amplify other genes, this method is less used.

2.3.4. Serology

Serology was found to be the more effective tool for diagnosing *Bartonella* endocarditis and cat-scratch diseases, with a sensitivity of 97% and 90%, respectively, as compared to combined molecular and culture-based methods (La Scola & Raoult, 1999). In 35 out of 38 patients with endocarditis, IgG antibody titers were found to be >1 : 1600 (La Scola & Raoult, 1999), demonstrating the strong antibody production in immuno-competent subjects (La Scola & Raoult, 1999). Serology was, however, shown to be inef-fective in diagnosing bacillary angiomatosis (La Scola & Raoult, 1999), probably because of the immunodeficiency of targeted patients (Koehler et al., 1997). Serology was also found to be a sensitive method to diagnose *B. bacilliformis* infection, as more than 90% of subjects presenting with fever, headache, and bone/joint pain demonstrated antibody reactivity by Western-blot (Kosek et al., 2000).

Although micro-agglutination and complement-fixation techniques have been used in the past to define the epidemiology of Trench fever (Kostrzewski, 1949), methods widely used nowadays includes immunofluorescence, enzyme-linked immunoassay and western-blotting. Cross-reactivities between *Bartonella* sp. are frequent, preventing accurate diag-nosis at the genus level and led to the development of genus specific tools, such as monoclonal antibodies (Liang et al., 2001; Slater et al., 1992). Western-blotting with antisera to *B. quintana*, *B. henselae*, *B. bacilliformis*, and *B. elizabethae* also enabled the differentiation of some *Bartonella* sp. including *B. quintana*, *B. henselae*, *B. bacilliformis*, *B. clarridgeiae*, *B. grahamii*, *B. taylorii*, and *B. vinsonii* (Liang & Raoult, 2000). Using whole-cell antigen, cross-reactivities were also demonstrated with *Chlamydia* sp. (Maurin et al., 1997) and *Coxiella burnetii* (La Scola & Raoult, 1996). Such cross-reactivities are important to detect, as these bacteria could manifest similar clinical presentation such as negative-culture endocarditis.

3. *BARTONELLA*-RELATED INFECTIONS IN HUMANS

3.1. Trench Fever

3.1.1. Historical Background

Though having probably existed since the middle-ages or at least during the Turkish war in the years 1877–1883, trench fever was only recognized as a clinical entity during World War I (Kostrzewski, 1949). At that time, trench fever was one of the largest sources of wastage of man power in the fighting armies, being the cause of more than 20% of disease in ill soldiers from both sides (Swift, 1920). In 1915, the disease was baptized "trench fever" as British troops from the trenches (and not those from the rear) suffered from it. At the same time, German medical officers saw the first cases in Wolhynia, which presented a five-day interval between relapses, explaining the other names of trench fever: "Wolhynian fever," "Five-day fever," and "Quintan fever." The disease had been reported among some civilians after the war; however, it reappeared as an epidemic disease only during World War II (Kostrzewski, 1949).

Though lice-mediated transmission was suspected already during World War I, adequate preventive measures were not applied, as trench fever was a nonfatal disease and as controversies remained on possible rat-mediated transmission. Lice was definitely proven to be the vector of that disease in 1920 by successful inoculation of trench fever to human volunteer, in applying the excreta of infected lice to scarified skin (Swift, 1920). The first successful isolation of the agent of trench fever, named at that time *Rickettsia quintana*, was reported in 1961 (Vinson & Fuller, 1961). Chronic bacteremia described in homeless people and alcoholics of modern cities (Brouqui et al., 1999; Spach et al., 1995) could be assimilated to the modern form of the trench fever (Stein & Raoult, 1995).

3.1.2. Epidemiology

It was shown that the human body louse, *P. humanus corporis*, become infected with *B. quintana* while feeding on bacteremic humans. The louse does not suffer from the infection as *B. quintana* does not cross the gut (Figure 2.4). *B. quintana* is passively excreted in

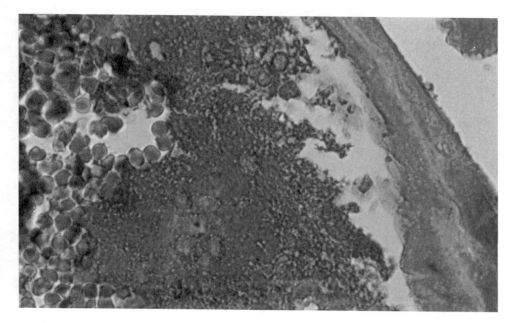

Figure 2.4. Immunohistology of the abdomen of *P. humanus corporis*. The peroxidase-stained *B. quintana* does not invade the digestive wall. Numerous red blood cells are seen within the dilated intestine (Original magnification 1000×). Courtesy of P. E. Fournier, Marseille.

the louse's feces, where it can survive for days. It is then inoculated back in to humans when the pruritic louse's bite is scratched. Interestingly, the infected lice migrate away from fevered hosts, thus spreading the disease to healthy people living in close contact (Kostrzewski, 1949). The transmission process explains why delousing procedures are effective in controlling outbreaks and why trench fever spread in winter, when due to cold weather, the soldiers cluster together, wearing multiple layers of clothes that are kept on for long periods.

3.1.3. Clinical Presentation

The incubation period for trench fever of 15–25 days could be reduced to 6–10 days when experimentally induced into volunteers (Maurin & Raoult, 1996; Mooser, 1959). The outstanding features of typical cases are the sudden onset of fever, headache, and general body pains, resembling the onset of influenza, but followed in a few days by pain and tenderness in the shins and relapsing fever; however, many subjects also present only with painful shins, which were often, in the absence of fever, wrongly attributed to flat feet or rheumatism due to prolonged standing in mud and water (Swift, 1920). Headache is often severe, mainly localized behind eyes. The acute phase could be accompanied by nausea, diarrhea or constipation, giddiness, frequent micturition, insomnia, restlesness, and shivering (Jacomo & Raoult, 2000; Maurin & Raoult, 1996). Fever is generally relapsing every 4–8 days, with 5 being the more frequently observed interval (Maurin & Raoult, 1996; Swift, 1920). Fever bouts, which last from 1 to 3 days, were observed 2–8 times and decreased in intensity over time (Mooser, 1959). Maculopapular eruption could be seen, especially on the trunk (Gluckman, 1996; Mooser, 1959). Enlarged spleen, conjunctival congestion, and furred tongue may be seen. Major polymorphonuclear leucocytosis often accompanies the episodes of fever, and anemia may occur, especially in chronic forms (Maurin & Raoult, 1996). Though being generally a self-limited disease, chronic bacteremia may be observed after up to 8 years (Kostrzewski, 1949).

3.1.4. Management

Eradication of infected louse should be achieved. Changing and washing clothes are effective, though Demetrin impregnation of clothes could be useful (Sholdt et al., 1989). Trench fever was reported to respond favorably to the prescription of tetracycline (Maurin & Raoult, 1996). However, to prevent relapses, prolonged treatment and combined therapy may be advocated, especially as aminoglycosides are the only antibiotics shown to be bactericidal for *Bartonella* sp. (Musso et al., 1995) and as chronic bacteremia in the homeless people is not controlled with doxycycline (Raoult, unpublished data).

3.2. Carrion's Disease

3.2.1. Historical Background

The chronic form of Carrion's disease was described initially in Peru in 1571, probably endemic in that region since pre-Columbian times (Amano et al., 1997; Jacomo & Raoult,

2001). This form was named verruaga peruana, as it is characterized by the presence of multiple wart-like vascular tumors of the skin called verrugas. The first cases of the acute form, named Oroya fever, occurred in 1869, during the construction of a railway intended to connect Lima to the mining town of Oroya. An estimated 8,000 workers, mostly nonnatives hired from Chile and the coastal plain of Peru, died of an epidemic febrile illness (Bass et al., 1997a). In 1885, the fatal experiment of Daniel Alcides Carrion, a 26-year-old medical student gave the first evidence that both clinical entities were due to the same agent (Bass et al., 1997a; Ihler, 1996; Schultz, 1968). He inoculated himself with blood taken from a skin lesion of a patient suffering from verruga peruana. Three weeks later, he presented with an acute febrile illness accompanied with chills, arthralgia, myalgia, abdominal pain, and died within 18 days of acute hemolysis. Subsequently, Alberto Barton described in detail the etiologic agent of the disease, which was subsequently named after him, *Bartonella bacilliformis*.

3.2.2. Epidemiology

As for every vector-borne disease, the vector repartition influences the geographical distribution of the disease. Thus, the vector of *B. bacilliformis* in Peru, *Lutzomyia verrucarum*, a weak flyer that cannot survive strong winds, is present mainly between an altitude of 1,100 and 3,000 m at the occidental flanks of the Andean valley (Caceres, 1993). This sand fly and its neighbor *L. peruensis* could be found at higher altitudes in intra-Andean areas (Caceres, 1993; Ellis et al., 1999), where 6,000 m high mountains protect the vector from strong winds, explaining the observed occurrence of an outbreak in the Urumbamba region near Cuzco (Ellis et al., 1999). Other sand flies related to *L. verrucarum* could account for the presence of the disease in other areas of South America, such as in Ecuador, where it was reported in Manabi at an altitude of 50–400 m only (Amano et al., 1997). So being also present in Colombia, Bolivia, Chile, and Guatemala, no proven endemic case was reported outside South America (Jacomo & Raoult, 2001). The prolonged (up to 5 months) asymptomatic bacteremic stage which occurs before the occurrence of the verruaga peruana lesions allows for infection of the sandflies, while feeding at night on infected humans. No other mammalian reservoir of the disease has been identified.

3.2.3. Clinical Presentation

Oroya fever, which correspond to the acute form of Carrion's disease, can be rapidly fatal due to major erythrocytes parasitism and subsequent severe hemolytic anemia, however, generally it is self-resolute and may be followed later by the localized form verruaga peruana. The most common findings of Oroya fever are fever (usually sustained, but with temperature no greater than 39°C), pallor, malaise, nonpainful hepatomegaly, and lymphadenopathy (Maguina et al., 2001). Headache (80%), cough (70%), emesis (65%), icterus (55%), myalgia (50%), and dyspnea (45%) are also reported frequently in the severe form defined by the presence of fever, anemia, and intra-erythrocytic cocco-bacillus seen on Giemsa stained smears (Ellis et al., 1999). *Salmonella* septicemia may occur as a significant contributor to Oroya mortality (Cuadra, 1956), potentially through blockage of the reticulo-endothelial system. This was confirmed recently with recovery of *Salmonella* from 5 (20%) out of 25 patients for whom blood cultures were done (Maguina et al., 2001). Additional infectious complications, highlighting the importance of the *Bartonella*-related immunosuppression, have been reported including five cases of toxoplasmosis, one case of disseminated histoplasmosis, one case of *Pneumocystis carinii* pneumonia, and three other cases with bacteremias (Maguina et al., 2001). In this recent study, the mortality of 9% was strongly associated with the presence of petechiae and anasarca at admission. The severe course, which affects mainly children or nonnative subjects, is however rare when taking into account an attack rate of 13.8%, estimated in a recent study (Kosek et al., 2000). Thus, most people present only with fever, gastrointestinal symptoms, bone and joint pain, and headache, with or without anemia. In endemic area, a presumptive diagnosis other than Oroya fever was reported at admission for 8 (12%) of 68 patients with acute bartonellosis; these included typhoid fever, malaria, brucellosis, viral hepatitis, tuberculosis, leptospirosis, meningitis, hematological malignancy, hemolytic anemia, and aplastic anemia (Maguina et al., 2001). Misdiagnoses rate will be probably much higher in nonendemic area, where doctors are less familiar with the disease, thus leading to delayed therapy initiation. The incubation period is about 3 weeks and fever lasts from 2 days to a few weeks. Asymptomatic bacteremias have been noticed following acute infection.

After recovery from the acute phase, patients may present with the chronic form, verruaga peruana, even after having treatment with penicillin or chloramphenicol. Verruaga peruana is characterized by angio-proliferative skin lesions, which can appear as (1) 2–3 cm subcutaneous nodules; (2) "miliary" eruption of millimetric lesions; and (iii) exophytic or pedonculated angiogenic centimetric lesions, or more rarely, bleeding ulcerations, probably resulting from opening of exophytic lesions (Bass et al., 1997; Kosek et al., 2000; Maguina et al., 2001). The miliary form, mainly localized to the extremities and often associated with pruritis is the commonest form (Maguina et al., 2001). Verruaga peruana generally resolve spontaneously within 1 month to a year.

3.2.4. Management

As nonnative subjects are especially susceptible to the acute form, preventive measures should be recommended to travelers to endemic region. These include the use of insect repellants and wearing long clothes at night to prevent sandfly bites.

Rapid introduction of antibiotic therapy led to dramatic decrease of the fatality rate of Oroya fever. Though the severe form was almost always fatal when untreated, only 1 subject died out of 50 presenting with acute bartonellosis and treated with chloramphenicol (Kosek et al., 2000). The effectiveness of chloramphenicol was also reported recently by Maguina et al. (2001). *B. bacilliformis* strains were shown to be highly susceptible to aminoglycosides, macrolides, doxycycline, rifampin, and most beta-lactams (except oxacillin, cephalothin, and cefotetan) (Sobraques et al., 1999). However, in view of frequent concomitant *Salmonella* infection, chloramphenicol has been widely used (Uertega & Payne, 1955). Verruaga peruana is usually treated by streptomycin or rifampicin (Maguina et al., 2001).

3.3. Bacillary Angiomatosis

3.3.1. Historical Background

Stoler et al. (1983) first reported an AIDS patient with multiple subcutaneous vascular nodules that contained numerous bacillary organism visualized by electron microscopy. Reports of similar skin lesions were reported in additional AIDS subjects (Cockerell et al.,

1987; Tappero et al., 1993), other immunosuppressed subjects (Cline et al., 1999; Kemper et al., 1990; Tappero et al., 1993), and immunocompetent individuals (Cockerell et al., 1990; Tappero et al., 1993). In view of the pathognomonic vasoproliferation and the high number of bacilli seen in the biopsies, the disease was named bacillary angiomatosis by Leboit et al. (1989), and they noted the presence of "bacilli similar to the agent of cat-scratch disease." However, the organism could not be cultivated from the lesions until 1990 (Slater et al., 1990); in the same issue of the *New England Journal of Medicine*, the 16s rRNA sequence homology of the causative organism to that of *B. quintana* (at that time still named *Rochalimea*) was established (Relman et al., 1990) and the morphological aspects of the peliosis bacterial agent described (Perkocha et al., 1990). The presumed agent of bacillary angiomatosis, now known as *B. henselae* was formally described by Regnery et al. (1992). The same year Koehler et al. (1992) demonstrated that both *B. henselae* and *B. quintana* can cause bacillary angiomatosis. Since the availability in 1995 of potent antiretroviral therapy, which considerably decreased the number of HIV-infected subjects with low CD4, the incidence of the disease decreased dramatically in the HIV-infected population, as did most other opportunistic infections (Ledergerber et al., 2001).

3.3.2. Epidemiology

Cat scratch and cat bite were found to be associated with bacillary angiomatosis in uni- and bivariate analysis (Tappero et al., 1993), demonstrating the role of cats as reservoir and humans as incidental host. Another study confirmed that contact with cats was a risk factor of *B. henselae* bacillary angiomatosis and has shown that homelessness or poor socioeconomic status were associated with *B. quintana* bacillary angiomatosis (Gasquet et al., 1998). No other animal exposures (including dogs, birds, and rodents) were found to be associated with this clinical entity (Tappero et al., 1993), confirming the strong host specificity for cats of *B. henselae*. In active intravenous drug-users, concern on potential transmission of *Bartonella* sp. by syringe exchange exist, in view of the bacteremia associated with bacillary angiomatosis reported for *B. quintana* in homeless subjects.

3.3.3. Clinical Presentation

Although any organ can be involved, skin lesions are the more frequently recognized. Bacillary angiomatosis is often characterized by a mild clinical course, explaining the long duration of signs or symptoms before diagnosis; however, fever, chills, malaise, anorexia, vomiting, headache, and multiple cutaneous lesions are frequent clinical presentations observed in AIDS patients with low CD4 counts (<100 CD4/mm^3).

Single or multiple (up to 100) red papules are the most common skin lesions. However, subcutaneous nodules, pedunculated lesions, and dry-hyperkeratotic plaques have been reported. After skin, bone is the second more frequent site involved. Bone lesions, characterized by well circumscribed osteolysis, is often painful and usually affects long bones (Baron et al., 1990). Lymph node involvement is frequent, though being generally associated with a lesion in the drainage area. Involvement of gastrointestinal or respiratory mucosa has been repeatedly described; lesions could be nodular, polypoid, or ulcerated. The latter could be associated with severe bleeding. Any organ could potentially be involved, with a symptomatology related to lesions' localization; thus, bacillary angiomatosis of the brain, penis, vulva, cervix, muscle, and bone marrow were also reported (Blanche et al., 1998; Eden et al., 1996; Fagan et al., 1995; Long et al., 1996; Spach et al.,

1992). Splenic and hepatic involvement, named bacillary peliosis, in view of their different histopathological characteristics, will be discussed below.

3.3.4. Management

The differential diagnosis of skin lesions, including Kaposi sarcoma, various skin tumors, and pyogenic granuloma, should prompt histopathological diagnostic confirmation. As bacillary angiomatosis occurs mainly in immunodeficient cases, the coexistence of another opportunistic disease, such as a Kaposi sarcoma should be kept in mind.

Erythromycin (500 mg four times a day per os) has been associated with a dramatic effect on the angiogenic lesions, which disappeared within hours (Koehler et al., 1997); however, recurrence is the rule after antibiotic interruption. Doxycycline was shown to be effective in several case reports (Koehler et al., 1998; Koehler & Tappero, 1993; Mui et al., 1990). Antimycobacterial drugs were also reported to be effective in treating bacillary angiomatosis (Perkocha et al., 1990), probably due to the strong bacteriostatic activity of rifampicin (Maurin & Raoult, 1998). In fact, the treatment duration may be more important than the antibiotic itself and prolonged therapy (more than 1 month) may be recommended (Maurin & Raoult, 1998).

3.4. Bacillary Peliosis

3.4.1. Historical Background

In the 1960s peliosis hepatis, which consists histologically of multiple blood-filled cystic spaces often communicating with the hepatic sinusoids, was thought to be induced by viruses (Bergs & Scotti, 1967). However, similar lesions were observed in mice or rats exposed to various drugs or toxins, including phalloidine and oxazepam (Fox & Lahcen, 1974; Tuchweber et al., 1973). The pathological process was then attributed to anabolic steroids and this entity was until the late 1980s mainly reported in patients with advanced cancer or receiving anabolic steroids.

Perkocha et al. (1990) first described the bacillary peliosis hepatis. The histology of peliosis hepatis associated with HIV infection differs from that of peliosis hepatis without HIV infection by the presence of a myxoid stroma and clumps of a granular purple material that on Warthin–Starry staining and electron microscopy proved to be bacilli. Perkocha et al. (1990) failed in culturing the bacilli and assumed that they were the same bacilli as those found in the skin lesions of bacillary angiomatosis. Their hypothesis was confirmed by Slater et al. (1992) two years later. However, bacillary peliosis hepatis was shown to be mainly associated with *B. henselae*, though cutaneous and lytic bone lesions were more frequently observed in *B. quintana*-associated bacillary angiomatosis (Koehler et al., 1997).

3.4.2. Epidemiology

Bacillary peliosis share a common epidemiology with bacillary angiomatosis, explaining why both entities are often associated. HIV-infected subjects with low CD4 counts are especially at risk.

3.4.3. Clinical Presentation

Abdominal pain, fever, hepatomegaly, and/or splenomegaly are the more common clinical presentation. The presence of concomitant bacillary angiomatosis skin lesions may facilitate a rapid diagnosis. In case of splenic peliosis, pancytopenia or thrombocytopenia are often observed, while increased hepatic enzymes is frequently associated with hepatic peliosis.

Ultrasound and computed tomography images show hepatic and/or splenic hypodense lesions, which raise a large differential diagnosis, especially in the targeted population, which is often severely immunocompromised. Complications include hepatic or splenic ruptures and massive intraperitoneal hemorrhages. Biliary duct obstruction has also been reported, secondary to obstruction of the duct by enlarged local lymphnodes (Krekorian et al., 1990).

3.5. Cat-Scratch Disease

3.5.1. Historical Background

In 1889, Parinaud reported three patients with follicular conjunctivitis, fever, and local lymphadenopathy (Parinaud, 1889). Parinaud's oculoglandular syndrome corresponds in fact to a particular localization of the cat-scratch disease, translation of its French name "maladie des griffes du chat," given by Debré et al. (1950). The first evidence that cat-scratch disease was due to a bacteria was found in 1983 by Wear et al. (1985) who demonstrated the presence of small pleomorphic organisms stained with Whartin–Starry silver. English et al. (1988) reported the successful culture of a bacteria, subsequently named *Afipia felis*, from lymphnodes taken from patients with cat-scratch disease. However, this bacteria was not subsequently confirmed to be the etiological agent of the disease. No or few serological reactions were noticed with this agent during cat-scratch disease (Amerein et al., 1996; Szelc-Kelly et al., 1995), which may be a water contaminant (La Scola & Raoult, 1999). Regnery et al. (1992) provided the first serological evidence that *B. henselae* was associated with cat-scratch disease. This was later confirmed by isolation (Dolan et al., 1993) and PCR (Anderson et al., 1994).

3.5.2. Epidemiology

Cat-scratch disease has been reported worldwide. Cats are the reservoirs of *B. henselae* and *B. clarridgae*, about half of the cats being infected (Chomel et al., 1995, 1999). Both species have been associated with cat-scratch disease. However, neither *B. clarridgeiae* nor other species were detected by PCR from specimens taken from 273 patients suspected of having cat-scratch disease, while 39% of them were found to be positive for *B. henselae* (Zeaiter et al., 2002b). Though cat fleas play a role in transmission from cats to cats (Chomel et al., 1999), its role in transmission to humans remains controversial; a cat scratch or cat bite being reported in most human cases. The disease occurs mainly in healthy subjects, mostly children, because they are at highest risk of being scratched or bitten by cats. Dog scratch or bite could also potentially cause cat-scratch disease (Keret et al., 1999; Tsukahara et al., 1998).

3.5.3. Clinical Presentation

The most frequent presentation is lymphadenopathy in the draining region of the cat scratch or bite (Fournier & Raoult, 1998). However, the first manifestation is a papular skin lesion at the inoculation site, which can be seen in about 50% of cases 3–10 days after injury (Bass et al., 1997b). Lymphadenopathy occur after about one additional week and generally resolves spontaneously within 1–3 months. About 10% of them will enlarge even more, fluctuate and potentially suppurate, if not drained (Bass et al., 1997b). Patients could also present with mild fever, anorexia, arthralgia, myalgia, and/or headache (Carithers, 1985). Atypical courses of cat-scratch disease, with the severity mainly related to the anatomic site involved include: (1) the Parinaud oculoglandular syndrome and other ocular involvement; (2) granulomatous hepatitis and other gastrointestinal cat-scratch diseases; (3) neurologic complications; (4) osteomyelitis; and (5) pulmonary manifestations.

3.5.3a. Ocular Involvement.   Ocular bartonella infections were mostly reported to be associated to *B. henselae*. However, *B. grahamii* was shown once to be associated with neuroretinitis (Kerkhoff et al., 1999) and serologic evidence of *B. elizabethae* infection in a case of neuroretinitis was provided (O'Halloran et al., 1998). Parinaud oculoglandular syndrome is the commonest ocular manifestation of cat-scratch disease. It is characterized by unilateral eye redness, foreign body sensation, and epiphora (Cunningham & Koehler, 2000). Ulceration of the conjunctiva and discharge are common, while swelling is usually mild. Regional lymphadenopathy is part of the syndrome definition (Parinaud, 1889). Neuroretinitis and retinochoroiditis are also infrequently associated with cat-scratch disease (1–2%). Typically, it is a stellar retinitis. Usually unilateral, it could also be bilateral or associated with Parinaud syndrome. Complications include branch retinal artery and vein occlusion and serous retinal detachment (Cunningham & Koehler, 2000). Papillitis, vitritis, uveitis, and focal choroiditis or vasculitis could also be seen.

3.5.3b. Gastrointestinal Involvement.   The hepatic involvement, which is frequently associated with splenic lesions could be recognized, especially in children presenting with hepatomegaly, fever, and a history of exposure to cat scratch or bite (Bass et al., 1997b). Other atypical gastrointestinal features include ileitis mimicking Crohn disease (Massei et al., 2000) and acute gastroenteritis (Liapi-Adamidou et al., 2000).

3.5.3c. Neurological Complications.   Neurological complications occur in 0.17–3% of cat-scratch disease (Noyola et al., 1999). Encephalopathy is the most common central nervous system manifestation of cat-scratch disease (Fournier & Raoult, 1998; Noyola et al., 1999). Its clinical manifestations may include fever, convulsions, status epilepticus, headache, malaise, behavior changes, lethargy, coma, respiratory depression, hemiplegia, aphasia, ataxia, facial nerve palsy, and hearing loss (Fournier & Raoult, 1998). Despite the severity of symptoms, patients fully recover within 2 weeks to 1 year (Fournier & Raoult, 1998). Arteritis and direct bacterial invasion have both been the proposed mechanisms of cat-scratch encephalitis (Carithers & Margileth, 1991; Selby & Walker, 1979). Two cases of transverse myelitis have also been reported (Pickerill & Milder, 1981; Salgado & Weisse, 2000).

3.5.3d. Osteomyelitis.   Osteomyelitis, observed in 0.3% of cases, generally results from extension of an adjacent lymphadenopathy (Fournier & Raoult, 1998). Fever and pain at the infected sites are the main features (Gregory & Decker, 1986; Hulzebos et al., 1999; Keret et al., 1998; Krause et al., 2000; Modi et al., 2001).

3.5.3e. Pulmonary Manifestations. Pulmonary manifestations, which occur in 0.2% of cat-scratch diseases, include pleural effusion and pneumonia, sometimes severe and requiring intubation (Abbasi & Chesney, 1995; Fournier & Raoult, 1998; Marseglia et al., 2001).

3.5.4. Management

In vitro, *B. henselae* was shown to be highly susceptible to penicillin G, aminopenicillins, third-generation cephalosporins, aminoglycosides, macrolides, tetracyclines, and rifampin (Maurin & Raoult, 1998). In vivo, erythromycin and doxycycline both have been shown to be effective in treating disseminated *Bartonella* infections in HIV-infected subjects. However, these data could not be extended to the treatment of cat-scratch disease. Indeed, Carithers (1985), has shown that penicillins, erythromycin, and doxycycline were ineffective. In view of the intracellular localization of *Bartonella* (Brouqui & Raoult, 1996), the frequent relapses after treatment interruption (Carithers, 1985) and the absence of bactericidal activity on *Bartonella* sp. of penicillin G, aminopenicillins, third-generation cephalosporins, macrolides, tetracyclines, and rifampin (Musso et al., 1995), combinations and prolonged therapies, including an aminoglycoside might be used, at least for visceral cat-scratch diseases (Maurin & Raoult, 1998). Though the majority of cat-scratch diseases occurring in normal hosts do not require antibiotic therapy for resolution of infection (Conrad, 2001), 5 days of oral azithromycin has been shown to afford some clinical benefit as compared to placebo (Bass et al., 1998). Actually, there is no consensus on the treatment of cat-scratch disease.

3.6. Chronic Bacteremia

3.6.1. Historical Background

Chronic *B. quintana* bacteremia was reported during World War I in soldiers presenting with trench fever; *B. bacilliformis* bacteremia has also been described for years and bacteremia is a common feature of bacillary angiomatosis (see above). However, the term chronic bacteremia applies to another clinical entity, first described by Spach et al. (1995), characterized by chronic *B. quintana* bacteremia in homeless, alcoholic subjects. Such chronic bacteremia was subsequently shown to be frequent (14% had positive blood cultures) in homeless people and potentially paucisymptomatic (6 out of 10 patients with bacteremia had no fever) (Brouqui et al., 1999).

3.6.2. Epidemiology

The various species of bartonella share the ability to cause chronic bacteremia and sustained infection of erythrocytes in their natural host. Such prolonged bacteremia probably facilitates the transmission of *B. quintana* to lice. The detection of *B. quintana* in lice from patients with bacteremia strongly suggests that body lice play the role of vector (Brouqui et al., 1999), as in trench fever. This explains the observed epidemiological association of chronic bacteremia with alcoholism and homelessness (Brouqui et al., 1999; Spach et al., 1995). Prolonged bacteremia may lead to *B. quintana* transmission by blood transfusion or sharing of syringe and needle.

3.6.3. Clinical Presentation

Though reported in only 40% of subjects with positive blood cultures, both fever and headache were the main symptoms found to be significantly associated with *B. quintana* infection in homeless people (Brouqui et al., 1999). Leg pain and thrombocytopenia are also part of the clinical feature. In fact, there are two main clinical presentations: (1) an acute form characterized by high-grade fever, leg pain, granulocytosis, and a rapid antibody response; and (2) a chronic form, without symptoms characterized by prolonged bacteremia and delayed antibody response (Brouqui et al., 1999).

3.6.4. Management

To accurately diagnose *B. quintana* bacteremia, blood cultures should be performed even in asymptomatic homeless people. The delay of seroconversion prevent the use of serology in diagnosing chronic bacteremia, though when positive, its high titers are associated with excellent specificity (Fournier et al., 2002). Eradication of infected louse could be achieved by changing and washing clothes. When impossible, impregnation of clothes with Demethrin is helpful.

Data on optimal therapeutic regimen are lacking. In vitro, *B. quintana* is sensitive to tetracyclines, macrolides, penicillins, aminoglycosides, and chloramphenicol (Maurin et al., 1995; Myers et al., 1984). Though trench fever was reported to respond favorably to the prescription of tetracycline (Maurin & Raoult, 1996), as chronic bacteremia in homeless people is not controlled with doxycycline (Raoult, unpublished data) and as aminoglycosides are the only antibiotics shown to be bactericidal on *Bartonella* sp. (Musso et al., 1995), a combined therapy may be more suitable.

3.7. Endocarditis

3.7.1. Historical Background

The first description of a *Bartonella* endocarditis was that due to *B. quintana*, published by Spach et al. (1993). The second case, and the only reported case due to *B. elisabethae* was published one month later (Daly et al., 1993). Since then endocarditis due to other *Bartonella* sp. has been reported including *B. henselae* (Fournier et al., 2001; Holmes et al., 1995; Raoult et al., 1996), *B. quintana* (Drancourt et al., 1995; Fournier et al., 2001; Guyot et al., 1999; Raoult et al., 1996; Spach et al., 1995), and *B. vinsonii* subsp. *berkhoffii* (Roux et al., 2000). Thus, a total of 50 cases has been reported between 1993 and 2001, including those due to *B. elisabethae* and *B. vinsonii* subsp. *berkhoffii* (Fournier et al., 2001).

3.7.2. Epidemiology

Bartonella endocarditis account for about 3% of blood culture negative endocarditis (Raoult et al., 1996). *B. henselae* was shown to occur mainly in subjects with previous history of valvular disease (90%) and history of cat bite or scratch ($p < 0.001$) (Fournier et al., 2001). Inversely, patients infected with *B. quintana* were less likely than controls to have a known valvular disease and more likely to be homeless and alcoholic; they were also more frequently infected with body lice (Fournier et al., 2001). *B. quintana* endocarditis could occur in the context of chronic bacteremia, even in the absence of previously known valvular disease; however, the absence of history of previous valvular disease may reflect the lack of medical care in homeless people before the diagnosis of endocarditis.

3.7.3. Clinical Presentation

Bartonella sp. cause subacute endocarditis. Fever above 38°C was observed in 85% and aortic valve was involved in 94% of the 33 cases reported until 1996 (Raoult et al., 1996). The insidious course and the fastidious nature of the etiological agent explain that diagnosis was frequently delayed and that most cases reported to date presented with dyspnea on exertion, bibasal lung rales, and cardiac murmur, all signs of cardiac failure (Brouqui & Raoult, 2001). The high frequency of vegetations (86%) and of embolic phenomena (41%) in the series reported by Raoult et al. (1996) may reflect the delay in diagnosing *Bartonella* endocarditis and the chronicity of the disease as confirmed by histologic examination (Lepidi et al., 2000). The white blood cell count is generally normal and thrombocytopenia is common. The initial clinical presentation is probably less severe and its specific symptoms and signs, if any, remain to be defined. In view of the insidious course of the disease, microbiological investigation of blood and/or valvular samples for the presence of signs of evolutive infection should be undertaken in patients with valvular abnormalities, especially those exposed (cat owners and homeless people), even in the absence of fever.

3.7.4. Management

Clinical data on the effectiveness of various therapeutic regimen are lacking. In vitro, *B. henselae* was shown to be highly susceptible to penicillin G, aminopenicillins, third-generation cephalosporins, aminoglycosides, macrolides, tetracyclines, and rifampin (Maurin & Raoult, 1998), and *B. quintana* was shown to be sensitive to tetracyclines, macrolides, penicillins, aminoglycosides, and chloramphenicol (Maurin et al., 1995; Myers et al., 1984). However, the possible intracellular localization of some *Bartonella* in human valve (Raoult et al., 1996), and the absence of bactericidal activity on *Bartonella* sp. of penicillin G, aminopenicillins, third-generation cephalosporins, macrolides, tetracyclines, and rifampin (Musso et al., 1995) suggest that use of an aminoglycoside, which was the only compound with a bactericidal activity, may be needed. Several patients were treated, most of them with a favorable outcome, with aminoglycosides (76%), beta-lactam compound (74%), and tetracycline (35%) (Brouqui & Raoult, 2001). Thus, based on these few data, a prolonged therapy including an aminoglycoside with either doxycycline, ampicillin, or ceftriaxone may be recommended. In addition to antibiotic therapy, surgery is often required in view of the frequency of vegetations and the extent of valvular damage. Thus, valvular surgery was performed in 96% of 48 cases (Fournier et al., 2001).

4. PATHOGENESIS AND NATURAL HISTORY OF
BARTONELLA INFECTIONS IN MAMMALS

Bartonella infections are vector-borne diseases characterized by a natural cycle, vectors and reservoir hosts (Table 2.1). The host specificity is high and *Bartonella* sp. colonize red blood cells of their specific healthy host, leading to asymptomatic chronic bacteremia. Human pathogenicity is either related to natural infection (*B. quintana* and *B. bacilliformis*) or to incidental infections (for other *Bartonella* sp.), acquired while being in contact with naturally-infected mammals. *Bartonella* sp. were shown to multiply and persist in red blood cells, sharing common persistence and dissemination strategies. Thus, *B. henselae* was found to infect cats' red blood cells, *B. tribochorum* rat cells, while *B. quintana* and *B. bacilliformis* were shown to invade human red blood cells. Bacteremias were described even in healthy mammals, thus being one established exception to one of Koch's basic tenet: "Bacteria do not occur in the blood or tissues of healthy animals or humans" (Brock, 1999). It was shown in rats' red blood cells that the bacterial replication was regulated and stopped at a maximum of eight bacteria per cell (Schülein et al., 2001). The mechanism of regulation is unknown, but prevents hemolysis and allows the persistence of *Bartonella* sp. within red blood cells. Disregulation of this mechanism, with uninterrupted multiplication of *B. bacilliformis* within red blood cells could explain, the rare acute hemolytic form of Carrion's disease (Oroya fever). In the rat model of *B. tribochorum* infection, Schulein et al. (2001) demonstrated the presence of periodic erythrocytes infection waves that echo the 5-days periodicity of the "Quintan fever." The fact that, with the exception of *B. bacilliformis*, *Bartonella* parasitize erythrocytes without inducing hemolysis, suggest that the periodic infection waves are due to the liberation of the bacteria from a distant sanctuary site (Dehio, 2001). This unknown sanctuary site might be the endothelial cells (Dehio, 2001) or bone marrow erythroblasts (Greub & Raoult, 2002). The presence of Bartonella within erythrocytes, a place where they are partially protected from the immune system, also explains the observation of disseminated diseases in alcoholic (chronic bacteremia in homeless people) or immunosupressed subjects (bacillary angiomatosis in AIDS patients) due to other *Bartonella* sp.

Apart from their tropism for red blood cells, a second typical pathogenic feature of *Bartonella* species is their ability to trigger angiogenesis. Such pathological angiogenesis is observed in verruaga peruana, explaining the propensity for bleeding of the ulcerated lesions, and in bacillary angiomatosis and peliosis. The first experimental evidence that *Bartonella*-related angiogenesis may be due to a protein was provided by Garcia et al. (1990). They demonstrated that *B. bacilliformis* extracts possess an activity that stimulates endothelial cell proliferation up to three times that of control. The factor, which was found to be specific for endothelial cells and was larger than 12–14 kDa (not dialyzed), was thought to be a protein as it was heat sensitive and precipitated with 45% ammonium sulfate (Garcia et al., 1990). *B. bacilliformis* extracts were also reported to stimulate the production of tissue plasminogen (Garcia et al., 1990). Live bacteria were later shown to increase both parameters (angiogenesis and tissue plasminogen production) in a fashion similar to the homogenates of *B. bacilliformis* (Garcia et al., 1992). In 1994, Conley et al. (1994) demonstrated in a similar in vitro model that *B. henselae* induces an angiogenic factor, the susceptibility of which to trypsin also suggests that the factor may be a protein.

More recently, it has been shown that this factor may be secreted by *B. henselae* (Maeno et al., 1999), indicating that *B. henselae* may induce endothelial cell proliferation independently of bacterial invasion. The dramatic effect of erythromycin on the cutaneous lesions of bacillary angiomatosis (Koehler et al., 1997; Koehler & Tappero, 1993) may be due to an inhibition of the production of the angiogenic factor, as erythromycin is known to interact with protein production at the ribosome level. An angiogenesis-based effect will better explain the rapidity of its effect and its lack of sustained response than a direct microbicidal one. Angiogenesis was not only characterized by cell proliferation, but also by altered spatial organization within the monolayer and changes in cell morphology due to cytoskeleton reorganization (Palmari et al., 1996).

The *Bartonella*–endothelial cell interaction is however not restricted to angiogenesis stimulation. Thus, (1) invasion of endothelial cells was described for *B. quintana* (Brouqui & Raoult, 1996), *B. henselae* (Dehio et al., 1997), and *B. bacilliformis* (Blumwald et al., 1985); and (2) a proinflammatory activation of endothelial cells was postulated, which is thought to result in receptor–ligand interactions between the activated endothelium and circulating neutrophils (Dehio, 2001). This is supported by the recent demonstration that *B. henselae* itself and *B. henselae*-derived outer membrane proteins induce an NF-κ B-dependant upregulation of E-selectin and ICAM-1 in endothelial cells, which in turn results in enhanced polymorphonuclear rolling and adhesion (Fuhrmann et al., 2001).

5. FUTURE DIRECTIONS

Bartonella sp. related infections were until recently under-recognized. Both the reemergence of older disease, such as the modern form of the trench fever that affects alcoholics and homeless people, and the emergence or recognition of new clinical entities due to *Bartonella* sp., pose major challenges for the next decades. Future researches should especially aim at (1) identifying potential new species of *Bartonella*, which could yet be overlooked by present diagnostic procedures; (2) defining the factors determining the host specificity (especially for human specific species); (3) determining the location in the host of a *Bartonella* sp. sanctuary, if any, which should be responsible for relapses of intraerythrocytic infections; (4) finding which protein or factor is involved in stimulating angiogenesis; (5) improving diagnostic procedures with better precision for specificity and sensitivity; (6) establishing the best therapeutic strategy for each clinical entity; and (7) developing vaccines.

References

Abbasi, S., & Chesney, P. J. (1995). Pulmonary manifestations of cat-scratch disease: A case report and review of the literature. *Pediatr Infect Dis J, 14,* 547–548.

Alexander, B. (1995). A review of bartonellosis in Ecuador and Colombia. *Am J Trop Med Hyg, 52,* 354–359.

Amano, Y., Rumbea, J., Knobloch, J., Olson, J., & Kron, M. (1997). Bartonellosis in Ecuador: Serosurvey and current status of cutaneous verrucous disease. *Am J Trop Med Hyg, 57,* 174–179.

Amerein, M. P., De Briel, D., Jaulhac, B., Meyer, P., Monteil, H., & Piemont, Y. (1996). Diagnostic value of the indirect immunofluorescence assay in cat scratch disease with *Bartonella henselae* and *Afipia felis* antigens. *Clin Diag Lab Immunol, 3*, 200–204.

Anderson, B., Sims, K., Regnery, R., Robinson, L., Schmidt, M. J., Goral, S., Hager, C., & Edwards, K. (1994). Detection of *Rochalimaea henselae* DNA in specimens from cat scratch disease patients by PCR. *J Clin Microbiol, 32*, 942–948.

Baron, A. L., Steinbach, L. S., Leboit, P. E., Mills, C. M., Gee, J. H., & Berger, T. G. (1990). Osteolytic lesions and bacillary angiomatosis in HIV infection: Radiologic differentiation from AIDS related Kaposi sarcoma. *Radiology, 177*, 77–81.

Bass, J. W., Freitas, B. C., Freitas, A. D., Sisler, C. L., Chan, D. S., Vincent, J. M., Person, D. A., Claybaugh, J. R., Wittler, R. R., Weisse, M. E., Regnery, R. L., & Slater, L. N. (1998). Prospective randomized double blind placebo-controlled evaluation of azithromycin for treatment of cat-scratch disease. *Pediatr Infect Dis J, 17*, 447–452.

Bass, J. W., Vincent, J. F., & Person, D. A. (1997a). The expanding spectrum of *Bartonella* infections: I. Bartonellosis and trench fever. *Pediatr Infect Dis J, 16*, 2–10.

Bass, J. W., Vincent, J. M., & Person, D. A. (1997b). The expanding spectrum of *Bartonella* infections: II. Cat scratch disease. *Pediatr Infect Dis J, 16*, 163–179.

Bereswill, S., Hinkelmann, S., Kist, M., & Sander, A. (1999). Molecular analysis of riboflavin synthesis genes in *Bartonella henselae* and use of the *ribC* gene for differentiation of *Bartonella* species by PCR. *J Clin Microbiol, 37*, 3159–3166.

Bergmans, A. M. C., Peeters, M. F., Schellekens, J. F. P., Vos, M. C., Sabbe, L. J. M., Ossewaarde, J. M., Verbakel, H., Hooft, H. J., & Schouls, L. M. (1997). Pitfalls and fallacies of cat scratch disease serology: Evaluation of *Bartonella henselae*-based indirect fluorescence assay and enzyme-linked immunoassay. *J Clin Microbiol, 35*, 1931–1937.

Bergs, V. V., & Scotti, T. M. (1967). Virus-induced peliosis hepatis in rats. *Science, 158*, 377–378.

Birtles, R. J., Harrison, T. G., Saunders, N. A., & Molyneux, D. H. (1995). Proposals to unify the genera *Grahamella* and B*artonella*, with descriptions of *Bartonella talpae* comb.nov., *Bartonella peromysci* comb. nov., and three new species, *Bartonella grahamii* sp. nov., *Bartonella taylorii* sp. nov., and *Bartonella doshiae* sp. nov. *Internat J Syst Bacteriol, 45*, 1–8.

Birtles, R. J., Hazel, S., Bown, K., Raoult, D., Begon, M., & Bennett, M. (2000). Subtyping of uncultured bartonellae using sequence comparison of 16 S/23 S rRNA intergenic spacer regions amplified directly from infected blood. *Mol Cell Probes, 14*, 79–87.

Birtles, R. J., & Raoult, D. (1996). Comparison of partial citrate synthase gene (*gltA*) sequences for phylogenetic analysis of *Bartonella* species. *Internat J Syst Bacteriol, 46*, 891–897.

Blanche, P., Bachmeyer, C., Salmon-Ceron, D., & Sicard, D. (1998). Muscular bacillary angiomatosis in AIDS. *J Infect, 37*, 193–193.

Blumwald, E., Fortin, M. G., Rea, P. A., Verma, D. P. S., & Poole, R. J. (1985). Presence of host-plasma membrane type H+-ATPase in the membrane envelope enclosing the bacteroids in soybean root nodules. *Plant Physiol, 78*, 665–672.

Borczuk, A. C., Niedt, G., Sablay, L. B., Kress, Y., Mannion, C. M., Factor, S. M., & Tanaka, K. E. (1998). Fibrous long-spacing collagen in bacillary angiomatosis [see comments]. *Ultrastruct Pathol, 22*, 127–133.

Breitschwerdt, E. B., Atkins, C. E., Brown, T. T., Kordick, D. L., & Snyder, P. S. (1999). *Bartonella vinsonii* subsp. *berkhoffii* and related members of the alpha subdivision of the *Proteobacteria* in dogs with cardiac arrhythmias, endocarditis, or myocarditis. *J Clin Microbiol, 37*, 3618–3626.

Brenner, D. J., O'Connor, S., Winkler, H. H., & Steigerwalt, A. G. (1993). Proposals to unify the genera *Bartonella* and *Rochalimaea*, with descriptions of *Bartonella quintana* comb. nov., *Bartonella vinsonii* comb. nov., *Bartonella henselae* comb. nov., and *Bartonella elizabethae* comb.nov., and to remove the family Bartonellaceae from the order Rickettsiales. *Internat J Syst Bacteriol, 43*, 777–786.

Brenner, S. A., Rooney, J. A., Manzewitsch, P., & Regnery, R. L. (1997). Isolation of *Bartonella (Rochalimae) henselae*: Effects of methods of blood collection and handling. *J Clin Microbiol, 35*, 544–547.

Brock, T. D. (1999). *Robert Koch, a life in medicine and bacteriology.* Washington: ASM Press.

Brouqui, P., La Scola, B., Roux, V., & Raoult, D. (1999). Chronic *Bartonella quintana* bacteremia in homeless patients. *N Engl J Med, 340*, 184–189.

Brouqui, P., & Raoult, D. (1996). *Bartonella quintana* invades and multiplies within endothelial cells in vitro and in vivo and forms intracellular blebs. *Res Microbiol, 147*, 719–731.

Brouqui, P., & Raoult, D. (2001). Endocarditis due to rare and fastidious bacteria. *Clin Microbiol Rev, 14*, 177–207.

Caceres, A. G. (1993). Distribucion geografica de Lutzomyia verrucarum (Townsend, 1913) (Diptera, Psychodidae, Phlebotominae), vector de la bartonellosis humana en el Peru. *Rev Inst Med Trop Sao Paulo, 35*, 485–490.

Carithers, H. A. (1985). Cat-scratch disease: An overview based on a study of 1200 patients. *Amer J Dis Child, 139*, 1124–1133.

Carithers, H. A., & Margileth, A. M. (1991). Cat scratch disease. Acute encephalopathy and other neurologic manifestations. *Am J Dis Child, 145*, 98–101.

Chang, C. C., Chomel, B., Kasten, R., Heller, R., Kocan, K. M., Ueno, H., Yamamoto, K., Bleich, V., Pierce, B., Gonzales, B., Swift, P., Boyce, W., Jang, S., Boulouis, H. J., & Piémont, Y. (2000). *Bartonella* spp. isolated from wild and domestic ruminants in North America. *Em Infect Dis, 6*, 306–311.

Chomel, B. B., Abbott, R. C., Kasten, R. W., Floydhawkins, K. A., Kass, P. H., Glaser, C. A., Pedersen, N. C., & Koehler, J. E. (1995). *Bartonella henselae* prevalence in domestic cats in California: Risk factors and association between bacteremia and antibody titers. *J Clin Microbiol, 33*, 2445–2450.

Chomel, B. B., Carlos, E. T., Kasten, R. W., Yamamoto, K., Chang, C. C., Carlos, R. S., Abenes, M. V., & Pajares, C. M. (1999). *Bartonella henselae* and *Bartonella clarridgeiae* infection in domestic cats from the Philippines. *Am J Trop Med Hyg, 60*, 593–597.

Clarridge, J. E., Raich, T. J., Pirwani, D., Simon, B., Tsai, L., Rodriguez-Barradas, M. C., Regnery, R., Zollo, A., Jones, D. C., & Rambo, C. (1995). Strategy to detect and identify *Bartonella* species in routine clinical laboratory yields *Bartonella henselae* from human immunodeficiency virus-positive patient and unique *Bartonella* strain from his cat. *J Clin Microbiol, 33*, 2107–2113.

Cline, M. S., Cummings, O. W., Goldman, M., Filo, R. S., & Pescovitz, M. D. (1999). Bacillary angiomatosis in a renal transplant recipient. *Transplantation, 67*, 296–298.

Cockerell, C. J., Bergstresser, P. R., Myrie-Williams, C., & Tierno, P. M. (1990). Bacillary epithelioid angiomatosis occuring in an immunocompetent individual. *Arch Dermatol, 126*, 787–790.

Cockerell, C. J., Tierno, P. M., Friedman-Kien, A. E., & Kim, K. S. (1991). Clinical, histologic, microbiologic, and biochemical characterization of the causative agent of bacillary (epithelioid) angiomatosis—a rickettsial illness with features of bartonellosis. *J Invest Dermatol, 97*, 812–817.

Cockerell, C. J., Whitlow, M. A., Webster, G. F., & Friedman-Kien, A. E. (1987). Epithelioid angiomatosis: A distinct vascular disorder in patients with the acquired immunodeficiency syndrome or AIDS-related complex. *Lancet, 2*, 654–656.

Conley, T., Slater, L., & Hamilton, K. (1994). *Rochalimaea* species stimulate human endothelial cell proliferation and migration in vitro. *J Lab Clin Med, 124*, 521–528.

Conrad, D. A. (2001). Treatment of cat-scratch disease. *Curr Opin Pediatr, 13*, 56–59.

Cuadra, M. C. (1956). Salmonellosis complications in human bartonellosis. *Tex Rep Biol Med, 14*, 97–113.

Cunningham, E. T., & Koehler, J. E. (2000). Ocular bartonellosis. *Am J Ophtalmol, 130*, 340–349.

Daly, J. S., Worthington, M. G., Brenner, D. J., Moss, W. C., Hollis, D. G., Weyant, R. S., Steigerwalt, A. G., Weaver, R. E., Daneshvar, M. I., & O'Connor, S. P. (1993). *Rochalimaea elizabethae* sp. nov. isolated from a patient with endocarditis. *J Clin Microbiol, 31*, 872–881.

Dauga, C., Miras, I., & Grimont, P. A. D. (1996). Identification of *Bartonella henselae* and *B. quintana* 16S rDNA sequences by branch-, genus-, and species-specific amplification. *J Med Microb, 45*, 192–199.

Debré, R., Lamy, M., Jammet, M. L., Costil, L., & Mozziconacci, P. (1950). La maladie des griffes du chat. *Société Médicale des Hôpitaux de Paris, 66*, 76–79.

Dehio, C. (2001). *Bartonella* interactions with endothelial cells and erythrocytes. *Trends Micobiol, 9*, 279–285.

Dehio, C., Lanz, C., Pohl, R., Behrens, P., Bermond, D., Piémont, Y., Pelz, K., & Sander, A. (2001). *Bartonella schoenbuchii* sp. nov., isolated from the blood of wild roe deer. *Int J Syst Evol Microbiol, 51*, 1557–1565.

Dehio, C., Meyer, M., Berger, J., Schwarz, H., & Lanz, C. (1997). Interaction of *Bartonella henselae* with endothelial cells results in bacterial aggregation on the cell surface and the subsequent engulfment and internalisation of the bacterial aggregate by a unique structure, the invasome. *J Cell Sci, 110*, 2141–2154.

Dolan, M. J., Wong, M. T., Regnery, R. L., Jorgensen, J. H., Garcia, M., Peters, J., & Drehner, D. (1993). Syndrome of *Rochalimaea henselae* adenitis suggesting cat scratch disease. *Ann Intern Med, 118*, 388–390.

Drancourt, M., Mainardi, J. L., Brouqui, P., Vandenesch, F., Carta, A., Lehnert, F., Etienne, J., Vigier, E., Goldstein, F., Acar, J., & Raoult, D. (1995). *Bartonella (Rochalimaea) quintana* endocarditis in homeless patients: Report of three cases. *N Engl J Med, 332*, 419–423.

Drancourt, M., & Raoult, D. (1993). Proposed tests for the routine identification of *Rochalimaea* species. *Eur J Clin Microbiol Infect Dis, 12*, 710–713.

Droz, S., Chi, B., Horn, E., Steigerwalt, A. G., Whitney, A. M., & Brenner, D. J. (1999). *Bartonella koehlerae* sp. nov., isolated from cats. *J Clin Microbiol, 37*, 1117–1122.

Eden, C. G., Marker, A., & Pryor, J. P. (1996). Human immunodeficiency virus-related bacillary angiomatosis of the penis. *Br J Urol, 77*, 323–324.

Ellis, B. A., Rotz, L. D., Leake, J. A., Samalvides, F., Bernable, J., Ventura, G., Padilla, C., Villaseca, P., Beati, L., Regnery, R., Childs, J. E., Olson, J. G., & Carrillo, C. P. (1999). An outbreak of acute bartonellosis (Oroya fever) in the Urubamba region of Peru, 1998. *Am J Trop Med Hyg, 61*, 344–349.

English, C. K., Wear, D. J., Margileth, A. M., Lissner, C. R., & Walsh, G. P. (1988). Cat-scratch disease: Isolation and culture of the bacterial agent. *J Am Med Assoc, 259*, 1347–1351.

Fagan, W. A., Skinner, S. M., Ondo, A., Williams, J. T., Anthony, K., De Villez, R. L., & Pulitzer, D. R. (1995). Bacillary angiomatosis of the skin and bone marrow in a patient with HIV infection. *J Am Acad Dermatol, 32*, 510–512.

Fournier, P. E., Lelievre, H., Eykyn, S. J., Mainardi, J. L., Marrie, T. J., Bruneel, F., Roure, C., Nash, J., Clave, D., James, E., Benoit-Lemercier, C., Deforges, L., Tissot-Dupont, H., & Raoult, D. (2001). Epidemiologic and clinical characteristics of *Bartonella quintana* and *Bartonella henselae* endocarditis—a study of 48 patients. *Medicine, 80*, 245–251.

Fournier, P. E., Mainardi, J. L., & Raoult, D. (2002). Value of microimmunofluorescence for the diagnosis and follow-up of *Bartonella* endocarditis. *Clin Diag Lab Immunol, 9*(4): 795–801.

Fournier, P. E., & Raoult, D. (1998). Cat scratch disease and an overview of other *Bartonella henselae* related infections. In A. Schmidt (Ed.), Bartonella *and* Afipia *species emphasizing* Bartonella henselae (pp. 32–62). Basel: Karger.

Fox, K. A., & Lahcen, R. B. (1974). Liver-cell adenomas and peliosis hepatis in mice associated with oxazepam. *Res Commun Chem Pathol Pharmacol, 8*, 481–483.

Fuhrmann, O., Arvand, M., Göhler, A., Schmid, S., Krüll, M., Hippenstiel, S., Seybold, J., Dehio, C., & Suttorp, N. (2001). *Bartonella henselae* induces NF-mB-dependent upregulation of adhesion molecules in cultured human endothelial cells: Possible role of outer membrane proteins as pathogenic factors. *Infect Immun, 69*, 5088–5097.

Garcia, F. U., Wojta, J., Broadley, K. N., Davidson, J. M., & Hoover, R. L. (1990). *Bartonella bacilliformis* stimulates endothelial cells in vitro, and is angiogenic in vivo. *Am J Pathol, 136*, 1125–1135.

Garcia, F. U., Wojta, J., & Hoover, R. L. (1992). Interactions between live *Bartonella bacilliformis* and endothelial cells. *J Infect Dis, 165*, 1138–1141.

Gasquet, S., Maurin, M., Brouqui, P., Lepidi, H., & Raoult, D. (1998). Bacillary angiomatosis in immunocompromised patients: A clinicopathological and microbiological study of seven cases and review of literature. *AIDS, 12*, 1793–1803.

Gluckman, S. J. (1996). Q fever and trench fever. *Clin Dermatol, 14*, 283–287.

Gregory, D. W., & Decker, M. D. (1986). Cat scratch disease: An infection beyond the lymph node. *Am J Med Sci, 292*, 389–390.

Greub, G., & Raoult, D. (2002). Bartonella: New explanations for old diseases. *J Med Microbiol* 51(11): 915–923.

Guyot, A., Bakhai, A., Fry, N., Merritt, J., Malnick, H., & Harrison, T. (1999). Culture-positive *Bartonella quintana* endocarditis. *Eur J Clin Microbiol Infect Dis, 18*, 145–147.

Heller, R., Kubina, M., Mariet, P., Riegel, P., Delacour, G., Dehio, C., Lamarque, F., Kasten, R., Boulouis, H. J., Monteil, H., Chomel, B., & Piemont, Y. (1999). *Bartonella alsatica* sp. nov., a new *Bartonella* species isolated from the blood of wild rabbits. *Int J Syst Bacteriol, 49*, 283–288.

Heller, R., Riegel, P., Hansmann, Y., Delacour, G., Bermond, D., Dehio, C., Lamarque, F., Monteil, H., Chomel, B., & Piémont, Y. (1998). *Bartonella tribocorum* sp. nov., a new *Bartonella* species isolated from the blood of wild rats. *Int J Syst Bacteriol, 48*, 1333–1339.

Holmes, A. H., Greenough, T. C., Balady, G. J., Regnery, R. L., Anderson, B. E., Oikeane, J. C., Fonger, J. D., & Mcrone, E. L. (1995). *Bartonella henselae* endocarditis in an immunocompetent adult. *Clin Infect Dis, 21*, 1004–1007.

Houpikian, P., & Raoult, D. (2001a). 16S/23S rRNA intergenic spacer regions for phylogenetic analysis, identification, and subtyping of *Bartonella* species. *J Clin Microbiol, 39*, 2768–2778.

Houpikian, P., & Raoult, D. (2001b). Molecular phylogeny of the genus *Bartonella*: What is the current knowledge? *FEMS Microbiol Lett, 200*, 1–7.

Hulzebos, C. W., Koetse, H. A., Kimpen, J. L., & Wolfs, T. F. (1999). Vertebral osteomyelitis associated with cat-scratch disease. *Clin Infect Dis, 28*, 1310–1312.

Ihler, G. M. (1996). *Bartonella bacilliformis*: Dangerous pathogen slowly emerging from deep background. *FEMS Microbiol Lett, 144*, 1–11.

Jacomo, V., & Raoult, D. (2000). Human infections caused by *Bartonella* spp. Part 1. *Clin Microbiol Newsletter, 22*, 1–8.

Jacomo, V., & Raoult, D. (2002). Natural history of *Bartonella* infections (an exception to Koch's postulate). *Clin Diag Lab Immun 9*, 8–18.

Joblet, C., Roux, V., Drancourt, M., Gouvernet, J., & Raoult, D. (1995). Identification of *Bartonella* (*Rochalimaea*) species among fastidious Gram-negative bacteria based on the partial sequence of the citrate-synthase gene. *J Clin Microbiol, 33*, 1879–1883.

Kelly, T. M., Padmalayam, I., & Baumstark, B. R. (1998). Use of the cell division protein FtsZ as a means of differentiating among Bartonella species. *Clin Diagn Lab Immunol, 5*, 766–772.

Kemper, C. A., Lombard, C. M., Deresinski, S. C., & Tompkins, L. S. (1990). Visceral bacillary epithelioid angiomatosis: Possible manifestations of disseminated cat scratch disease in the immunocompromised host: A report of two cases. *Am J Med, 89*, 216–222.

Keret, D., Giladi, M., Kletter, Y., & Wientroub, S. (1999). Cat-scratch disease osteomyelitis from a dog scratch. *J Bone Joint Surg Br, 80*, 766–767.

Kerkhoff, F. T., Bergmans, A. M. C., van der Zee, A., & Rothova, A. (1999). Demonstration of *Bartonella grahamii* DNA in ocular fluids of a patient with neuroretinitis. *J Clin Microbiol, 37*, 4034–4038.

Koehler, J. E., LeBoit, P. E., Egbert, B. M., & Berger, T. G. (1998). Cutaneous vascular lesions and disseminated cat-scratch disease in patients with the acquired immunodeficiency syndrome (AIDS) and AIDS-related complex. *Ann Intern Med, 109*, 449–455.

Koehler, J. E., Quinn, F. D., Berger, T. G., Leboit, P. E., & Tappero, J. W. (1992). Isolation of *Rochalimaea* species from cutaneous and osseous lesions of bacillary angiomatosis. *N Engl J Med, 327*, 1625–1631.

Koehler, J. E., Sanchez, M. A., Garrido, C. S., Whitfeld, M. J., Chen, F. M., Berger, T. G., Rodriguez-Barradas, M. C., Leboit, P. E., & Tappero, J. W. (1997). Molecular epidemiology of *Bartonella* infections in patients with bacillary angiomatosis-peliosis. *N Engl J Med, 337*, 1876–1883.

Koehler, J. E., & Tappero, J. W. (1993). Bacillary angiomatosis and bacillary peliosis in patients infected with human immunodeficiency virus. *Clin Infect Dis, 17*, 612–624.

Kordick, D. L., Hilyard, E. J., Hadfield, T. L., Wilson, K. H., Steigerwalt, A. G., Brenner, D. J., & Breitschwerdt, E. B. (1997). *Bartonella clarridgeiae*, a newly recognized zoonotic pathogen causing inoculation papules, fever, and lymphadenopathy (cat scratch disease). *J Clin Microbiol, 35*, 1813–1818.

Kordick, D. L., Swaminathan, B., Greene, C. E., Wilson, K. H., Whitney, A. M., O'Connor, S., Hollis, D. G., Matar, G. M., Steirgerwalt, A. G., Malcolm, G. B., Hayes, P. S., Hadfield, T. L., Breitschwerdt, E. B., & Brenner, D. J. (1996). *Bartonella vinsonii* subsp. *berkhofii* subsp. nov., isolated from dogs; *Bartonella vinsonii* subsp. *vinsonii*; and amended description of *Bartonella vinsonii*. *Int J Syst Bacteriol, 46*, 704–709.

Kosek, M., Lavarello, R., Gilman, R. H., Delgado, J., Maguina, C., Verastegui, M., Lescano, A. G., Mallqui, V., Kosek, J. C., Recavarren, S., & Cabrera, L. (2000). Natural history of infection with *Bartonella bacilliformis* in a nonendemic population. *J Infect Dis, 182*, 865–872.

Kostrzewski, J. (1949). The epidemiology of Trench fever. *Bul de l'Académie polonaise des sciences et des lettres Classe de Médecine 7*, 233–263.

Krause, K., Wenish, C., Fladerer, P., Daxbock, F., Krejs, G. J., & Reisinger, E. C. (2000). Osteomyelitis of the hip joint associated with systemic cat-scratch disease in an adult. *Eur J Clin Microbiol Infect Dis, 19*, 781–783.

Krekorian, T. D., Radner, A. B., Alcorn, J. M., Haghighi, P., & Ang, F. C. (1990). Biliary obstruction caused by epitheloïd angiomatosis in a patient with AIDS. *Am J Med, 89*, 820–822.

Larson, A. M., Dougherty, M. J., Nowowiejski, D. J., Welch, D. F., Matar, G. M., Swaminathan, B., & Coyle, M. B. (1994). Detection of *Bartonella (Rochalimaea) quintana* by routine acridine orange staining of broth blood cultures. *J Clin Microbiol, 32*, 1492–1496.

La Scola, B., & Raoult, D. (1996). Serological cross reactions between *Bartonella quintana*, *Bartonella henselae*, and *Coxiella burnetii*. *J Clin Microbiol, 34*, 2270–2274.

La Scola, B., & Raoult, D. (1999a). *Afipia felis* is a hospital water supply in association with free-living amoebae. *Lancet, 353*, 1330.

La Scola, B., & Raoult, D. (1999b). Culture of *Bartonella quintana* and *Bartonella henselae* from human samples: A 5-year experience (1993 to 1998). *J Clin Microbiol, 37*, 1899–1905.

Leboit, P. E. (1995). Bacillary angiomatosis. *Mod Pathol, 8*, 218–222.

Leboit, P. E., Berger, T. G., Egbert, B. M., Beckstead, J. H., Yen, T. S., & Stoler, M. H. (1989). Bacillary angiomatosis. The histopathology and differential diagnosis of a pseudoneoplastic infection in patients with human immunodeficiency virus disease. *Am J Surg Pathol, 13*, 909–920.

Ledergerber, B., Egger, M., Erard, V., Weber, R., Hirschel, B., Furrer, H., Battegay, M., Vernazza, P., Bernasconi, E., Opravil, M., Kaufmann, D., Sudre, P., Francioli, P., & Telenti, A. (2001). AIDS-related opportunistic illnesses occurring after initiation of potent antiretroviral therapy: The Swiss HIV Cohort Study. *JAMA, 282,* 2220–2226.

Lepidi, H., Fournier, P. E., & Raoult, D. (2000). Quantitative analysis of valvular lesions during Bartonella endocarditis. A case control study. *Am J Clin Pathol, 114,* 880–889.

Liang, Z., La Scola, B., Lepidi, H., & Raoult, D. (2001). Production of *Bartonella* genus-specific monoclonal antibodies. *Clin Diag Lab Immunol, 8,* 847–849.

Liang, Z., & Raoult, D. (2000). Differentiation of *Bartonella* species by a microimmunofluorescence assay, sodium dodecyl sulfate–polyacrylamide gel electrophoresis, and Western immunoblotting. *Clin Diag Lab Immunol 7,* 617–624.

Liapi-Adamidou, G., Tsolia, M., Magiakou, A. M., Zeis, P. M., Theodoropoulos, V., & Karpathios, T. (2000). Cat-scratch disease in 2 siblings presenting as acute gastroenteritis. *Scand J Infect Dis, 32,* 317–319.

Long, S. R., Whitfeld, M. J., Eades, C., Koehler, J. E., Korn, A. P., & Zaloudek, C. J. (1996). *Bacillary angiomatosis* of the cervix and vulva in a patient with AIDS. *Ob Gyne, 88,* 709–711.

Maeno, N., Oda, H., Yoshiie, K., Rezwanul Whahid, M., Fujimura, T., & Matayoshi, S. (1999). Live *Bartonella henselae* enhances endothelial cell proliferation without direct contact. *Microb Pathog, 27,* 419–427.

Maguina Vargas, C. (1998). *Bartonellosis o enfermedad de carrion. Nuevos aspectos de una vieja enfermedad,* Lima, Peru.

Maguina, C., Garcia, P. J., Gotuzzo, E., Cordero, L., & Spach, D. H. (2001). Bartonellosis (Carrion's disease) in the modern era. *Clin Infect Dis, 33,* 772–779.

Marseglia, G. L., Monafo, V., Marone, P., Meloni, F., Martini, A., & Burgio, G. R. (2001). Asymptomatic persistent pulmonary infiltrates in an immunocompetent boy with cat-scratch disease. *Eur J Pediatr, 160,* 260–261.

Marston, E. L., Sumner, J. W., & Regnery, R. L. (1999). Evaluation of intraspecies genetic variation within the 60 kDa heat-shock protein gene (*groEL*) of *Bartonella* species. *Int J Syst Bacteriol, 49,* 1015–1023.

Massei, F., Massimetti, M., Messina, F., Macchia, P., & Maggiore, G. (2000). *Bartonella henselae* and inflammatory bowel disease. *Lancet, 356,* 1245–1246.

Matar, G. M., Koehler, J. E., Malcolm, G., Lambert-Fair, M. N., Tappero, J., Hunter, S. B., & Swaminathan, B. (1999). Identification of *Bartonella* species directly in clinical specimens by PCR-restriction fragment length polymorphism analysis of a 16S rRNA gene fragment. *J Clin Microbiol, 37,* 4045–4047.

Maurin, M., Eb, F., Etienne, J., & Raoult, D. (1997). Serological cross-reactions between *Bartonella* and *Chlamydia* species: Implications for diagnosis. *J Clin Microbiol, 35,* 2283–2287.

Maurin, M., Gasquet, S., Ducco, C., & Raoult, D. (1995). MICs of 28 antibiotic compounds for 14 *Bartonella* (formerly *Rochalimaea*) isolates. *Antimicrob Agents Chemother, 39,* 2387–2391.

Maurin, M., & Raoult, D. (1996). *Bartonella (Rochalimaea) quintana* infections. *Clin Microbiol Rev, 9,* 273–292.

Maurin, M., & Raoult, D. (1998). Minimal inhibitory concentration determination in *Bartonella henselae*. In A. Schmidt (Ed.), Bartonella *and* Afipia *species emphazing* Bartonella henselae (pp. 164–175). Basel: Karger.

Modi, S. P., Eppes, S. C., & Klein, J. D. (2001). Cat-scratch disease presenting as multifocal osteomyelitis with thoracic abscess. *Pediatr Infect Dis J, 20,* 1006–1007.

Mooser, H. (1959). The etiology of trench fever. *Proceedings of the 6th International Congress of Tropical Medicine and Malaria, Lisbon, 1958, 5,* 631–635.

Mui, B. S., Mulligan, M. E., & George, W. L. (1990). Response of HIV-associated disseminated cat-scratch disease to treatment with doxycycline. *Am J Med, 89,* 229–231.

Musso, D., Drancourt, M., & Raoult, D. (1995). Lack of bactericidal effect of antibiotics except aminoglycosides on *Bartonella (Rochalimaea) henselae. J Antimicrob Chemother, 36,* 101–108.

Myers, W. F., Grossman, D. M., & Wisseman, C. L., Jr. (1984). Antibiotic susceptibility patterns in *Rochalimaea quintana,* the agent of trench fever. *Antimicrob Agents Chemother, 25,* 690–693.

Noyola, D. E., Holder, D. L., Fishman, M. A., & Edwards, M. S. (1999). Recurrent encephalopathy in cat-scratch disease. *Pediatr Infect Dis J, 18,* 567–568.

O'Halloran, H. S., Draud, K., Minix, M., Rivard, A. K., & Pearson, P. A. (1998). Leber's neuroretinitis in a patient with serologic evidence of *Bartonella elizabethae. Retina, 18,* 276–278.

Palmari, J., Teysseire, N., Dussert, C., & Raoult, D. (1996). Image cytometry and topographical analysis of proliferation of endothelial cells in vitro during *Bartonella (Rochalimaea)* infection. *Analyt Cell Path, 11,* 13–30.

Parinaud, H. (1889). Conjonctivite infectieuse transmise par les animaux. *Ann Ocul, 101,* 252–253.

Perkocha, L. A., Geaghan, S. M., Yen, T. S., Nishimura, S. L., Chan, S. P., Garcia-Kennedy, R., Honda, G., Stoloff, A. C., Klein, H. Z., Goldman, R. L., Van Meter, S., Ferrel, L., & Leboit, P. E. (1990). Clinical and pathological features of bacillary peliosis hepatis in association with human immunodeficiency virus infection. *N Engl J Med, 323,* 1581–1586.

Pickerill, R. G., & Milder, J. E. (1981). Transverse myelitis associated with cat-scratch disease in an adult. *JAMA, 246,* 2840–2841.

Raoult, D., Fournier, P. E., Drancourt, M., Marrie, T. J., Etienne, J., Cosserat, J., Cacoub, P., Poinsignon, Y., Leclercq, P., & Sefton, A. M. (1996). Diagnosis of 22 new cases of *Bartonella* endocarditis. *Ann Intern Med, 125,* 646–652.

Regnery, R. L., Anderson, B. E., Clarridge, J. E., Rodriguez-Barradas, M. C., Jones, D. C., & Carr, J. H. (1992). Characterization of a novel *Rochalimaea* species, *R. henselae* sp. nov., isolated from blood of a febrile, human immunodeficiency virus-positive patient. *J Clin Microbiol, 30,* 265–274.

Relman, D. A., Loutit, J. S., Schmidt, T. M., Falkow, S., & Tompkins, L. S. (1990). The agent of bacillary angiomatosis: An approach to the identification of uncultured pathogens. *N Engl J Med, 323,* 1573–1580.

Renesto, P., Gautheret, D., Drancourt, M., & Raoult, D. (2001a). Determination of the *rpoB* gene sequences of *Bartonella henselae* and *Bartonella quintana* for phylogenic analysis. *Res Microbiol, 151,* 831–836.

Renesto, P., Gouvernet, J., Drancourt, M., Roux, V., & Raoult, D. (2001b). Use of *rpoB* gene analysis for detection and identification of *Bartonella* species. *J Clin Microbiol, 39,* 430–437.

Roux, V., Eykyn, S. J., Wyllie, S., & Raoult, D. (2000). *Bartonella vinsonii* subsp. *berkhoffii* as an agent of afebrile blood culture-negative endocarditis in a human. *J Clin Microbiol, 38,* 1698–1700.

Roux, V., & Raoult, D. (1995). Inter- and intraspecies identification of *Bartonella (Rochalimea)* species. *J Clin Microbiol, 33,* 1573–1579.

Salgado, C. D., & Weisse, M. E. (2000). Transverse myelitis associated with probable cat-scratch disease in a previously healthy pediatric patient. *Clin Infect Dis, 31,* 609–611.

Sander, A., & Penno, S. (1999). Semiquantitative species-specific detection of *Bartonella henselae* and *Bartonella quintana* by PCR-enzyme immunoassay. *J Clin Microbiol, 37,* 3097–3101.

Sander, A., Posselt, M., Böhm, N., Ruess, M., & Altwegg, M. (1999). Detection of *Bartonella henselae* DNA by two different PCR assays and determination of the genotypes of strains involved in histologically defined cat scratch disease. *J Clin Microbiol, 37,* 993–997.

Schmidt, H. U., Kaliebe, T., Poppinger, J., Buhler, C., & Sander, A. (1996). Isolation of *Bartonella quintana* from an HIV-positive patient with bacillary angiomatosis. *Eur J Clin Microbiol Infect Dis, 15,* 736–741.

Schultz, M. G. (1968). Daniel Carrion's experiment. *N Engl J Med, 278,* 1323–1326.

Schülein, R., Seubert, A., Gilles, C., Lanz, C., Hansmann, Y., Piemont, Y., & Dehio, C. (2001). Invasion and persistent intracellular colonization of erythrocytes: A unique parasite strategy of the emerging pathogen *Bartonella. J Exp Med, 193,* 1077–1086.

Selby, G., & Walker, G. K. (1979). Cerebral arteritis in cat-scratch disease. *Neurology, 29*, 1413–1418.

Sholdt, C., Rogers, E., Gerberg, E., & Shreck, C. (1989). Effectiveness of permethrin-treated military uniform fabric against human body lice. *Military Med, 154*, 90–93.

Slater, L. N., Coody, D. W., Woolridge, L. K., & Welch, D. F. (1992). Murine antibody responses distinguish *Rochalimaea henselae* from *Rochalimaea quintana*. *J Clin Microbiol, 30*, 1722–1727.

Slater, L. N., Welch, D. F., Hensel, D., & Coody, D. W. (1990). A newly recognized fastidious Gram-negative pathogen as a cause of fever and bacteremia. *N Engl J Med, 323*, 1587–1593.

Slater, L. N., Welch, D. F., & Min, K. W. (1992). *Rochalimaea henselae* causes bacillary angiomatosis and peliosis hepatis. *Arch Intern Med, 152*, 602–606.

Sobraques, M., Maurin, M., Birtles, R., & Raoult, D. (1999). In vitro susceptibilities of four *Bartonella baciliformis* strains to 30 antibiotic compounds. *Antimicrob Agents Chemother, 43*, 2090–2092.

Spach, D. H., Callis, K. P., Paauw, D. S., Houze, Y. B., Schoenknecht, F. D., Welch, D. F., Rosen, H., & Brenner, D. J. (1993). Endocarditis caused by *Rochalimaea quintana* in a patient infected with human immunodeficiency virus. *J Clin Microbiol, 31*, 692–694.

Spach, D. H., Kanter, A. S., Dougherty, M. J., Larson, A. M., Coyle, M. B., Brenner, D. J., Swaminathan, B., Matar, G. M., Welch, D. F., Root, R. K., & Stamm, W. E. (1995). *Bartonella (Rochalimaea) quintana* bacteremia in inner-city patients with chronic alcoholism. *N Engl J Med, 332*, 424–428.

Spach, D. H., Panther, L. A., Thorning, D. R., Dunn, J. E., Plorde, J. J., & Miller, R. A. (1992). Intracerebral bacillary angiomatosis in a patient infected with human immunodeficiency virus. *Ann Méd Inte(Paris), 116*, 740–742.

Stein, A., & Raoult, D. (1995). Return of trench fever. *Lancet, 345*, 450–451.

Stoler, M. H., Bonfiglio, T. A., Steigbigel, R. T., & Pereira, M. (1983). An atypical subcutaneous infection associated with acquired immune deficiency syndrome. *Am J Clin Pathol, 80*, 714–718.

Swift, H. F. (1920). Trench fever. *Harvey Lect Ser XV*, 58–86.

Szelc-Kelly, C. M., Goral, S., Perez-Perez, G. I., Perkins, B. A., Regnery, R. L., & Edwards, K. M. (1995). Serologic responses to *Bartonella* and *Afipia* antigens in patients with cat scratch disease. *Pediatrics, 96*, 1137–1142.

Tappero, J. W., Koehler, J. E., Berger, T. G., Cockerell, C. J., Lee, T. H., Busch, M. P., Stites, D. P., Mohle-Boetani, J. C., Reingold, A. L., & Leboit, P. E. (1993). Bacillary angiomatosis and bacillary splenitis in immunocompetent adults. *Ann Intern Med, 118*, 363–365.

Tierno, P. M., Inglima, K., & Parisi, M. T. (1995). Detection of *Bartonella (Rochalimaea) henselae* bacteremia using BacT/Alert blood culture system. *Am J Clin Pathol, 104*, 530–536.

Tsukahara, M., Tsuneoka, H., Iino, H., Ohno, K., & Murano, I. (1998). *Bartonella henselae* infection from a dog. *Lancet, 352*, 1682.

Tuchweber, B., Kovacs, K., Khandekar, J. D., & Garg, B. D. (1973). Peliosis-like changes induced by phalloidin in the rat liver: A light and electon microscopic study. *J Med, 4*, 327–345.

Uertega, O., & Payne, E. H. (1955). Treatment of the acute febrile phase of Carrion's disease with chloramphenicol. *Am J Trop Med Hyg, 4*, 507–511.

Vinson, J. W., & Fuller, H. S. (1961). Studies on trench fever. 1. Propagation of rickettsia-like organisms from a patient's blood. *Pathol Microbiol, 24*, S152–S166.

Walter, E., & Mockel, J. (1997). Peliosis hepatis. *N Engl J Med, 337*, 1603.

Wear, D. J., Malaty, R. H., Zimmerman, L. E., Hadfield, T. L., & Margileth, A. M. (1985). Cat scratch disease bacilli in the conjunctiva of patients with Parinaud's oculoglandular syndrome. *Ophtalmology, 92*, 1282–1287.

Welch, D., Carrol, K., Hofmeister, E., Persing, D., Robison, D., Steigerwalt, A., & Brenner, D. (1999). Isolation of a new subspecies, *Bartonella vinsonii* subsp. *arupensis*, from a cattle rancher: Identify with isolates found in conjunction with *Borrelia burgdorferi* and *Babesia microti* among naturally infected mice. *J Clin Microbiol, 37*, 2598–2601.

Wilck, M. B., Wu, Y., Howe, J. G., Crough, J. Y., & Edberg, S. C. (2001). Endocarditis caused by culture-negative organisms visible by brown and brenn staining: Utility of PCR and DNA sequencing for diagnosis. *J Clin Microbiol, 39*, 2025–2027.

Wong, M. T., Dolan, M. J., Lattuada, C. P., Regnery, R. L., Garcia, M. L., Mokulis, E. C., Labarre, R. C., Ascher, D. P., Delmar, J. A., Kelly, J. W., Leigh, D. R., Mcrae, A. C., Reed, J. B., Smith, R. E., & Melcher, G. P. (1995). Neuroretinitis, aseptic meningitis, and lymphadenitis associated with *Bartonella (Rochalimaea) henselae* infection in immunocompetent patients and patients infected with human immunodeficiency virus type 1. *Clin Infect Dis, 21*, 352–360.

Wong, R., Tappero, J., & Cockerell, C. J. (1997). Bacillary angiomatosis and other *Bartonella* species infections. *Semin Cutan Med Surg, 16*, 188–199.

Zeaiter, Z., Fournier, P. E., Ogata, H., & Raoult, D. (2002a). Phylogenetic classification of *Bartonella* species by comparing *groEL* sequences. *Int J Syst Evol Microbiol, 52*, 165–171.

Zeaiter, Z., Fournier, P. E., & Raoult, D. (2002b). Genomic variation of *Bartonella henselae* detected in lymph nodes from patients with cat-scratch disease. *J Clin Microbiol, 40*, 1023–1030.

Section II

Resistant Bacteria and Resurgence

3

Antibiotic-Resistant *Streptococcus pneumoniae*: Implications for Management in the 21st Century

Cynthia G. Whitney and Nina E. Glass

1. INTRODUCTION

Streptococcus pneumoniae, or pneumococcus, is a common cause of upper respiratory tract infections, such as sinusitis and otitis media. Pneumococci cause about 7 million episodes of otitis media each year in the United States alone (Dowell et al., 1999a). The bacteria also cause severe syndromes such as pneumonia, meningitis, peritonitis, endocarditis, and septic arthritis. Pneumococci are the most common cause of hospitalized community-acquired pneumonia in the United States (Marston et al., 1997); worldwide, an estimated 1 million children die of pneumococcal pneumonia each year, most in developing countries (Mulholland, 1999). In the United States, where vaccines are routinely used to prevent disease due to *Haemophilus influenzae* type B, pneumococcus is the most common cause of bacterial meningitis (Schuchat et al., 1997). Before antibiotic therapy, about 80% of people with pneumococcal bacteremia died of the infection (Austrian & Gold, 1964). Recent reports indicate that case-fatality rates for pneumococcal bacteremia are about 10.0%, although this figure is higher among the elderly and persons with chronic illnesses (Robinson et al., 2001). The emergence of strains resistant to antibiotics has become a major concern and has made treating pneumococcal disease much more difficult.

 S. pneumoniae resistant to antibiotics have been reported since the early 1940s, when pneumococci resistant to sulfonamides were first identified (Frisch et al., 1943). As new classes of antibiotics have been introduced, resistance has developed. In the 1960s and 1970s, the first reports of pneumococci resistant to tetracycline (Evans & Hansman, 1963), erythromycin and lincomycin (Kislak, 1967), and chloramphenicol (Cybulska et al., 1970) were published. The first case of *S. pneumoniae* partially resistant to penicillin was reported in Australia in 1967 (Hansman & Bullen, 1967). Strains of *S. pneumoniae* resistant to these drugs are now found throughout the world. Multiply-resistant strains of

Reemergence of Established Pathogens in the 21st Century
Edited by Fong and Drlica, Kluwer Academic/Plenum Publishers, New York, 2003

S. pneumoniae, seen first in South Africa in the late 1970s (Jacobs et al., 1978), have also become more prevalent. Recently, fluoroquinolone resistance has been reported not long after those agents became widely available (Chen et al., 1999; Ho et al., 2001c).

In this chapter, we will review the ways in which pneumococci have adapted to defend themselves against antimicrobial agents, how resistant pneumococci have spread throughout the world, and factors associated with a higher risk of infection with a resistant strain. We will also review current treatment recommendations in light of resistance and evidence of whether resistance contributes to poor treatment outcomes. Finally, we will explore mechanisms for preventing disease due to resistant strains and future trends in antibiotic resistance.

2. MICROBIOLOGY AND DEFINITIONS OF RESISTANCE

S. pneumoniae is a Gram-positive coccus that reproduces in chains and is catalase-negative. On blood agar, pneumococcal colonies appear α-hemolytic (i.e., colonies on blood agar are surrounded by a green zone). For routine identification in the microbiology laboratory, the organism is differentiated from other non-β-hemolytic, catalase-negative organisms by susceptibility to optochin and solubility in bile. Other tests can be used to identify the organism but are not routinely used. One such technique, the Quellung reaction, is a specific method for microscopic detection of pneumococci that utilizes anticapsular antisera to enhance visualization of the pneumococcal capsule. A nucleic acid probe for identification of pneumococci is also commercially available (Geslin et al., 1997).

Most pneumococcal strains isolated from ill persons contain a characteristic polysaccharide capsule. The capsule is a major virulence factor, allowing the bacteria to evade phagocytosis by neutrophils. Ninety pneumococcal serotypes, distinguishable by the structure of the polysaccharide capsule, have been identified as causing disease. Because serotype information is no longer used in the treatment of individual patients, this procedure is only performed in a limited number of reference laboratories. Serotypes are often linked to particular resistance patterns (Whitney et al., 2000); therefore data on serotypes are useful for tracking trends in antibiotic resistant pneumococci. Unencapsulated pneumococci are not uncommon in studies of nasopharyngeal carriage of well individuals and have been associated with outbreaks of conjunctivitis (Barker et al., 1999; Ertugrul et al., 1997; Shayegani et al., 1982).

The reservoir for pneumococci is the human upper respiratory tract, where the organism often can be found in persons without any symptoms of disease. Pneumococci are transmitted in respiratory droplets. Carriage of pneumococcus is more common in children than in adults, and children may be responsible for introducing carriage into many households (Gray et al., 1980; Hendley et al., 1975). A study in the United States found that infants acquired their first pneumococcus at a mean age of 6 months; duration of carriage varied by serotype between 2.5 and 4.5 months (Gray et al., 1980). Duration of carriage decreased with age. In a Swedish study with more frequent assessments of carriage, reported duration of carriage was shorter but remained longer in children (median 30 days in children <1 year of age) than in adults (median 14 days) (Ekdahl et al., 1997). Carriage rates may be higher in some developing country settings. Reported carriage rates range from 10% to 76%, but reports in the range of 40–50% for children and 10–30% for adults are most common (Ghaffar et al., 1999).

2.1. Defining Resistance

Antimicrobial resistance can be defined in several ways. From a clinical point of view, resistance is an organism's ability to survive exposure to an antimicrobial agent to the extent that the agent is ineffective for treating a patient's illness. From an epidemiologic or microbiologic perspective, resistance can refer to an organism's ability to survive exposure to a higher concentration of an antimicrobial agent than it typically has in the past. Resistance using this latter definition may not describe a level high enough to be of concern clinically.

In the laboratory, microbiologists can determine the amount of antibiotic needed to inhibit growth of a bacterial strain; this amount of antibiotic is referred to as the strain's minimum inhibitory concentration (MIC). If MIC testing is to be useful for guiding therapy, studies are needed to determine at what MIC organisms are not likely to be effectively treated with a particular antibiotic. Several methods are used to bridge this gap between in vitro MIC results and likely in vivo effectiveness. These include: (1) examining the frequency distribution of an organism's MICs; (2) comparing an organism's MICs when a known mechanism of resistance is present to MICs when the mechanism is absent; (3) relating the in vitro activity of an antimicrobial agent to its known pharmacokinetics, also known as pharmacodynamic analysis; and (4) comparing MIC values to outcomes in clinical studies (Doern, 1995). Once these studies are conducted, an MIC level above which an organism is resistant, or conversely, below which an organism is considered susceptible, can be determined. These levels are known as MIC interpretive criteria or "breakpoints."

Worldwide, multiple groups have developed and disseminated MIC interpretive criteria (Brown, 1994). In North America, most clinical microbiologists follow recommendations made by NCCLS, formerly called the National Committee for Clinical Laboratory Standards (Table 3.1). NCCLS interpretive criteria are updated annually; changes to breakpoints in the last few years have included the addition of breakpoints for linezolid and certain oral cephalosporins and changing the breakpoint values for amoxicillin and erythromycin. In response to a growing body of data on the need for higher concentrations of drug to effectively treat meningitis compared to other clinical syndromes, NCCLS has included in their 2002 standards two categories of breakpoints for intravenous cephalosporins for meningitis and non-meningitis patients. Like all new NCCLS standards, this change is considered tentative for 1 year.

2.2. Susceptibility Testing Methods

With the emergence of antibiotic resistance in pneumococci over the last decade, increasing attention is now paid to appropriate susceptibility testing methods. Pneumococci are fastidious organisms, requiring specific supplemented media for optimal growth in the laboratory; therefore, certain procedures must be followed to obtain accurate

Table 3.1

Summary of 2002 NCCLS Guidelines: Antimicrobial Agents Recommended for Testing and Interpretive Criteria for Susceptibility Results for *Streptococcus pneumoniae* (NCCLS, 2002). Test and Report Categories are Defined as: (A) Agents that Should be Tested and the Results Reported to Clinicians; (B) Agents that should be Tested but the Results Reported Selectively; and (C) Supplemental Agents that should be Considered for Testing Based on Local Need and the Results Reported Selectively

Antimicrobial agent	Disk diffusion zone diameter				Minimum inhibitory concentration[a]			
	Test and report category	Breakpoints, mm			Test and report category	Breakpoints, µg/ml		
		Susceptible	Intermediate	Resistant		Susceptible	Intermediate	Resistant
Oxacillin	A	≥20	—	—	A	—	—	—
Penicillin	—	—	—	—	A	≤0.06	0.12–1	≥2
Erythromycin	A	≥21	16–20	≤15	A	≤0.25	0.5	≥1
Trimethoprim-sulfamethoxazole	A	≥19	16–18	≤15	A	≤0.5/9.5	1/19–2/38	≥4/76
Clindamycin	B	≥19	16–18	≤15	B	≤0.25	0.5	≥1
Levofloxacin[b]	B	≥17	14–16	≤13	B	≤2	4	≥8
Tetracycline	B	≥23	19–22	≤18	B	≤2	4	≥8
Vancomycin[b]	B	≥17	—	—	B	≤1	—	—
Cefotaxime[b]								
Meningitis[c]	—	—	—	—	B	≤0.5	1	≥2
Non-meningitis[c]	—	—	—	—	B	≤1	2	≥4
Meropenem	—	—	—	—	B	≤0.25	0.5	≥1
Chloramphenicol	C	≥21	—	≤20	C	≤4	—	≥8
Linezolid	C[c]	≥21	—	—	C	≤2	—	—
Rifampin	C	≥19	17–18	≤16	C	≤1	2	≥4
Imipenem	—	—	—	—	C	≤0.12	0.25–0.5	≥1
Amoxicillin (non-meningitis)[b,c]	—	—	—	—	C	≤2	4	≥8
Cefuroxime sodium	—	—	—	—	C	≤0.5	1	≥2

[a] Appropriate methods include broth microdilution, agar dilution, or antimicrobial gradient strips.

[b] Alternative agents can be tested for these drug classes, based on the local situation. For levofloxacin: gatifloxacin, moxifloxacin, sparfloxacin, or ofloxacin. For cefotaxime: ceftriaxone and cefepime. For amoxicillin: amoxicillin-clavulanic acid.

[c] This is a tentative NCCLS recommendation in 2002.

susceptibility results. NCCLS-recommended methods for MIC testing include broth microdilution and antimicrobial gradient strips (Etest®, AB BIODISK, Solna, Sweden); for several agents, disk diffusion testing provides an acceptable approximation of the MIC result (Table 3.1) (NCCLS, 2000). In the early- and mid-1990s, laboratories conducting susceptibility testing on pneumococci routinely screened isolates for resistance to penicillin using an oxacillin disk diffusion test; MIC testing was performed only on isolates with reduced susceptibility to oxacillin. According to current NCCLS recommendations, all pneumococcal strains from patients with life-threatening infections such as bacteremia or meningitis should undergo susceptibility testing using a method that directly determines the MIC to avoid any delay due to screening with an oxacillin disk.

In July 1997, the American College of Pathologists sent a pneumococcal strain to 4,202 clinical laboratories as part of their proficiency testing program. Among respondents providing MIC results, about half were using antimicrobial gradient strips and about half various broth microdilution techniques (Doern et al., 1999). Many of the laboratories performed susceptibility testing using inappropriate agents; 5% of MIC results and 20% of disk diffusion results were for drugs with no existing NCCLS breakpoint. Relying on clinical laboratory information to detect new resistance patterns may be difficult; for example, few laboratories participating in recent studies were routinely testing for resistance to fluoroquinolone agents (Barrett et al., 2002; Doern et al., 1999).

3. MECHANISMS OF RESISTANCE

The presence of pneumococci in the nasopharynx has fostered development of resistance. The location means that pneumococci are in relatively close proximity to oral bacteria, which has allowed for transfer of genetic material from resistant closely related species such as *Streptococcus mitis* or *Streptococcus oralis*. Uptake of new genetic material has occurred either through transformation (uptake and incorporation of free genetic material), most commonly, or through conjugative transposons (large DNA segments encoding resistance that have self-transfer capability). Point mutations leading to resistance are less common. In addition, the ability of pneumococci to reside in the nasopharynx for extended periods of time allows for selection of resistant strains during antibiotic use, either through new acquisition of a resistant strain during therapy or unmasking of a resistant strain that might have been present in lower numbers than a susceptible strain before therapy.

Since the 1940s, penicillin and other β-lactam agents have been the mainstay of therapy for pneumococcal infections. β-lactams work by binding to cell wall synthesizing enzymes called penicillin binding proteins (PBPs). The main mechanism of resistance in clinical pneumococcal strains involves alteration of the PBP structure so that β-lactams bind less well. Six PBPs have been identified: 1a, 1b, 2x, 2a, 2b, and 3 (Charpentier & Tuomanen, 2000; Tillotson & Watson, 2001). Transformational changes in PBP2x and PBP2b confer low-level resistance; subsequent transformations in other PBPs (most often PBP1a) confer high-level resistance. In addition to changes in PBPs, other, less common, resistance mechanisms have been identified (Filipe et al., 2002; Grebe et al., 1997).

Alterations in drug binding targets can confer resistance for a number of other drugs (Table 3.2) in addition to the β-lactam agents. For macrolides, the gene *ermAM* encodes

Table 3.2

Primary Mechanisms of Resistance of *Streptococcus pneumoniae* for Commonly-Used Therapeutic Agents (Charpentier & Tuomanen, 2000; Filipe et al., 2002; Schrag et al., 2000)

Antibiotic class	Antibiotic agent(s)	Resistance mechanism	Genes involved	Phenotype
β-lactams	Penicillin	Altered drug target (penicillin binding proteins, PBPs)	*pbp1a, pbp2x,* and *pbp2b*	Intermediate- or high-level resistance
		Changes in cell wall structure	*murMN*	High-level resistance
	Cephalosporins	Altered drug target (PBPs)	*pbp1a, pbp2x*	Intermediate- or high-level resistance
Macrolides	Erythromycin	Drug efflux	*mefE*	Intermediate resistance
		Altered drug target (ribosome)	*ermAM*	High-level resistance
Tetracyclines	Tetracycline	Altered drug target (ribosome)	*tetM, tetO*	High-level resistance
Fluoroquinolones	Ciprofloxacin, sparfloxacin, levofloxacin	Altered drug target (DNA topoisomerase IV)	*parC, parE*	Low- or intermediate level resistance; high-level resistance in the presence of *gyrA* or *gyrB* mutation
		Altered drug target (DNA gyrase)	*gyrA, gyrB*	Low- or intermediate-level resistance; high-level resistance in the presence of *parC* or *parE* mutation
Phenicols	Chloramphenicol	Enzymatic alteration of drug	*cat*	High-level resistance
Diaminopyrimidines	Trimethoprim	Altered drug target (dihydrofolate reductase)	*dhf*	Mostly high-level resistance
Sulphonamides	Sulfamethoxazole	Altered drug target (dihydropteroate reductase)	*sulA*	Mostly high-level resistance

an enzyme that methylates an adenine residue in the peptidyl transferase domain of the 23s rRNA; this methylation may lead to a conformational change in the ribosome, which reduces the affinity of macrolides (such as erythromycin, azithromycin, clarithromycin), lincosamides (such as clindamycin), and streptogramins (such as quinupristin–dalfopristin). This type of macrolide resistance is known as the macrolides–lincosamides–streptogramins (MLS) phenotype and results in very high MIC values (≥ 16 µg/ml) for erythromycin. For the quinolone agents, such as ciprofloxacin, levofloxacin, and gatifloxacin, the main resistance mechanisms identified to date are modifications to the drug binding sites on DNA gyrase (most commonly *gyrA*) and topoisomerase IV (most commonly *parC*). As with PBPs, a single mutation in these genes can result in low level resistance with sequential changes in the targets resulting in high level resistance to fluoroquinolones (Charpentier & Tuomanen, 2000).

Drug efflux is another resistance mechanism used by pneumococci for macrolide and fluoroquinolone agents. The gene *mefE* encodes a transmembrane protein that serves as a macrolide efflux pump. Pneumococci with *mefE* do not have associated resistance to lincosamides and streptogramins and are said to exhibit the M phenotype. Although M phenotype strains tend to have macrolide MICs that are lower than MLS phenotype strains, the erythromycin MICs in M phenotype strains have been increasing. In 1999, the erythromycin MIC_{50} among M phenotype isolates was 8.0 µg/ml (Hyde et al., 2001). Recently, clinical and laboratory pneumococcal strains have been found that appear to accumulate lower concentrations of fluoroquinolone agents inside the cell compared to wild-type strains, suggestive of the presence of an efflux pump (Tillotson & Watson, 2001). This efflux pump has been associated with the *pmrA* gene in pneumococci (Brenwald et al., 1998). Strains with this efflux phenotype exhibited ciprofloxacin MICs of 4–8 µg/ml in a study from the United Kingdom (Brenwald et al., 1998).

Glycopeptide antibiotics, such as vancomycin and teicoplanin, work by preventing cell wall synthesis. Resistance to this class of antibiotics has not yet been identified in clinical pneumococcal isolates. In the last few years, however, a phenomenon known as tolerance, in which the bacteria can survive but not reproduce in the presence of vancomycin, has been described (Novak et al., 1999). Antibiotics that disrupt cell wall synthesis in pneumococci act by triggering the autolysin protein LytA to cause cell wall digestion and cell death; inactivation of the *lytA* gene encoding the autolysin protein results in tolerance. Vancomycin tolerance was found in 3% of 116 clinical isolates from Sweden and the United States (Normark et al., 2001). Whether vancomycin tolerance contributes to poor patient outcomes is unclear.

4. EPIDEMIOLOGY AND DISTRIBUTION OF RESISTANT STRAINS

A number of factors have been associated with an increased risk of pneumococcal disease caused by a strain resistant to one or more antimicrobial agents. Penicillin-, macrolide-, and multidrug-resistant pneumococci are most common among pneumococcal infections in young children (Clavo-Sanchez et al., 1997; Hyde et al., 2001; Whitney et al., 2000). Among adults, penicillin-resistant infections are more common in the elderly (Whitney et al., 2000). In the United States, persons of white race are more likely to have a resistant infection than are black persons (Whitney et al., 2000). Daycare attendance, recent otitis media or pneumonia, alcoholism, and recent hospitalization also have been associated with penicillin-resistant infections (Clavo-Sanchez et al., 1997; Hofmann et al., 1995; Levine et al., 1999; Pallares et al., 1987). Risk factors for disease caused by fluoro-quinolone-resistant strains differ somewhat from risk factors for disease with β-lactam- or macrolide-resistant strains. Disease caused by a fluoroquinolone-resistant strain has been linked to recent fluoroquinolone use, a recent stay in a long-term care facility, and recent hospitalization (Ho et al., 2001a). In addition, fluoroquinolone-resistant strains are almost exclusively isolated from adults (Chen et al., 1999). Patterns of antimicrobial use may be the underlying explanation for the associations of all these factors with drug-resistant infections.

A number of studies have attempted to evaluate the association between recent antibi-otic use and either disease with or carriage of a resistant pneumococcal strain; results have been mixed. In a review of studies addressing the association of use and resistance in per-sons with pneumococcal disease, 9 of 14 studies found that recent antibiotic use was sig-nificantly more common among those with disease caused by a resistant infection than among those with disease due to a susceptible strain (Lipsitch, 2001). Among 17 studies examining antimicrobial use and carriage, nearly all found that recent antimicrobial use was more common among persons carrying a resistant strain compared with persons car-rying a susceptible strain. Caution should be used when interpreting these findings, how-ever. Use of antimicrobial agents may reduce carriage of susceptible strains or prevent progression to culture-confirmed disease for those with susceptible strains; outside the set-ting of an outbreak, few studies suggest that persons treated with antibiotics have a higher risk of carriage or disease caused by a resistant strain than untreated persons have (Lipsitch, 2001).

4.1. Geographic Variation in the Prevalence of Resistant Strains

Marked geographic variation is seen in the prevalence of antibiotic-resistant pneu-mococci. Even isolates from different institutions within one city can show substantial differences in the proportion of strains resistant to various agents (Schrag et al., 2002). Therefore, studies that use data from a single institution to represent the prevalence of resistance in a country should be interpreted with caution. Likewise, reports of resistance based on carriage studies or disease in children may not be representative of the prevalence of resistance among pneumococci from the general population, given that children tend to have a higher proportion of strains resistant to many agents than adults.

In the last few years, reports from an increasing number of countries suggest that few areas remain unaffected by the problem of drug-resistance in pneumococci (Figure 3.1). Isolates with intermediate or full resistance to penicillin accounted for <10% of pneumo-coccal strains in recent reports from Morocco, Austria, Germany, and Norway (Benbachir et al., 2001; Georgopoulos et al., 1998; Kristiansen et al., 2001; Sahm et al., 2000). In con-trast, over half of the isolates had reduced susceptibility to penicillin in recent reports from Senegal, Uganda, Hong Kong, Japan, France, Spain, Kuwait, and Saudi Arabia (Benbachir et al., 2001; Ho et al., 2001c; Mokaddas et al., 2001; Perez-Trallero et al., 2001; Sahm et al., 2000; Shibl et al., 2000; Yoshimine et al., 2001). In the United States, isolates from

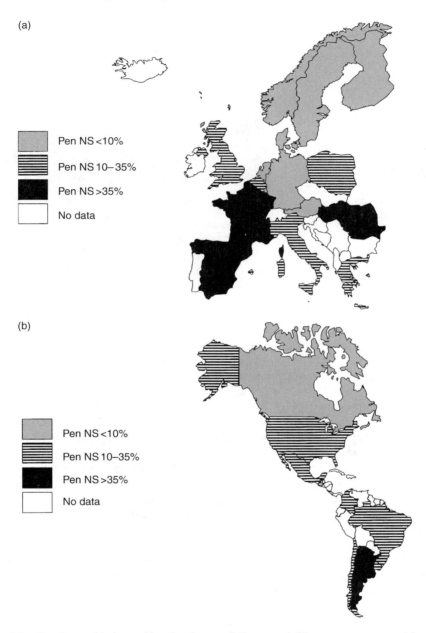

Figure 3.1. Prevalence of isolates with reduced susceptibility to penicillin among pneumococci by region: (a) Europe, (b) the Americas, and (c) Asia. Figures include data from studies published since 1996 that include isolates from both children and adults (Araj et al., 1999; di Fabio et al., 2001; Georgopoulos et al., 1998; Gur et al., 2001; Hermans et al., 1997; Ho et al., 2001b; Hoban et al., 2001; Kamme et al., 1999; Konradsen & Kaltoft, 2002; Kristiansen et al., 2001; Kyaw et al., 2002; Maraki et al., 2001; Marchese et al., 2001; Marton & Meszner, 1999; Melo-Cristino et al., 2001; Mokaddas et al., 2001; Overweg et al., 1999; Pana et al., 1997; Perez-Trallero et al., 2001; Sahm et al., 2000; Sankilampi et al., 1997; Shibl et al., 2000; Song et al., 1999; Thornsberry et al., 2002; Verhaegen et al., 2000).

(c)

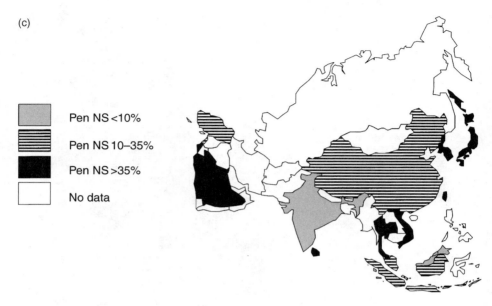

Pen NS <10%

Pen NS 10–35%

Pen NS >35%

No data

Figure 3.1.   Continued

the southeast tend to be penicillin-resistant more often than isolates from other regions. In the United States overall, 24–35% of pneumococcal strains are resistant to penicillin, with most resistant strains having high-level (MIC ≥ 2 μg/ml) rather than intermediate resistance (MIC 0.12–1 μg/ml) (Doern et al., 2001; Whitney et al., 2000). Pneumococci that are resistant to penicillin are more likely to be resistant to other agents than are pneumococci that are penicillin-susceptible (Whitney et al., 2000).

In some areas, macrolide resistance has rapidly become more common since the introduction of azithromycin and other newer macrolides. Between 1993 and 1999, macrolide prescriptions increased 13% overall and 320% among children <5 years in the United States due to increased use of azithromycin and clarithromycin (Hyde et al., 2001). Between 1995 and 1999, the proportion of isolates from blood and cerebrospinal fluid that were resistant to erythromycin increased from 11% to 20%. The increase in macrolide resistance was entirely caused by an increase in the frequency of isolates with the M phenotype (erythromycin resistant and clindamycin susceptible). M-phenotype isolates accounted for 82% of macrolide-resistant strains in the United States in 1999 (Hyde et al., 2001). An increase in erythromycin-resistant strains exhibiting the M phenotype was also noted in South Africa during the 1990s (Huebner et al., 2000; Widdowson & Klugman, 1998).

Wide variation can be found among reports that assess the proportion of pneumococcal isolates that are resistant to macrolides. Macrolide resistance has been notably common among pneumococcal isolates in recent studies from Italy (26–32%), Spain (35–36%),

(Marchese et al., 2001; Oteo et al., 2001; Perez-Trallero et al., 2001) and Hong Kong (68%) (Ho et al., 2001c). The proportion of macrolide-resistant strains with the M phenotype or the MLS phenotype also differs geographically. In North America, the M phenotype is more common among erythromycin-resistant pneumococci (Hyde et al., 2001); in Europe and South Africa, the MLS phenotype is predominant (Lagrou et al., 1999; Marchese et al., 1999; Tait-Kamradt et al., 2000; Widdowson & Klugman, 1998).

Although fluoroquinolones are a relatively new class of drugs, fluoroquinolone resistance is an increasing concern. An increase in fluoroquinolone resistance that mirrored the increase in use of fluoroquinolone agents was documented in Canada (Chen et al., 1999). Fluoroquinolone resistance may be most prevalent in Hong Kong. In a 2001 report, 12–13% of pneumococcal strains had reduced susceptibility to levofloxacin, sparfloxacin, or gatifloxacin and 18% had reduced susceptibility to ciprofloxacin (Ho et al., 2001c). Most of the fluoroquinolone-resistant strains in Hong Kong were related to a multiply-resistant Spanish 23F pneumococcal clone that has been found on multiple continents (Ho et al., 2001b). In contrast to the high proportion of isolates with fluoroquinolone resistance observed in Hong Kong, reports from elsewhere suggest that <2% of pneumococci are resistant to levofloxacin (Bell et al., 2002; Brueggemann et al., 2002; Doern et al., 2001; Hoban et al., 2001; Koeth et al., 2002; Maraki et al., 2001; Marchese et al., 2001; Oteo et al., 2001; Perez-Trallero et al., 2001; Sahm et al., 2000; Thornsberry et al., 2002).

4.2. Resistant Pneumococcal Clones

Although over 90 pneumococcal serotypes have been identified, some serotypes are more likely to cause disease than others. Only a small number of serotypes (6B, 9V, 19F, 14, and 23F) are responsible for the majority of disease due to drug-resistant strains (Figure 3.2) (Whitney et al., 2000). This suggests that development of resistance among pneumococci is not a random event. In fact, the spread of a few highly successful resistant pneumococcal clones, rather than multiple strains developing new resistance mutations, has mainly been responsible for the rapid emergence of penicillin- and macrolide-resistant pneumococci.

The Pneumococcal Molecular Epidemiology Network (PMEN) was established in 1997 in order to standardize the nomenclature and classification of resistant clones. For a strain to be included in the network, investigators must show that the strain: (1) has wide distribution throughout a country; (2) has been established over a number of years; (3) is resistant to one or more antimicrobial agents in wide clinical use; (4) has been described in a publication; and (5) is available for deposit into the American Type Culture Collection of clones (Pneumococcal Molecular Epidemiology Network, 2001). Proposals for admission of new clones into PMEN are reviewed at annual meetings; to date, the group has accepted a number of clones into their network (Table 3.3) (McGee et al., 2001). Some of the resistant clones, most notably Spanish[23F]-1 and Spain[9V]-3, have been found in multiple countries around the world.

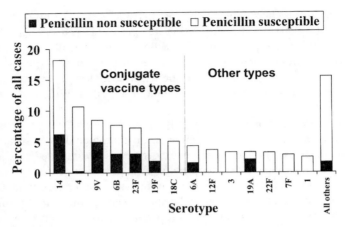

Figure 3.2. Distribution of penicillin-resistance among isolates from patients with invasive pneumococcal disease in the United States by serotype. Data are from Centers for Disease Control and Prevention's (CDC) Active Bacterial Core Surveillance, 1998 (Whitney et al., 2000).

5. CLINICAL RELEVANCE OF RESISTANCE

Assessing whether resistance to antimicrobial agents contributes to a poor outcome for patients is difficult. For otitis media and meningitis, available evidence suggests that treatment failures can occur for patients with pneumococcal strains with MICs in the intermediate range for agents of choice. For pneumonia, studies have provided conflicting results. Studies of pneumonia patients that compared the outcome of persons with susceptible strains to persons with pneumococcal strains with intermediate-level penicillin resistance (MICs 0.1–1.0 μg/ml) found no influence of resistance on outcome (Friedland, 1995; Friedland & Klugman, 1992; Pallares et al., 1995). Results of studies on resistance and outcome that included patients with MICs in the fully resistant range (MICs ≥2.0 μg/ml) have not been consistent (Buckingham et al., 1998; Choi & Lee, 1998; Deeks et al., 1999; Dowell et al., 1999b; Feikin et al., 2000; Turett et al., 1999). Most evidence suggests that standard treatment with a β-lactam agent is effective for pneumococcal pneumonia caused by strains with MICs ≤1.0 μg/ml.

For macrolide agents, some have postulated that pneumonia caused by macrolide-resistant isolates with the M phenotype may be successfully treated with the newer agents, as the MICs of pneumococci exhibiting the M phenotype are lower than MICs of MLS-phenotype strains (Amsden, 1999). The MICs of M-phenotype isolates may be increasing, however. In the United States, the MIC_{50} among M-phenotype strains increased from 4.0 μg/ml in 1995 to 8.0 μg/ml in 1999 (Hyde et al., 2001). Case reports suggest that treatment failures have occurred at MICs of 8.0 or 16 μg/ml (Kelley et al., 2000). Therefore, most pneumococcal isolates with the M phenotype may have MICs in the range in which treatment failures have been reported.

Table 3.3

Resistance Patterns and Countries of Isolation for Resistant Clones Included in the Pneumococcal Molecular Epidemiology Network as of September 2000 (Koornhof et al., 2001; McGee et al., 2001)

Clone name[a]	Type strain resistance pattern[b]							Countries where identified
	PEN	CTX	ERY	CLI	CHL	TET	SXT	
CSR14-10	R	I	R	R	R	R	S	Slovakia, Czech Republic
CSR19A-11	R	I	R	R	R	R	R	Czech Republic
England14-9	S	S	R	S	S	S	S	United Kingdom
Finland6B-12	I		R	R	S	R	R	Finland
Hungary19A-6	R	S	R	R	R	R	I	Hungary, Czech Republic, Slovakia
Poland23F-16	R	R	R	S	R	R	R	Poland
South Africa6B-8	I	S	S	S	S	S	I	South Africa
South Africa19F-7	I	S	S	S	S	S	R	South Africa
South Africa19F-13	R	R	R	R	R	R	R	South Africa
Spain6B-2	R	I	S	S	R	R	R	France, Finland, Germany, Spain, Iceland, United States, United Kingdom, Taiwan, Chile, Hong Kong
Spain9V-3	R	I	S	S	S	S	R	France, Spain, Portugal, Bulgaria, Italy, Germany, Sweden, United Kingdom, United States, Canada, Colombia, Chile, Argentina, Uruguay, Brazil, Mexico, Taiwan, Korea, Thailand
Spain14-5	R	I	S	S	R	R	I	Spain
Spain23F-1	R	S	S	S	R	R	R	Spain, France, Iceland, Portugal, Bulgaria, the Netherlands, Croatia, Finland, Belgium, Italy, Germany, United Kingdom, United States, Canada, Colombia, Argentina, Uruguay, Chile, Mexico, Taiwan, Korea, Thailand, Hong Kong, South Africa
Taiwan19F-14	R	I	R	S	S	R	R	Taiwan, other countries in Asia
Taiwan23F-15	I or R	I	R	R	S	R	S	Taiwan
Tennessee23F-4	I	R	R	S	S	S	R	United States

[a] Clone names are composed of the country where the clone was first identified, the primary serotype of the clone in superscript, a dash, the order the clone was included in the network, a second dash (if needed) and other identified serotypes.

[b] MIC interpretation according to 2002 NCCLS guidelines (NCCLS, 2002). Abbreviations: S = susceptible, I = intermediate, R = resistant, PEN = penicillin, CTX = cefotaxime, ERY = erythromycin, CLI = clindamycin, CHL = chloramphenicol, TET = tetracycline, SXT = trimethoprim sulfamethoxazole.

For the fluoroquinolone agents, evidence is mounting that treatment failures can occur in patients with pneumonia caused by a fluoroquinolone-resistant pneumococcus (Davidson et al., 2002; Wortmann & Bennett, 1999). A recent report describing four patients included two patients who developed resistant strains while on oral levofloxacin therapy (initial levofloxacin MICs 1.0 and 4.0 μg/ml, subsequent MICs 8.0 and 16 μg/ml) and who had progression of their pneumonia on therapy (Davidson et al., 2002). Two other patients included in the report may have had resistant strains at the time levofloxacin therapy was initiated. Both of these patients also had progression of their pneumonia and one patient died; pneumococcal MICs to levofloxacin from strains collected while on therapy were 16 μg/ml.

6. DIAGNOSIS AND TREATMENT IN THE ERA OF RESISTANCE

Treating disease syndromes that are commonly caused by pneumococci, such as pneumonia, otitis media, and meningitis, has been challenging. With pneumonia and otitis media, *S. pneumoniae* is just one of the multiple possible causes, and rarely is the precise etiology determined. With severe pneumonia and meningitis, starting optimal therapy immediately may be critical for a patient's survival. An etiology often can be determined for patients with meningitis, but therapy must begin before the etiology can be confirmed and well before results of antibiotic susceptibility testing are available. The emergence of resistance in pneumococci has complicated treatment decisions even further.

Since the mid-1990s, professional and governmental organizations have developed treatment guidelines to assist clinicians with therapy decisions and to help improve patient outcomes. Several groups have published guidelines for therapy of community-acquired pneumonia (Table 3.4) (American Thoracic Society, 2001; Bartlett et al., 2000; British Thoracic Society Standards of Care Committee, 2001; Mandell et al., 2000). Although the mainstays of pneumonia therapy—β-lactams, macrolides, tetracyclines, and fluoroquinolones—appear in most guidelines, differences exist between recommendations from the various groups.

For pneumonia patients, antimicrobial susceptibility testing can be very helpful in therapy decisions for those cases in which a pathogen can be isolated. For most pneumonia patients, however, an etiology cannot be determined, even with extensive diagnostic testing. Guidelines differ on the recommended approach to obtaining an etiologic diagnosis. For example, recommendations from the Infectious Diseases Society of America recommend routine collection of sputum for Gram stain and culture whereas recommendations from the American Thoracic Society do not (American Thoracic Society, 2001; Bartlett et al., 2000; Heffelfinger et al., 2000). In all situations, however, treatment should not be delayed in order to obtain an etiologic diagnosis, as studies suggest that starting therapy early can improve outcome in patients with pneumonia.

Otitis media is the most common clinical syndrome caused by pneumococci. In the United States, otitis media accounted for 11% of office visits and 37% of outpatient prescriptions for children <15 years during 1999–2000 (McCaig et al., 2002). *S. pneumoniae* is just one of the three main pathogens that cause otitis media; the other two main causes are *Haemophilus influenzae* and *Moraxella catarrhalis*. Treatment options are limited to

Table 3.4
Summary of Recommendations from Selected Guidelines for
Empiric Antimicrobial Therapy of Community-Acquired Pneumonia[a]

Guideline	Outpatients	Empiric antibiotic therapy recommendations	
		Inpatients not requiring intensive care	Inpatients requiring intensive care
Infectious Diseases Society of America, 2000	(1) Doxycycline (2) Macrolide (3) Fluoroquinolone	(1) Extended-spectrum cephalosporin + macrolide (2) β-Lactam/β-lactamase inhibitor + macrolide (3) Fluoroquinolone	Extended-spectrum cephalosporin or β-lactam/β-Lactamase inhibitor + either a fluoroquinolone or a macrolide
American Thoracic Society, 2001	(1) Azithromycin (2) Clarithromycin (3) Doxycycline	(1) High-dose ampicillin, extended-spectrum cephalosporin, or β-lactam/β-lactamase inhibitor + either macrolide or doxycycline (2) Fluoroquinolone with pneumococcal activity	Extended-spectrum cephalosporin + either azithromycin or fluoroquinolone
Canadian Community-Acquired Pneumonia Working Group, 2000	(1) Erythromycin (2) Azithromycin (3) Alarithromycin Alternative: Doxycycline	Fluoroquinolone with pneumococcal activity Alternative: Extended spectrum cephalosporin + macrolide	Fluoroquinolone with pneumococcal activity + extended-spectrum cephalosporin or β-lactam/ β-lactamase inhibitor Alternative: Macrolide + extended-spectrum cephalosporin, or β-lactam/ β-lactamase inhibitor
British Thoracic Society, 2001	Amoxicillin Alternative: (1) Erythromycin (2) Clarithromycin	(1) Amoxicillin + macrolide (2) Ampicillin or penicillin + macrolide Alternative: Fluoroquinolone with pneumococcal activity	β-Lactam/β-lactamase inhibitor or extended-spectrum cephalosporin + macrolide (± rifampin) Alternative: Fluoroquinolone with pneumococcal activity + penicillin

[a]American Thoracic Society, 2001; Bartlett et al., 2000; British Thoracic Society Standards of Care Committee, 2001; Mandell et al., 2000; recommendations for special groups of patients with conditions that may require therapy modifications are not included in the table.

agents available in oral form that are safe to use in children; amoxicillin, in standard dose, in high dose, or in combination with clavulanic acid, remains the drug of choice for otitis media (American Academy of Pediatrics, 2000; Dowell et al., 1999a; Kellner, 2001).

In contrast to the situation for patients with otitis media or pneumonia, diagnostic tests for patients with bacterial meningitis are often helpful. Cultures of cerebrospinal fluid frequently yield an etiologic agent; therefore, antimicrobial susceptibility testing results can be used to guide therapy decisions. Some antimicrobial agents that are used for pneumonia, such as the macrolides, tetracyclines, and fluoroquinolones, may not reach sufficient concentrations in cerebrospinal fluid to be useful for treating meningitis. Therefore, treatment choices are limited for empiric therapy of meningitis. In the United States, where pneumococcus is the most common cause of bacterial meningitis and resistance to β-lactam agents is common, treatment recommendations are to administer cefotaxime or ceftriaxone plus vancomycin until susceptibility results are available or until diagnostic evidence strongly suggests an etiology other than pneumococcus (American Academy of Pediatrics, 2000).

7. PREVENTING RESISTANT PNEUMOCOCCAL INFECTIONS

Selective pressure from antibiotic use is the driving force behind emerging antibiotic resistance in pneumococci. Therefore, optimizing and reducing antibiotic use is a logical approach to reducing or preventing antibiotic resistance among pneumococci. Studies are underway to determine if alternative methods of antibiotic use, such as drug cycling and use of multiple drugs at the same time, can improve on standard prescribing practices for preventing development of resistance. For example, a trial of short-course, high-dose amoxicillin versus traditional dosing for respiratory tract infections found that children randomized to the new regimen were less likely to carry penicillin-resistant pneumococci 28 days after starting therapy (Schrag et al., 2001).

7.1. Reducing Inappropriate Antibiotic Use

Prescribing antibiotics for conditions for which they may not be helpful is a widespread practice; in the United States, studies indicate that clinicians frequently prescribe antibiotics for viral upper respiratory infections (Gonzales et al., 1997; Nyquist et al., 1998). Campaigns to reduce inappropriate antibiotic use are underway in several countries. In the United States, recommendations for improving antibiotic use for upper respiratory infections for both children and adults have been published (Dowell et al., 1998; Gonzales et al., 2001). These documents focus on means for determining situations in which antibiotic therapy is not likely to be useful. The appropriate use campaigns in the United States along with media attention on antibiotic resistance are leading to less antibiotic use; a recent report suggests that the average rate of antibiotic prescriptions in children <15 years decreased from 838 per 1,000 children in 1989–1990 to 503 per 1,000 children in 1999–2000 (McCaig et al., 2002). How much reducing antibiotic use can do to reduce the risk of antibiotic resistant infections is unclear.

7.2. Pneumococcal Vaccines

The emergence of antibiotic resistance has placed renewed emphasis on preventing pneumococcal disease through use of pneumococcal vaccines. Currently available pneumococcal polysaccharide vaccines include 25 μg of purified capsular polysaccharide antigens from each of 23 different serotypes; the vaccine induces production of serotype-specific antibodies. A recent review of data from around the world found regional differences in distribution of serogroups, but 11 serogroups accounted for at least 75% of the isolates causing invasive disease in adults in each geographic region (Hausdorff et al., 2000). In the United States, serotypes included in the 23-valent vaccine account for at least 85–90% of strains causing invasive disease in adults (Centers for Disease Control and Prevention, 1997; Robinson et al., 2001).

Pneumococcal polysaccharide vaccine is recommended for use in adults in many industrialized countries (Fedson, 1998). Vaccines comprised of polysaccharide antigens alone produce weak or short-lived immune responses in infants and toddlers (Koskela et al., 1986), so the vaccine is generally not used in children <2 years of age. In North America, use of pneumococcal polysaccharide vaccines is recommended by the U.S. Centers for Disease Control and Prevention's Advisory Committee on Immunization Practices (ACIP), the U.S. Preventive Services Task Force, Canada's National Advisory Committee on Immunization, as well as several professional organizations (Centers for Disease Control and Prevention, 1997; National Advisory Committee on Immunization, 2002; U.S. Preventive Services Task Force, 1996). Although there are some minor differences in the recommendations, all recommend vaccination for adults ≥65 years and for persons 2–64 years who have certain chronic illnesses or immunocompromising conditions.

Post-licensure epidemiological studies have documented the effectiveness of pneumococcal polysaccharide vaccines for prevention of invasive infection (bacteremia and meningitis) among the elderly and younger adults with certain chronic medical conditions (Butler et al., 1993; Farr et al., 1995; Shapiro et al., 1991; Sims et al., 1988). Studies of vaccine effectiveness in immunocompetent persons ≥65 years suggest that the pneumococcal polysaccharide vaccine is 75% effective against bacteremic disease caused by vaccine serotypes (Butler et al., 1993). Vaccine effectiveness against invasive disease is lower in persons with immunocompromising conditions.

Data on vaccine efficacy and effectiveness against pneumonia are less clear. Randomized, controlled trials of a single dose of pneumococcal polysaccharide vaccine were conducted in the 1970s among young, healthy South African gold miners, a group with high rates of pneumococcal pneumonia. Protective efficacy against pneumococcal pneumonia in these trials ranged from 76% to 92% (Austrian et al., 1976; Smit et al., 1977). In non-epidemic situations in industrialized countries, most pneumococcal disease in adults occurs in the elderly or in persons with chronic medical conditions. Studies in these groups suggest that the vaccine does not provide protection against non-bacteremic pneumococcal pneumonia (Gaillat et al., 1985; Honkanen et al., 1999; Kaufman, 1947; Koivula et al., 1997; Örtqvist et al., 1998; Simberkoff et al., 1986). The pneumococcal polysaccharide vaccine does not reduce nasopharyngeal carriage.

In February 2000, a protein–polysaccharide conjugate vaccine (Prevnar,™ Wyeth Lederle Vaccines, Pearl River, New York) was licensed for use in infants and young children in the United States. In the United States, the pneumococcal conjugate vaccine is recommended for all children under 2 years of age. In addition, children 2–4 years old who have immunocompromising conditions or certain chronic illnesses putting them at high risk for disease should receive vaccine (Centers for Disease Control and Prevention, 2000). The vaccine is licensed in several other countries in addition to the United States and efforts are underway to speed introduction of pneumococcal conjugate vaccines into developing countries.

The conjugate vaccine includes polysaccharide antigens for the seven most common serotypes occurring in children in the United States and in many other industrialized countries. These seven vaccine serotypes account for over 80% of strains resistant to penicillin in the United States (Whitney et al., 2000). All resistant clones currently in the PMEN are serotypes included in the vaccine.

Studies indicate that the conjugate vaccine is highly effective against invasive pneumococcal disease (Black et al., 2000) and somewhat effective against otitis media and pneumonia (Black et al., 2000; Shinefield & Black, 2000). Studies of nasopharygeal carriage of pneumococci indicate that conjugate vaccines reduce nasopharyngeal carriage of vaccine-type strains by about one-half (Dagan et al., 1996, 1997, 2002; Mbelle et al., 1999; Obaro et al., 1996, 2000). Field trials are ongoing to examine the efficacy of a 9-valent vaccine formulation, which would include serotypes more appropriate for developing countries.

If vaccinating children reduces pneumococcal carriage which in turn reduces transmission of resistant strains to adults, vaccinating children <5 years may markedly reduce the overall number of infections caused by penicillin-nonsusceptible strains. Not only are young children at highest risk for disease due to drug-resistant strains, but this group may serve as the reservoir for drug-resistant infections in the community. The frequency of nasopharyngeal carriage is usually highest in young children and is higher in adults with young children than in other adults (Hendley et al., 1975). Case-control studies of risk factors for invasive pneumococcal disease in adults have found that adults with invasive disease were much more likely to have close contact with a child than control adults (Breiman et al., 2000; Nuorti et al., 2000).

8. THE FUTURE OF DRUG-RESISTANT *STREPTOCOCCUS PNEUMONIAE*

The next few years bring both challenges and opportunities in the ongoing struggle against antibiotic resistance in pneumococci. Human travel will foster the spread of resistant pneumococcal clones and new resistant clones will be identified. The current widespread use of the newer macrolides will continue to provide selective pressure for strains resistant to those agents. Vancomycin-resistant pneumococci may appear. And with the rapidly increasing use of fluoroquinolone agents, fluoroquinolone-resistant pneumococci are likely to become common in many more countries.

Pneumococcal resistance in developing countries provides a particular challenge. In developing countries, pneumonia is a major cause of childhood mortality; estimates suggest that as many as 1 million children die each year of pneumococcal pneumonia, with most of the deaths occurring in developing countries (Mulholland, 1999). Many developing countries lack the data needed to assess local pneumococcal resistance patterns. Therefore, determining the optimal therapy among available antibiotics can be difficult. In some cases, resources may not be available to change recommended antibiotics if resistance data suggest more expensive drugs are needed. The World Health Organization and other agencies are expanding efforts to address the problem of antibiotic resistance in developing countries.

New agents are needed to provide treatment options for strains that are resistant to multiple antibiotics and to avoid overuse of antibiotics that are commonly prescribed for standard empiric therapy. Some of the new drugs under evaluation as potential therapies for pneumococcal disease include new macrolide and fluoroquinolone formulations, a penem (faropenem), a ketolide (telithromycin), a combination of streptogramins (quinupristin/dalfopristin), and an oxazolidinone (linezolid). In a sample of pneumococcal strains resistant to erythromycin, tetracycline, ciprofloxacin, or trimethoprim/sulfamethoxazole from throughout Europe, ≥90% of strains resistant to these drugs were susceptible to faropenem, gatifloxacin, moxifloxacin, gemifloxacin, telithromycin, quinopristin/dalfopristin, vancomycin, and linezolid (Schmitz et al., 2001). Whether these drugs will compare favorably to standard therapies in terms of tolerability and effectiveness against disease is unknown.

New pneumococcal vaccines provide the best opportunity for reducing infections caused by resistant pneumococci. The new protein–polysaccharide conjugate vaccine for children is effective against disease and can prevent carriage and transmission of vaccine-type strains. A limitation of the vaccine is that it only covers a few pneumococcal serotypes. Although those serotypes are the ones most often resistant, new pneumococcal serotypes are likely to become resistant. In addition, non-vaccine serotypes may begin to cause more disease. Ongoing research is evaluating the addition of more serotypes to the 7-valent vaccine formulation and the possibility of using conjugate vaccines in other age groups. A new generation of pneumococcal vaccines based on proteins common to all pneumococci is also being evaluated.

New therapies, new vaccines, and new attention to appropriate use of antimicrobial agents appear promising for addressing the problem of pneumococcal resistance. To date, however, pneumococci have repeatedly shown their ability to adapt to changes in their environment, and the organisms continue to cause substantial morbidity and mortality. The search for optimal prevention measures and therapies will remain an ongoing process.

References

American Academy of Pediatrics. (2000). Pneumococcal infections. In L. K. Pickering (Ed.), *2000 red book: Report of the Committee on Infectious Diseases* (p. 460). Elk Grove Village, IL: Author.

American Thoracic Society. (2001). Guidelines for the management of adults with community-acquired pneumonia. *Am J Respir Crit Care Med, 163*, 1730–1754.

Amsden, G. W. (1999). Pneumococcal macrolide resistance—myth or reality? *J Antimicrob Chemother, 44*, 1–6.

Araj, G. F., Bey, H. A., Itani, L. Y., & Kanj, S. S. (1999). Drug-resistant *Streptococcus pneumoniae* in the Lebanon: Implications for presumptive therapy. *Int J Antimicrob Agents, 12*, 349–354.

Austrian, R., Douglas, R. M., Schiffman, G., Coetzee, A., Koornhof, H., Hayden-Smith, S., & Reid, R. (1976). Prevention of pneumococcal pneumonia by vaccination. *Trans Assoc Am Physicians, 89*, 184–189.

Austrian, R., & Gold, J. (1964). Pneumococcal bacteremia with especial [sic] reference to bacteremic pneumococcal pneumonia. *Ann Intern Med, 60*, 759–776.

Barker, J. H., Musher, D. M., Silberman, R., Phan, H. M., & Watson, D. A. (1999). Genetic relatedness among nontypeable pneumococci implicated in sporadic cases of conjunctivitis. *J Clin Microbiol, 37*, 4039–4041.

Barrett, N., Reingold, A., Gershman, K., McCombs, K., Harrison, L., Johnson, S., Hibbs, J., Cassidy, M., Cieslak, P., Craig, A., Jorgensen, J., Feikin, D., Whitney, C., & Chuang, I. (2002). Assessment of susceptibility testing practices for *Streptococcus pneumoniae*—United States, February 2000. *Morb Mortal Wkly Rep, 51*, 392–394.

Bartlett, J. G., Dowell, S. F., Mandell, L. A., File, T. M., Jr., Musher, D. M., & Fine, M. J. (2000). Practice guidelines for the management of community-acquired pneumonia in adults. *Clin Infect Dis, 31*, 347–382.

Bell, J. M., Turnidge, J. D., Jones, R. N., & The Sentry Regional Participants Group. (2002). Antimicrobial resistance trends in community-acquired respiratory tract pathogens in the Western Pacific Region and South Africa: Report from the SENTRY antimicrobial surveillance program, (1998–1999) including an in vitro evaluation of BMS284756. *Int J Antimicrob Agents, 19*, 125–132.

Benbachir, M., Benredjeb, S., Boye, C. S., Dosso, M., Belabbes, H., Kamoun, A., Kaire, O., & Elmdaghri, N. (2001). Two-year surveillance of antibiotic resistance in *Streptococcus pneumoniae* in four African cities. *Antimicrob Agents Chemother, 45*, 627–629.

Black, S., Shinefield, H., Fireman, B., Ray, P., Hansen, J. R., Elvin, L., Ensor, K. M., Hackell, J., Siber, G., Malinoski, F., Madore, D., Chang, I., Kolberger, R., Watson, W., & Austrian, R. (2000). Efficacy, safety and immunogenicity of heptavalent conjugate pneumococcal vaccine in children. Northern California Kaiser Permanente Study Center Group. *Pediatr Infect Dis J, 19*, 187–195.

Breiman, R. F., Keller, D. W., Phelan, M., Sniadack, D. H., Stephens, D. S., Rimland, D., Farley, M. M., Schuchat, A., & Reingold, A. L. (2000). Evaluation of effectiveness of the 23-valent pneumococcal capsular polysaccharide vaccine for HIV-infected patients. *Arch Intern Med, 160*, 2633–2638.

Brenwald, N., Gill, M., & Wise, R. (1998). Prevalence of a putative efflux mechanism among fluoroquinolone-resistant clinical isolates of *Streptococcus pneumoniae*. *Antimicrob Agents Chemother, 42*, 2032–2035.

British Thoracic Society Standards of Care Committee. (2001). BTS guidelines for the management of community-acquired pneumonia in adults. *Thorax, 56*, iv1–iv64.

Brown, D. F. J. (1994). Developments in antimicrobial susceptibility testing. *Rev Med Microbiol, 5*, 65–75.

Brueggemann, A. B., Coffman, S. L., Rhomberg, P., Huynh, H., Almer, L., Nilius, A., Flamm, R., & Doern, G. V. (2002). Fluoroquinolone resistance in *Streptococcus pneumoniae* in United States since 1994–1995. *Antimicrob Agents Chemother, 46*, 680–688.

Buckingham, S. C., Brown, S. P., & Joaquin, V. H. (1998). Breakthrough bacteremia and meningitis during treatment parenterally with cephalosporins for pneumococcal pneumonia. *J Pediatr, 132*, 174–176.

Butler, J. C., Breiman, R. F., Campbell, J. F., Lipman, H. B., Broome, C. V., & Facklam, R. R. (1993). Polysaccharide pneumococcal vaccine efficacy: An evaluation of current recommendations. *JAMA, 270*, 1826–1831.

Centers for Disease Control and Prevention. (1997). Prevention of pneumococcal disease: Recommendations of the Advisory Committee on Immunization Practices (ACIP). *Morb Mortal Wkly Rep, 46*, 1–24.

Centers for Disease Control and Prevention. (2000). Prevention of pneumococcal disease among infants and young children: Recommendations of the Advisory Committee on Immunization Practices. *Morb Mortal Wkly Rep, 49*(No. RR-9), 1–35.

Charpentier, E., & Tuomanen, E. (2000). Mechanisms of antibiotic resistance and tolerance in *Streptococcus pneumoniae*. *Microbes Infect, 2*, 1855–1864.

Chen, D. K., McGeer, A., de Azavedo, J. C., & Low, D. E. (1999). Decreased susceptibility of *Streptococcus pneumoniae* to fluoroquinolones in Canada. *N Engl J Med, 341*, 233–239.

Choi, E., & Lee, H. (1998). Clincial outcome of invasive infections by penicillin-resistant *Streptococcus pneumoniae* in Korean children. *Clin Infect Dis, 26*, 1346–1354.

Clavo-Sanchez, A. J., Giron-Gonzalez, J. A., Lopez-Prieto, D., Canueto-Quintero, J., Sanchez-Porto, A., Vergara-Campos, A., Marin-Casanova, P., & Cordoba-Dona, J. A. (1997). Multivariate analysis of risk factors for infection due to penicillin-resistant and multidrug-resistant *Streptococcus pneumoniae*: A multicenter study. *Clin Infect Dis, 24*, 1052–1059.

Cybulska, J., Jeljaszewicz, J., Lund, E., & Munksgaard, A. (1970). Prevalence of types of *Diplococcus pneumoniae* and their susceptibility to 30 antibiotics. *Chemotherapy, 15*, 304–316.

Dagan, R., Givon-Lavi, N., Zamir, O., Sikuler-Cohen, M., Guy, L., Janco, J., Yagupsky, P., & Fraser, D. (2002). Reduction of nasopharyngeal carriage of *Streptococcus pneumoniae* after administration of a 9-valent pneumococcal conjugate vaccine to toddlers attending day care centers. *J Infect Dis, 185*, 927–936.

Dagan, R., Melamed, R., Muallem, M., Piglansky, L., Greenberg, D., Abramson, O., Mendelman, P. M., Bohidar, N., & Yagupsky, P. (1996). Reduction of nasopharyngeal carriage of pneumococci during the second year of life by a heptavalent conjugate vaccine. *J Infect Dis, 174*, 1271–1278.

Dagan, R., Muallem, M., Melamed, R., Leroy, O., & Yagupsky, P. (1997). Reduction of pneumococcal nasopharyngeal carriage in early infancy after immunization with tetravalent pneumococcal vaccines conjugated to either tetanus toxoid or diphtheria toxoid. *Pediatr Infect Dis J, 16*, 1060–1064.

Davidson, R., Cavalcanti, R., Brunton, J. L., Bast, D. J., de Azavedo, J. C., Kibsey, P., Fleming, C., & Low, D. E. (2002). Resistance to levofloxacin and failure of treatment of pneumococcal pneumonia. *N Engl J Med, 346*, 747–750.

Deeks, S. L., Palacio, R., Ruinsky, R., et al. (1999). Risk factors and course of illness among children with invasive penicillin-resistant *Streptococcus pneumoniae*. *Pediatrics, 103*, 409–413.

di Fabio, J. L., Castaneda, E., Agudelo, C. I., de la Hoz, F., Hortal, M., Camou, T., Echaniz-Aviles, G., Noemi, M., Barajas, C., Heitmann, I., Hormazabal, J. C., Brandileone, M. C., Dias Vieira, V. S., Regueira, M., Ruvinski, R., Corso, A., Lovgren, M., Talbot, J. A., & de Quadros, C. (2001). Evolution of *Streptococcus pneumoniae* serotypes and penicillin susceptibility in Latin America, Sireva-Vigia Group, 1993 to 1999. PAHO Sireva-Vigia Study Group. Pan American Health Organization. *Pediatr Infect Dis J, 20*, 959–967.

Doern, G. V. (1995). Interpretive criteria for *in vitro* antimicrobial susceptibility testing. *Rev Med Microbiol, 6*, 126–136.

Doern, G. V., Brueggemann, A. B., Pfaller, M. A., & Jones, R. N. (1999). Assessment of laboratory performance with *Streptococcus pneumoniae* antimicrobial susceptibility testing in the United States: A report from the College of American Pathologists Microbiology Proficiency Survey Program. *Arch Path Lab Med, 123*, 285–289.

Doern, G. V., Heilmann, K. P., Huynh, H. K., Rhomberg, P. R., Coffman, S. L., & Brueggemann, A. B. (2001). Antimicrobial resistance among clinical isolates of *Streptococcus pneumoniae* in the United States during 1999–2000, including a comparison of resistance rates since 1994–1995. *Antimicrob Agents Chemother, 45*, 1721–1729.

Dowell, S. F., Butler, J. C., Giebink, S., Jacobs, M. R., Jernigan, D., Musher, D., Rakowsky, A., Schwartz, B., & Drug-resistant *Streptococcus pneumoniae* Therapeutic Working Group. (1999a). Acute otitis media: Management and surveillance in an era of pneumococcal resistance—A report from the Drug-Resistant *Streptococcus pneumoniae* Therapeutic Working Group. *Pediatr Infect Dis J, 18*, 1–9.

Dowell, S. F., Marcy, S. M., Phillips, W. R., Gerber, M. A., & Schwartz, B. (1998). Principles of judicious use of antimicrobial agents for pediatric upper respiratory tract infections. *Pediatrics, 101*, 163–165.

Dowell, S. F., Smith, T., Leversedge, K., & Snitzer, J. (1999b). Pneumonia treatment failure associated with highly-resistant pneumococci. *Clin Infect Dis, 29*, 462–463.

Ekdahl, K., Ahlinder, I., Hansson, H. B., Melander, E., Molstad, S., Soderstrom, M., & Persson, K. (1997). Duration of nasopharyngeal carriage of penicillin-resistant *Streptococcus pneumoniae*: Experiences from the South Swedish Pneumococcal Intervention Project. *Clin Infect Dis, 25*, 1113–1117.

Ertugrul, N., Rodriguez-Barradas, M. C., Musher, D. M., Ryan, M. A. K., Agin, C. S., Murphy, S. J., Shayegani, M., & Watson, D. A. (1997). BOX-polymerase chain reaction-based DNA analysis of nonserotypeable *Streptococcus pneumoniae* implicated in outbreaks of conjunctivitis. *J Infect Dis, 176*, 1401–1405.

Evans, W., & Hansman, D. (1963). Tetracycline-resistant pneumococcus. *Lancet, i*, 451.

Farr, B. M., Johnston, B. L., Cobb, D. K., Fisch, M. J., Germanson, T. P., Adal, K. A., & Anglim, A. M. (1995). Preventing pneumococcal bacteremia in patients at risk: Results of a matched case–control study. *Arch Intern Med, 155*, 2336–2340.

Fedson, D. S. (1998). Pneumococcal vaccination in the United States and 20 other developed countries. *Clin Infect Dis, 26*, 1117–1123.

Feikin, D. R., Schuchat, A., Kolczak, M., Barrett, N. L., Harrison, L. H., Lefkowitz, L., McGeer, A., Farley, M. M., Vugia, D. J., Lexau, C., Stefonek, K. R., Patterson, J. E., & Jorgensen, J. H. (2000). Mortality from invasive pneumococcal pneumonia in the era of antibiotic resistance, 1995–1997. *Am J Public Health, 90*, 223–229.

Filipe, S. R., Severina, E., & Tomasz, A. (2002). The *murMN* operon: A functional link between antibiotic resistance and antibiotic tolerance in *Streptococcus pneumoniae. Proc Natl Acad Sci USA, 99*, 1550–1555.

Friedland, I. R. (1995). Comparison of the response to antimicrobial therapy of penicillin-resistant and penicillin-susceptible pneumococcal disease. *Pediatr Infect Dis J, 14*, 885–890.

Friedland, I. R., & Klugman, K. P. (1992). Antibiotic-resistant pneumococcal disease in South African children. *Am J Dis Child, 146*, 920–923.

Frisch, A., Price, A., & Myers, G. (1943). Type VIII pneumococcus: Development of sulfadiazine resistance, transmission by cross infection, and persistence in carriers. *Ann Intern Med, 18*, 271–278.

Gaillat, J., Zmirou, D., Mallaret, M. R., Rouhan, D., Bru, J. P., Stahl, J. P., Delormas, P., & Micoud, M. (1985). Essai clinique du vaccin antipneumococcique chez des personnes âgées vivant en institution. *Rev Épidémiol Santé Publique, 33*, 437–444.

Georgopoulos, A., Buxbaum, A., Straschil, U., & Graninger, W. (1998). Austrian national survey of prevalence of antimicrobial resistance among clinical isolates of *Streptococcus pneumoniae* 1994–96. *Scand J Infect Dis, 30*, 345–349.

Geslin, P., Fremaux, A., Spicq, C., Sissia, G., & Georges, S. (1997). Use of a DNA probe test for identification of *Streptococcus pneumoniae* nontypable strains. *Adv Exp Med Biol, 418*, 383–385.

Ghaffar, F., Friedland, I. R., & McCracken, G. H., Jr. (1999). Dynamics of nasopharyngeal colonization by *Streptococcus pneumoniae. Ped Infect Dis J, 18*, 638–646.

Gonzales, R., Bartlett, J. G., Besser, R. E., Cooper, R. J., Hickner, J. M., Hoffman, J. R., & Sande, M. A. (2001). Principles of appropriate antibiotic use for treatment of acute respiratory tract infections in adults: Background, specific aims, and methods. *Ann Intern Med, 134*, 479–486.

Gonzales, R., Steiner, J. F., & Sande, M. A. (1997). Antibiotic prescribing for adults with colds, upper respiratory tract infections, and bronchitis by ambulatory care physicians. *JAMA, 278*, 901–904.

Gray, B., Converse, 3rd, G., & Dillon, H., Jr. (1980). Epidemiologic studies of *Streptococcus pneumoniae* in infants: Acquisition, carriage, and infection during the first 24 months of life. *J Infect Dis, 142*, 923–933.

Grebe, T., Paik, J., & Hakenbeck, R. (1997). A novel resistance mechanism against beta-lactams in *Streptococcus pneumoniae* involves CpoA, a putative glycosyltransferase. *J Bacteriol, 179*, 3342–3349.

Gur, D., Guciz, B., Hascelik, G., Esel, D., Sumerkan, B., Over, U., Soyletir, G., Ongen, B., Kaygusuz, A., & Toreci, K. (2001). *Streptococcus pneumoniae* penicillin resistance in Turkey. *J Chemother, 13*, 541–545.

Hansman, D., & Bullen, M. (1967). A resistant pneumococcus. *Lancet, ii*, 264–265.

Hausdorff, W. P., Bryant, J., Paradiso, P. R., & Siber, G. R. (2000). Which pneumococcal serogroups cause the most invasive disease: Implication for conjugate vaccine formulation and use, part 1. *Clin Infect Dis, 30*, 100–121.

Heffelfinger, J. D., Dowell, S. F., Jorgensen, J. H., Klugman, K. P., Mabry, L. R., Musher, D. M., Plouffe, J. F., Rakowsky, A., Schuchat, A., Whitney, C. G., & Drug-Resistant *Streptococcus pneumoniae* Therapeutic Working Group. (2000). Management of community-acquired pneumonia in the era of pneumococcal resistance: A report from the Drug-Resistant *Streptococcus pneumoniae* Therapeutic Working Group. *Arch Intern Med, 160*, 1399–1408.

Hendley, J. O., Sande, M. A., Stewart, P. M., & Gwaltney, J. M. J. (1975). Spread of *Streptococcus pneumoniae* in families. I. Carriage rates and distribution of types. *J Infect Dis, 132*, 55–61.

Hermans, P. W., Sluijter, M., Elzenaar, K., van Veen, A., Schonkeren, J. J., Nooren, F. M., van Leeuwen, W. J., de Neeling, A. J., van Klingeren, B., Verbrugh, H. A., & de Groot, R. (1997). Penicillin-resistant *Streptococcus pneumoniae* in the Netherlands: Results of a 1-year molecular epidemiologic survey. *J Infect Dis, 175*, 1413–1422.

Ho, P. L., Tse, W. S., Tsang, K. W., Kwok, T. K., Ng, T. K., Cheng, V. C., & Chan, R. M. (2001a). Risk factors for acquisition of levofloxacin-resistant *Streptococcus pneumoniae*: A case–control study. *Clin Infect Dis, 32*, 701–707.

Ho, P. L., Yam, W. C., Cheung, T. K., Ng, W. W., Que, T. L., Tsang, D. N., Ng, T. K., & Seto, W. H. (2001b). Fluoroquinolone resistance among *Streptococcus pneumoniae* in Hong Kong linked to the Spanish 23F clone. *Emerg Infect Dis, 7*, 906–908.

Ho, P. L., Yung, R. W., Tsang, D. N., Que, T. L., Ho, M., Seto, W. H., Ng, T. K., Yam, W. C., & Ng, W. W. (2001c). Increasing resistance of *Streptococcus pneumoniae* to fluoroquinolones: Results of a Hong Kong multicentre study in 2000. *J Antimicrob Chemother, 48*, 659–665.

Hoban, D. J., Doern, G. V., Fluit, A. C., Roussel-Delvallez, M., & Jones, R. N. (2001). Worldwide prevalence of antimicrobial resistance in *Streptococcus pneumoniae, Haemophilus influenzae,* and *Moraxella catarrhalis* in the SENTRY Antimicrobial Surveillance Program, 1997–1999. *Clin Infect Dis, 32*, S81–93.

Hofmann, J., Cetron, M. S., Farley, M. M., Baughman, W. S., Facklam, R. R., Elliott, J. A., Deaver, K. A., & Breiman, R. F. (1995). The prevalence of drug-resistant *Streptococcus pneumoniae* in Atlanta. *N Engl J Med, 333*, 481–486.

Honkanen, P. O., Keistinen, T., Miettinen, L., Herva, E., Sankilampi, U., Laara, E., Leinonen, M., Kivela, S. L., & Makela, P. H. (1999). Incremental effectiveness of pneumococcal vaccine on simultaneously-administered influenza vaccine in preventing pneumonia and pneumococcal pneumonia among persons aged 65 years or older. *Vaccine, 17*, 2493–2500.

Huebner, R. E., Wasas, A. D., & Klugman, K. P. (2000). Trends in antimicrobial resistance and serotype distribution of blood and cerebrospinal fluid isolates of *Streptococcus pneumoniae* in South Africa, 1991–1998. *Int J Infect Dis, 4*, 214–218.

Hyde, T. B., Gay, K., Stephens, D. S., Vugia, D. J., Pass, M., Johnson, S., Barrett, N. L., Schaffner, W., Cieslak, P. R., Maupin, P. S., Zell, E. R., Jorgensen, J. H., Facklam, R. R., Whitney, C. G., & Active Bacterial Core Surveillance/Emerging Infections Program Network. (2001). Macrolide resistance among invasive *Streptococcus pneumoniae* isolates. *JAMA, 286*, 1857–1862.

Jacobs, M., Koornhoof, H., Robins-Browne, R., Stevenson, C., Vermaak, Z., Frieman, I., Miller, G., Witcomb, M., Isaacson, M., Ward, J., & Austrian, R. (1978). Emergence of multiply resistant pneumococci. *N Engl J Med, 299*, 735–740.

Kamme, C., Ekdahl, K., & Molstad, S. (1999). Penicillin-resistant pneumococci in southern Sweden, 1993–1997. *Microb Drug Res, 5*, 31–36.

Kaufman, P. (1947). Pneumonia in old age: Active immunization against pneumonia with pneumo-coccus polysaccharide: Results of a six year study. *Arch Intern Med, 79*, 518–531.

Kelley, M., Weber, D., Gilligan, P., & Cohen, M. (2000). Breakthrough pneumococcal bacteremia in patients being treated with azithromycin and clarithromycin. *Clin Infect Dis, 31*, 1008–1011.

Kellner, J. D. (2001). Drug-resistant *Streptococcus pneumoniae* infections: Clinical importance, drug treatment, and prevention. *Semin Respir Infect, 16*, 186–195.

Kislak, J. (1967). Type 6 pneumococcus resistant to erythromycin and lincomycin. *N Engl J Med, 276*, 852.

Koeth, L. M., Jacobs, M. R., Bajaksouzian, S., Zilles, A., Lin, G., & Appelbaum, P. C. (2002). Comparative in vitro activity of gemifloxacin to other fluoroquinolones and non-quinolone agents against *Streptococcus pneumoniae, Haemophilus influenzae* and *Moraxella catarrhalis* in the United States in 1999–2000. *Int J Antimicrob Agents, 19*, 33–37.

Koivula, I., Stén, M., Leinonen, M., & Mäkelä, P. H. (1997). Clinical efficacy of pneumococcal vaccine in the elderly: A randomized, single-blind population-based trial. *Am J Med, 103*, 281–290.

Konradsen, H. B., & Kaltoft, M. S. (2002). Invasive pneumococcal infections in Denmark from 1995 to 1999: Epidemiology, serotypes, and resistance. *Clin Diagn Lab Immunol, 9*, 358–365.

Koornhof, H. J., Keddy, K., & McGee, L. (2001). Clonal expansion of bacterial pathogens across the world. *J Travel Med, 8*, 29–40.

Koskela, M., Leinonen, M., Häivä, V.-M., Timonen, M., & Mäkelä, P. H. (1986). First and second dose antibody responses to pneumococcal polysaccharide vaccine in infants. *Pediatr Infect Dis J, 5*, 45–50.

Kristiansen, B. E., Sandnes, R. A., Mortensen, L., Tveten, Y., & Vorland, L. (2001). The prevalence of antibiotic resistance in bacterial respiratory pathogens from Norway is low. *Clin Microbiol Infect, 7*, 682–687.

Kyaw, M. H., Clarke, S., Jones, I. G., & Campbell, H. (2002). Incidence of invasive pneumococcal disease in Scotland, 1988–99. *Epidemiol Infect, 128*, 139–147.

Lagrou, K., Peetermans, W., Verhaegen, J., Lierde, S., Verbist, L., & Eldere, J. (1999). Macrolide resistance in Belgian *Streptococcus pneumoniae*. *J Antimicrob Chemother, 44*, 119–121.

Levine, O. S., Farley, M., Harrison, L. H., Lefkowitz, L., McGeer, A., & Schwartz, B. (1999). Risk factors for invasive pneumococcal disease in children: A population-based case–control study in North America. *Pediatrics, 103*, E28.

Lipsitch, M. (2001). Measuring and interpreting associations between antibiotic use and penicillin resistance in *Streptococcus pneumoniae*. *Clin Infect Dis, 32*, 1044–1054.

Mandell, L. A., Marrie, T. J., Grossman, R. F., Chow, A. W., & Hyland, R. H. (2000). Canadian guidelines for the initial management of community-acquired pneumonia: An evidence-based update by the Canadian Infectious Diseases Society and the Canadian Thoracic Society. The Canadian Community-Acquired Pneumonia Working Group. *Clin Infect Dis, 31*, 383–421.

Maraki, S., Christidou, A., & Tselentis, Y. (2001). Antimicrobial resistance and serotype distribution of *Streptococcus pneumoniae* isolates from Crete, Greece. *Int J Antimicrob Agents, 17*, 465–469.

Marchese, A., Mannelli, S., Tonoli, E., Gorlero, F., Toni, M., & Schito, G. C. (2001). Prevalence of antimicrobial resistance in *Streptococcus pneumoniae* circulating in Italy: Results of the Italian Epidemiological Observatory Survey (1997–1999). *Microb Drug Resist, 7*, 277–287.

Marchese, A., Tonoli, E., Debbia, E. A., & Schito, G. C. (1999). Macrolide resistance mechanisms and expression of phenotypes among *Streptococcus pneumoniae* circulating in Italy. *J Antimicrob Chemother, 44*, 461–464.

Marston, B. J., Plouffe, J. F., File, T. M., Jr., Hackman, B. A., Salstrom, S. J., Lipman, H. B., Kolczak, M. S., & Breiman, R. F. (1997). Incidence of community-acquired pneumonia requiring hospitalization. Results of a population-based active surveillance study in Ohio. The Community-Based Pneumonia Incidence Study Group. *Arch Intern Med, 157*, 1709–1718.

Marton, A., & Meszner, Z. (1999). Epidemiological studies on drug resistance in *Streptococcus pneumoniae* in Hungary: An update for the 1990s. *Microb Drug Res, 5*, 201–205.

Mbelle, N., Huebner, R. E., Wasas, A. D., Kimura, A., Chang, I., & Klugman, K. P. (1999). Immunogenicity and impact on nasopharyngeal carriage of a nonavalent pneumococccal conjugate vaccine. *J Infect Dis, 180*, 1171–1176.

McCaig, L. F., Besser, R. E., & Hughes, J. M. (2002). Trends in antimicrobial prescribing rates for children and adolescents. *JAMA, 287*, 3096–3102.

McGee, L., McDougal, L., Zhou, J., Spratt, B. G., Tenover, F. C., George, R., Hakenbeck, R., Hryniewicz, W., Lefevre, J. C., Tomasz, A., & Klugman, K. P. (2001). Nomenclature of major antimicrobial-resistant clones of *Streptococcus pneumoniae* defined by the pneumococcal molecular epidemiology network. *J Clin Microbiol, 39*, 2565–2571.

Melo-Cristino, J., Fernandes, M. L., Serrano, N., & The Portuguese Surveillance Group for the Study of Bacterial Respiratory Pathogens. (2001). A multicenter study of the antimicrobial susceptibility of *Haemophilus influenzae, Streptococcus pneumoniae,* and *Moraxella catarrhalis* isolated from patients with community-acquired lower respiratory tract infections in 1999 in Portugal. *Microb Drug Res, 7*, 33–38.

Mokaddas, E. M., Wilson, S., & Sanyal, S. C. (2001). Prevalence of penicillin-resistant *Streptococcus pneumoniae* in Kuwait. *J Chemother, 13*, 154–160.

Mulholland, K. (1999). Strategies for the control of pneumococcal diseases. *Vaccine, 17*, S79–S84.

National Advisory Committee on Immunization. (2002). Pneumococcal vaccine. In *Canadian immunization guide* (6th ed., pp. 177–184). Ottawa: Canadian Medical Association.

NCCLS. (2000). Methods for dilution antimicrobial susceptibility tests for bacteria that grow aerobically; approved standard (5th ed.). In *NCCLS document M7-A5* (Vol. 20). Wayne, PA: Author.

NCCLS. (2002). Performance standards for antimicrobial susceptibility testing: Twelfth informational supplement. In *NCCLS document M100-S12* (Vol. 22). Wayne, PA: Author.

Normark, B., Novak, R., Örtqvist, Å., Källenius, G., Tuomanen, E., & Normark, S. (2001). Clinical isolates of *Streptococcus pneumoniae* that exhibit tolerance of vancomycin. *Clin Infect Dis, 32*, 552–558.

Novak, R., Henriques, B., Charpentier, E., Normark, S., & Tuomanen, E. (1999). Emergence of vancomycin tolerance in *Streptococcus pneumoniae*. *Nature, 399*, 590–593.

Nuorti, J. P., Butler, J. C., Farley, M. M., Harrison, L. H., McGeer, A., Kolczak, M. S., Breiman, R. F., & Active Bacterial Core Surveillance Team. (2000). Cigarette smoking and invasive pneumococcal disease. *N Engl J Med, 342*, 681–689.

Nyquist, A. C., Gonzales, R., Steiner, J. F., & Sande, M. A. (1998). Antibiotic prescribing for children with colds, upper respiratory tract infections, and bronchitis. *JAMA, 279*, 875–877.

Obaro, S. K., Adegbola, R. A., Banya, W. A. S., & Greenwood, B. M. (1996). Carriage of pneumococci after pneumococcal vaccination. *Lancet, 348*, 271–272.

Obaro, S. K., Adegbola, R. A., Chang, I., Banya, W. A. S., Jaffar, S., McAdam, K. W. J. P., & Greenwood, B. M. (2000). Safety and immunogenicity of a nonavalent pneumococcal vaccine conjugated to CRM_{197} administered simultaneously but in a separate syringe with diphtheria, tetanus and pertussis vaccines in Gambian infants. *Pediatr Infect Dis J, 19*, 463–469.

Örtqvist, Å., Hedlund, J., Burman, L. Å., Elbel, E., Hofer, M., Leinonen, M., Lindblad, I., Sundelof, B., & Kalin, M. (1998). Randomized trial of 23-valent pneumococcal capsular polysaccharide vaccine in prevention of pneumonia in middle-age and elderly people. *Lancet, 351*, 399–403.

Oteo, J., Alos, J. I., & Gomez-Garces, J. L. (2001). Antimicrobial resistance of *Streptococcus pneumoniae* isolates in 1999 and 2000 in Madrid, Spain: A multicentre surveillance study. *J Antimicrob Chemother, 47*, 215–218.

Overweg, K., Hermans, P. W., Trzcinski, K., Sluijter, M., de Groot, R., & Hryniewicz, W. (1999). Multidrug-resistant *Streptococcus pneumoniae* in Poland: Identification of emerging clones. *J Clin Microbiol, 37*, 1739–1745.

Pallares, R., Gudiol, F., Linares, J., Ariza, J., Rufi, G., Murgui, L., Dorca, J., & Viladrich, P. (1987). Risk factors and response to antibiotic therapy in adults with bacteremic pneumonia caused by penicillin-resistant pneumococci. *N Engl J Med, 317*, 18–22.

Pallares, R., Linares, J., Vadillo, M., et al. (1995). Resistance to penicillin and cephalosporin and mortality from severe pneumococcal pneumonia in Barcelona, Spain. *N Engl J Med, 333*, 474–480.

Pana, M., Ungureanu, V., Mihalcu, F., Vereanu, A., & Stanescu, C. (1997). Study of resistant pneumococci in Romania between 1973–1995. *Adv Exp Med Biol, 418*, 471–473.

Perez-Trallero, E., Fernandez-Mazarrasa, C., Garcia-Rey, C., Bouza, E., Aguilar, L., Garcia-de-Lomas, J., Baquero, F., & Spanish Surveillance Group for Respiratory Pathogens. (2001). Antimicrobial susceptibilities of 1,684 *Streptococcus pneumoniae* and 2,039 *Streptococcus pyogenes* isolates and their ecological relationships: Results of a 1-year (1998–1999) multicenter surveillance study in Spain. *Antimicrob Agents Chemother, 45*, 3334–3340.

Pneumococcal Molecular Epidemiology Network, 2001. (2002, August 6). http://pneumo.com/physician/html/pmen/history/history.asp

Robinson, K. A., Baughman, W., Rothrock, G., Barrett, N. L., Pass, M., Lexau, C., Damaske, B., Stefonek, K., Barnes, B., Patterson, J., Zell, E. R., Schuchat, A., Whitney, C. G., & Active Bacterial Core Surveillance/Emerging Infections Program Network. (2001). Epidemiology of invasive *Streptococcus pneumoniae* infections in the United States, 1995–1998: Opportunities for prevention in the conjugate vaccine era. *JAMA, 285*, 1729–1735.

Sahm, D. F., Jones, M. E., Hickey, M. L., Diakun, D. R., Mani, S. V., & Thornsberry, C. (2000). Resistance surveillance of *Streptococcus pneumoniae, Haemophilus influenzae* and *Moraxella catarrhalis* isolated in Asia and Europe, 1997–1998. *J Antimicrob Chemother, 45*, 457–466.

Sankilampi, U., Herva, E., Haikala, R., Liimatainen, O., Renkonen, O. V., & Leinonen, M. (1997). Epidemiology of invasive *Streptococcus pneumoniae* infections in adults in Finland. *Epidemiol Infect, 118*, 7–15.

Schmitz, F.-J., Verhoef, J., Milatovic, D., & Fluit, A. C. (2001). Treatment options for *Streptococcus pneumoniae* strains resistant to macrolides, tetracycline, quinolones, or trimethoprim/sulfamethoxazole. *Eur J Clin Microbiol Infect Dis, 20*, 827–829.

Schrag, S. J., Beall, B., & Dowell, S. F. (2000). Limiting the spread of resistant pneumococci: Biological and epidemiologic evidence for the effectiveness of alternative interventions. *Clin Microbiol Rev, 13*, 588–601.

Schrag, S. J., Pena, C., Fernandez, J., Sanchez, J., Gomez, V., Perez, E., Feris, J. M., & Besser, R. E. (2001). Effect of short-course, high-dose amoxicillin therapy on resistant pneumococcal carriage: A randomized trial. *JAMA, 286*, 49–56.

Schrag, S. J., Zell, E. R., Schuchat, A., & Whitney, C. G. (2002). Sentinel surveillance: A reliable way to track antibiotic resistance in communities? *Emerg Infect Dis, 8*, 496–502.

Schuchat, A., Robinson, K., Wenger, J. D., Harrison, L. H., Farley, M., Reingold, A. L., Lefkowitz, L., & Perkins, B. A. (1997). Bacterial meningitis in the United States in 1995. *N Engl J Med, 337*, 970–976.

Shapiro, E. D., Berg, A. T., Austrian, R., Schroeder, D., Parcells, V., Margolis, A., Adair, R. K., & Clemens, J. D. (1991). The protective efficacy of polyvalent pneumococcal polysaccharide vaccine. *N Engl J Med, 325*, 1453–1460.

Shayegani, M., Malmberg Parsons, L., Gibbons Jr., W. E., & Campbell, D. (1982). Characterization of nontypable *Streptococcus pneumoniae*-like organisms from outbreaks of conjunctivitis. *J Clin Microbiol, 16*, 8–14.

Shibl, A. M., Al Rasheed, A. M., Elbashier, A. M., & Osoba, A. O. (2000). Penicillin-resistant and -intermediate *Streptococcus pneumoniae* in Saudi Arabia. *J Chemother, 12*, 134–137.

Shinefield, H. R., & Black, S. (2000). Efficacy of pneumococcal conjugate vaccines in large scale field trials. *Pediatr Infect Dis J, 19*, 394–397.

Simberkoff, M. S., Cross, A. P., Al-Ibrahim, M., Baltch, A. L., Geiseler, P. J., Nadler, J., Richmond, A. S., Smith, R. P., Schiffman, G., & Shepard, D. S. (1986). Efficacy of pneumococcal vaccine in high-risk patients. Results of a Veterans Administration Cooperative Study. *N Engl J Med, 315*, 1318–1327.

Sims, R. V., Steinmann, W. C., McConville, J. H., King, L. R., Zwick, W. C., & Schwartz, J. S. (1988). The clinical effectiveness of pneumococcal vaccine in the elderly. *Ann Intern Med, 108*, 653–657.

Smit, P., Oberholzer, D., Hayden-Smith, S., Koornhof, H. J., & Hilleman, M. R. (1977). Protective efficacy of pneumococcal polysaccharide vaccines. *JAMA, 238*, 2613–2616.

Song, J. H., Lee, N. Y., Ichiyama, S., Yoshida, R., Hirakata, Y., Fu, W., Chongthaleong, A., Aswapokee, N., Chiu, C. H., Lalitha, M. K., Thomas, K., Perera, J., Yee, T. T., Jamal, F., Warsa, U. C., Vinh, B. X., Jacobs, M. R., Appelbaum, P. C., & Pai, C. H. (1999). Spread of drug-resistant *Streptococcus pneumoniae* in Asian countries: Asian Network for Surveillance of Resistant Pathogens (ANSORP) Study. *Clin Infect Dis, 28*, 1206–1211.

Tait-Kamradt, A., Davies, T., Appelbaum, P., Depardieu, F., Courvalin, P., Petitpas, J., Wondrack, L., Walker, A., Jacobs, M. R., & Sutcliffe, J. (2000). Two new mechanisms of macrolide resistance in clinical strains of *Streptococcus pneumoniae* from Eastern Europe and North America. *Antimicrob Agents Chemother, 44*, 3395–3401.

Thornsberry, C., Sahm, D. F., Kelly, L. J., Critchley, I. A., Jones, M. E., Evangelista, A. T., & Karlowsky, J. A. (2002). Regional trends in antimicrobial resistance among clinical isolates of *Streptococcus pneumoniae, Haemophilus influenzae*, and *Moraxella catarrhalis* in the United States: Results from the TRUST Surveillance Program, 1999–2000. *Clin Infect Dis, 34*, S4–S16.

Tillotson, G. S., & Watson, S. J. (2001). Antimicrobial resistance mechanisms: What's hot and what's not in respiratory pathogens. *Semin Respir Infect, 16*, 155–168.

Turett, G. S., Blum, S., Fazal, B. A., Justman, J. E., & Telzak, E. E. (1999). Penicillin resistance and other predictors of mortality in pneumococcal bacteremia in a population with high human immunodeficiency virus seroprevalence. *Clin Infect Dis, 29*, 321–327.

U.S. Preventive Services Task Force. (1996). *Guide to clinical preventive services* (2nd ed.). Baltimore: Williams & Wilkins.

Verhaegen, J., Van De Ven, J., Verbiest, N., Van Eldere, J., & Verbist, L. (2000). Evolution of *Streptococcus pneumoniae* serotypes and antibiotic resistance in Belgium—update (1994–98). *Clin Microbiol Infect, 6*, 308–315.

Whitney, C. G., Farley, M. M., Hadler, J., Harrison, L. H., Lexau, C., Reingold, A., Lefkowitz, L., Cieslak, P. R., Cetron, M., Zell, E. R., Jorgensen, J. H., & Schuchat, A. (2000). Increasing prevalence of multidrug-resistant *Streptococcus pneumoniae* in the United States. *N Engl J Med, 343*, 1917–1924.

Widdowson, C. A., & Klugman, K. P. (1998). Emergence of the M phenotype of erythromycin-resistant pneumococci in South Africa. *Emerg Infect Dis, 4*, 277–281.

Wortmann, G., & Bennett, S. (1999). Fatal meningitis due to levofloxacin-resistant *Streptococcus pneumoniae*. *Clin Infect Dis, 29*, 1599–1600.

Yoshimine, H., Oishi, K., Mubiru, F., Nalwoga, H., Takahashi, H., Amano, H., Ombasi, P., Watanabe, K., Joloba, M., Aisu, T., Ahmed, K., Shimada, M., Mugerwa, R., & Nagatake, T. (2001). Community-acquired pneumonia in Ugandan adults: Short-term parenteral ampicillin therapy for bacterial pneumonia. *Am J Trop Med Hyg, 64*, 172–177.

4

MRSA in the 21st Century: Emerging Challenges

Ignatius W. Fong and Maria Kolia

1. INTRODUCTION

Since the first clinical observations and laboratory studies published by Ogston (1882) about staphylococcal disease and its role in sepsis and abscess formation, *Staphylococcus aureus* remains an important and dangerous pathogen in humans. In addition to causing both community-acquired and nosocomial infections with increasing frequency, it has also presented the problem of drug resistance. By the end of 1950s, at least 85% of *S. aureus* strains were resistant to penicillin in the United States and France (Wenzel et al., 1991). In 1959, methicillin and semisynthetic penicillin oxacillin were introduced. They were not inactivated by penicillinase and were expected to solve the problem of penicillin resistance. Two years later, strains resistant to methicillin had already been isolated.

No antibiotic resistance marker has distinguished a species more than methicillin resistance has for *S. aureus*. And it is no wonder, since it renders the antistaphylococcal penicillins useless, namely a whole class of bactericidal and relatively nontoxic drugs. Methicillin Resistant *S. aureus* (MRSA) is the term used to refer to strains of *S. aureus* that possess intrinsic resistance to methicillin, oxacillin, nafcillin, cephalosporins, imipenem, and other β-lactams. The rapidity, with which methicillin resistance spread throughout Europe, and subsequently to the rest of the world, has created therapeutic problems, patient management difficulties, confusion regarding infection control practices, and resource allocation uncertainties. Given the capacity of *S. aureus* to colonize, combined with its virulence, it becomes apparent why the MRSA are prevalent virtually everywhere, from large tertiary university hospitals to nursing care units and outpatient populations, such as intravenous drug addicts.

When considering the huge burden for the entire health care system that MRSA represent, as well as the implications for individual patients, a number of questions and issues need to be separately addressed. A thorough understanding of the microbiology and the mechanisms by which this resistance has developed, evolved and spread, is crucial for

Reemergence of Established Pathogens in the 21st Century
Edited by Fong and Drlica, Kluwer Academic/Plenum Publishers, New York, 2003

preventing further dissemination, as well as for exploring treatment possibilities. A constant epidemiological surveillance is also necessary, in order to evaluate the extent of the problem and the efficacy of our efforts to contain it, as well as for the identification of emerging trends and the formulation of future strategies. Moreover, knowledge of the different clinical entities where the MRSA are encountered, and guidelines for their management, need to be founded on basic therapeutic principles, but also constantly refreshed. That is not only because MRSA infections are frequent and diverse, or because the patient population is characterized by increasingly complex clinical problems. It is also due to the fact that the pharmaceutical industry research is not likely to yield any brand new category of antistaphylococcal agents for clinical use in the near future. So, we have to find new roles for old agents and define the role of the newer ones.

The significance of colonization as a means of spreading those strains, as a precursor to invasive disease, and the factors that either enhance the appearance or sustain invasive disease, must be further explored. Furthermore, the means of prevention and isolation that should be applied against both colonization and invasive disease, have always been sources of controversy and confusion. But these difficulties have also provided us with a better understanding of the MRSA problem.

Finally, as the MRSA landscape is always changing in the light of new data, and as new problems emerge, such as the Vancomycin Intermediately Resistant *S. aureus* (VISA), we have to adapt our therapeutics accordingly, in order to keep abreast with the microorganism's novel survival strategies.

2. MICROBIOLOGY AND MECHANISM OF RESISTANCE

S. aureus is a member of the *Bacillaceae* family, and belongs to the *Staphylococcus* genus. Staphylococci are nonmotile, nonspore-forming, usually catalase positive and facultative anaerobes. Under the microscope, the organisms appear as Gram-positive cocci in clusters. *S. aureus* is distinguished from other species on the basis of gold pigmentation of colonies and positive results of coagulase, acetoin production, and heat—stable nuclease tests (many automated commercial identification systems are also available) (Franklin, 1998; Humphreys, 1997; Kloos & Bannerman, 1999).

S. aureus is part of the flora of humans and mammals. It prefers the anterior nares as a habitat, especially in the human adult.

2.1. Genome

The staphylococcal genome consists of a circular chromosome (of approximately 2,800 base-pairs), with prophages, plasmids, and transposons (Franklin, 1998). Genes governing virulence and resistance to antibiotics are found both on the chromosome and on the extrachromosomal elements. They can be transferred between staphylococcal strains, species, or other Gram-positive bacteria through the extrachromosomal elements (Chambers, 1997).

Approximately 30–50 kb of additional chromosomal DNA, *mec*, not found in susceptible strains, is present in methicillin-resistant strains. *Mec* is always found on the *S. aureus* chromosome. *Mec* contains *mecA*, the structural gene for penicillin-binding protein 2a (PBP 2a); also *mecI* and *mecRI*, regulatory elements controlling *mecA* transcription, and 20–40 kb of *mec*-associated DNA. *mecA* encodes PBP 2a (also called PBP 2′), an inducible 76 kDa PBP that determines methicillin resistance. There is no homologue to *mecA* in methicillin susceptible strains, and it is highly conserved among staphylococcal species. The origins of *mec* remain obscure. A *mecA* homologue with 88% amino acid similarity has been identified in *Staphylococcus sciuri*, interestingly a species with a susceptible phenotype, although this gene is ubiquitous in it. These data support the hypothesis that the *mecA* originated in a coagulase-negative *Staphylococcus* species, possibly an evolutionary relative of *S. sciuri* (Wu et al., 1996). All MRSA are clonal descendents from the few ancestral strains that acquired *mecA* (Kreiswirth et al., 1993), possibly through transposition. Studies of the *mec* sequences suggest that *mecA* and its associated DNA are novel mobile elements. *mec* is designated as staphylococcal cassette chromosome *mec* (*SCCmec*). The MRSA have gradually become resistant to many antibiotics, such as carbapenems, new quinolones, minocycline, etc. It seems that they accumulate the multiple resistance genes around the *mecA* gene inside the *SCCmec* (Ito & Hiramatsu, 1998). *mecA* and the regulatory genes *mecRI* and *mecI* are surrounded by this additional 25–50 kb DNA, containing transposons and insertion sequences, where plasmids carrying a variety of resistance determinants can be integrated into the staphylococcal chromosome (Archer & Niemeyer, 1994; Hiramatsu et al., 1996). Two genes, cassette chromosome recombinase genes A and B (ccr AB) can mobilize *mec*. They encode proteins that catalyze precise excision and precise site- specific and orientation- specific integration of *mec* into *S. aureus* chromosome (Katayama et al., 2000). Because the prevalence of MRSA and the *mec* gene has increased worldwide, and because *mec* is mobile, it is possible that new MRSA strains are being generated by horizontal transmission of resistance. The transmission of *mecA* in vivo from a *S. epidermidis* strain to a methicillin-susceptible *S. aureus* (MSSA) strain of the same patient has been shown (Wielders et al., 2001).

The *mecA* promoter region and the first 300 nucleotides of *mecA* are similar in sequence to the analogous regions of the staphylococcal β-lactamase. The *mecI* and *mecRI* are regulatory genes, similar in molecular organization, structure, function, and mechanism of regulation to plasmid- borne β-lactamase regulatory elements. This similarity suggests that they originated from the regulatory region of a β-lactamase gene (Maranan et al., 1997). Intact and fully functional *mec* regulatory genes appear to strongly repress the production of PBP 2a, but when they contain certain deletions, its production is constitutive. If the strains contain an inducible β-lactamase, the production of PBP 2a is also inducible, co-regulated by the β-lactamase regulatory genes (which is usually the case, because almost all MRSA produce β-lactamases as well). However, regulatory elements other than *mecI* and *mecRI* are also required for strong repression of PBP 2a, and still some PBP 2a is produced. It seems likely, that the polymorphism exhibited by *mecI*, *mecRI*, and *mecA* promoter of the MRSA, reflects the selective pressure of β-lactam antibiotics for lack of strong repression, so that sufficient PBP 2a is produced to offer a survival advantage (Chambers, 1997). Six *fem* or *aux* chromosomal genes (A through F), distinct from *mec*, as well as others, also seem to regulate the expression of resistance (Hryniewitcz, 1999).

2.2. Other Staphylococcal Components and Products

The cell wall of staphylococci is 50% by weight composed of peptidoglycan. Peptidoglycan chains consist of alternating polysaccharide subunits of *N*-acetylglucosamine and *N*-acetylmuramic acid. These chains are cross-linked by tetrapeptide chains bound to *N*-acetylmuramic acid and by pentaglycine bridges specific for *S. aureus*. Peptidoglycan may exhibit endotoxin properties, and differences in its structure among strains may account for variations in their ability to cause disseminated intravascular coagulation. Most staphylococci produce microcapsule that contains various polysaccharides. Of the 11 known polysaccharide serotypes, types 5 and 8 are involved in 75% of human infections. Most MRSA are type 5 (Franklin, 1998).

S. aureus is equipped with a large number of virulence factors and exotoxins. They enable the species to evade body's defenses, in order to adhere to tissues and colonize, invade, cause, and sustain infection. These are cell wall polymers, (peptidoglycan and techoic acid), cell surface proteins (protein A which reacts with the Fc of IgG, clumping factor, fibronectin-binding protein and collagen- binding protein), or exoproteins (α-, β-, γ-, δ-lysins, Panton–Valentine leucocidin, epidermolytic toxins, enterotoxins, toxic shock syndrome toxin, coagulase, hyaluronidase, staphylokinase, lipase, phospholipases, deoxyribonuclease, and proteases). No single virulence factor is solely responsible for overcoming a particular host defense, but specific exotoxins cause the symptoms of distinct syndromes. For example, exfoliative toxin A, a serine protease, has recently been found to specifically cleave and disrupt the function of Desmoglein 1, a desmosomal cadherin that maintains keratinocyte cell–cell adhesion in the superficial living epidermis. This way exfoliative toxin A mediates blister formation in bullous impetigo and in Staphylococcal Scalded Skin Syndrome (Amagai et al., 2000). There is no evidence that the MRSA differ in possession of virulence factors from the methicillin susceptible strains. Some MRSA strains are more likely than others to spread into hospitals and cause epidemics, but that is also true for different susceptible strains (Boyce, 1992).

The whole genome of a MRSA strain and a related vancomycin resistant MRSA has been sequenced. It is a complex mixture of genes; many seem to be acquired by lateral transfer, which reveals the ability of the organism to acquire useful genes from various organisms. Plasmids or mobile genetic elements carry most antibiotic resistance genes. Three classes of new pathogenicity islands were identified: a toxic-shock-syndrome toxin island family, exotoxin islands, and enterotoxin islands. Clusters of exotoxin and enterotoxin genes were found closely linked with other gene clusters encoding putative pathogenetic factors. Repeated duplication of genes encoding superantigens may explain why *S. aureus* is capable of infecting humans of diverse genetic backgrounds, causing severe immune reactions. Some 70 candidate genes for new virulence factors were revealed (Kuroda et al., 2001).

2.3. Mechanism of Resistance to Methicillin

"Intrinsic" or "methicillin" resistance is resistance to β-lactams that are not hydrolyzed by staphylococcal β-lactamase, such as methicillin, oxacillin, nafcillin, oxacillin, and dicloxacillin. The main targets of the β-lactam antibiotics in *S. aureus* are the PBPs. The PBPs are cell wall enzymes with transpeptidase and carboxylase activities that produce cross-linking of the peptidoglycan chains that constitute the backbone of the bacterial cell wall. Their substrate is acyl-D- alanyl- D- alanine and β-lactams act as its analogue, forming covalent bonds. Thus, they disrupt cell wall synthesis, resulting eventually in cell cycle-dependent (probably at the time of cell division) death and lysis (Maranan et al., 1997). To the latter events, there seems to be an important contribution of the cell's own membrane enzymes (autolysins), that cleave peptidoglycan bonds in the process of cell growth and cell wall repair; these enzymes are left to act unopposed (Chambers, 2000). The MRSA, as well as the coagulase-negative methicillin-resistant staphylococci, possess the *mecA* gene whose product is PBP 2a. It is a unique PBP with low affinity to β-lactam antibiotics, allowing it to operate in high concentrations of β-lactams that inhibit normal PBPs. Under such "lethal" conditions, PBP 2a retains its transpeptidase activity and assumes the role of normal PBPs in cell wall synthesis (Michel & Gutmann, 1997).

The phenotype of methicillin resistance is greatly variable. The methicillin MICs (minimal inhibitory concentrations) vary from 3 to 200 µg/ml, and the resistance phenotype can be either homogenous or heterogeneous. Heterogeneous resistance, described from the first MRSA clinical isolates, is the most common phenotype (Tomasz et al., 1991). In such a bacterial population, a minority of cells expresses the phenotype of resistance, although the whole population carries the genetic markers for it (Hartman & Tomasz, 1986). The proportion of the population that demonstrates resistance at high concentrations of methicillin varies from 10^{-2} to 10^{-8}, and is a genetic trait of each strain (De Lencastre et al., 1993; Hartman & Tomasz, 1986; Tomasz et al., 1991). One mechanism is through the *fem* (and other) genes, which modifies cell wall peptidoglycan synthesis or cross-links, influencing the phenotype of heterogeneous resistance (Chambers, 1997). It is suggested that, because PBP 2a is exogenous, it results in deficient cell wall cross-linkage (De Jonge & Tomasz, 1993), making additional genes, whose enzyme products are also involved in cell wall synthesis, necessary for enhanced expression of methicillin resistance (Kondo et al., 2001). There are culture conditions that totally suppress the expression of resistance, for example, addition of EDTA (ph 5.2) or incubation at 37–40°C. There are also conditions that enhance it (culture medium containing high concentration of a β-lactam). Such changes are totally transient and reversible, apparently attributable to the inducible nature of PBP 2a production. There are also rare clinically- and laboratory-derived strains that show a homogenous pattern of methicillin resistance (Chambers, 1997).

There are strains of *S. aureus* that show reduced susceptibility to methicillin, the "borderline oxacillin resistant *S. aureus*" (BORSA), with an oxacillin MIC between 2 and 4 µg/ml. This is not the same as the "intrinsic" resistance of MRSA (these strains are *mecA* negative), but it can be hard to distinguish in the laboratory (Mulligan et al., 1992). Suggested mechanisms are: (1) Very high levels of staphylococcal β-lactamase production, which can slowly hydrolyze even compounds that are stable to β-lactamase (Kernodle et al., 1989). Culture conditions that favor expression of methicillin resistance also enhance β-lactamase overproduction. These strains show susceptibility when a β-lactamase inhibitor is added, or when the β-lactamase plasmid is eliminated (McDougal & Thornsberry, 1986). (2) Alterations in PBPs resulting in lower rate of penicillin binding and faster rate of release than in susceptible strains (Chambers et al., 1994). (3) Overproduction of PBP 4, so that more enzyme can be available for cell wall synthesis in the presence of a β-lactam antibiotic (conferring low-level resistance) (Henze & Berger-Baechi, 1996).

Another peculiar phenotype of *S. aureus* is the Small Colony Variants. They are associated with very persistent infections, they grow slowly and have atypical colonies and unusual biochemical profiles, causing detection and identification problems. Because of their special nutrient needs, they produce energy deficiently, resulting in reduced susceptibility to cell wall active substances and to aminoglycosides (which need active transfer into the cell). Antibiotic effects are further compromised by their propensity for intracellular survival. Their susceptibility profiles become apparent only after careful isolation and use of dilution methods (Proctor et al., 1998).

2.4. Culture and Sensitivity Testing

The best methods for detecting MRSA use either molecular probes for the *mecA* gene, or detect the production of PBP 2a (Boyce, 1992; van Leeuwen et al., 1999), provided that the microorganism has been identified to the species level first. The "gold standard" for methicillin resistance is any test that utilizes either polymerase chain reaction (PCR) or DNA hybridization for detecting of the *mecA* gene (Tokue et al., 1992; Unal et al., 1994; van Leeuwen et al., 1999). But these methods are too expensive for routine use in the clinical laboratory, so other, less costly techniques are extensively used. Given the heterogeneity of methicillin resistance, culture conditions that enhance its expression have been developed and standardized for susceptibility testing. These methods of susceptibility testing are empirically derived and stand several steps apart from the biochemical or genetic determinants of methicillin resistance. These methods must utilize either oxacillin, or nafcillin, or methicillin. Oxacillin is usually preferred due to its chemical stability. The use of other β-lactam antibiotics, especially cephalosporins, is not recommended because methicillin-resistant strains are often missed (Hackbarth & Chambers, 1989). All staphylococci resistant to methicillin, nafcillin, or oxacillin, should be reported as resistant to all penicillins, cephalosporins, carbacephems, carbapenems, and β-lactamase inhibitor combinations irrespective of any apparent in vitro susceptibility (Ferraro et al., 2001). The most standardized and accurate among these susceptibility testing methods are:

1. *Disk diffusion.* The National Committee of Clinical Laboratory Standards (NCCLS) (Ferraro et al., 2001) recommend using 1 μg oxacillin disc on Mueller–Hinton agar, inoculum prepared directly from a plate instead of a broth culture, and incubation for 24 hr at 35°C. This is the least specific method (~80%) (Unal et al., 1994; York et al., 1996).

2. *Dilution tests.* The NCCLS recommend cation-adjusted Mueller–Hinton broth supplemented with 2% NaCl, an inoculum of 0.5×10^8 CFU/ml, prepared directly from a plate, and a 24 hr incubation at 35°C. Under these conditions, the breakpoints for oxacillin are ≤ 2 and ≥ 4 μg/ml for susceptibility and resistance, respectively. Alternatively, agar dilution testing performed by using Mueller–Hinton agar that contains 2% NaCl and incubation at 35°C for 24 hr can be used. These methods have $\geq 95\%$ sensitivity.

Staphylococcal isolates with MIC values close to the limits of susceptibility (4 and 2 μg of methicillin and oxacillin/ml, respectively), termed "BORSA," have a reported prevalence from 0.9 to 12.5% (Maranan et al., 1997) (such wide variation is due to adoption of various breakpoints and techniques and lack of standard criteria). Some of these isolates turn out to be extremely heteroresistant MRSA after more careful evaluation, or even still elude, because the detection limit of PCR for *mecA* gene is above 1,000 bacterial cells (Schentag et al., 1998). Other strains are truly "borderline resistant," lacking PBP 2a and possessing other mechanisms of β-lactam resistance. Nevertheless, it is suggested that these strains be considered resistant to β-lactam antibiotics, even with the addition of β-lactamase inhibitors (Mulligan et al., 1992).

Some strains of *S. aureus* also exhibit the phenomenon of tolerance, defined as a ratio of MIC/MBC (minimal bactericidal concentration) equal or greater than 1/32, whereas non-tolerant strains have an MIC/MBC ratio equal or less than 1/4. In a given strain, tolerance to one β-lactam is reproducible when it is tested against other β-lactams as well. Its clinical relevance probably lies with infections where we depend mainly on antibiotic action for the killing of bacteria (e.g., endocarditis).

3. *The agar screen test.*   It is performed by inoculating 0.5×10^8 CFU/ml of the isolate on Mueller–Hinton agar supplemented with 4% NaCl and 6 μg/ml oxacillin, and incubating at 35°C for 24 hr. The presence of more than one colony is indicative of resistance. This method approaches 100% sensitivity for detection of MRSA (Chambers, 1993).

Except the above mentioned, there are also rapid automated methods (e.g., Vitek GPS-SA card or Microscan) for the detection of MRSA, and they have had variable accuracy (Chambers, 1993). The newer Alamar panel, E-test (with 2% NaCl agar), and the BBL MRSA ID system show promising accuracy for detection of MRSA, but are less accurate with testing of coagulase-negative staphylococci (as is the case with other methods). The MRSA screen latex agglutination test has shown potential, with high specificity and sensitivity, provided the coagulase-negative staphylococci (CNS) have been ruled out (van Leeuwen et al., 1999). A multiplex PCR on colonies picked directly from agar plates, which detects both the coagulase gene (*coa*) and the *mecA* in 4 hr has been developed for concomitant *S. aureus* identification and methicillin susceptibility reporting. The first studies show 100% sensitivity and specificity for identification and 98% sensitivity for methicillin resistance (Schmitz et al., 1997). In general, laboratories using the rapid automated methods should confirm the results with a second test, such as the agar screen, before reporting a strain susceptible. Alternatively, a trial comparing the commercial method with a reference test, to document its sensitivity and specificity for the particular strains of their hospital or community could be performed (Chambers, 1997). Laboratories should also periodically re-evaluate the automated system they use with additional testing, otherwise gross misclassification may result in unnecessary infection control measures and vancomycin use (Ender et al., 1999). Finally, as many contemporary strains of MRSA are also resistant to multiple other classes of antimicrobials, this "multi-resistance" (although genetically distinct from β-lactam resistance) could be a useful marker for clinical laboratories (Morgan et al., 1999; Mulligan et al., 1992). *S. aureus* isolates that appear susceptible to oxacillin by an automated method but are multidrug resistant should be additionally tested with a reference method.

2.5. Typing

As MRSA became more prevalent over the years, the need for typing emerged. Typing is important when trying to define an epidemic, locate sources of different strains, or determine the significance of endemic strains and human carriers. The perfect typing system would be capable of typing all MRSA isolates, and would be discriminatory enough (too low discrimination would not separate different strains; too high discrimination would cause confusion by separating subpopulations of the same strain on the basis of minor differences). It would also be reproducible, fast, easily performed and interpreted, and cost effective. Apparently, such a system does not exist, but numerous methods have been utilized. Conventional methods are based on phenotypic characteristics of the bacteria, while newer molecular techniques apply directly to the genetic material.

Most handy among typing systems (apparently phenotypic) is the susceptibility profile. It is available in every laboratory and hospital for a quick assessment by the clinician or epidemiologist. It can suggest the existence of a need for further evaluation, but it has low discrimination, because different strains can show similar susceptibility patterns, while microorganisms of the same origin can acquire or lose plasmids and thereby change susceptibilities. Another widely used and recognized phenotypic method is susceptibility to bacteriophages (Walker et al., 1999). Its disadvantages are that it is time consuming, not all strains are typeable, it is not always reproducible among laboratories, and it is less discriminatory than molecular methods. These and other phenotypic typing systems (serotyping, biotyping) are being used as screening tools. Techniques based on DNA are replacing their role in definite typing.

Among current molecular techniques, the genomic DNA restriction fragment length polymorphism (RFLP) involving the pulsed field gel electrophoresis (PFGE) has become the gold standard of MRSA genotyping (Tang et al., 2000), as it randomly samples the entire genome. It offers best discrimination and reproducibility when utilizing the *SmaI* restriction enzyme (Hryniewitcz, 1999). PFGE restriction fragment profiles also allow assessment of the genetic relatedness of different strains according to criteria by Tenover et al. (1995). However, the method is considerably complex and time-consuming, while not entirely free of interpretation ambiguities, and not perfectly reproducible between laboratories (Hryniewitcz, 1999; Tang et al., 2000). Recently, improvements of the method have been developed, such as the GenePath, a standardized PFGE typing system with better reproducibility (Walker et al., 1999). Nevertheless, some investigators argue that PFGE may be too discriminatory for following long-term outbreaks, because it detects minor changes that the microbial genome undergoes in the course of time (Hryniewitcz, 1999; Tang et al., 2000).

Other RFLP methods utilize PCR amplification, or the newer variation of arbitrarily primed PCR (AP-PCR), also termed rapid amplified polymorphic DNAs (RAPD) (faster and less costly method for evaluating large numbers of strains, but not highly reproducible; Hryniewitcz, 1999). By PCR, specific genes, such as the protein A (*spa*) gene, or coagulase (*coa*) gene can be sequenced (Tang et al., 2000) (method still too costly, discrimination depends on how ubiquitous, preserved, or variable the gene is). The multilocus sequence typing (MLST) scheme (Enright et al., 2000) has been developed for *S. aureus*. Sequence analysis of five to seven housekeeping genes provides a database from which to infer relationships between loosely related isolates that have had substantial time to diversify. The method is too labor-intensive and costly. Sequencing a single gene (such as the *spa*) is more feasible. Genome sequencing has the advantage of objectivity: the genetic code is highly portable, easily stored, and compared.

In order to overcome restrictions and disadvantages of each method, combinations of two molecular methods have been utilized, such as *spa* sequencing with PFGE (Shopsin et al., 2000a; Tang et al., 2000), *spa* with *coa* sequencing (Hryniewitcz, 1999), *mecA* locus with transposon Tn554 sequencing (Melter et al., 1999), *coa* sequencing with PFGE (Udo & Jacob, 2000), etc. Also combinations of a molecular with a phenotypic method, such as phage typing with PFGE (Walker et al., 1999) have been useful. All these systems, as well as newer ones, such as fluorescent amplified fragment length polymorphism (fAELP) (Hookey et al., 1999) show promising features, but still need further systematic evaluation.

2.6. Antibiotics against MRSA: Mechanisms of Action and Mechanisms of Resistance

Once resistance has excluded the use of β-lactam antibiotics, it is the task of clinicians to find alternative treatments for staphylococcal infections. But it is also characteristic of the MRSA to develop resistance to multiple drugs. There are two reasons for this: First, they are subjected to greater selective pressure than the MSSA, because different antibiotics are tried against them. Also, they survive as flora in the hospital environment, where multiple antibiotics are being used. Second, the *mec* gene itself, which encodes for methicillin resistance, is also a locus intended for insertion of mobile resistance genes.

Mechanisms of action of different antibiotic classes used against MRSA, as well as mechanisms of resistance, are briefly explained below. Ranges of MRSA and MSSA resistance to these antibiotics (from various specimen sources and settings) are depicted in Table 4.1 (Charlebois et al., 2000; Cookson, 1998; Diekema et al., 2001; Dowzicky et al., 1998; Guerin et al., 2000; Herold et al., 1998; Herwald, 1999; Johnson & Speller, 1997; Luh et al., 2000; Paradisi et al., 2001; Roberts et al., 1998; Santos Sanches et al., 2000; Schmitz et al., 2001; Simor et al., 2001; Udo & Jacob, 2000).

2.6.1. Macrolide–Lincosamide–Streptogramin (MLS) Group

The MLS agents belong to protein synthesis inhibitors. Protein synthesis takes place on the bacterial ribosome in three stages, namely initiation (30S subunit joins mRNA and tRNA), elongation (joining of amino acids with peptide bonds), and termination (release of complete protein). The key reaction of this pathway, peptide bond formation, is catalyzed by the peptidyl transferase in the center of 50S subunit. The MLS group and chloramphenicol block this enzyme. Type A streptogramins (e.g., dalfopristin) interfere with substrate attachment with the donor and acceptor sites of peptidyl transferase, thus blocking the earliest stage of elongation. Macrolides (erythromycin, clarithromycin, azithromycin, etc.), lincosamides (clindamycin, lincomycin), and type B streptogramins (e.g., quinupristin) constitute the MLS_B group. Each of these categories of compounds has a distinct binding site on the 50S, where they prevent the extension and cause the release

Table 4.1
Resistance of MSSA and MRSA to Non-β-Lactam Antibiotics

Antimicrobial	% MSSA resistant	% MRSA resistant
Macrolides	12–94	30–97
Clindamycin	<8	5[a]–98
Chloramphenicol	<5	4.7–58
Tetracycline	4–10	15–82
Aminoglycosides	<5	7–91
Rifampin	<3	4.5–45
TMP/SMX	<3	5[1]–100
Ciprofloxacin	≤8.4	10–97
Gatifloxacin	<0.5	4–26
Fusidic acid	S	2–18
Mupirocin	<4	3–63
Vancomycin	S	S
Teicoplanin	S	≤0.3
Linezolid	S	S
Quinupristin-Dalfopristin	0.1	0–31

Note: S: susceptible (100%).
[a] From community isolates.

of incomplete polypeptide chains. These compounds are bacteriostatic, while the combination of streptogramin A and streptogramin B (quinupristin/dalfopristin) is synergistic and bactericidal (Vanuffel & Cocito, 1996). This happens because the conformational change that type A streptogramins cause on the peptidyl transferase center, increases ribosomal affinity for type B streptogramins, resulting in non-reversible blockage of protein synthesis.

There are three phenotypes of resistance to these agents. The MLS$_B$ phenotype, namely reduced binding of the MLS$_B$ group drugs, is produced by enzymes that methylate the target rRNA. These enzymes are inducible or constitutive, and they are located on plasmids or on the chromosome. This type of resistance can either be dissociated (resistance to a single antibiotic) or undissociated (resistance to macrolides, lincosamides and type B streptogramins, but not type A streptogramins and their synergic mixture with B compounds). MS phenotype concerns macrolides and streptogramin B resistance only, is attributable to an efflux pump, and is encoded by a plasmid-borne gene. There is a similar efflux pump that confers resistance to streptogramin type A antibiotics, also encoded by a plasmid (mostly found in CNS). A third mechanism of resistance to lincosamides and/or streptogramins, but not macrolides, is the inactivation of each of these agents by various enzymes (Cocito et al., 1997; Maranan et al., 1997). The constitutive MLS$_B$ type of resistance makes the combination quinupristin–dalfopristin bacteriostatic against staphylococci (Lamb et al., 1999).

2.6.2. Chloramphenicol

Chloramphenicol entrance to the cell is energy-dependent. It binds to the 50S subunit of the ribosome and blocks transpeptidation by inhibiting the attachment of aminoacyl–tRNA.

Resistant *S. aureus* acquire a plasmid, which encodes for an inducible modifying enzyme (acetyltransferase).

2.6.3. Aminoglycosides (Gentamicin, Netilmicin, Amikacin, etc.)

Aminoglycosides are bactericidal compounds, whose entrance into the cell through the bacterial cell wall and cytoplasmic membrane is energy-dependent (and they require aerobic conditions for optimal activity). They bind to 30S subunit of ribosomes and inhibit protein synthesis (they cause misreading of mRNA codons). Bacteria acquire resistance by altering the target site (chromosomal for streptomycin), or by reducing uptake, but most commonly by modifying the aminoglycoside molecule and rendering it incapable of binding to the ribosome. These modifying enzymes are acetyltransferases, adenyltransferases, and phosphotransferases encoded by transposons, which are found on plasmids or on the chromosome. There are modifying enzymes for every aminoglycoside, and one resistant strain can simultaneously carry many of them.

2.6.4. Tetracyclines

Tetracyclines are bacteriostatic, and they are actively transported into the cell. They act on the 30S ribosomal subunit, blocking the binding of aminoacyl–tRNA, and therefore, inhibiting protein synthesis. There are two mechanisms of resistance, which can coexist, in the same strain. One is an inducible efflux pump encoded by a plasmid. The second is a protein that protects the ribosome and prevents tetracycline binding, which is encoded either by the chromosome or by a transposon (Schmitz et al., 2001).

2.6.5. Trimethoprim–Sulfamethoxazole (TMP–SMX)

Trimethoprim and sulfonamides both inhibit the synthesis of tetrahydrofolic acid, which is essential in protein and nucleotide synthesis in the microorganism. TMP inhibits the enzyme dihydrofolate reductase, and SMX inhibits dihydropteroate synthetase. Sequential blocking of the same pathway by those two compounds is the reason of their synergism. Resistance to TMP is conferred by a transposon-borne enzyme that reduces target site affinity for the drug. Resistance to SMX is due to a chromosomal mutation, which results in para-amino benzoic acid (PABA)—the normal substrate of dihydropteroate synthetase—overproduction, thus effectively competing SMX enzyme blockade.

2.6.6. Rifampin

Rifampin is a DNA-dependent RNA polymerase inhibitor, preventing initiation of transcription. Resistance occurs when a mutation produces an altered polymerase, which exhibits reduced affinity for rifampin. The rate of appearance of this mutation is high.

2.6.7. Fluoroquinolones (Ciprofloxacin, Ofloxacin, Norfloxacin, etc.)

Fluoroquinolones target the bacterial DNA gyrase (topoisomerase II) and topoisomerase IV, thus inhibiting DNA replication and cell segregation. Their primary target in

S. aureus is the A subunit of topoisomerase IV (Blanche et al., 1996). Mutations in topoisomerase IV gene of the staphylococcal chromosome confer low-level resistance. Point mutations in the chromosomal structural gene of DNA gyrase A or B subunit follow, conferring high level resistance (Ferrero et al., 1994, 1995). Nevertheless, it still remains to be determined which of the two enzymes is the primary fluoroquinolone target for some of the newer compounds, such as clinafloxacin, sitafloxacin, and gatifloxacin (Hooper, 2000). A chromosomal, inducible or constitutive, multidrug efflux pump results in reduced accumulation in the cell, affecting mostly the hydrophilic (e.g., ciprofloxacin, norfloxacin), among these compounds (Kaatz & Seo, 1997). Each of these resistance mechanisms arises in a single step (Kaatz & Seo, 1997).

2.6.8. Fusidic Acid

Fusidic acid inhibits the ribosomal GTPase, thus blocking the elongation phase of protein synthesis. Resistance occurs with alteration of target site, which is encoded by the chromosome or by plasmids.

2.6.9. Mupirocin

Mupirocin is bacteriostatic, but appears bactericidal at lower pH, such as that of many parts of the skin. Its target is isoleucyl–tRNA synthetase (IleS), as it is an analogue of isoleucyl–tRNA. There are certain difficulties in defining mupirocin resistance, as it is a topical agent, and correlation between MIC, local concentrations, and clinical outcome are problematic. Nevertheless, low-level resistance seems to be due to a chromosomally encoded mutant IleS, or to an altered tRNA synthetase protein complex that inhibits mupirocin access to IleS. While high-level resistance is conferred by an acquired novel IleS, which is encoded by plasmids (Cookson, 1998).

2.6.10. Glycopeptides (Vancomycin, Teicoplanin)

Glycopeptides are high molecular weight antibiotics that act on the cell wall synthesis. They bind to the D-alanyl-D-alanine terminal of a four-peptide chain that stems out from the peptidoglycan backbone, thus sterically inhibiting the addition of more subunits to peptidoglycan. As with β-lactams, the microorganism's own cell wall repairing enzymes, the autolysins, play a role in cell lysis and death. Resistant enterococci have acquired plasmid-encoded enzymes that produce a different terminal for the stem chains, where the glycopeptides cannot bind. Such a mechanism of resistance has not been found in clinical staphylococcal isolates, but it has been successfully transferred from enterococci to staphylococci in vitro (Noble et al., 1992). MRSA with intermediate vancomycin resistance (VISA) seem to owe this to accelerated cell wall turnover, thicker cell wall, and increased production of PBP 2 (Hanaki et al., 1998).

2.6.11. Oxazolidinones (Linezolid)

Oxazolidinones are a novel category of compounds that act at the initiation phase of protein synthesis, by inhibiting the formation of initiation complex. A specific binding site at the 50S ribosomal subunit has been determined. In vitro resistance develops only very slowly. Resistant clinical isolates (mostly enterococci, but also MRSA) have been reported; mutations in the 23S ribosomal RNA are responsible (Tsiodras et al., 2001). Resistance mechanisms to other drug categories that bind to the 50S ribosomal subunit do not interfere with oxazolidinone activity (Fines & Leclercq, 2000). Linezolid is bacteriostatic against *S. aureus* (Clemett & Markham, 2000).

3. EPIDEMIOLOGY

Humans are a natural reservoir of *S. aureus*. A large proportion of healthy adults are transiently or persistently colonized, and colonization is a predisposing factor to infection. *S. aureus* is transmitted most commonly through personal contact, and rarely through environmental sources, such as inanimate objects or the air (in burn units).

Gram-positive bacterial infections have become an increasing problem in recent years, especially in hospitals. Among these pathogens, *S. aureus* is the most commonly isolated from nosocomial pneumonia and surgical wound infections, and the second most common, after CNS, from bacteremias (Emori & Gaynes, 1993). When both nosocomial and community-acquired blood stream infections are taken into account, *S. aureus* is the most commonly isolated pathogen (Diekema et al., 2001). Factors that have contributed to the dominant role of Gram-positive pathogens in hospitals are the high proportion of immunocompromised patients, along with changing anti-cancer regimens and increased mucositis (Livermore, 2000), the increased use of intravascular devices (Steinberg et al., 1996), and the expanded use of agents directed against Gram-negative bacilli (Cormican & Jones, 1996). Another, still more alarming trend, is the increase of antibiotic resistance among these pathogens. This latter trend clearly applies to the MRSA, as well.

3.1. Tools of Epidemiology

When the MRSA first emerged as a nosocomial pathogen, an increase in the incidence or prevalence of MRSA in a given institution was due to the spread of one or two strains. However, in recent years, such an increase could be attributable to newly admitted patients infected by or colonized with one or more MRSA strains, to nosocomial transmission, or to both. According to a consensus panel's definition (Wenzel et al., 1998), "an outbreak of MRSA is an increase in the rate of MRSA cases or a clustering of new cases due to the transmission of a single microbial strain in a health care institution, including long-term care facilities." A case is defined as either a colonized or infected patient. An increased case rate has a statistical definition, by incidence or incidence density: number of new cases per 100 admissions/time or per 100 patient-days. Alternatively, an acceptable definition of an increased rate can utilize one of the following: (1) monthly 25% increase above baseline, (2) an increase in new nosocomial cases compared with hospitals of similar size, (3) one case per month in a high-risk unit or an MRSA-free unit, and (4) three or more nosocomial cases per month in any unit (Wenzel et al., 1998).

In order to use the most appropriate measures against the spread of MRSA, it is important to determine each time whether new cases are due to several different strains or a single strain. The clinical microbiology laboratory must save MRSA isolates, in order to compare their phenotypic or genotypic characteristics. The susceptibility test is the most widely available, easy and fast among typing methods. It is also highly reproducible and under strict quality control. However, it is only useful as an initial screening method (Guerin et al., 2000), because of its low discriminatory power. Other typing methods, either phenotypic (phage type, capsular type, immunoblots of whole cell polypeptides or exported proteins (Boyce, 1992), etc.), or newer genotypic methods that analyze chromo-somal or plasmid DNA, should be employed. These new genetic techniques are replacing the phenotypic ones, because they are far more reliable. The choice of method depends on available resources, the specific resistance or virulence characteristics of the strain(s) under study, or the time frame of the probable outbreak (short- or long-term) (Tang et al., 2000). For best discrimination, combinations of methods have often been applied. It should be stressed, however, that typing is not enough by itself, but it must be combined with all the epidemiological data, in order to accurately depict the MRSA problem in any given situation.

3.2. MRSA in the Hospital

MRSA are usually introduced into health care institutions by colonized or infected patients who serve as reservoirs and rarely by colonized health care workers. They are usu-ally transmitted, however, via transient colonization of the hands of personnel after contact with the colonized or infected patient (Mulligan et al., 1992; Thompson et al., 1982).

MRSA is usually isolated from the lower respiratory tract (*S. aureus* accounts for 20% of nosocomial pneumonias (Emori & Gaynes, 1993)), surgical wound infections, skin and soft tissue infections, and bacteremias or intravascular devices, while few come from the urinary tract or other sources (Boyce, 1992; Roberts et al., 1998; Simor et al., 2001).

S. aureus and *Escherichia coli* are the commonest nosocomial pathogens. MRSA are, therefore, among the most prevalent pathogens in the hospital, and a dramatic increase of MRSA nosocomial infections has taken place over the last 25 years. For example, in the U.S. hospitals, the percentage of MRSA among *S. aureus* infections rose from 2.1% in 1975 to 29% (and 50% of associated deaths) in 1995 (Panlilio et al., 1992; Roberts et al., 1998), while 1999 data indicate that it has reached 36% (Staples et al., 2000), with non-Intensive Care Unit (ICU) MRSA being above 30% (Archibald et al., 1997; Livermore, 2000). Another striking example of increasing proportions of MRSA is offered by England and Wales, where the bacteremias due to these pathogens rose from 1–2% in 1993 to 32% in 1997 (Anonymous, 1999). This particular increase was attributable to two clones mainly, depicting the fact that methicillin resistance "spreads" rather than "emerges," following the rules of an outbreak. Generally, MRSA are usually found to be a few clones within a restricted area, whereas MSSA are usually multiple clones. A pattern usually encountered is the coexistence of multiple divergent MRSA clones (termed endemic) with one or two dominant ones that are causing an increase from baseline incidence (termed epidemic), especially wherever MRSA have been prevalent for some time (Flournoy, 1997; Melter et al., 1999; Roberts et al., 1998; Simor et al., 2001). In accordance with this concept are the wide geographic differences of MRSA incidence. They vary from 50% to 70% in Japanese hospitals (Arakawa et al., 2000; Diekema et al., 2001) and over 50% in Italy and Portugal, to <1% in Scandinavia (Kotilainen et al., 2001), and 2% in Switzerland and the Netherlands (Diekema et al., 2001). However, even in countries of previous low incidence, such as Canada, the MRSA seem to be on the rise (from <1% in 1995 (Suh et al., 1998), to 6.1% in 1999 (Simor et al., 2001)).

MRSA seem to be prevalent in hospitals all over the world (Table 4.2; Diekema et al., 2001). In the Middle East, reported rates vary from ~20% in Palestinian to ~60% in Saudi Arabian hospitals (Alghaithy et al., 2000; Essawi et al., 1998). In Asia, the MRSA problem is present wherever it has been sought: 30–87% of *S. aureus* from surveillance studies in India (Verma et al., 2000), and reported (but of unknown frequency) from Thailand (Wongwanich et al., 2000). High percentages of MRSA are also encountered in Hong Kong (74%), Taiwan (61%), and Singapore (62%) (Diekema et al., 2001). In South America, there is a widely disseminated multi-resistant MRSA clone in Brazilian hospitals (Teixeira et al., 1995) (rates 34–66%; Diekema et al., 2001; Moraes et al., 2000; Sadoyama & Gontijo Filho, 2000; da Silva Coimbra et al., 2000). This epidemic strain, the "Brazilian clone" has also spread to Uruguay, Chile (Aires de Sousa et al., 2001), Argentina and Portugal (da Silva Coimbra et al., 2000). In South Africa, 43% of *S. aureus* from invasive infections are MRSA (Diekema et al., 2001). There have been sparse reports of MRSA from the rest of the African continent (Ben Hassen et al., 1995; Geyid & Lemeneh, 1991; Hayanga et al., 1997).

It also seemed, at least in some instances, that the MRSA were not simply replacing the MSSA, but that they were causing additional morbidity, being largely responsible for the increase in total *S. aureus* infections (Boyce et al., 1983; Chaix et al., 1999; Tam & Yeung, 1988).

Nevertheless, the spread of MRSA cannot be accounted for solely by unknown factors of virulence or colonization that render a strain more successful. Hospital hygiene

Table 4.2
Rates of MRSA Isolates, by Nation, at SENTRY Centers, 1997–1999

European country	No. of *S. aureus* isolates (% resistant to methicillin)	Western Hemisphere country	No. of *S. aureus* isolates (% resistant to methicillin)	Western Pacific country	No. of *S. aureus* isolates (% resistant to methicillin)
Austria	117 (9.4)	Argentina	424 (42.7)	Australia	606 (23.6)
Belgium	82 (25.6)	Brazil	814 (33.7)	Hong Kong	172 (73.8)
England	131 (27.5)	Chile	428 (45.3)	Japan	289 (71.6)
France	718 (21.4)	Colombia	139 (8.6)	Singapore	122 (62.3)
Germany	347 (4.9)	Mexico	88 (11.4)	South Africa	77 (42.9)
Greece	128 (34.4)	Canada	1410 (5.7)	Taiwan	90 (61.1)
Italy	297 (50.5)	United States	7169 (34.2)		
The Netherlands	147 (2.0)				
Poland	159 (25.8)				
Portugal	318 (54.4)				
Spain	352 (19.3)				
Switzerland	114 (1.8)				
Turkey	104 (37.5)				

Note: Adapted from (Diekema et al., 2001) with permission from the publisher.

and/or infection control measures are also important, as implied by sharp differences observed between neighboring European countries in the past (Peters & Becker, 1996; Voss et al., 1994) and more recently (Table 4.2; Diekema et al., 2001). A similar example is offered by the different MRSA rates between United States and Canada (Table 4.2). Nosocomial MRSA strains are also often resistant to many other classes of antibiotics. The patterns of this multi-resistance show great geographic variation, perhaps reflecting the different antibiotic pressures that selected these strains (Santos Sanches et al., 2000).

Some studies have found that larger hospitals have higher percentages of MRSA (Emori & Gaynes, 1993; Panlilio et al., 1992). Excess use of antibiotics, particularly β-lactams, in the hospital, certainly favors MRSA. Moreover, once MRSA are introduced into hospitals, they usually persist (Maranan et al., 1997). For an individual patient, the risk of acquiring MRSA increases, as the proportion of other patients with MRSA in the same unit increases (colonization pressure) (Merrer et al., 2000). Furthermore, some predisposing factors for MRSA acquisition are also markers of severity of illness and debility, and thus, of increased need for care. So, it is not clear how much these predisposing factors are confounded by increased contact with personnel hands, which carry the MRSA (Luh et al., 2000).

Among host risk factors for acquisition and selection of MRSA are the prior or current use of antibiotics (especially multiple or broad-spectrum), previous or prolonged hospitalization, decubitus ulcers, and intravascular devices (Rao, 1998; Steinberg et al., 1996). Patients with severe underlying illnesses and poor functional status, trauma or prior surgery are more vulnerable. Neurological damage seems to be a particular risk factor (Mylotte et al., 2000). Generally, states of compromised immune defenses and/or need for frequent vascular access, such as diabetes mellitus, peripheral vascular disease, renal failure and hemodialysis (Chow & Yu, 1989; Terpenning et al., 1994), HIV infection (Conterno et al., 1998; Nguyen et al., 1999), and intravenous drug abuse (Fleisch et al., 2001), predispose to MRSA colonization and infection. Finally, admission to the ICU is among the most common ways of acquiring MRSA (Roberts et al., 1998).

The ICU, with its severely ill patients and high antibiotic use, is an environment where MRSA are more common (as is the case with multi-resistant microbes in general), and where they present a particularly difficult problem, because they cause higher mortality than other multi-resistant pathogens (Albrich et al., 1999). MRSA, along with other resistant bacteria, also spread from the ICU to the rest of the hospital, and, subsequently, to other hospitals. S. aureus infections doubled from 1987 to 1997 in U.S. ICUs and MRSA reached 45% among them, 56.2% of which were susceptible only to vancomycin (Franklin, 1998). In other words, one fourth of S. aureus were susceptible only to vancomycin, showing that the MRSA of ICUs are alarmingly multi-resistant. The finding of frequent MRSA co-infection among patients colonized or infected with Vancomycin-Resistant Enterococci (VRE) in one hospital study (Poduval et al., 2000), illustrates the catastrophic consequences of this restriction of therapeutic choices to vancomycin alone. From infections in European ICUs, S. aureus accounted for 30.1% (most common pathogen), and 60% were MRSA (~80% in French and Italian ICUs) (Vincent et al., 1995). The MRSA from bacteremias were 72.4% (Johnson & Speller, 1997). Some risk factors, common for all ICU infections, seem to be the use of intravascular devices, mechanical ventilation, length of stay in the ICU, antecedent trauma and stress ulcer prophylaxis (Johnson & Speller, 1997; Vincent et al., 1995). For staphylococcal bacteremias, aseptic technique when inserting and manipulating catheters is important (Albrich et al., 1999), while in mechanically ventilated patients, coma is a particular risk factor for airway colonization and pulmonary infection with *S. aureus* (Rello et al., 1992).

The consequences of MRSA acquisition in the ICU are also noteworthy. They do not only result from prolonged ICU and hospital stay, increased use of antibiotics, and increased use of invasive interventions. They also cause, in comparison with MSSA, prolonged ICU and hospital stay, increased use of antibiotics, increased use of invasive interventions, and 250% increased hospital costs (Carbon, 1999). MRSA infections in the ICU are also associated with decreased chances of survival (Ibelings & Bruining, 1998). Similarly, higher mortality and longer hospital stay than MSSA infections, have been caused by MRSA infections outside the ICU (hospital or community acquired) (Carbon, 1999).

Another favorable environment for the spread of MRSA is the Nursing Home. It shares many features with the hospital, such as a vulnerable population with comorbid conditions, open wounds and prosthetic devices, and high antibiotic use (prevalence ~8%—Nicolle et al., 1996). Moreover, patients stay for long periods, colonization is persistent because decubitus ulcers and other wounds are frequent, there is a higher patient to personnel ratio, plus a limited access to infection control training and resources. There is no systematic surveillance data, but studies have shown that 5–80% of residents can have their nares, their pharynx, or, more often, their wounds, colonized with MRSA (Bradley, 1999; Nicolle et al., 1996; Washio et al., 1998). Furthermore, 10–24% of newly arriving residents can acquire MRSA in the facility (Bradley et al., 1991; Giret et al., 2001). Colonization seems to result in infection more rarely than in the hospital (Bradley et al., 1991) (1.6 MRSA infections per 100 residents per year in one facility; Drinka et al., 2001). But it has also been found that MRSA colonize the most seriously ill and debilitated, and, therefore, result in infection more often than MSSA (Muder et al., 1991). Long-term care facilities have also been recognized as reservoirs for hospital MRSA outbreaks (Aeilts et al., 1982; Kotilainen et al., 2001).

3.3. MRSA in the Community

The definition of community versus hospital acquired MRSA is problematic, because MRSA colonization can persist for months or years after discharge (Sanford et al., 1994; Thompson et al., 1982). Most of the MRSA found in the first 72 hr of hospital admission come from patients that have been hospitalized again in the past 6 months to 1 year (Boyce, 1998; Suh et al., 1998) or have been residing in a nursing home. There are certain populations, vulnerable to *S. aureus* colonization or infection, among which MRSA can spread and persist. Such are the intravenous drug users (Fleisch et al., 2001), or the dialysis patients (Chow & Yu, 1989), or individuals, in general, in frequent contact with the health care system (children with cystic fibrosis have been recently recognized among them [Herold et al., 1998]).

But MRSA have also been recovered from individuals "with no predisposing risk factor" for their acquisition. The incidence of MRSA in such populations is low, from 0% (Shopsin et al., 2000b) to 6% (Charlebois et al., 2000) in studies from U.S. urban populations. Their susceptibility profiles are also different from MRSA isolated from nosocomial or high-risk community cases: they are usually susceptible to most antistaphylococcal drugs, except β-lactams. These community MRSA are, therefore, totally distinct strains from their nosocomial counterparts. MRSA prevalence is suspected to be on the rise in pediatric populations (Adcock et al., 1998; Centers for Disease Control and Prevention, 1999; Herold et al., 1998; Hussain et al., 2000), where β-lactams are frequently used. Studies have found 0–3% colonization with MRSA among children "with no predisposing risk factor" (Suggs et al., 1999), but it can rise up to 24% after contact with a case of disease (Adcock et al., 1998; Shahin et al., 1999). In a tertiary care U.S. hospital, half of the children with a community-acquired MRSA infection had no predisposing risk factor (Hussain et al., 2000). In a survey of such community- acquired MRSA infections, most patients were healthy children and young adults (median age 16 years), 84% were initially treated by a regimen that did not cover MRSA, and most infections were caused by a single clone with wide dissemination, that was unrelated to nosocomial strains (Naimi et al., 2001).

The origin of these community strains is unknown since they are of different clonal type from nosocomial strains. Horizontal transfer of the *mec* gene, which is a large chromosomal element, is considered rare; it is possible through the cassette chromosome recombinase genes A and B, whose protein products can precisely excise and integrate *mec*. As the prevalence of MRSA and, therefore, *mec* increases, chances that it gets transferred to methicillin susceptible strains also increase (Chambers, 2001). Whether these "community" MRSA strains originate from hospital strains after multiple changes or from MSSA strains through transfer of the resistance gene, implications for prevention remain the same: the force driving their spread is the increased antibiotic use.

While MRSA remain largely a nosocomial problem, we may soon be compelled to recognize it as a community infection problem as well. Spread of MRSA can increase the complexity and costs of treating community-acquired staphylococcal infections. There is also a potential for adverse outcome in the rare community acquired infection without predisposing risk factors, simply because MRSA is not expected and covered for by empiric regimens.

4. CLINICAL ENTITIES

S. aureus is a widespread pathogen. The range of its relationship with the human host extends from uneventful coexistence to rapidly fatal infection. While this variety of clinical entities has been extensively studied for more than a century and powerful antibiotics have been invented, the spread of the MRSA is threatening to limit our therapeutic options. Thus, we are prompted to re-evaluate the significance of those well-known clinical entities in the context of evolving antibiotic resistance.

4.1. Colonization

4.1.1. Colonization and Transmission

The most usual site from which *S. aureus* can be cultured in healthy adults is the anterior nares. Other proposed sites are the oropharynx, axillae, groin, and anal area, but the yield is lower. Some individuals, approximately 20% of the general population, have their nares persistently colonized with the same strain, while the majority (~60%) are colonized intermittently with different strains, and another ~20% are almost never colonized. In cross-sectional surveys, the percentage of the general population colonized with *S. aureus* has varied from 20% to 55% (Kluytmans et al., 1997). Children have higher rates than adults (Shopsin et al., 2000b), while the throat and perianal area have been suggested as better sites for exposing colonization of children (Shahin et al., 1999).

How and why *S. aureus* adheres preferentially to human nasal mucosa is not fully understood. *S. aureus* binds to both anterior nasal epithelial cells covered with mucus and to the glycoprotein component of mucus (mucin), but not to ciliated cells of the airway epithelium. Two staphylococcal cell wall surface proteins seem to bind to mucin, while different strains of *S. aureus* differ in avidity of adherence (Shuter et al., 1996). There is also variation among individuals, with higher rates of *S. aureus* binding to cells from carriers than non-carriers (Kluytmans et al., 1997).

The rate of *S. aureus* colonization does not differ significantly between the general population and health care workers, patients upon hospital admission or during hospitalization (Kluytmans et al., 1997). Certain conditions favor *S. aureus* nasal carriage, such as insulin dependent diabetes mellitus, hemodialysis or continuous ambulatory peritoneal dialysis (CAPD), intravenous drug abuse, and HIV infection or AIDS. Local conditions affecting the nasal mucosa, such as influenza A virus infection (Kluytmans et al., 1997), inhalation of illegal drugs (Holbrook et al., 1997), and perennial allergic rhinitis (Shiomori et al., 2000), have been proposed to play a role.

Sites of MRSA colonization other than the nose are also very important. Patients with dermatitis, skin infection, or wounds and chronic ulcers, and generally any skin break, have a significantly higher rate of *S. aureus* colonization, which is usually persistent on these lesions (Kotilainen et al., 2001; Scanvic et al., 2001). Such patients are often a reservoir of MRSA in an institution. Antibiotic use has been found to protect from *S. aureus* colonization (Holbrook et al., 1997), but, on the other hand, previous or current antibiotic use is among the most common predisposing factors for MRSA colonization. Interestingly, previous fluoroquinolone use has been found to be an independent risk factor for persistent MRSA colonization (Harbarth et al., 2000).

When a *S. aureus*-colonized individual is admitted to the hospital and given antibiotics, two series of events may lead to MRSA colonization. Either the MSSA strain, along with all susceptible flora, is eradicated and replaced by a hospital MRSA strain (Kluytmans et al., 1997) (usually multi-resistant); or the apparently MSSA population already contains a low number of *mecA* positive microorganisms, namely MRSA, which are then selected by β-lactams and predominate (Schentag et al., 1998).

In addition to the anterior nares, also the wounds, decubitus and vascular ulcers, burns, sputum, tracheostomy and gastrostomy sites, and urine from indwelling catheters should be cultured from patients when looking for MRSA. Implant devices in general are very important sites of persistent colonization, because MRSA can form a very persevering biofilm on them (Jones et al., 2001). Moreover, some investigators have proposed the perineum as the major site of carriage (Brady et al., 1990). In previously or repeatedly hospitalized patients, MRSA carriage (usually, but not always the same strain), can persist for years, with a half-life of up to 40 months, as described by Sanford et al. (1994).

MRSA can also be recovered from the hands and nares of hospital staff, usually transiently. While personnel rarely, but particularly when they have dermatitis lesions, are persistent carriers, such carriers can spread MRSA and become clinically significant in the setting of an outbreak (Bartzokas et al., 1984). During an outbreak 2–5% of staff usually are

MRSA carriers (Haley, 1991). Inanimate objects and surfaces in the hospital are not usually positive for MRSA. Surface contamination has been found more frequently around a patient with wound- or urine- derived MRSA than with nasal colonization (Bartzokas et al., 1984; Herwald, 1999). In burn units, where transmission through air-borne microorganisms does occur, especially when ventilation is poor, the surfaces and gowns can be heavily contaminated (Farrington et al., 1990). Even contaminated breast milk from milk banks has been implicated in the spread of epidemic MRSA in neonatal units (Novak et al., 2000).

The primary mode of MRSA transmission is through the hands of health care workers, who become transiently colonized after contact with colonized or infected patients, or contaminated material, and subsequently transfer the bacteria to the next patient(s) (Mulligan et al., 1992). Nasal carriage contributes to transmission because it results in hand carriage of MRSA (Boyce, 1992). Therefore, increased workload and staff shortage in a unit is a risk factor for an MRSA outbreak (Haley et al., 1995). It has been shown that each day of substandard nurse to patient ratio in an ICU increases the chance of each patient acquiring MRSA by 5% (Grundmann et al., 2002).

4.1.2. Colonization and Infection

Colonized individuals suffer *S. aureus* infection more frequently than non-colonized. Among hemodialysis patients, for example, up to 62% of whom can be *S. aureus* carriers, carriage has been proven to increase the frequency of infection (Chow & Yu, 1989). Nasal carriage of *S. aureus* serves as a reservoir of skin colonization and subsequent infection when a breach of skin integrity (or compromise of other defense mechanisms, such as in comatose intubated patients) offers a portal of entry. The colonizing strain is usually isolated from the subsequent infection (von Eiff et al., 2001; Pujol et al., 1996). The rate at which colonization results to infection varies among populations, according to their vulnerability: underlying illness, immune status, prosthetic devices, type of surgery and perioperative prophylaxis, antisepsis, preoperative length of hospitalization, etc. Among *S. aureus* colonized individuals, those with MRSA have often been found to be at higher risk of infection (Muder et al., 1991; Sadoyama & Gontijo Filho, 2000), a finding supported by epidemiological data of increased *S. aureus* infection rate after the introduction of MRSA in an institution (Pujol et al., 1996). In hospital outbreaks, the ratio of MRSA infected to colonized patients can be as high as 40% (Mulligan et al., 1992), while among candidates for abdominal surgery, 46% of MRSA colonized suffered a systemic postoperative infection in one study (Eyraud et al., 2000). In another study, among hospitalized patients with chronic ulcers, those colonized with MRSA had a several-fold increase of risk for MRSA bacteremia, particularly after the insertion of a central venous catheter (Roghmann et al., 2001).

4.2. Invasive Disease

4.2.1. Skin and Soft Tissue Infections

In the SENTRY study, skin and soft tissue infections caused by MRSA ranged from less than 10% to almost 40% of *S. aureus* infections in different geographic regions (Diekema et al., 2001).

MRSA is a nosocomial pathogen, usually acquired during current or previous hospital stay, or in the operating theater. Therefore, the soft tissue infections that cause more concern are clean surgical wound and traumatic wound infections. Peri-operative antimicrobial prophylaxis does not usually cover methicillin resistance. On the contrary, prolonged administration of a third generation cephalosporin after surgery, has been correlated with increase of MRSA infections, without reduction of other infection rates, when compared to shorter duration of less "advanced" regimens (Fukatsu et al., 1997). While most surgical patients will develop superficial localized infection of subcutaneous tissues, a substantial proportion can have deep-seated infection requiring debridement and reconstruction surgery. MRSA can become endemic (Brady et al., 1990) or cause an outbreak (Jelic et al., 1996) in a surgical unit, with catastrophic results in some settings, such as cardiothoracic or vascular surgery. When a vascular graft is infected with MRSA, the outcome is amputation, sepsis, or death (Chalmers et al., 1999). MRSA can also cause the whole spectrum of *S. aureus* skin and soft tissue infections, such as cellulitis and fasciitis, or impetigo, furuncle, etc. Community skin and soft tissue infections in patients without predisposing risk factors caused by MRSA (rare overall) have mostly been encountered among children. A significant aspect of these latter superficial infections is that they can facilitate the spread of MRSA in the community.

4.2.2. Bone and Joint Infections

S. aureus causes bone and joint infections that are both destructive and persistent. They are hard to eradicate and can recur after long periods of apparent remission. There are many reasons for this. First, the pharmacokinetics of many antimicrobials in bone are poor, partly due the poor perfusion of bone, especially when pus disrupts the periosteum and occludes Haver's channels forming necrotic bone and sequestra. It is also possible that the bacteria survive in latent forms, such as the Small Colony Variants (Proctor et al., 1998). In addition to the above, osteomyelitis often occurs in the context of the diabetic foot, with all its neuropathy and vascular compromise, or adjacent to foreign bodies, such as joint prostheses or internal fixation materials, where *S. aureus* can form a biofilm. Moreover, *S. aureus* osteomyelitis can be the source of sepsis and seeding of other organs. Given all those perils and limitations, it is easily understood how methicillin resistance can compromise the chances to cure such an infection, and is one of the reasons why in some centers vancomycin is routinely used as prophylaxis when inserting a joint prosthesis.

4.2.3. Lung Infections

Nosocomial pneumonia, which is associated with increased morbidity and mortality, is the second most common nosocomial infection (Emori & Gaynes, 1993). *S. aureus* not only predominates among Gram-positive etiologic agents, but has become the primary pathogen isolated from hospital–acquired respiratory infections in recent years (Fagon et al., 1998). This is true both for non-ICU and ICU pneumonias.

In the SENTRY study, almost 50% of lung *S. aureus* isolates were MRSA in the United States (Diekema et al., 2001). One should suspect MRSA even in a mild to moderate pneumonia, when particular risk factors are present, namely coma, head trauma, diabetes, and renal failure; or when severe disease occurs in a patient without risk factors after the fifth day in the hospital (American Thoracic Society, 1995). MRSA can also cause hematogenous pneumonia secondary to right-sided endocarditis, infected intravascular devices, or septic phlebitis. Moreover, acquisition of MRSA pneumonia outside the hospital can occur among nursing home residents or recently hospitalized individuals, when it follows an influenza infection (Bradley, 1999).

In the ICU, pneumonia and lower respiratory tract infections account for more than 50% of total infections, with a mortality rate of pneumonia ranging from 31% to 46% (Vincent et al., 1995). Although it is problematic to differentiate between infection and colonization when assessing lower respiratory tract culture results from intubated patients, it seems that *S. aureus* is the most common isolate—32% in a large cross-sectional survey (Albrich et al., 1999; Vincent et al., 1995). MRSA is more common in the ICU than in other areas of the hospital. In one study, risk factors for MRSA (as opposed to MSSA) pneumonia among mechanically ventilated patients included previous treatment with antibiotics, steroid use, prolonged mechanical ventilation prior to infection, history of chronic obstructive pulmonary disease, and older age. Furthermore, MRSA pneumonia resulted more frequently in bacteremia and septic shock, and mortality directly attributable to the pneumonia was significantly higher (Rello et al., 1994).

4.2.4. Bloodstream Infections

Bloodstream infections can be divided into primary bacteremia, secondary (to another focus of infection) bacteremia, and catheter colonization and infection. *S. aureus* bacteremia accounts for 50–87% of nosocomial bacteremias, with mortality rate from 16% to 43% (Conterno et al., 1998). The proportion of MRSA infections among them varies according to hospital prevalence of MRSA and to whether an outbreak is going on. Nevertheless, it has been suggested that MRSA bacteremias receive more often inadequate therapy than MSSA episodes, and that they carry a higher mortality risk, even when therapy is appropriate (Conterno et al., 1998). Whether this is due to the underlying conditions predisposing to MRSA infection rather than the nature of the bacteria itself is not clear. Case control studies of MRSA and MSSA bacteremia found no difference in mortality but longer hospital stay with MRSA infections (Cosgrove et al., 2001).

Endocarditis can be a cause of *S. aureus* bacteremia, and it is critical to differentiate between those two entities in an individual patient (Turnidge & Grayson, 1993). *S. aureus* is among the commonest pathogens isolated from both native and prosthetic valve endocarditis. MRSA endocarditis occurs in patients who are predisposed to introduce this bacterium into their circulation, such as hemodialysis patients, hospitalized patients with intravascular devices, and patients who have prosthetic valves. However, it has been most commonly encountered and studied among intravenous drug abusers, who often have right-sided endocarditis (Crane et al., 1986; Levine et al., 1991). In patient populations consisting exclusively or mainly of intravenous drug abusers, MRSA endocarditis resulted in a slower than expected rate of clearance of bacteremia (Levine et al., 1991). Furthermore, when compared to MSSA endocarditis that received the same treatment (vancomycin), MRSA endocarditis showed higher mortality and lower microbiologic response. Patients with right-sided MRSA disease did not have the favorable prognosis

($>$90% response) described in similar populations with MSSA disease (Gentry et al., 1997). Another factor that contributes to this inferior outcome is the lesser bactericidal activity of vancomycin against *S. aureus*, compared to penicillinase-resistant penicillins, such as nafcillin (Small & Chambers, 1990).

4.2.5. Toxin-Induced Syndromes (Staphylococcal Scalded Skin Syndrome, Toxic Shock Syndrome, and Enteritis)

Staphylococcal Scalded Skin Syndrome (SSSS) is a rare clinical entity usually seen in neonates and young children, which is caused by *S. aureus* strains producing exfoliative toxin A or exfoliative toxin B. There have been reports of MRSA causing SSSS, both in children and adults. Those strains produced Exfoliative Toxin or Toxic Shock Syndrome Toxin-1 (TSST-1) and enterotoxin (Ackland et al., 1999; Ansai et al., 2000; Farrel, 1999; Sakata, 2001). There have also been reports of MRSA strains producing TSST-1 and/or enterotoxin that colonized health care workers (Horikawa et al., 2001; Soares et al., 1997), or caused nosocomial infections accompanied by the characteristic syndromes (Kodama et al., 1997; Takahashi et al., 1998). These strains have mainly been reported from Japan.

A new clinical entity, also described in Japan, is termed Neonatal Toxic-shock-syndrome-like Exanthematous Disease (NTED). It is caused by MRSA producing TSST-1, and the affected neonates suffer, along with the MRSA infection or colonization, thrombocytopenia and an exanthem that does not fulfill criteria for toxic shock syndrome (it does not desquamate and it is not accompanied by shock), and resolves spontaneously (Okada et al., 2000; Takahashi et al., 1998, 2000).

4.3. Are MRSA More Virulent?

The association of MRSA infection with prolonged hospitalization, increased need for invasive interventions, and adverse outcomes, plus the fact that MRSA seem to add to *S. aureus* morbidity, pose the question if these strains are more virulent.

MRSA can survive in environments of increased antibiotic use (being usually resistant to many other agents in addition to β-lactams), where more seriously ill patients are found. Therefore, selective pressure favors the colonization of the most seriously ill and vulnerable with MRSA. Furthermore, adverse outcomes can sometimes be attributed to resistance to the original β-lactam regimen (Centers for Disease Control and Prevention, 1999; French et al., 1990), or to the fact that vancomycin is a less potent compound than penicillinase-resistant penicillins (Small & Chambers, 1990). In addition to that, severity of underlying illness or debility is a measure of the intensity of care requirements and frequency of contact with personnel, who potentially carry the MRSA (Luh et al., 2000). Moreover, Cosgrove et al. (2001) demonstrated in a retrospective study that MRSA bacteremia was associated with similar mortality compared to MSSA bacteremia, when they adjusted for confounding factors. In conclusion, there is no data to support the idea that MRSA might be more virulent than MSSA.

5. PREVENTION AND TREATMENT OF MRSA INFECTIONS

5.1. Prevention

5.1.1. The Benefits of Preventing MRSA Spread

MRSA have been a long-standing situation in many countries and hospitals. Since they are no more virulent than MSSA and vancomycin is available for their treatment, many have suggested that we accept them as part of the hospital flora and abandon special efforts to contain them, because these efforts are labor–intensive and costly. But there are many good reasons why containing the MRSA in a hospital should be attempted and why this containment, once achieved, should be maintained. First, the rate of nosocomial MRSA transmission is a good marker of the quality of infection control practices in a given hospital. Indeed, the measures used to control MRSA transmission are also effective against the transmission of other nosocomial multi-resistant pathogens (Eveillard et al., 2001), so an overall reduction in the rate of nosocomial infections can be anticipated (even more so because MRSA do not just replace MSSA, but they cause additional morbidity). Second, MRSA infections result in more prolonged hospital stay and more invasive interventions, thus increasing costs substantially. A third reason is that MRSA are usually resistant to many other classes of antimicrobials too, often limiting treatment options to vancomycin. In the European SENTRY study, 87% of MRSA were resistant to five or more antibiotic classes, compared to only 2% of MSSA. Furthermore, only 3% of MRSA were resistant to β-lactam antibiotics alone (Fluit et al., 2001). If MRSA are highly prevalent in an institution, empiric use of vancomycin increases, as well as vancomycin surgical prophylaxis in certain instances. Vancomycin has disadvantages compared to β-lactams, namely inferior efficacy, more toxicity, exclusively intravenous administration, and higher cost. Finally, extensive use of vancomycin selects for vancomycin-resistant strains of enterococci, CNS, and possibly for *S. aureus* strains with reduced susceptibility to vancomycin.

The costs of MRSA surveillance and control measures can be substantial. While the costs caused by the presence of MRSA in a hospital cannot be directly calculated, control programs have been studied in several hospitals. The amounts saved by their success in reducing MRSA infections have been calculated for the specific program in the given hospital or unit (Chaix et al., 1999; Herwaldt, 1999; Nettleman et al., 1991; Papia et al., 1999). Such programs, besides high cost-effectiveness, have also demonstrated that MRSA infections are preventable, meaning that it would be unethical not to try to prevent them. It is, therefore, the duty of the epidemiologist or infectious diseases expert or clinician to persuade hospital authorities that the proposed measures are feasible, efficacious, and cost-effective. Thus, necessary funding and resources for their implementation can be acquired.

5.1.2. Control Measures

5.1.2a. Surveillance.   The extent and location of the MRSA problem in a hospital must be known, if the kind and targeting of control measures is to be chosen. Since it is neither possible nor desirable to culture all patients at all times, selected high-risk populations and high-risk units should be the focus of surveillance. Frequent reviewing of routine microbiology laboratory results and applying the definitions of an outbreak (see p. 8 and Wenzel et al., 1998) is a method of keeping constant awareness, as well as deciding for further surveillance strategies. Some of these strategies that have often been proposed and successfully utilized are:

1. "Flagging" or otherwise locating and identifying patients known to carry MRSA from previous hospital admission, when they are readmitted or transferred to a different unit.
2. Maintaining a list of known MRSA cases in the hospital, along with their demographic characteristics, location, length of stay, sites of positive cultures, and antibiogram or other typing information. If the number of cases increases, this information can lead to probable sources of transmission (Boyce et al., 1994; Wenzel et al., 1998).
3. Screening all new admissions and transfers to high-risk units (Chaix et al., 1999), namely units where MRSA acquisition can be easy and/or disastrous. Such are the organ transplantation, orthopedic, cardiothoracic, and vascular surgery departments, the ICUs, and the burn unit (Rubinovitch & Pitet, 2001).
4. Prospective screening surveys in high-risk units at pre-set time intervals (Wenzel et al., 1991), or during an outbreak.
5. Screening high-risk patients (see Table 4.3) on admission.
6. Screening patient contacts of an index case (e.g., roommates or all patients in the same ICU) (Cohen et al., 1991; Wenzel et al., 1998).
7. Screening health care workers, if epidemiologically linked to a cluster of cases or an outbreak.
8. Routine surveillance cultures after decolonization/treatment of MRSA infection and discontinuation of any special precaution (Suh et al., 1998).

Various combinations and modifications of the above procedures can be adjusted to the particular needs and resources of each hospital, for example, screening all admissions

Table 4.3
Screening Recommendations for MRSA Carriage

Patient screening recommended	Consider patient screening
• Known previous MRSA carriage/disease	• Receiving care at home
• Not coming from home (coming from hospital, rehabilitation center, nursing home, etc.)	• Receiving treatment with injections
• Hospitalized in the past 6 months	• Intravenous drug abuse
• Frequent contact with the health care system in the past 2 years	• Coming from country or region with high MRSA prevalence
• Chronic wounds/ulcers and skin breaks in general	• Multiple antibiotic courses during the last year
	• Chronic prosthetic device (urinary catheter, gastrostomy, etc.)

to the hospital, or screening only high-risk patients on admission to a high-risk unit. Cultures of inanimate objects, such as equipment, gowns, surfaces, or foods, are not warranted, except for research purposes or in extraordinary circumstances, when there is epidemiological evidence of their role in the transmission of MRSA.

5.1.2b. Containment Measures. There are two general categories of measures against MRSA: those that prevent transmission, and those that eliminate the organism from an individual. The former are an indispensable component of any control program, while the latter can be part of an effort either to contain or to eradicate MRSA ("search and destroy" strategy). Eradication of MRSA can also be aimed at preventing an infection in the individual patient, while measures that hinder MRSA transmission may also be effective against other nosocomial pathogens.

No matter what combination of surveillance and containment measures one chooses to implement, cooperation of the hospital staff is indispensable. One cannot simply announce measures and expect the problem to be solved. A campaign must be undertaken to explain the correct infection control practices, for example, the correct technique of hand washing, as well as the rationale and necessity of their constant use. Education and feedback, namely informing staff of positive and negative changes of MRSA infection rates in their unit, have been proven highly effective, even when only the simplest measures were implemented (Nettleman et al., 1991). Observing and encouraging adherence to the measures, for instance through assigning an infection control nurse, is also desirable, and it leads to long-term compliance and sustaining of any success (Haley et al., 1995). Moreover, observation can reveal potential causes of failure or non- compliance to simple measures, preventing one from adding new, more complicated, and unnecessary procedures (Herwaldt, 1999). Nevertheless, blaming the staff of incorrectly applying or abandoning the measures is not enough; they may be facing problems which should be dealt with, such as overcrowding, understaffing, or shortage of appropriate material. In conclusion, healthcare workers should be educated, persuaded, constantly reminded, and assisted in applying any infection control measures. Any MRSA control project should take that aspect into account.

Measures that have been used to prevent MRSA transmission, and their features, are briefly listed and explained below:

Hand washing after each patient contact. Since the hands of personnel are the most important means of MRSA transmission, the significance of hand washing cannot be stressed enough. Compliance to hand washing is crucial in attaining and maintaining any positive result. Moreover, the success of some other measures is probably mediated, at least partly, by their reinforcing effect on hand washing. It should be accompanied, however, by moisturizing and good skin care, because frequently washed hands can suffer contact dermatitis, which favors MRSA colonization.

Rinsing hands with a chlorhexidine disinfectant solution or alcohol (CIDA-RINSE) gel after each patient contact. This measure is effective and can partly replace hand washing, which is more time-consuming, thereby increasing compliance to hand disinfection (Hugonnet et al., 2002; Parienti et al., 2002; Pittet, 2000).

Environmental cleaning. Contaminated surfaces are not an important source of MRSA transmission, so no special measures are warranted. On the other hand, good cleaning has been good hospital practice for almost a century, and it has been known for a long time to reduce the numbers of microbes in the environment.

Gloves for patient care.   Gloves provide a physical barrier and prevent soiling, but hands contamination occurs through intact gloves at the rate of 15% of contacts with MRSA colonized patients (Grundmann et al., 2002). Therefore, after each patient contact the hands must still be washed.

Gowns for patient care.   Transmission of MRSA through personnel clothes has not been documented. When soiling occurs or is expected, gowns should be changed regardless of patient MRSA status.

Masks when caring for patients with MRSA pneumonia or contaminated wounds. Air borne transmission of MRSA has not been documented, except in burn units. Masks can prevent health care workers from touching their nose with contaminated hands. Nevertheless, MRSA nasal carriage is usually transient among personnel, so the contribution of masks to preventing transmission should not be essential.

Cleaning of equipment after patient contact.   Stethoscopes, blood pressure cuffs, tourniquets, etc., should either not be shared or cleaned after they are used for an MRSA infected or colonized patient. Material that cannot be cleaned should not be shared.

Isolation room.   It is useful because it discourages staff and visitors from leaving without washing their hands, as well as sharing equipment between patients, but it is not available and practical in all hospitals. A more feasible alternative is placing MRSA patients together in the same room. If none of these is possible, at least one should avoid placing an MRSA patient next to a patient with open wounds, ostomies, or prosthetic devices (Mylotte, 1994). The same precautions should apply to candidates for high- risk surgery (organ transplantation or insertion of foreign materials). Again, MRSA transmission will not be avoided, if hands are not washed.

Cohorting.   Placing all MRSA patients of a unit to a separate area and dedicating equipment and staff exclusively to them is expensive (because of personnel needs), and requires a large number of such patients, usually in the setting of an outbreak (Darouiche et al., 1991). Nevertheless, it has been tried during outbreaks with varying success. It is certainly warranted (and feasible) in the ICU setting (Grundmann et al., 2002).

Strict isolation precautions.   They were tried in the early years of MRSA emergence. They were not more effective than simpler barrier precautions and they were very labor-intensive, often hampering patient care. Consequently, they were abandoned (Ribner et al., 1986).

Control of antibiotic use.   Prior use of antibiotics, especially broad-spectrum or in multiple courses, is a major risk factor for MRSA acquisition. Moreover, reducing the duration and antimocrobial spectrum of surgical prophylaxis has been shown to reduce the rate of MRSA infections (Brady et al., 1990; Fukatsu et al., 1997; Kusachi et al., 1999). Therefore, the results of rational and justified use of antibiotics should be beneficial in the long term. There are, however, certain settings, such as the ICU, where a reduction in antibiotic use appears difficult.

Decolonization of personnel.   Nasal colonization of personnel is usually transient, and special measures are not warranted. In the case, however, of a persistent carrier, who is epidemiologically linked to an outbreak, eliminating MRSA from that carrier can help ending the outbreak. Staff who receive decolonization treatment should be followed with cultures after its completion to ensure that it has been successful (at least three negative cultures one week apart from each other). Whether or not they should be removed from patient care during that time, remains controversial (Boyce et al., 1994; Mylotte, 1994).

Decolonization of patients. Except from measures that hinder MRSA transmission, thus indirectly reducing the burden of the organism in a hospital, one can pursue a direct reduction of this burden, by decolonizing all patients who carry MRSA. This approach necessitates the widespread use of antibiotics for eradication, which can promote resistance to the agents used. It should, therefore, be reserved for situations of an outbreak or when MRSA have become highly endemic (Boyce et al., 1994). Decolonization of patients can also be attempted when trying to eradicate newly introduced MRSA in a previously MRSA- free facility (Kotilainen et al., 2001). Arguments for attempting eradication from patients, however, include that reducing the burden of patient "reservoir" in hospitals or in the community may reduce the incidence of disease attributable to MRSA. Clearly more studies are needed in this area to clarify the role and cost-effectiveness of routine decolonization.

Topical agents and systemic regimens used to eradicate MRSA from a carrier are separately discussed below.

5.1.2c. Mupirocin.

Mupirocin, also called pseudomonic acid, is produced by submerged fermentation of Pseudomonas fluorescens. Its antibacterial spectrum includes staphylococci, streptococci, and some Gram-negative organisms. It acts by inhibiting bacterial IleS, thus blocking protein synthesis. Its mode of action and its structure are both unique, perhaps explaining the absence of cross-resistance with other classes of antibiotics. When it is administered systemically, it is rapidly converted to an inactive metabolite. These properties make mupirocin an ideal candidate for topical use. Indeed, after a special nasal formulation was released to the market, mupirocin was successfully used to eradicate nasal carriage of *S. aureus* from both health-care workers and patients during outbreaks. It was also demonstrated that intranasal mupirocin substantially reduced hand carriage of *S. aureus*, and that relapse (usually with a different strain) was delayed (Reagan et al., 1991), features desirable when managing an outbreak. Compared with systemic regimens, nasal mupirocin ointment 2% was found equally effective and easier to administer (Parras et al., 1995). No other agent has been found appropriate for topical use (Chow & Yu, 1989). Definitely, mupirocin is the agent of choice for nasal carriage eradication of both MSSA and MRSA (Hudson, 1994). It is usually applied twice daily for 5–7 days or three times daily for 3–7 days.

Besides controlling an outbreak or reducing high rates of endemic MRSA, intranasal mupirocin has also been used in patients at high risk of developing a systemic *S. aureus* infection as a preventive measure. Hemodialysis patients have long been known not only to have a high rate of nasal *S. aureus* carriage and to be at risk for subsequent *S. aureus* bacteremia, but also to be protected by systemic regimens that eradicate this carriage (Chow & Yu, 1989). In such a population, mupirocin treatment and maintenance (once to thrice weekly application) greatly decreases *S. aureus* bacteremia (Boelaert et al., 1991, 1993). However, this long-term use would likely encourage development of mupirocin resistant strains. Preventive mupirocin treatment was also successful in cardiothoracic surgery candidates, where it reduced postoperative sternotomy infections (Kluytmans et al., 1996). Nasal decolonization with mupirocin is also recommended when an infected central venous catheter with *S. aureus* is removed, prior to insertion of a new one (Mermel et al., 2001). However, such conclusions cannot be generalized. For example, in liver transplant candidates, nasal mupirocin not only did not reduce subsequent *S. aureus* infections, but most patients' colonization relapses were with MRSA, while previously colonized with

MSSA (Paterson et al., 2000). Further study is needed to determine prophylactic decolonization indications and contraindications in surgical candidates. A preoperative prophylactic measure that can be recommended, not only against MRSA (Brady et al., 1990), but any pathogen of wound infection, is a whole-body washing with a disinfectant soap. Another subset of patients that benefits from *S. aureus* decolonization is those who suffer recurrent superficial infections (furuncles, carbuncles, etc.), as a familial or idiopathic condition. Intranasal mupirocin in combination with disinfectant soap washings is highly efficacious (Leigh & Joy, 1993). Studying the potential benefits of *S. aureus* eradication for HIV patients has also been suggested (Nguyen et al., 1999), but these patients, especially when their immunocompromised state has progressed, will receive prophylactic regimens with antistaphylococcal activity (cotrimoxazole, azithromycin).

There is a paucity of randomized controlled studies with mupirocin for eradication of MRSA, however, and most of the data are based on observational studies. Recent controlled studies using mupirocin twice daily for 5 days, found no benefit over placebo (Harbarth et al., 1999). Further controlled studies are needed with longer duration of therapy (i.e., 10 days), alone or combined with systemic therapy.

There are also some restrictions to the use of mupirocin. One very important concern is the emergence of resistance. There are two distinct types of mupirocin resistance: low level and high level. Low level resistance (MIC: 6.25–256 mg/L) is conferred by a mutation of the IleS which is located on the chromosome. It emerges and spreads among MRSA shortly after the introduction of mupirocin to clinical use, mostly in patients who have repeatedly used mupirocin. It does not, however, preclude *S. aureus* elimination (especially with MIC $\leq$ 50 mg/L), because the local concentration of mupirocin is 20,000 mg/L (Watanabe et al., 2001). When eradication failure is encountered, other causes could be plausible, such as extranasal sites of colonization, re-acquisition of the same strain during hospitalization, or incorrect application of the ointment (nasal massage is recommended to facilitate penetration to the posterior nasopharynx) (Cookson, 1998). Despite this, low-level mupirocin resistance has indeed been associated with persistent carriage of MRSA (Harbarth et al., 2000). On the other hand, high-level mupirocin resistance (MIC > 256 mg/L) definitely means that the strain cannot be eradicated by mupirocin. This type of resistance is due to a novel IleS encoded by various plasmids, which can also carry other resistance determinants, such as for tetracycline, erythromycin, gentamicin, triclosan, etc. (Cookson, 1998; Pawa et al., 2000). It is rarely encountered, but it was found in 2.4% of MRSA in New Zealand, where mupirocin was made available without prescription (Hefferman et al., 1995). It is, therefore, apparent that mupirocin, being a valuable tool in containing MRSA outbreaks, should be preserved from resistance by targeted and judicious use. Prolonged, frequent, or indiscriminate use should be avoided, and susceptibility of *S. aureus*, and especially MRSA, should be monitored.

Another problem, which is closely associated to mupirocin resistance, is the colonization of extranasal sites. Mupirocin should not be used alone, when additional sites of *S. aureus* are suspected or documented, such as wounds, ostomies, throat, or anus, because failure (Harbarth et al., 2000) and subsequent development of resistance is threatened. In such patients mupirocin should be combined with a systemic regimen and/or disinfectant soap washings. Routine combination of intranasal mupirocin with a whole-body wash with disinfectant soap can also be recommended for optimal decolonization results. Decolonization should not, however, be attempted with any regimen, when there are colonized indwelling devices, such as a urinary catheter, endotracheal tube, etc., because the bacteria cannot be eliminated when they are protected in a biofilm (Jones et al., 2001; Pujol et al., 1996).

5.1.2d. Other Decolonization Agents. Besides mupirocin, two other kinds of treatment can be used for decolonization: whole-body washings with disinfectant soaps and systemically administered antibiotics.

Disinfectant soaps commonly used both for hand washing of hospital staff and whole-body washing of patients and staff carriers of *S. aureus* (usually MRSA) contain triclosan or chlorhexidine. They are applied in conjunction with a systemic course or with intranasal mupirocin (Leigh & Joy, 1993; Parras et al., 1995). They have also been successfully used as sole agents for decolonization and infection rate reduction in surgical patients (Bartzokas et al., 1984; Brady et al., 1990). About 1% triclosan has better activity against MRSA, while 4% chlorhexidine is better against Gram-negative bacteria (Faoagali et al., 1999). A recent concern, however, is the potential for development of resistance. Multi-resistant *S. aureus* strains have demonstrated low-level triclosan resistance, but its clinical significance remains unknown. Strains of both MRSA and MSSA with enhanced MICs to triclosan have also been isolated. Nevertheless, biocides act on multiple sites, rendering MICs of little value in assessing their bactericidal activity (Suller & Russell, 2000). Elevated MICs to chlorhexidine and the quarternary ammonium compounds among MRSA, in comparison to MSSA, have also been found, but they were still in the susceptible range (Suller & Russell, 1999). Thus, resistance of MRSA to disinfectants does not seem impending.

Extranasal sites' colonization with MRSA, particularly wounds and extensive skin lesions are a common source of persistent carriage and they cause mupirocin treatment to fail. In this case, a brief course of systemic antibiotics is warranted, combined with disinfectant soap washings, with or without mupirocin applied intranasally and on the affected lesions. Rifampin has shown the best results in eradicating *S. aureus* carriage, but resistance develops quickly. Therefore, a 5 days per os regimen containing rifampin in combination with another per os non-β-lactam agent, such as tetracycline, minocycline, cotrimoxazole, fusidic acid, or clindamycin is warranted in such patients (Arathoon et al., 1990; Chow & Yu, 1989; Darouiche et al., 1991; Kotilainen et al., 2001; Mulligan et al., 1992; Parras et al., 1995). Ciprofloxacin is not recommended, due to the high proportion of failure and the finding that its use predisposes to MRSA acquisition. The regimen should be tailored according to the susceptibilities of the hospital's MRSA and the side effects most anticipated and/or feared in the particular patient population.

In the face of mupirocin resistance development and eradication failures, other compounds and strategies are being investigated. Povidone–iodine cream, in comparison to mupirocin, is highly and rapidly bactericidal, but it is partly inactivated by nasal secretions. The balance between its antibacterial activity and its clearance by nasal secretions has to be studied further (Hill & Casewell, 2000). A different strategy, that of bacterial interference, that is, colonizing with one microbe in order to prevent colonization by another, was tried in the 1960s, using a less virulent strain of *S. aureus*, with some success. Occasional serious infections caused its abandonment (Kluytmans et al., 1997). The interest towards bacterial interference has recently been renewed by the observation that *Lactobacillus fermentum* hinders *S. aureus* adherence. Studies are underway to determine the mechanism and/or products of *Lactobacillus* which confer such protection (Strauss, 2000).

5.1.3. MRSA Containment in Special Settings

5.1.3a. MRSA in the Nursing Home.   There are certain differences between the population and mission of the nursing home as compared to the hospital. First of all, residents stay for prolonged periods of time and often require permanent devices, such as urinary catheters, or have chronic ulcers, creating thus a population that can serve as a constant reservoir of the organism and that cannot be decolonized. Second, the various barrier and isolation precautions that are applied in the hospital setting, such as cohorting and isolation rooms, are not practical in the nursing home and would compromise the quality of life of MRSA-colonized residents. A third consideration is that nursing home residents are not acutely ill and colonization is not expected to result in infection as often. Finally, nursing homes have limited resources to devote to infection surveillance and control measures.

Therefore, simple and efficient measures ought to be given priority, such as changing of gloves and hand washing after each patient contact, proper wound care and dressing, good housekeeping, and changing of gowns when soiling is expected. If the MRSA status of residents is known, such information should be used to determine baseline occurrence of infection and spot an outbreak, or to avoid transmission, for example, by placing a patient with large colonized wounds next to one with a prosthetic device. Empiric treatment of infections should also take into account such information. Surveillance cultures of residents and personnel are too costly and labor intensive to be recommended, except perhaps during an outbreak. Since antibiotic use is a major predisposing factor for MRSA acquisition (as well as for other multi-resistant pathogens), the need for their rational and judicious empiric use cannot be stressed enough. Culture-guided rather than empiric treatment of infections should be encouraged, with the dual benefit of optimal individual therapy (e.g., avoiding to treat MRSA infections with β-lactams) and of decreasing selection pressure by narrowing the spectrum of regimens.

Efforts of eradication of MRSA from such a facility are also too costly and too difficult to implement. Containment and prevention of transmission should rather be the goal. Additionally, measures that improve general and specific immunity and decrease susceptibility to infection should be vigorously pursued. These include adequate nutrition, optimal management of chronic conditions (e.g., care of neuropathic feet and prevention of decubitus ulcers), use of immunizing agents such as influenza vaccine, and limiting of invasive devices to those absolutely necessary for patient care.

5.1.3b. MRSA in the Burn Unit.   In a burn unit, MRSA can be found in the air or on inanimate objects in great numbers and can be transmitted through them in addition to the hands of personnel. Burn patients can be the source of an MRSA hospital outbreak, and permanent eradication can often be very difficult, especially when controlled ventilation is not available, because air-borne organisms can be the primary mode of transmission. The only way to stop an outbreak of MRSA in a burn unit seems to be to close it until all MRSA positive patients are discharged, and then terminally disinfect it. Additionally, colonized staff should be treated or removed. Continuous surveillance of new admissions is also necessary in order to prevent MRSA outbreaks.

5.1.3c. MRSA in the Neonatal ICU.   *S. aureus* infections' outbreaks have long been a problem in neonatal ICUs, but MRSA have significantly contributed to their morbidity.

Two main features of such outbreaks are that a single clone is usually responsible, and that patients are almost never colonized or infected upon admission, but acquire MRSA in the unit. These facts highlight the importance of adherence to standard infection control practices. They also explain why measures that limit hand-borne transmission, such as staff education, avoidance of overcrowding (i.e., adherence to guidelines for patient to staff and space ratios), hand washing, patient scrub bathing, and cohorting have usually been successful in terminating outbreaks (Farrington et al., 1990; Haley et al., 1995). Application of the triple dye to the umbilical stump after its catheterization has been proposed as an effective measure against an MRSA infection (Haley et al., 1995).

5.2. Treatment

When the MRSA rate in the particular hospital is very high, nosocomial severe infections suspected to be due to *S. aureus* should be empirically treated as MRSA, awaiting culture and sensitivity testing results. The same is true for community- acquired infections when the patient has risk factors (see Table 4.3). When blood stream isolates of *S. aureus* in a particular hospital or region are 10% or less due to MRSA, it is reasonable to use a β-lactamase-resistant penicillin for empiric treatment of *S. aureus* sepsis. However, there is no good data that delayed appropriate treatment of MRSA (namely initial empiric treatment with a β-lactam agent) increases mortality compared to early empirical treatment with vancomycin. Whether a regimen covering MRSA should be initiated in community-acquired severe *S. aureus* pediatric infections remains to be further studied.

5.2.1. Vancomycin

The drug of choice for systemic MRSA infections is vancomycin. Vancomycin has a half-life of 4–6 hr and the primary route of elimination is by glomerular filtration. It has a large volume of distribution, achieving adequate concentrations in ascitic, pericardial, pleural, and synovial fluids. It does not penetrate the meninges, except when they are inflamed, when CSF levels can reach ~20% of serum—but they vary. CSF levels of vancomycin are usually adequate (~25 μg/ml), but occasionally intrathecal administration of 4–20 mg/day may be necessary. Concentration in bile reaches 50% of serum. The usual adult daily dose is 30 mg/kg, divided in two doses—roughly 1 g every 12 hr. Depending on patient weight and severity of illness (e.g., meningitis) doses up to 1 g every 8 hr can be given when renal function is normal. Dose adjustment is necessary in the presence of renal insufficiency. Vancomycin is administered intravenously. The infusion should last 1 hr or more, in order to avoid the common side effect of head and neck flushing, with or without hypotension (known as the "red man syndrome"). When this occurs, administration can be safely resumed at a slower rate. The gastrointestinal tract does not absorb vancomycin; intramuscular administration results in severe pain at the injection site. In patients with continuous ambulatory peritoneal dialysis (CAPD), it can be given intraperitoneally (50 mg/L in the dialysate) and achieve therapeutic serum levels, enabling the treatment of CAPD-related Gram-positive infections via this route (but it can also cause peritoneal irritation) (Lundstrom & Sobel, 2000; Morse et al., 1987). Vancomycin is not removed by hemodialysis, but peritoneal dialysis can reduce serum levels by 35–40% (Lundstrom & Sobel, 2000).

The most common side effects are fever, chills, and phlebitis at the infusion site. Among vancomycin side effects, the "red man syndrome," which results from non-immunological histamine release, is also common, especially if the drug is infused quickly. Nephrotoxicity and ototoxicity (which is reversible and very rare) can also occur (Cantu et al., 1994). More commonly, when vancomycin is combined with an aminoglycoside, it can enhance the oto-toxicity and nephrotoxicity caused by these compounds. Reversible neutropenia can rarely occur after prolonged high-dose therapy. Skin rash is not uncommon.

Vancomycin is indicated for all systemic, life-threatening infections caused by MRSA, such as bacteremia and sepsis, endocarditis, osteomyelitis and arthritis, cellulitis, pneumonia, etc. Supurative foci should be removed, namely abscesses drained and foreign bodies removed. The duration of treatment is the same as with methicillin-susceptible *S. aureus*.

Regarding vancomycin use in surgical prophylaxis, it should be considered when the prevalence of MRSA and MRSE is high in the hospital and the results of an infection would be catastrophic (e.g., when prosthetic material is inserted). However, use of pro-phylactic vancomycin is not encouraged and has to be weighed against the risk of colo-nization and infection with vancomycin-resistant enterococci.

Susceptibility of *S. aureus*, and particularly MRSA, to any other antimicrobial except vancomycin cannot be taken for granted (Table 4.1). Sensitivity testing should validate their use as alternative treatment.

5.2.2. Teicoplanin

Teicoplanin, like vancomycin, is a glycopeptide antibiotic. Its mechanism of action and its antimicrobial spectrum are similar to vancomycin. Its pharmacokinetics, however, are different. It is not absorbed after per os administration, but intramuscular injection is well tolerated and absorption is quick. It is not significantly metabolized, and it is elimi-nated by glomerular filtration. Its half-life is 83–168 hr. It is significantly bound by serum proteins. Its penetration to tissues and fluids of interest in the treatment of serious infec-tions needs more study. The daily doses that are recommended vary between 6 and 15 mg/kg/day, while doses of less than 6 mg/kg/day have yielded inferior outcomes. Adjustment according to renal function is necessary (Lundstrom & Sobel, 2000). Loading doses of 12–15 mg/kg/day for up to 10 days, or 12 mg/kg every 12 hr for three doses have been utilized in most studies, followed by subsequent lesser doses for the rest of treatment. Satisfactory results have been obtained from the treatment of *S. aureus* endocarditis (12 mg/kg/day as monotherapy or 6 mg/kg/day in combinations), intravenous catheter bacteremia, skin and soft tissue infections (400 mg/day), acute and chronic osteomyelitis and septic arthritis (6 mg/kg/day after initial loading or continuous 12 mg/kg/day) (Grueneberg, 1997).

The safety profile of teicoplanin resembles that of vancomycin, with a few excep-tions: Intramuscular injection is well tolerated, the "red man syndrome" is rare, and drug fever is more common.

The pharmacokinetic and administration properties enable once daily intramuscular dosing. Thus, teicoplanin is an effective alternative to vancomycin when treating mild and

chronic MRSA infections, such as chronic osteomyelitis, because prolonged hospitalization and/or use of central venous lines is not necessary.

5.2.3. Linezolid

Linezolid belongs to oxazolidinones, compounds that inhibit protein synthesis by
inhibiting initiation complex formation in the bacterial ribosome. This mode of action is
different from any other antimicrobial agents'. There is, therefore, no cross-resistance with
other known compounds (Fines & Leclercq, 2000). Oxazolidinones are active against
Gram-positive cocci and other Gram-positive organisms, as well as some anaerobic bacteria. Of great interest is their activity against staphylococci, including MRSA and VISA,
penicillin-resistant *S. pneumoniae*, and vancomycin-resistant enterococci. The other
representative of this class is eperezolid, which is not approved for human use yet. In vitro
linezolid is bacteriostatic against *S. aureus*, and also inhibits expression of some of its virulence factors. Linezolid has activity in vitro and in animal models of severe infections
equivalent to that of vancomycin against *S. aureus* (Clemett & Markham, 2000; Hamel
et al., 2000). A moderate post-antibiotic effect is observed with most susceptible organisms (Munckhof et al., 2001).

The usual adult dose of linezolid is 600 mg twice daily (400 mg for skin infections),
and the pediatric dose is 10 mg/kg. It is rapidly and completely absorbed after oral administration. Plasma protein binding is low (31%) and volume of distribution is 50 L. It penetrates well into tissues and compartments, such as the CSF, the kidney and urine, bile,
synovial fluid and bone (Bouza & Munoz, 2001). Elimination half-life is 4.5–5.5 hr. It is
eliminated, mostly intact (small proportion metabolized by oxidation), by both the kidney
and liver. Metabolites accumulate with renal impairment, with unknown implications.
Dose adjustment in renal insufficiency and in mild to moderate liver disease is not needed.
Linezolid is removed by dialysis. Gastrointestinal side effects, headache and dizziness,
rash and reversible thrombocytopenia are common. Tongue discoloration and taste perver-
sion have also been observed (Bouza & Munoz, 2001). Dose-dependent reversible myelosuppression and acquired sideroblastic anemia have also been reported (Green & Maddox,
2001). Linezolid is a weak inhibitor of monoamine oxidase. Tyramine intake restriction is
not warranted (Antal et al., 2001), but the clinical significance of drug interactions is not
clarified yet (Bouza & Munoz, 2001; Hendershot et al., 2001).

Linezolid is an alternative to vancomycin for the treatment of MRSA infections,
such as uncomplicated and complicated skin and soft tissue infections, and nosocomial
pneumonia.

Since it has shown efficacy and safety comparable to that of vancomycin (Bouza &
Munoz, 2001; Rubinstein et al., 2001; Stevens et al., 2000), an important advantage of
linezolid is the ability to administer orally, which can reduce intravenous catheter use and
hospital stay (Li et al., 2001).

Resistance of MRSA to linezolid develops very slowly in vitro. It has also developed
in a patient after prolonged treatment of MRSA peritonitis without removal of the peritoneal dialysis catheter, and in several cases of enterococcal infection (Tsiodras et al.,
2001). A second linezolid resistant MRSA was recently described in a patient treated for
empyrmia, mutations and increasing resistance developed in a stepwise manner during
21 day therapy of a susceptible strain (Wilson et al., 2003). This is worrisome so soon

after marketing of the drug and raises the possibility of future increased resistance with more widespread use of this agent.

5.2.4. Quinupristin–Dalfopristin

The drug is composed of two semi-synthetic streptogramin molecules: quinupristin (a group B or type I streptogramin) and dalfopristin (a group A or type II streptogramin). The combination of the two in a 30/70 (w/w) mixture has synergistic antibacterial activity against many Gram-positive organisms, notably multi-resistant pathogens such as methicillin resistant staphylococci and vancomycin-resistant *Enterococcus faecium*. Its mechanism of action is through protein synthesis inhibition. Dalfopristin binding on the bacterial ribosome causes a conformational change that subsequently increases the binding of quinupristin. Thus, a stable drug-ribosome complex is created that inhibits protein synthesis. In vitro the drug is bactericidal against *S. aureus*, but is rendered bacteriostatic in the presence of constitutive MLS_B phenotype of resistance (quinupristin resistance) (Fuchs et al., 2001), which is not uncommon among MRSA. Resistance by MRSA is found 1–31% in surveys (Dowzicky et al., 1998, 2000; Luh et al., 2000). Prior use of streptogramin antibiotics in animal husbandry seems to be associated with resistant organisms (Hayes et al., 2001; Luh et al., 2000). MRSA have also been shown to exhibit tolerance to quinupristin–dalfopristin (higher MBC than MIC) (Sambatakou et al., 1998). Resistance of MRSA and vancomycin-resistant *E. faecium* also emerges during human use (Dowzicky et al., 2000), but staphylococci resistant to macrolides and lincosamides are commonly susceptible to quinupristin–dalfopristin. Mechanisms of resistance to both compounds must develop, in order to inactivate the combination (Dowzicky et al., 2000; Vanuffel & Cocito, 1996).

Quinupristin–dalfopristin is administered intravenously in an adult dose of 7.5 mg/kg every 8 hr. It undergoes non-enzymatic metabolism and the active metabolites are excreted through the gastrointestinal tract. Elimination half-life is 0.7–1.5 hr. No dose adjustment is needed for renal impairment. It is not removed by peritoneal dialysis. Hepatic insufficiency increases concentrations, but there are no specific recommendations for dose adjustment. Common side effects include infusion site reactions and thrombophlebitis, arthralgia and myalgia, gastrointestinal side effects, elevated hepatic enzymes, elevated conjugated bilirubin, and rash (Allington & Rivey, 2001). Thrombocytopenia and *Clostridium difficile* colitis have also been reported. Quinupristin–dalfopristin is an inhibitor of cytochrome P450 3A4 enzyme pathway and can, therefore, increase concentrations of agents that are metabolized by this enzymatic pathway, such as cyclosporine, diazepam, and many others (Allington & Rivey, 2001).

Quinupristin–dalfopristin has shown comparable efficacy and safety to vancomycin in the treatment of *S. aureus* catheter-related bacteremia, skin and soft tissue infections, and nosocomial pneumonia (Allington & Rivey, 2001). Good success rates against MRSA were also observed during compassionate use (patients intolerant of or failing all other treatment options) (Drew et al., 2000). It is, therefore, an acceptable alternative to vancomycin for treatment of MRSA infections.

Against MRSA, in vitro combinations of quinupristin–dalfopristin with cefepime, ceftazidime, imipenem, and piperacillin–tazobactam have shown antagonism (Fuchs et al., 2001). Combinations with ofloxacin and gentamicin were indifferent (Kang et al., 1997), while with vancomycin and ciprofloxacin both antagonism and synergism have been shown (Fuchs et al., 2001; Kang et al., 1997; Sambatakou et al., 1998). In vivo synergism with rifampin was shown against quinupristin-susceptible, but not quinupristin-resistant *S. aureus* (Zarrouk et al., 2001). Use of quinupristin–dalfopristin in combination with other compounds, cannot, therefore, be recommended.

5.2.5. Other Non-β-Lactam Antimicrobials

Rifampin has excellent antistaphylococcal activity and can also penetrate into tissues and leukocytes and kill intracellular organisms. Because resistance develops quickly, it is used in combination with the glycopeptides, as well as other drugs. Synergy has been demonstrated in vitro and in animal models of *S. aureus* infection with clindamycin, erythromycin, trimethoprim, and ciprofloxacin (Bamberger et al., 1991; Hackbarth et al., 1986). Addition of rifampin (300 mg every 8 hr per os—if MRSA is susceptible) to a 6 weeks vancomycin regimen is recommended when treating MRSA prosthetic valve endocarditis (Wilson et al., 1995), or other serious MRSA infections in the presence of foreign bodies that cannot be removed. This recommendation is based on animal data and experience from coagulase-negative staphylococci (Wilson et al., 1995). In native valve MRSA endocarditis, adding rifampin to vancomycin has not shown any clinical benefit (Levine et al., 1991).

Addition of gentamicin (1 mg/kg every 8 hr—if MRSA is susceptible) enhances nephrotoxicity and it should be limited to 3–5 days in cases of native valve endocarditis; two weeks are recommended in prosthetic valve endocarditis, based on animal experiments (Kobasa et al., 1983) and data from coagulase-negative staphylococcal prosthetic valve endocarditis (Wilson et al., 1995).

The addition of rifampin and gentamicin is also recommended when treatment of serious MRSA infections with vancomycin alone has failed (Fekety, 2000).

Cotrimoxazole and rifampin or doxycycline/minocycline with rifampin may be used for minor skin and soft tissue infections, and even for follow-up therapy for osteomyelitis, if the MRSA is known to be susceptible in vitro to both agents in the combination. We have had good results with these combined agents for minor and even moderate soft tissue infections (author's personal experience, unpublished data). At St. Michael Hospital, Toronto, Canada, from January to October 2001 (a 10 month period) there were 1138 *S. aureus* isolates (including screening for carriage) of which 189 (16.6%) were MRSA. However, only 12 (6.3%) were cultured from the bloodstream. Approximately, 95% were susceptible to tetracycline/doxycycline, 76.6% to cotrimoxazole, 71.8% to gentamicin, 94.1% to rifampin, 93.8% to fusidic acid, 88.8% to mupirocin, but only 6.3% were susceptible to clindamycin and 5.3% to ciprofloxacin (unpublished data).

The fluoroquinolones were initially active against *S. aureus*, but resistance develops quickly, especially among MRSA, both in vitro and in clinical practice. This is also true for the newer compounds (sparfloxacin, moxifloxacin, clinafloxacin, and levofloxacin) that have enhanced activity against Gram-positive cocci (Boos et al., 2001; Gilbert et al., 2001). They have better activity than older fluoroquinolones against MRSA for the time being.

Trimethoprim–sulfamethoxazole can treat mild susceptible MRSA infections as an alternative to vancomycin. For serious infections, it has been shown less effective than vancomycin (Markowitz et al., 1992).

6. VANCOMYCIN INTERMEDIATE-RESISTANT *S. AUREUS*

S. aureus strains against which vancomycin has a MIC of 8 or 16 mg/L are considered to be intermediately resistant (MICs equal or greater than 32 mg/L characterize resistance) according to U.S. and French criteria, while resistance is MIC ≥ 8 mg/L according to British and Japanese* criteria. These strains are also resistant to teicoplanin, and they are called VISA or GISA (glycopeptide intermediate resistant *S. aureus*). The term VISA is preferred because it points out the analogy with VRE (vancomycin resistant enterococci). The VISA strains are also methicillin-resistant and have been linked with clinical failures of vancomycin treatment (Fridkin, 2001; Tenover et al., 2001).

S. aureus strains with vancomycin MICs in the susceptible range (≤4, usually 1–4 mg/L) that contain cells that grow on brain–heart infusion screening agar (contains vancomycin, usually 4–6 μg/ml) are termed hetero-VISA. Many of these strains have been identified in retrospect from collections of MRSA and their clinical significance is unknown. For that reason, hetero-VISA need not be reported (Fridkin, 2001; Tenover et al., 2001).

VISA strains cannot be detected by disc diffusion methods. Depending on local needs and resources, laboratories should use a screening procedure, for example, vancomycin-containing agar, to test all *S. aureus* or all MRSA isolates; or *S. aureus* with vancomycin MIC ≥ 4 should be subjected to confirmatory testing (Fridkin, 2001; Tenover et al., 2001). A MIC susceptibility testing method is necessary to confirm VISA. E-test on brain–heart infusion agar with 2.0 McFarland inoculum with vancomycin and teicoplanin strips gives the best specificity and sensitivity (Walsh et al., 2001). When colonies grow on vancomycin-containing agar, the MIC of the parent strain (and not of these colonies) should be reported.

VISA strains have been reported from Japan, the United States, United Kingdom, France and Germany (Tenover et al., 2001). They seem to be overall very rare, although few systematic surveillance data exist. In Japan, where they were first described, they have not disseminated (Ike et al., 2001). Between 1995 and 1997, *S. aureus* bloodstream isolates from U.S. hospitals with a vancomycin MIC of 4 mg/L (susceptibility breakpoint) rose from 0% to 0.4%, perhaps indicating a trend (Sahm et al., 1999). VISA have been linked with clinical failures of vancomycin therapy, usually in patients with the following characteristics or potential risk factors: dialysis, prolonged central venous line (or other foreign body) infection with MRSA, and prolonged administration of vancomycin (Boyle-Vavra et al., 2001a; Tenover et al., 2001). A case of VISA emerging during exclusively oral administration of vancomycin has also been described (Paton et al., 2001). The VISA strains were resistant to many antimicrobials, including methicillin. In many instances, the VISA strain seemed to have developed from the MRSA that was persistently infecting the patient (Boyle-Vavra et al., 2001a; Paton et al., 2001; Tenover et al., 2001). Evolution of a clinical VISA isolate from hetero-VISA has also been shown (Chesneau et al., 2000).

Hetero-VISA have been reported from many countries after retrospective testing of MRSA isolates (Tenover et al., 2001). Methicillin susceptible hetero-VISA has also been

---

* Strains that grow on brain–heart infusion screening agar containing 4 μg/ml vancomycin and have a vancomycin MIC ≥ 8 mg/L are termed vancomycin-resistant by Japanese investigators.

described (Bobin-Dubreux et al., 2001). They seem to have disseminated in French hospitals during the late 1990s (0.6% of *S. aureus* in one survey) (Chesneau et al., 2000; Guerin et al., 2000; Reverdy et al., 2001). The clinical significance of heterogeneous intermediate vancomycin resistance is unknown, but the potential of being a precursor to homogeneous intermediate resistance is alarming.

The mechanism of resistance to glycopeptides does not seem to be the same in the different VISA isolates from around the world, as changes in their peptidoglycan composition are not uniform (Boyle-Vavra et al., 2001b). The *van* genes that confer vancomycin resistance to enterococci have not been found in staphylococci. Studies of the prototype Japanese VISA strain have shown increased cell wall thickness and increased cell wall turnover, increased production of PBP 2 and 2a (Hanaki et al., 1998), and decreased production of PBP 4 (Finan et al., 2001). Other VISA strains have shown absence of PBP 4 and decreased cell wall cross-linking (Finan et al., 2001), or increased cross-linking (Boyle-Vavra et al., 2001a). Increased cell wall thickness (a common feature of many VISA strains) and decreased cross-linking are ways of trapping more vancomycin molecules on D-alanyl-D-alanine residues in the peptidoglycan before they reach their site of action below the peptidoglycan, where its synthesis takes place (Hiramatsu, 2001). Multiple mechanisms of vancomycin resistance seem to be emerging all around the world as a response to selective pressure from the use of the antibiotic.

Regarding hetero-VISA, it has been observed that broad-spectrum cephalosporin pressure, which can convert hetero- to homo-resistance to methicillin, can also produce hetero-VISA (Hiramatsu, 2001).

Because VISA could spread as easily as MRSA did in the past, and because they represent a major threat, infection control measures with the aim of quick detection and eradication are warranted. Judicious use of vancomycin is even more important, because they currently seem to "emerge" rather than "spread," probably from a background of multiply resistant MRSA that have developed some degree of heterogeneous intermediate resistance to vancomycin.

In terms of therapeutic options, VISA have usually had a susceptibility profile of multiresistant MRSA. The recently approved linezolid and quinupristin–dalfopristin are valuable options to treat such infections. Nevertheless, MRSA strains resistant to quinupristin–dalfopristin from the European SENTRY study were also hetero-VISA (Werner et al., 2001). Therefore, one should not forget that resistance to these compounds is already developing. The arms race with *S. aureus* is continuing, and, as always, prevention is better (more desirable, more feasible, and less expensive) than cure.

7. VANCOMYCIN RESISTANT *S. AUREUS*

As of June 2002, eight patients with clinical infections caused by VISA have been confirmed in the United States, and the first vancomycin-resistant *S. aureus* (VRSA) (vancomycin MIC $\geq$ 32 μg/ml) was reported (Sievert et al., 2002). In April 2002, a patient with diabetes, peripheral vascular disease, and chronic renal failure underwent amputation of a gangrenous toe and subsequently developed MRSA bacteremia from an infected arteriovenous hemodialysis graft. The infection was treated with vancomycin, rifampin, and removal of the infected graft. In June, cultures of an infected dialysis catheter tip and exit site grew *S. aureus* resistant to oxacillin (MIC $\geq$ 16 μg/ml) and vancomycin (MIC $\geq$ 128 μg/ml). The isolate contained the *van A* vancomycin resistance gene from enterococci and the oxacillin-resistance gene *mecA*. The isolate was susceptible to champherical, line-zolid, minocycline, tetracycline, quinupristin-dalfopristin, and trimethoprim/sulfamethoxazole.

The presence of *van A* in this VRSA suggests that the resistance determinant might have been acquired through exchange of genetic material from a vancomycin-resistant enterococcus. To date, there has been no documented spread of this microorganism to other patients or health care workers, but it is likely that more reports of VRSA will be forth-coming in the near future.

8. FUTURE DIRECTIONS

The increasing resistance of Gram-positive pathogens has prompted the search for new compounds active against them and renewed interest in the modification of old. New glycopeptides and higher doses of vancomycin are under in vitro study for VISA (Aeschliman et al., 2000). Daptomycin is a lipopeptide antibiotic that interferes with cell membrane transport. It has shown activity and pharmacodynamic properties against MRSA comparable to that of vancomycin in vitro, in vivo, and in two small human stud-ies (Akins & Rybak, 2001; Kaatz et al., 1990; Rybak et al., 1992). A novel minocycline derivative (a glycylcycline) has also shown good in vitro activity against MRSA (Patel et al., 2000).

New classes of antimicrobials are also being developed. Evernimicin belongs to everninomycins, a novel class of oligosaccharide compounds. Its mode of action is to block protein synthesis initiation by interacting with the 23S ribosomal RNA. Its binding site is different from that of other antibiotics that target the ribosome (Belova et al., 2001). It is highly active against MRSA in vitro and bacteriostatic in vivo (Boucher et al., 2001; Jones et al., 2001). The hetero-aromatic polycycles (HARP) are compounds that bind to ds-DNA and block replication and transcription. They display activity against Gram-positive pathogens (Burli et al., 2001; Ge et al., 2001).

Natural antibacterial substances are also under investigation. Small cationic peptides derived from the skin of frogs (the temporin A analogs and others) can disrupt cell mem-brane barriers and have shown anti-staphylococcal activity (Mangoni et al., 2000; Wade et al., 2000). Likewise, a unique antibacterial peptide termed dermcidin was found in the human sweat; interestingly, it is slightly anionic. It displays anti-staphylococcal activity (Schittek et al., 2001). These natural peptides may play a role against colonization and/or infection with *S. aureus*. Since they already exist in nature, one can hope that development of resistance to these peptides will not be easy.

Because *S. aureus* has exhibited a remarkable ability to acquire resistance, other strategies, besides developing new drugs, are needed. Prevention of colonization would be an attractive means of reducing nosocomial infections due to *S. aureus*, and particularly due to MRSA, since it is already known which patients are at risk. Bacterial interference can be achieved by colonizing with one microbe in order to prevent colonization by another. It has been observed that *Lactobacillus fermentum* hinders *S. aureus* adherence.

It would be interesting to determine the mechanism and/or products of *Lactobacillus* which confer such protection (Strauss, 2000). Another interesting experimental anticolonization strategy is the use of cell wall hydrolases produced by bacteriophages: because they are specific for the host of the phage, they would not interfere with normal flora (Nelson et al., 2001). So far, they have only been studied against streptococci, but they have a broad antibacterial potential (Nelson et al., 2001).

Development of a vaccine against *S. aureus* has been a goal for decades. Candidate targets for vaccines that have shown some protection in animals are: (1) *S. aureus* adhesins, such as fibronectin-binding protein, fibrinogen-binding protein, collagen-binding protein (Lee, 1998; Rennermalm et al., 2001), and capsular polysaccharides (Burgeot et al., 2001; Lee, 1998; Mckenney et al., 2000), (2) RNAIII-activating protein (RNAIII is a regulatory RNA molecule that controls many virulence factors) (Balaban et al., 1998), and (3) The *mecA* gene, in an effort to target specifically MRSA (Ohwada et al., 1999). A vaccine consisting of conjugated capsular polysaccharides type 5 and type 8 (85% of *S. aureus* infections, including most MRSA and VISA) reduced by 57% *S. aureus* infections in hemodialysis patients for 10 months, after which protection and antibody levels waned. Addition of a newly described type 336 polysaccharide is expected to increase efficacy (Shinefield et al., 2002).

Regarding MRSA infection prevention and treatment, a number of issues need to be clarified. The role of screening and eradicating MRSA from contacts of patients in the household and in other settings, such as daycare, dormitory, and the like, in order to prevent spread in the community, needs to be urgently explored. Spread of MRSA in some communities has already occurred, and an outbreak of skin and soft tissue infections in a prison was recently reported (Centers for Disease Control, 2001). Furthermore, because MRSA have varying susceptibility profiles, and the efficacy of glycopeptides may soon cease to be certain, the role of various combinations of antistaphylococcal compounds in serious infections should be investigated.

References

Ackland, K. M., Darvay, A., Griffin, C., Aali, S. A., & Russel-Jones, R. (1999). Staphylococcal scalded skin syndrome in an adult associated with methicillin-resistant *Staphylococcus aureus*. *Br J Dermatol, 140,* 518–520.

Adcock, P. M., Pastor, P., Medley, F., Patterson, J. E., & Murphy, T. V. (1998). Methicillin-resistant *Staphylococcus aureus* in two child care centers. *J Infect Dis, 178,* 577–580.

Aeilts, G. D., Sapico, F. L., Ganawati, H. N., Malik, G. M., & Montgomerie, J. Z. (1982). Methicillin-resistant *Staphylococcus aureus* colonization and infection in a rehabilitation facility. *J Clin Microbiol, 16,* 218–223.

Aeschliman, J. R., Allen, G. P., Hershberger, E., & Rybak, M. J. (2000). Activities of LY333328 and vancomycin administered alone or in combination with gentamicin against three strains of vancomycin-intermediate *Staphylococcus aureus* in an in vitro pharmacodynamic infection model. *Antimicrob Agents Chemother, 44,* 2991–2998.

Aires de Sousa, M., Miragaia, M., Santos Sanches, I., Avila, S., Adamson, I., Casagrande, S. T., Brandileone, M. C. C., Palacio, R., Dell'Aqua, L., Hortal, M., Camou, T., Rossi, A., Velasquez-Meza, M. E., Echaniz-Avilles, G., Solorzano-Santos, F., Heitmann, I., & de Lencastre, H. (2001).

Three-year assessment of methicillin-resistant *Staphylococcus aureus* clones in Latin America from 1996 to 1998. *J Clin Microbiol, 39,* 2197–2205.

Akins, R. L., & Rybak, M. J. (2001). Bactericidal activities of two daptomycin regimens against clinical strains of glycopeptide-intermediate resistant *Staphylococcus aureus*, vancomycin-resistant *Enterococcus faecium*, and methicillin-resistant *Staphylococcus aureus* isolates in an in vitro pharmacodynamic model with simulated endocardial vegetations. *Antimicrob Agents Chemother, 45,* 454–459.

Albrich, W. C., Angstwurm, M., Bader, L., & Gaertner, R. (1999). Drug resistance in Intensive Care Units. *Infection, 27*(Suppl. 2), S19–S22.

Alghaithy, A. A., Bilal, N. E., Gebedou, M., & Weily, A. H. (2000). Nasal carriage and antibiotic resistance of *Staphylococcus aureus* isolates from hospital and non-hospital personnel in Abha, Saudi Arabia. *Trans R Soc Trop Med Hyg, 94,* 504–507.

Allington, D. R., & Rivey, M. P. (2001). Quinupristin/dalfopristin: A therapeutic review, *Clin Ther, 23,* 24–44.

Amagai, M., Matsuyoshi, N., Wang, Z. H., Andl, C., & Stanley, J. R. (2000). Toxin in bullous impetigo and staphylococcal scalded-skin syndrome targets desmoglein 1. *Nature Med, 6,* 1275–1277.

American Thoracic Society Consensus Statement. (1995). Hospital-acquired pneumonia in adults: Diagnosis, assessment of severity, initial antimicrobial therapy and preventive strategies. *Am J Respir Crit Care Med, 153,* 1711–1725.

Anonymous. (1999). Methicillin resistance in *Staphylococcus aureus* isolated from blood in England and Wales: 1994 to 1998. *Commun Dis Rep CDR Weekly, 9,* 65–68.

Ansai, S. I., Shimauki, T., Uchino, H., Nakamura, C., & Arai, S. (2000). Staphylococcal scalded skin syndrome with prosthetic valve endocarditis. *Eur J Dermatol, 10,* 630–632.

Antal, A. J., Hendershot, P. E., Batts, D. H., Sheu, W. P., Hopkins, N. K., & Donaldson, K. M. (2001). Linezolid, a novel oxazolidinone antibiotic: Assessment of monoamine oxidase inhibition using pressor response to oral tyramine. *J Clin Pharmacol, 41,* 552–562.

Arakawa, Y., Ike, Y., Nagasawa, M., Shibata, N., Doi, Y., Shibayama, K., Yagi, T., & Kurata, T. (2000). Trends in antimicrobial-drug resistance in Japan. *Emerging Infect Dis, 6,* 572–575.

Arathoon, E. G., Hamilton, J. R., Hench, C. E., & Stevens, D. A. (1990). Efficacy of short courses of oral novobiocin-rifampin in eradicating carrier state of methicillin-resistant *Staphylococcus aureus* and *in vitro* killing studies of clinical isolates. *Antimicrob Agents Chemother, 34,* 1665–1659.

Archer, G. L., & Niemeyer, D. M. (1994). Origin and evolution of DNA associated with resistance to methicillin in staphylococci. *Trends Microbiol, 2,* 343–347.

Archer, G. L., & Pennell, E. (1990). Detection of methicillin resistance in staphylococci by using a DNA probe. *Antimicrob Agents Chemother, 34,* 1720–1724.

Archibald, L., Phillips, L., Monnet, D., McGowan, J. E., Tenover, F., & Gaynes, R. (1997). Antimicrobial resistance in isolates from inpatients and outpatients in the United States: Increasing importance of the intensive care unit. *Clin Infect Dis, 24,* 211–215.

Balaban, N., Goldkorn, T., Nhan, R. T., Dang, L. B., Scott, S., Ridgley, R. M., Rasooly, A., Wright, S. C., Larrick, J. W., Rasooly, R., & Carlson, J. R. (1998). Autoinducer of virulence as a target for vaccine and therapy against *Staphylococcus aureus. Science, 280,* 438–440.

Bamberger, D. M., Fields, M. T., & Herndon, B. L. (1991). Efficacies of various antimicrobial agents in treatment of *Staphylococcus aureus* abscesses and correlation with in vitro tests of antimicrobial activity and neutrophil killing. *Antimicrob Agents Chemother, 35,* 2335–2339.

Bartzokas, C. A., Paton, J. H., Gibson, M. F., Graham, R., McLoughlin, G. A., & Croton, R. S. (1984). Control and eradication of methicillin-resistant *Staphylococcus aureus* on a surgical unit. *N Engl J Med, 311,* 1422–1425.

Belova, L., Tenson, T., Xiong, L., McNicholas, P. M., & Mankin, A. S. (2001). A novel site of antibiotic action in the ribosome: Interaction of evernimicin with the large ribosomal subunit. *Proc Natl Acad Sci USA, 98,* 3726–3731.

Ben Hassen, A., Bouabdallah, F., Ben Abdallah, T., Matri, A., Ben Maiz, H., & Ben Redjeb, S. (1995). Methicillin resistant *Staphylococcus aureus*. Decreased incidence in a medical resuscitation unit at C. H. U. Charles-Nicolle in Tunis. *Bull Soc Pathol Exot, 88*, 257–259 (abstract at: http://www.ncbi.nlm.nih.gov/entrez/query.fcgi?cmd=Retrieve&db=Pubmed&list_uids=864).

Blanche, F., Cameron, B., Bernard, F. X., Maton, L., Macse, B., Ferrero, L., Ratet, N., Lecoq, C., Goniot, A., Bisch, D., & Crouzet, J. (1996). Differential behaviors of *Staphylococcus aureus* and *Escherichia coli* type II DNA topoisomerases. *Antimicrob Agents Chemother, 40*, 2714–2720.

Bobin-Dubreux, S., Reverdy, M. E., Nervi, C., Rougier, M., Bolmstrom, A., Vandenesch, F., & Etienne, J. (2001). Clinical isolate of vancomycin-heterointermediate *Staphylococcus aureus* susceptible to methicillin and in vitro selection of a vancomycin-resistant derivative. *Antimicrob Agents Chemother, 45*, 349–352.

Boelaert, J. R., De Baere, Y. A., Geenaert, M. A., Godard, C. A., & Van Landuyt, H. W. (1991). The use of nasal mupirocin ointment to prevent *Staphylococcus aureus* bacteraemias in haemodialysis patients: An analysis of cost-effectiveness. *J Hosp Infect, 19*(Suppl. B), 41–46.

Boelaert, J. R., Van Landuyt, H. W., Godard, C. A., Daneels, R. F., Schurgers, M. L., Matthys, E. G., De Baere, Y. A., Gheyle, D. W., Gordts, B. Z., & Herwaldt, L. A. (1993). Nasal mupirocin ointment decreases the incidence of *Staphylococcus aureus* bacteraemias in haemodialysis patients. *Nephrol Dial Transplant, 8*, 235–239.

Boos, M., Mayer, S., Fischer, A., Koehrer, K., Scheuring, S., Heisig, P., Verhoef, J., Fluit, A. C., & Schmitz, F. J. (2001). In vitro development of resistance to six quinolones in *Streptococcus pneumoniae, Streptococcus pyogenes*, and *Staphylococcus aureus*. *Antimicrob Agents Chemother, 45*, 938–942.

Boucher, H. W., Thauvin-Eliopoulos, C., Loebenberg, D., & Eliopoulos, G. M. (2001). In vivo activity of evernimicin (SCH 27899) against methicillin-resistant *Staphylococcus aureus* in experimental infective endocarditis. *Antimicrob Agents Chemother, 45*, 208–211.

Bouza, E., & Munoz, P. (2001). Linezolid: Pharmacokinetic characteristics and clinical studies. *Clin Microbiol Infect, 7*(suppl. 4), 75–82.

Boyce, J. M. (1992). Methicillin-resistant *Staphylococcus aureus* in hospitals and long-term care facilities: Microbiology, epidemiology, and preventive measures, Special Review. *Infect Contr Hosp Epidemiol, 13*, 725–737.

Boyce, J. M. (1998). Editorial comment: Are the epidemiology and microbiology of methicillin-resistant *Staphylococcus aureus* changing? *JAMA, 279*, 623–624.

Boyce, J. M., Jackson, M. M., Pugliese, G., Batt, M. D., Fleming, D., Garner, J. S., Hartstein, A. I., Kauffman, C. A., Simmons, M., Weinstein, R., O'Boyle Williams, C., & the AHA Technical Panel on Infections Within Hospitals. (1994). Methicillin-resistant *Staphylococcus aureus* (MRSA): A briefing for acute care hospitals and nursing facilities. *Infect Contr Hosp Epidemiol, 15*, 105–115.

Boyce, J. M., White, R. L., & Spruill, E. Y. (1983). Impact of methicillin-resistant *Staphylococcus aureus* on the incidence of nosocomial infections. *J Infect Dis, 148*, 763–767.

Boyle-Vavra, S., Carey, R. B., & Daum, R. S. (2001a). Development of vancomycin and lysostaphin resistance in a methicillin-resistant *Staphylococcus aureus* isolate. *J Antimicrob Chemother, 48*, 617–625.

Boyle-Vavra, S., Labischinski, H., Ebert, C. C., Ehlert, K., & Daum, R. S. (2001b). A spectrum of changes occurs in peptidoglycan composition of glycopeptide-intermediate clinical *Staphylococcus aureus* isolates. *Antimicrob Agents Chemother, 45*, 280–287.

Bradley, S. F. (1999). Methicillin-resistant *Staphylococcus aureus*: Long-term care concerns. *Am J Med, 106*(Suppl. 5A), 2S–10S.

Bradley, S. F., Terpenning, M. S., Ramsey, M. A., Zarins, L. T., Jorgensen, K. A., Schaberg, D. R., & Kauffman, C. A. (1991). Methicillin-resistant *Staphylococcus aureus*: Colonization and infection in a long-term care facility. *Ann Intern Med, 148*, 417–422.

Brady, L. M., Thomson, M., Palmer, M. A., & Harkness, J. L. (1990). Successful control of endemic MRSA in a cardiothoracic surgical unit. *Med J, 152*, 240–245.

Burgeot, C., Gilbert, F. B., & Poutrel, B. (2001). Immunopotentiation of *Staphylococcus aureus* type 5 capsular polysaccharide co-entrapped in liposomes with α-toxin. *Vaccine, 19*, 2092–2099.

Burli, R., Taylor, M., Ge, Y., Baird, E., Touami, S., & Moser, H. (2001). HARP: A novel class of antibiotics, 41st Annual Interscience Conference on Antimicrobial Agents and Chemotherapy (Chicago 2001), Abstract No. 1685, p. 241.

Cantu, T. G., Yamanaka-Yuen, N. A., & Lietman, P. S. (1994). Serum vancomycin concentrations: Reappraisal of their clinical value. *Clin Infect Dis, 18*, 533–543.

Carbon, C. (1999). Costs of treating infections caused by methicillin-resistant staphylococci and vancomycin-resistant enterococci. *J Antimicrob Chemother, 44*, 31–36.

Centers for Disease Control and Prevention. (1999). Four pediatric deaths from community-acquired methicillin-resistant *Staphylococcus aureus*—Minnesota and North Dakota, 1997–1999. *JAMA, 282*, 1123–1125.

Centers for Disease Control and Prevention. (2001). Methicillin-resistant *Staphylococcus aureus* skin and soft tissue infections in a state prison—Mississippi 2000. *MMWR Morb Mortal Wkly Rep, 50*, 919–922.

Chaix, C., Durand-Zaleski, I., Alberti, C., & Brun-Buisson, C. (1999). Control of endemic methicillin-resistant *Staphylococcus aureus*: A cost-benefit analysis in an intensive care unit. *JAMA, 282*, 1745–1751

Chalmers, R. T. A., Wolfe, J. H. N., Chesire, N. J. W., Stansby, G., Nicolaides, A. N., Mansfield, A. O., & Barrett, S. P. (1999). Improved management of infrainguinal bypass graft infection with methicillin-resistant *Staphylococcus aureus*. *Br J Surg, 86*, 1433–1436.

Chambers, H. F. (1993). Detection of methicillin resistant staphylococci. *Infect Dis Clin North Am, 7*, 425–433.

Chambers, H. F. (1997). Methicillin resistance in Staphylococci: molecular and biochemical basis and clinical implications. *Clin Microbiol Rev, 10*, 781–791.

Chambers, H. F. (2000). Penicillins. In G. L. Mandell, J. A. Bennett, & R. Dolin (Eds.), *Principles and practice of infectious diseases* (5th ed., Vol. 1, pp. 261–262). Philadelphia: Churchill Livingston.

Chambers, H. F. (2001). The changing epidemiology of *Staphylococcus aureus? Emerging Infect Dis, 7*, 178–182.

Chambers, H. F., Sachdeva, M. J., & Hackbarth, C. J. (1994). Kinetics of penicillin binding to penicillin binding proteins of *Staphylococcus aureus*. *Biochem J, 301*, 139–144.

Charlebois, E. D., Bangsberg, D. R., Moss, N., & Perdreau-Remington, F. (2000). Community prevalence of resistant *Staphylococcus aureus*, 40th Interscience Conference on Antimicrobial Agents and Chemotherapy (Toronto 2000), Abstract No. 160, p. 70.

Chesneau, O., Morvan, A., & El Solh, N. (2000). Retrospective screening for heterogeneous vancomycin resistance in diverse *Staphylococcus aureus* clones disseminated in French hospitals. *J Antimicrob Chemother, 45*, 887–890.

Chien, J. W., Kucia, M. L., & Salata, R. A. (2000). Use of linezolid, an oxazolidinone, in the treatment of multidrug-resistant Gram-positive bacterial infections. *Clin Infect Dis, 30*, 146–151.

Chow, J. W., & Yu, V. L. (1989). *Staphylococcus aureus* nasal carriage in hemodialysis patients. *Arch Intern Med, 149*, 1258–1262.

Clemett, D., & Markham, A. (2000). Linezolid. *Drugs, 59*, 815–827.

Cocito, C., Di Giambatista, M., Nyssen, E., & Vanuffel, P. (1997). Inhibition of protein synthesis by streptogramins and related antibiotics. *J Antimicrob Chemother, 39*(Suppl. A), 7–13.

Cohen, S. H., Morita, M. M., & Bradford, M. (1991). A seven-year experience with methicillin-resistant *Staphylococcus aureus*. *Am J Med, 91*(Suppl. 3B), 233–237.

Conterno, L. O., Wey, S. B., & Castelo, A. (1998). Risk factors for mortality in *Staphylococcus aureus* bacteremia. *Infect Contr Hosp Epidemiol, 19*, 32–37.

Cookson, B. D. (1998). The emergence of mupirocin resistance: a challenge to infection control and antibiotic prescribing practice. *J Antimicrob Chemother, 41*, 11–18.

Cormican, M. G., & Jones, R. N. (1996). Emerging resistance to antimicrobial agents in Gram-positive bacteria. *Drugs, 51*(Suppl. 1), 6–12.

Cosgrove, S. E., Qi, Y., Kaye, K. S., Harbarth, S., Karchmer, A. W., & Carmeli, I. (2001). The impact of methicillin resistance in *Staphylococcus aureus* bacteremia on patient outcomes: Mortality, length of stay, and hospital charge, 41st Annual Interscience Conference on Antimicrobial Agents and Chemotherapy (Chicago 2001), Abstract No. 1686, p. 415.

Crane, L. R., Levine, D. P., Zervos, M. J., & Cummings, G. (1986). Bacteremia in narcotic addicts at the Detroit Medical Center. I. Microbiology, epidemiology, risk factors, and empiric therapy. *Rev Infect Dis, 8*, 364–373.

da Silva Coimbra, M. V., Teixeira, L. A., Ramos, R. L., Predari, S. C., Castello, L., Famiglietti, A., Vay, C., Klan, L., & Figueiredo, A. M. (2000). Spread of the Brazilian epidemic clone of a multi-resistant MRSA in two cities in Argentina. *J Med Microbiol, 49*, 187–192.

Darouiche, R., Wright, C., Hamill, R., Koza, M., Lewis, D., & Markowski, J. (1991). Eradication of colonization by methicillin-resistant *Staphylococcus aureus* by using oral mincycline-rifampin and topical mupirocin. *Antimicrob Agents Chemother, 35*, 1612–1615.

De Jonge, B. L. M., & Tomasz, A. (1993). Abnormal peptidoglycan produced in a methicillin-resistant strain of *Staphylococcus aureus* grown in the presence of methicillin: functional role of penicillin binding protein 2a in cell wall synthesis. *Antimicrob Agents Chemother, 37*, 342–346.

De Lencastre, H., Figueiredo, A. M. S., & Tomasz, A. (1993). Genetic control of population structure in heterogeneous strains of methicillin resistant *Staphylococcus aureus*. *Eur. J Clin Microbiol. Infect Dis, 12*(Suppl. 1), S13–S18.

Diekema, D. J., Pfaller, M. A., Schmitz, F. J., Smayevsky, J., Bell, J., Jones, R. N., Beach, M., & the SENTRY participants group. (2001). Survey of infections due to *Staphylococcus* species: Frequency of occurrence and antimicrobial susceptibility of isolates collected in the United States, Canada, Latin America, Europe and the Western Pacific Region for SENTRY antimicrobial surveillance program, 1997–1999. *Clin Infect Dis, 32*(Suppl. 2), S114–S132.

Dowzicky, M., Nadler, H. L., Feger, C., Talbot, G., Bompart, F., & Pease, M. (1998). Evaluation of in vitro activity of Quinupristin/Dalfopristin and comparator antimicrobial agents against worldwide clinical trial and other laboratory isolates. *Am J Med, 104*(Suppl. 5A), 34S–42S.

Dowzicky, M., Talbot, G. H., Feger, C., Prokocimer, P., Etienne, J., & Leclercq, R. (2000). Characterization of isolates associated with emerging resistance to quinupristin/dalfopristin (Synercid) during a worldwide clinical program. *Diagn Microbiol Infect Dis, 37*, 57–62.

Drew, R. H., Perfect, J. R., Srinath, L., Kurkimilis, E., Dowzicky, M., & Talbot, G. H., for the Synercid emergency-use study group. (2000). Treatment of methicillin-resistant *Staphylococcus aureus* infections with quinupristin–dalfopristin in patients intolerant of or failing prior therapy. *J Antimicrob Chemother, 46*, 775–784.

Drinka, P., Faulks, J. T., Gauerke, C., Goodman, B., Stemper, M., & Reed, K. (2001). Adverse events associated with methicillin-resistant *Staphylococcus aureus* in a nursing home. *Arch Intern Med, 161*, 2371–2377.

Emori, T. G., & Gaynes, R. P. (1993). An overview of nosocomial infections, including the role of the microbiology laboratory. *Clin Microbiol Rev, 6*, 428–442.

Ender, P. T., Durning, S. J., Woelk, W. K., Brockett, R. M., Astroga, A., Reddy, R., & Meier, P. A. (1999). Pseudo-outbreak of methicillin-resistant *Staphylococcus aureus*. *Mayo Clin Proc, 74*, 885–889.

Enright, M. C., Day, N. P., Davies, C. E., Peacock, S. J., & Spratt, B. G. (2000). Multilocus sequence typing for characterization of methicillin-resistant and methicillin-susceptible clones of *Staphylococcus aureus*. *J Clin Microbiol, 38*, 1008–1015.

Essawi, T., Na'was, T., Hawwari, A., Wadi, S., Doudin, A., & Fattom, A. I. (1998). Molecular, antibiogram and serological typing of *Staphylococcus aureus* isolates recovered from Al-Makased Hospital in East Jerusalem. *Trop Med Int Health, 3*, 576–583.

Eveillard, M., Eb, F., Tramier, B., Schmit, J. L., Lescure, F. X., Biendo, M., Canarelli, B., Daoudi, F., Laurans, G., Rousseau, F., & Thomas, D. (2001). Evaluation of the contribution of isolation precautions in prevention and control of multi-resistant bacteria in a teaching hospital. *J Hosp Infect, 47*, 116–124.

Eyraud, D., Vezinet, C., Robbert, J., Richard, O., Movschin, M., Borie, D., Jarlier, V., Hannoun, L., & Coriat, P. (2000). Efficiency of selective screening at admission of methicillin-resistant *Staphylococcus aureus* (MRSA) nasal carriers in abdominal surgery, 40th Interscience Conference on Antimicrobial Agents and Chemotherapy (Toronto 2000), Abstract No. 719, p. 408.

Fagon, J. Y., Maillet, J. M., & Novara, A. (1998). Hospital-acquired pneumonia: methicillin resistance and Intensive Care Unit Admission. *Am J Med, 104*(Suppl. 5A), 17S–23S.

Faoagali, J. L., George, N., Fong, J., Davy, J., & Dowser, M. (1999). Comparison of the antibacterial efficacy of 4% chlorhexidine gluconate and 1% triclosan handwash products in an acute clinical ward. *Am J Infect Control, 24*, 320–326.

Farrel, A. M. (1999). Staphylococcal scalded skin syndrome. *Lancet, 354*, 880–881.

Farrington, M., Ling, J., Ling, T., & French, G. L. (1990). Outbreaks of infection with methicillin-resistant *Staphylococcus aureus* on neonatal and burns units of a new hospital. *Epidemiol Infect, 105*, 215–228.

Fekety, R. (2000). Vancomycin. In G. L. Mandell, J. E. Bennett, & R. Dolin, (Eds.), *Principles and practice of infectious diseases* (5th ed., Vol. 1, pp. 382–387). Philadelphia: Churchill Livingstone.

Ferraro, M. J., Craig, W. A., Dudley, M. N., Eliopoulos, G., Hecht, D. W., Hindler, J. F., Reller, L. B., Sheldon, A. T., Swenson, J. M., Tenover, F. C., Testa, R. T., Weinstein, M. P., & Wikler, M. A. (2001). *Performance Standards for Antimicrobial Susceptibility Testing*; Eleventh Informational Supplement, NCCLS, Wayne, Pennsylvania, *21*, 48–49, 90–93.

Ferrero, L., Cameron, B., Manse, B., Lagneaux, D., Crouzet, J., Famechon, A., & Blanche, F. (1994). Cloning and primary structure of *Staphylococcus aureus* DNA topoisomerase IV: A primary target of fluoroquinolones. *Mol Microbiol, 13*, 641–653.

Ferrero, L., Cameron, B., & Crouzet, J. (1995). Analysis of *gyrA* and *grlA* mutations in stepwise selected ciprofloxacin-resistant mutants of *S aureus*. *Antimicrob Agents Chemother, 39*, 1554–1558.

Finan, J. E., Archer, G. L., Pucci, M. J., & Climo, M. W. (2001). Role of penicillin-binding protein 4 in expression of vancomycin resistance among clinical isolates of oxacillin-resistant *Staphylococcus aureus*. *Antimicrob Agents Chemother, 45*, 3070–3075.

Fines, M., & Leclercq, R. (2000). Activity of linezolid against Gram-positive cocci possessing genes conferring resistance to protein synthesis inhibitors. *J Antimicrob Chemother, 45*, 797–802.

Fleisch, F., Zbinden, R., Vanoli, C., & Ruef, C. (2001). Epidemic spread of a single clone of methicillin-resistant *Staphylococcus aureus* among injection drug users in Zurich, Switzerland. *Clin Infect Dis, 32*, 581–586.

Flournoy, D. J. (1997). Methicillin-resistant *Staphylococcus aureus* at a Veterans Affairs Medical Center (1986–96). *J Oklahoma State Med Assoc, 90*, 228–235.

Fluit, A. C., Wielders, C. L. C., Verhoef, J., & Schmitz, F. J. (2001). Epidemiology and susceptibility of 3,051 *Staphylococcus aureus* isolates from 25 university hospitals participating in the European SENTRY study. *J Clin Microbiol, 39*, 3727–3732.

Franklin, D. L. (1998). *Staphylococcus aureus* infections. *N Engl J Med, 339*, 520–532.

French, G. L., Cheng, A. F. B., Ling, J. M. L., Mo, P., & Donnan, S. (1990). Hong Kong strains of methicillin-resistant and methicillin-sensitive *Staphylococcus aureus* have similar virulence. *J Hosp Infect, 15*, 117–125.

Fridkin, S. K. (2001). Vancomycin-intermediate and -resistant *Staphylococcus aureus*: What the infectious disease specialist needs to know. *Clin Infect Dis, 32*, 108–115.

Fuchs, P. C., Barry, A. L., & Brown, S. D. (2001). Interactions of quinupristin-dalfopristin with eight other antibiotics as measured by time-kill studies with 10 strains of *Staphylococcus aureus* for which quinupristin-dalfopristin alone was not bactericidal. *Antimicrob Agents Chemother, 45,* 2662–2665.

Fukatsu, K., Saito, H., Matsuda, T., Ikeda, S., Furukawa, S., & Muto, T. (1997). Influences of type and duration of antimicrobial prophylaxis on an outbreak of methicillin-resistant *Staphylococcus aureus* and on the incidence of wound infection. *Arch Surg, 132,* 1320–1325.

Ge, Y., Wu, J., & White, S. (2001). Mechanistic study of a new class antibiotic HARP, 41st Annual Interscience Conference on Antimicrobial Agents and Chemotherapy (Chicago 2001), Abstract No. F-1686, p. 241.

Gentry, C. A., Rodvold, K. A., Novak, R. M., Hershow, R. C., & Naderer, O. J. (1997). Retrospective evaluation of therapies for *Staphylococcus aureus* endocarditis. *Pharmacotherapy, 17,* 990–997.

Gerberding, J. L., Miick, C., Liu, H. H., & Chambers, H. F. (1991). Comparison of conventional susceptibility tests with direct detection of penicillin-binding protein 2a in borderline oxacillin-resistant strains of *Staphylococcus aureus. Antimicrob Agents Chemother, 35,* 2574–2579.

Geyid, A., & Lemeneh, Y. (1991). The incidence of methicillin resistant *S. aureus* strains in clinical specimens in relation to their beta- lactamase producing and multiple-drug resistance properties in Addis Abeba. *Ethiop Med J, 29,* 149–161.

Gilbert, D. N., Kohlhepp, S. J., Slama, K. A., Grunkemeier, G., Lewis, G., Dworkin, R. J., Slaughter, S. E., & Leggett, J. E. (2001). Phenotypic resistance of *Staphylococcus aureus,* selected *Enterobacteriaceae,* and *Pseudomonas aeruginosa* after single and multiple in vitro exposures to ciprofloxacin, levofloxacin, and trovafloxacin. *Antimicrob Agents Chemother, 45,* 883–892.

Giret, P., Roblot, F., Poupet, J. Y. , Thomas, P., Lussier-Bonneau, M. D., Pradere, C., Becq-Giraudon, B., Fauchere, J. L., & Castel, O. (2001). Study of methicillin-resistant *Staphylococcus aureus* colonization among intermediate-care facility patients. *Rev Med Interne, 22,* 715–722 (abstract at: http://www.ncbi.nlm.nih.gov/entrez/query.fcgi?CMD=Text&DB=Pubmed).

Green, S. L., & Maddox, J. C. (2001). Linezolid and reversible myelosuppression. *JAMA, 286,* 1974.

Grueneberg, R. N. (1997). Anti-Gram-positive agents: what we have and what we would like. *Drugs, 54*(Suppl. 6), 29–38.

Grundmann, H., Hori, S., Winter, B., Tami, A., & Austin, D. J. (2002). Risk factors for the transmission of methicillin-resistant *Staphylococcus aureus* in an adult intensive care unit: fitting a model to the data. *J Infect Dis, 185,* 481–488.

Guerin, F., Buu-Hoi, A., Mainardi, J. L., Kac, G., Colardelle, N., Vaupre, S., Gutmann, L., & Podglajen, I. (2000). Outbreak of methicillin-resistant *Staphylococcus aureus* with reduced susceptibility to glycopeptides in a Parisian hospital. *J Clin Microbiol, 38,* 2985–2988.

Hackbarth, C. J., & Chambers, H. F. (1989). Methicillin-resistant staphylococci: Detection methods and treatment of infections. *Antimicrob Agents Chemother, 33,* 995–999.

Hackbarth, C. J., Chambers, H. F., & Sande, M. A. (1986). Serum antibacterial activity of rifampin an combination with other antimicrobial agents against *Staphylococcus aureus. Antimicrob Agents Chemother, 29,* 611–613.

Haley, R. W. (1991). Methicillin-resistant *Staphylococcus aureus*: Do we just have to live with it? *Ann Intern Med, 114,* 162–165.

Haley, R. W., Cushion, N. B., Tenover, F. C., Bannerman, T. L., Dryer, D., Ross, J., Sanchez, P. J., & Siegel, J. D. (1995). Eradication of endemic methicillin-resistant *Staphylococcus aureus* infections from a Neonatal Intensive Care Unit. *J Infect Dis, 171,* 614–624.

Hamel, J. C., Stapert, D., Moerman, J. K., & Ford, C. W. (2000). Linezolid, critical characteristics. *Infection, 28,* 60–64.

Hanaki, H., Kuwahara-Arai, K., Boyle-Vavra, S., Daum, R. S., Labischinski, H., & Hiramatsu, K. (1998). Activated cell-wall synthesis is associated with vancomycin resistance in methicillin-resistant *Staphylococcus aureus* clinical strains Mu3 and Mu50. *J Antimicrob Chemother, 42,* 199–209.

Harbarth, S., Dharan, S., Liassine, N., Herrault, P., Auckenthaler, R., & Pittet, D. (1999). Randomized, placebo-controlled, double-blind trial to evaluate the efficacy of mupirocin for eradicating carriage of methicillin-resistant *Staphylococcus aureus. Antimicrob Agents Chemother, 43,* 1412–1416.

Harbarth, S., Liassine, N., Dharan, S., Herrault, P., Auckenthaler, R., & Pittet, D. (2000). Risk factors for persistent carriage of methicillin-resistant *Staphylococcus aureus. Clin Infect Dis, 31,* 1380–1385.

Hartman, B. J., & Tomasz, A. (1986). Expression of methicillin resistance in heterogeneous strains of *Staphylococcus aureus. Antimicrob Agents Chemother, 29,* 85–92.

Hayanga, A., Okello, A., Hussein, R., & Nyong'o, A. (1997). Experience with methicillin resistant *Staphylococcus aureus* at the Nairobi Hospital. *East Afr Med J, 74,* 203–204.

Hayes, J. R., McIntosh, A. C., Qaiyumi, S., Johnson, J. A., English, L. L., Carr, L. E., Wagner, D. D., & Joseph, S. W. (2001). High frequency recovery of quinupristin-dalfopristin-resistant *Enterococcus faecium* isolates from the poultry production environment. *J Clin Microbiol, 39,* 2298–2299.

Hefferman, H., Davies, H., & Brett, M. (1995). MRSA increasing in New Zealand. *NZ Public Health Rep, 2,* 97–99.

Hendershot, P. E., Antal, E. J., Welshman, I. R., Batts, D. H., & Hopkins, N. K. (2001). Linezolid: Pharmacokinetic and pharmacodynamic evaluation of coadministration with pseudoephedrine HCl, phenylpropanolamine HCl, and dextromethorphan HBr. *J Clin Pharmacol, 41,* 563–572.

Henze, U. U., & Berger-Baechi, B. (1996). Penicillin-binding protein 4 overproduction increases β-lactam resistance in *Staphylococcus aureus. Antimicrob Agents Chemother, 40,* 2121–2125.

Herold, B. C., Immergluck, L. C., Maranan, M. C., Lauderdale, D. S., Gaskin, R. E., Boyle-Vavra, S., Leitch, C. D., & Daum, R. S. (1998). Community-acquired methicillin-resistant *Staphylococcus aureus* in children with no identified predisposing risk. *JAMA, 279,* 593–598.

Herwaldt, L. (1999). Control of methicillin-resistant *Staphylococcus aureus* in the hospital setting. *Am J Med, 106*(Suppl. 1), S11–S18.

Hill, R. L. R., & Casewell, M. W. (2000). The in-vitro activity of povidone-iodine cream against *Staphylococcus aureus* and its bioavailability in nasal secretions. *J Hosp Infect, 45,* 148–205.

Hiramatsu, K. (2001). Vancomycin-resistant *Staphylococcus aureus*: A new model of antibiotic resistance. *Lancet Infect Dis, 1,* 147–155.

Hiramatsu, K., Konodo, N., & Ito, T. (1996). Genetic basis for molecular epidemiology of MRSA. *J Infect Chemother, 2,* 117–129.

Holbrook, K. A., Klein, R. S., Hartel, D., Elliott, D. A., Barsky, T. B., Rothschild, L. H., & Lowy, F. D. (1997). *Staphylococcus aureus* nasal colonization in HIV-seropositive and HIV-seronegative drug users. *J Acquir Immun Def Syndr Human Retrovirol, 16,* 301–306.

Hookey, J. V., Edwards, V., Patel, S., Richardson, J. F., & Cookson, B. D. (1999). Use of fluorescent amplified fragment length polymorphism (fAELP) to characterize methicillin-resistant *Staphylococcus aureus. J Microbiol Methods, B37,* 7–15.

Hooper, D. C. (2000). Mechanisms of action and resistance of older and newer Fluoroquinolones. *Clin Infect Dis, 31*(Suppl. 2), S24–S28.

Horikawa, K., Murakami, K., & Kawano, F. (2001). Isolation and characterization of methicillin-resistant *Staphylococcus aureus* strains from nares of nurses and their gowns. *Microbiol Res, 155,* 345–349.

Hryniewitcz, W. (1999). Epidemiology of MRSA. *Infection, 27*(Suppl. 2), S13–S16.

Hudson, I. R. B. (1994). The efficacy of intranasal mupirocin ointment in the prevention or staphylococcal infections: A review of recent experience. *J Hosp Infect, 27,* 81–98.

Hugonnet, S., Perneger, T. V., & Pittet, D. (2002). Alcohol-based handrub improves compliance with hand hygiene in intensive care units, *Arch Intern Med, 162,* 1037–1043.

Humphreys, H. (1997). Staphylococcus. In D. Greenwood, R. Slack, & J. Peutherer (Eds.), *Medical microbiology,* (pp. 168–170) New York: Churchill Livingston.

Hussain, F. M., Boyle-Vavra, S., Bethel, C. D., & Daum, R. S. (2000). Current trends in community-acquired methicillin-resistant *Staphylococcus aureus* at a tertiary care pediatric facility. *Pediatr J Infect Dis, 19*, 1163–1166.

Ibelings, M. M., & Bruining, H. A. (1998). Methicillin-resistant *Staphylococcus aureus*: Acquisition and risk of death in the intensive care unit. *Eur J Surg, 164*, 411–418.

Ike, Y., Arakawa, Y., Ma, X., Tatewaki, K., Nagasawa, M., Tomita, H., Tanimoto, K., & Fujimoto, S. (2001). Nationwide survey shows that methicillin-resistant *Staphylococcus aureus* strains heterogeneously and intermediately resistant to vancomycin are not disseminated throughout Japanese hospitals. *J Clin Microbiol, 39*, 4445–4451.

Ito, D., & Hiramatsu, K. (1998). Acquisition of methicillin resistance and progression of multiantibiotic resistance in methicillin-resistant *Staphylococcus aureus*. *Yonsei Med J, 39*, 526–533.

Jelic I., Anic, D., Alfirevic, I., Kalinic, S., Ugljen, R., Letica, D., Ante Korda, Z., Vucemilo, I., Bulat, C., Predrijevac, M., Coric, V., Husar, J., Jelic, M., Hulin, D., Depina, I., & Dadic, D. (1996). Wound infection after median sternotomy during the war in Croatia. *J Cardiovasc Surg (Torino), 37*(Suppl. 1), 183–187.

Johnson, A. P., & Speller, D. C. E. (1997). Epidemiology of antibiotic resistance: Blood and cerebrospinal fluid (CSF). *J Med Microbiol, 46*, 445–447.

Jones, R. N., Hare, R. S., Sabatelli, F. J., & the Ziracin Susceptibility Testing Group. (2001). *In vitro* Gram-positive antimicrobial activity of evernimicin (SCH 27899), a novel oligosaccharide, compared with other antimicrobials: A multicentre international trial. *J Antimicrob Chemother, 47*, 15–25.

Jones, S. M., Morgan, M., Humphrey, T. J., & Lappin-Scott, H. (2001). Effect of vancomycin and rifampicin on meticillin-resistant *Staphylococcus aureus* biofilms. *Lancet, 357*, 40–41.

Kaatz, G. W., & Seo, S. M. (1997). Mechanisms of Fluoroquinolone resistance in genetically related strains of *Staphylococcus aureus*. *Antimicrob Agents Chemother, 41*, 2733–2737.

Kaatz, G. W., Seo, S. M., Reddy, V. N., Bailey, E. M., & Rybak, M. J. (1990). Daptomycin compared with teicoplanin and vancomycin for therapy of experimental *Staphylococcus aureus* endocarditis. *Antimicrob Agents Chemother, 34*, 2081–2985.

Kang, S. L., & Rybak, M. J. (1997). In vitro bactericidal activity of quinupristin/dalfopristin alone and in combination against resistant strains of *Enterococcus* species and *Staphylococcus aureus*. *J Antimicrob Chemother, 39* (Suppl. A), 33–39.

Katayama, Y., Ito, T., & Hiramatsu, K. (2000). A new class of genetic element, staphylococcus cassette chromosome mec, encodes methicillin resistance in *Staphylococcus aureus*. *Antimicrob Agents Chemother, 44*, 1549–1555.

Kernodle, D. S., Stratton, C. S., McMurray, L. W., Chipley, J. R., & McGraw, P. A. (1989). Differentiation of beta-lactamase variants in *Staphylococcus aureus* by substrate hydrolysis profiles. *J Infect Dis, 159*, 103–108.

Kloos, W. S., & Bannerman, T. (1999). *Staphylococcus* and *Micrococcus*. In P. R. Murray, E. J. Baron, M. A. Pfaller, F. C. Tenover, & R. H. Yolken (Eds.), *Manual of clinical microbiology* (7th ed., pp. 264–282) Washington, DC: American Society of Microbiology Press.

Kluytmans, J. A., Mouton, J. W., VandenBergh, M. F., Manders, M. J., Maat, A. P., Wagenvoort, J. H., Michel, M. F., & Verbrugh, H. A. (1996). Reduction of surgical-site infections in cardiothoracic surgery by elimination of nasal carriage of *Staphylococcus aureus*. *Infect Contr Hosp Epidemiol, 17*, 780–785.

Kluytmans, J., van Belkum, A., & Verbrugh, H. (1997). Nasal carriage of *Staphylococcus aureus*: Epidemiology, underlying mechanisms, and associated risks. *Clin Microbiol Rev, 10*, 505–520.

Kobasa, W. D., Kaye, K. L., Shapiro, T., & Kaye, D. (1983). Therapy for experimental endocarditis due to *Staphylococcus epidermidis*. *Rev Infect Dis, 5*(Suppl. 3), S533–S537.

Kodama, T., Santo, T., Yokohama, T., Takesue, Y., Hiyama, E., Imamura, Y., Murakami, Y., Tsumura, H., Shinbara, K., Tatsumoto, N., & Matsuura, Y. (1997). Postoperative infection caused by methicillin-resistant *Staphylococcus aureus*. *Surg Today, 27*, 816–825.

Kondo, N., Kuwahara-Arai, K., Kuroda-Murakami, H., Tateda-Suzuki, E., & Hiramatsu, K. (2001). Eagle-type methicillin resistance: New phenotype of high methicillin resistance under *mec* regulator gene control. *Antimicrob Agents Chemother, 45*, 815–824.

Kotilainen, P., Routamaa, M., Peltonen, R., Evesti, P., Eerola, E., Salmenlinna, S., Vuopio-Varkila, J., & Rossi, T. (2001). Eradication of methicillin-resistant *Staphylococcus aureus* from a Health Center Ward and associated Nursing Home. *Arch Intern Med, 161*, 859–863.

Kreiswirth, B., Kornblum, J., Arbeit, R. D., Eisner, W., Marlow, J. N., Mc Geer, A., Low, D. E., & Novick, R. P. (1993). Evidence of clonal origin of methicillin resistance in *Staphylococcus aureus*. *Science, 259*, 227–230.

Kuroda, M., Ohta, T., Uchiyama, I., Baba, T., Yuzawa, H., Kobayashi, I., Cui, L., Oguchi, A., Aoki, K., Nagai, Y., Lian, J., Ito, T., Kanamori, M., Matsumaru, H., Maruyama, A., Murakami, H., Hosoyama, A., Mizutani-Ui, Y., Takahashi, N. K., Sawano, T., Inoue, R., Kaito, C., Sekimizu, K., Hirakawa, H., Kuhara, S., Goto, S., Yabuzaki, J., Kanehisa, M., Yamashita, A., Oshima, K., Furuya, K., Yoshino, C., Shiba, T., Hattori, M., Ogasawara, N., Hayashi, H., & Hiramatsu, K. (2001). Whole genome sequencing of methicillin-resistant *Staphylococcus aureus*. *Lancet, 357*, 1225–1240.

Kusachi, S., Sumiyama, Y., Nagao, J., Kawai, K., Arima, Y., Yoshida, Y., Kajiwara, H., Saida, Y., & Nakamura, Y. (1999). New methods of control against postoperative methicillin-resistant *Staphylococcus aureus* infection. *Surg Today, 29*, 724–729.

Lamb, H. M., Figgit, D. P., & Faulds, D. (1999). Quinupristin/Dalfopristin: A review of its use in the management of serious Gram-positive infections. *Drugs, 58*, 1061–1097.

Lee, J. C. (1998). An experimental vaccine that targets staphylococcal virulence. *Trends Microbiol, 6*, 461–463.

Leigh, D. A., & Joy, C. (1993). Treatment of familial staphylococcal infection: Comparison of mupirocin nasal ointment and chlorhexidine/neomycin (Naseptin) cream in eradication of nasal carriage. *J Antimicrob Chemother, 31*, 909–917.

Levine, D. P., Fromm, B. S., & Reddy, B. R. (1991). Slow response to vancomycin or vancomycin plus rifampin in methicillin-resistant *Staphylococcus aureus* endocarditis. *Ann Intern Med, 115*, 674–680.

Li, Z., Willke, R. J., Rittenhouse, B. E., Pleil, A. M., Hafkin, B., Crouch, C. W., Pinto, L. A., Rybak, M., J., & Glick, H., A. (2001). Comparison of length of hospital stay for patients with known or suspected methicillin-resistant staphylococcus species infections treated with linezolid or vancomycin: A randomized, multicenter trial. *Pharmacotherapy, 21*, 263–274.

Ligozzi, M., Rossolini, G. M., Tonin, E. A., & Fontan, R. (1991). Nonradioactive DNA probe for detection of gene for methicillin resistance in *Staphylococcus aureus*. *Antimicrob Agents Chemother, 35*, 575–578.

Livermore, D. M. (2000). Epidemiology of antibiotic resistance. *Intensive Care Med, 26* (Suppl. 1), S14–S21.

Luh, K.-T., Hsueh, P.-R., Teng, L.-J., Pan, H.-J., Chen, Y.-C., Lu, J.-J., Wu, J.-J., & Ho, S.-W. (2000). Quinupristin–dalfopristin resistance among Gram-positive bacteria in Taiwan. *Antimicrob Agents Chemother, 44*, 3374–3380.

Lundstrom, T. S., & Sobel, J. D. (2000). Antibiotics for Gram-positive bacterial infections. *Infect Dis Clin North Am, 14*, 463–474.

Mangoni, M. L., Rinaldi, A. C., Di Giulio, A., Mignogna, G., Bozzi, A., Barra, D., & Simmaco, M. (2000). Structure-function relationships of temporins, small antimicrobial peptides from amphibian skin. *Eur J Biochem, 267*, 1447–1454.

Maranan, M. C., Moreira, B., Boyle-Vavra, S., & Daum, R. S. (1997). Antimicrobial resistance in staphylococci: Epidemiology, Molecular Mechanisms, and Clinical Relevance, Review. *Infect Dis Clin North Am, 11*, 813–849.

Markowitz, N., Quinn, E. L., & Saravolatz, L. D. (1992). Trimethoprim-sulfamethoxazole compared with vancomycin for treatment of *Staphylococcus aureus* infection. *Ann Intern Med, 117*, 390–398.

McDougal, L. K., & Thornsberry, C. (1986). The role of β-lactamase in staphylococcal resistance to penicillinase-resistant penicillin and cephalosporin. *J Clin Microbiol, 23*, 832–839.

Mckenney, D., Pouliot, K., Wang, Y., Murthy, V., Ulrich, M., Doring, G., Lee, J. C., Goldmann, D. A., & Pier, G. B. (2000). Vaccine potential of poly-1-6 β-D-*N*-succinylglucosamine, an immunoprotective surface polysaccharide of *Staphylococcus aureus* and *Staphylococcus epidermidis. Biotechnology, 83*, 37–44.

Melter, O., Santos Sanches, I., Schindler, J., Aires de Sousa, M., Mato, R., Kovarova, V., Zemlickova, H., & de Lencastre, H. (1999). Methicillin-resistant *Staphylococcus aureus* clonal types in the Czech Republic. *J Clin Microbiol, 37*, 2798–2803.

Mermel, A. L., Farr, B. M., Sherertz, R. J., Raad, I. I., O'Grady, N., Harris, J. S., & Craven, D. E. (2001). Guidelines for the management of intravascular catheter-related infections. *Clin Infect Dis, 32*, 1249–1272.

Merrer, J., Santoli, F., Apperre-De Vecchi, C., Tran, B., De Jonghe, B., & Outin, H. (2000). "Colonization pressure" and risk of acquisition of methicillin-resistant *Staphylococcus aureus* in a medical Intensive Care Unit. *Infect Contr Hosp Epidemiol, 21*, 718–723.

Michel, M., & Gutmann, L. (1997). Methicillin-resistant staphylococci and vancomycin-resistant enterococci: Therapeutic realities and possibilities, Review article. *Lancet, 349*, 1901–1906.

Moraes, B. A., Cravo, C. A., Loureiro, M. M., Solari, C. A., & Asensi, M. D. (2000). Epidemiological analysis of bacterial strains involved in hospital infections in a university hospital in Brazil. *Rev Inst Med Trop Sao Paolo, 42*, 201–207.

Morgan, M., Salmon, R., Keppie, N., Evans-Williams, D., Hosein, I., & Looker, D. N. (1999). All Wales surveillance of methicillin-resistant *Staphylococcus aureus* (MRSA): The first year's results. *J Hosp Infect, 41*, 173–179.

Morse, G. D., Nairn, D. K., & Walshe, J. J. (1987). Once weekly intraperitoneal therapy for Gram-positive peritonitis. *Am J Kidney Dis, 4*, 300–305.

Muder, R. R., Brennen, C., Wagener, M. M., Vickers, R. M., Rihs, J. D., Hancock, G. A., Yee, Y. C., Miller, J. M., & Yu, V. L. (1991). Methicillin-resistant staphylococcal colonization and infection in a long-term care facility. *Ann Intern Med, 114*, 107–112.

Mulligan, M. E., Murray-Leisure, K. A., Ribner, B. S., Standiford, H. C., John, J. F., Korvick, J. A., Kauffman, C. A., & Yu, V. L. (1992). Methicillin-resistant *Staphylococcus aureus*: A consensus review on the microbiology, pathogenesis, and epidemiology with implications for prevention and management. *Am J Med, 94*, 313–328.

Munckhof, W. J., Giles, C., & Turnidge, J. D. (2001). Post-antibiotic growth suppression of linezolid against Gram-positive bacteria. *J Antimicrob Chemother, 47*, 879–883.

Murakami, K., Minamide, W., Wada, K., Nakamura, E., Teraoka, H., & Watanabe, S. (1991). Identification of methicillin-resistant strains of staphylococci by polymerase chain reaction. *J Clin Microbiol, 29*, 2240–2244.

Mylotte, J. M. (1994). Control of methicillin-resistant *Staphylococcus aureus*: The ambivalence persists. *Infect Contr Hosp Epidemiol, 15*, 73–77.

Mylotte, J. M., Graham, R., Kahler, L., Young, L., & Goodnough, S. (2000). Epidemiology of nosocomial infection and resistant organisms in patients admitted for the first time to an Acute Rehabilitation Unit. *Clin Infect Dis, 30*, 425–432.

Naimi, T. S., LeDell, K. H., Boxrud, D. J., Groom, A. V., Steward, C. D., Johnson, S. K., Besser, J. M., O'Boyle, C., Danila, R. N., Cheek, J. E., Osterholm, M. T., Moore, K. A., & Smith, K. E. (2001). Epidemiology and clonality of community-acquired methicillin-resistant *Staphylococcus aureus* in Minnesota, 1996–1998. *Clin Infect Dis, 33*, 990–996.

Nelson, D., Loomis, L., & Fischetti, V. A. (2001). Prevention and elimination of upper respiratory colonization of mice by group A streptococci by using a bacteriophage lytic enzyme. *Proc Nat Acad Sci, 98*, 4107–4112.

Nettleman, M. D., Trilla, A., Fredrickson, M., & Pfaller, M. (1991). Assigning responsibility: Using feedback to achieve sustained control of methicillin-resistant *Staphylococcus aureus*. *Am J Med*, *91*(Suppl. 1), S228–S232.

Nguyen, M. H., Kauffman, C. A., Goodman, R. P., Squier, C., Arbeit, R. B., Singh, N., Wagener, M. M., & Yu, V. L. (1999). Nasal carriage of and infection with *Staphylococcus aureus* in HIV- infected patients. *Ann Intern Med*, *130*, 221–225.

Nicolle, L. E., Strausbaugh, L. J., & Garibaldi, R. A. (1996). Infections and antibiotic resistance in Nursing Homes. *Clin Microbiol Rev*, *9*, 1–17.

Noble, W. C., Virani, Z., & Cree, R. G. (1992). Co-transfer of vancomycin and other resistance genes from *Enterococcus faecalis* NCTC 12201 to *Staphylococcus aureus*. *FEMS Microbiol Lett*, *72*, 195–198.

Novak, F. R., Da Silva, A. V., Hagler, A. N., & Figueiredo, A. M. (2000). Contamination of expressed human breast milk with an epidemic multi-resistant *Staphylococcus aureus* clone. *J Med Microbiol*, *49*, 1109–1117.

Ogston, A. (1882). Micrococcus poisoning. *J Anat*, *17*, 24–58.

Ohwada, A., Sekiya, M., Hanaki, H., Arai, K. K., Nagaoka, I., Hori, S., Tominaga, S., Hiramatsu, K., & Fukuchi, Y. (1999). DNA vaccination by *mecA* sequence evokes an antibacterial response against methicillin-resistant *Staphylococcus aureus*. *J Antimicrob Chemother*, *44*, 767–774.

Okada, T., Makimoto, A., Kitamura, A., Furukawa, S., Miwa, K., & Sakai, R. (2000). A new exanthematous disease in newborn infants caused by exotoxins producing methicillin-resistant *Staphylococcus aureus*; pathology from viewpoints of local and systemic levels of exotoxin and cytokine. *Kansenshogaku Zasshi*, *74*, 573–579 (abstract at: http://www.ncbi.nlm.nih.gov:80/entrez/query.fcgi?CMD=Text&DB=PubMed).

Panlilio, A. L., Culver, D. H., Gaynes, R. P., Banerjee, S., Henderson, T. S., Tolson, J. S., & Martone, D. J. (1992). Methicillin-resistant *Staphylococcus aureus* in US hospitals, 1975–1991. *Infect Contr Hosp Epidemiol*, *13*, 582–586.

Papia, G., Louie, M., Tralla, A., Johnson, C., Collins, V., & Simor, A. E. (1999). Screening high-risk patients for methicillin-resistant *Staphylococcus aureus* on admission to the hospital: Is it cost-effective? *Infect Contr Hosp Epidemiol*, *20*, 473–477.

Paradisi, F., Corti, G., & Messeri, D. (2001). Antistaphylococcal (MSSA, MRSA, MSSE, MRSE) Antibiotics. *Med Clin North Am*, *85*, 1–17.

Parienti, J. J., Thibon, P., Heller, R., LeRoux, Y., Von Theobald, P., Bensadoun, H., Bouvet, A., Lemarchand, F., Le Coutour, X., & For members of the Antisepsie Chirurgicale des Mains Study Group. (2002). Hand-rubbing with an aqueous alcohol solution vs. traditional surgical hand-scrubbing and 30 day surgical site infection rates. A randomized equivalence study. *JAMA*, *288*, 722–727.

Parras, F., Guerrero, C., Bouza, E., Blazquez, M. J., Moreno, S., Menarguez, M. C., & Cercenado, E. (1995). Comparative study of mupirocin and oral co-trimoxazole plus topical fusidic acid in eradication of nasal carriage of methicillin-resistant *Staphylococcus aureus*. *Antimicrob Agents Chemother*, *39*, 175–179.

Patel, R., Rouse, M. S., Piper, K. E., & Steckelberg, J. M. (2000). In vitro activity of GAR-936 against vancomycin-resistant enterococci, methicillin-resistant *Staphylococcus aureus* and penicillin-resistant *Streptococcus pneumoniae*. *Diagn Microbiol Infect Dis*, *38*, 177–179.

Paterson, D. L., Singh, N., Gayowski, T., Marino, I. R., & Wagener, M. M. (2000). Lack of clinical efficacy of nasal mupirocin in preventing *Staphylococcus aureus* infections in liver transplant recipients, 40th Interscience Conference on Antimicrobial Agents and Chemotherapy (Toronto 2000), Abstract No. 487, p. 405.

Paton, R., Snell, T., Emmanuel, F. X. S., & Miles, R. S. (2001). Glycopeptide resistance in an epidemic strain of methicillin-resistant *Staphylococcus aureus*. *J Antimicrob Chemother*, *48*, 941–942.

Pawa, A., Noble, W. C., & Howell, S. A. (2000). Co-transfer of plasmids in association with conjugative transfer of mupirocin or mupirocin and penicillin resistance in methicillin-resistant *Staphylococcus aureus*. *J Med Microbiol, 49*, 1103–1107.

Peters, G., & Becker K. (1996). Epidemiology, Control and treatment of methicillin-resistant *Staphylococcus aureus*. *Drugs, 52*(Suppl. 2), 50–54.

Pittet, D. (2000). Improving compliance with hand hygiene in hospitals, *Infect Control Hosp Epidemiol, 21*, 381–386.

Poduval, R. D., Kamath, R. P., Norkus, E. P., & Corpuz, M. (2000). Vancomycin-resistant *Enterococcus* (VRE) and methicillin-resistant *Staphylococcus aureus* (MRSA)—new superbug alliance, 40th Interscience Conference on Antimicrobial Agents and Chemotherapy (Toronto 2000), Abstract No. 725 p. 410.

Proctor, R. A., Kahl, B., von Eiff, C., Vaudaux, P. E., Lew, D. P., & Peters, G. (1998). Staphylococcal Small Colony Variants have novel mechanisms of antibiotic resistance. *Clin Infect Dis, 27*(Suppl. 1), S68–S74.

Pujol, M., Pena, C., Pallares, R., Ariza, J., Ayats, J., Domingues, M. A., & Gudiol, F. (1996). Nosocomial *Staphylococcus aureus* bacteremia among nasal carriers of methicillin-resistant and methicillin-susceptible strains. *Am J Med, 100*, 509–516.

Rao, G. G. (1998). Risk factors for the spread of antibiotic-resistant bacteria. *Drugs, 55*, 323–330.

Reagan, D. R., Doebbeling, B. N., Pfaller, M. A., Sheetz, C. T., Houston, A. K., Hollis, R. J., & Wenzel, R. P. (1991). Elimination of coincident *Staphylococcus aureus* nasal and hand carriage with intranasal application of mupirocin calcium ointment. *Ann Intern Med, 114*, 101–106.

Rello, J., Ausina, V., Castelia, J., Net, A., & Prats, G. (1992). Nosocomial respiratory tract infections in multiple trauma patients. *Chest, 102*, 525–529.

Rello, J., Torres, A., Ricart, M., Valles, J., Gonzales, J., Artigas, A., & Rodriguez-Roisin, R. (1994). Ventilator-associated pneumonia by *Staphylococcus aureus*: Comparison of methicillin-resistant and methicillin-sensitive episodes. *Am J Respir Crit Care Med, 150*, 1545–1549.

Rennermalm, A., Li, Y. H., Bohaufs, L., Jarstrand, C., Brauner, A., Brennan, F. R., & Flock, J. I. (2001). Antibodies against a truncated *Staphylococcus aureus* fibronectin-binding protein protect against dissemination of infections in the rat. *Vaccine, 19*, 3376–3383.

Reverdy, M. E., Jarraud, S., Bobin-Dubreux, S., Burel, E., Girardo, P., Lina, G., Vandenesch, F., & Etienne, J. (2001). Incidence of *Staphylococcus aureus* with reduced susceptibility to glycopeptides in two French hospitals. *Clin Microbiol Infect, 7*, 267–272.

Ribner, B. S., Landry, M. N., & Gholson, G. L. (1986). Strict versus modified isolation for prevention of nosocomial transmission of methicillin-resistant *Staphylococcus aureus*. *Infect Control, 7*, 317–320.

Roberts, R. B., de Lencastre, A., Eisner, W., Severina, E., Shopsin, B., Kreiswirth, B. N., Tomasz, A., & the MRSA Collaborative Study Group. (1998). Molecular epidemiology of methicillin-resistant *Staphylococcus aureus* in 12 New York hospitals. *J Infect Dis, 178*, 164–171.

Roghmann, M. C., Siddiqui, A., Plaisance, K., & Standiford, H. (2001). MRSA colonization and the risk of MRSA bacteremia in hospitalized patients with chronic ulcers. *J Hosp Infect, 47*, 98–103.

Rubinovitch, B., & Pittet, D. (2001). Screening for methicillin-resistant *Staphylococcus aureus* in the endemic hospital: What have we learned? *J Hosp Infect, 47*, 9–18.

Rubinstein, E., Cammarata, S. K., Oliphant, T. H., Wunderink, R. G., & the Linezolid Nosocomial Pneumonia Study Group. (2001). Linezolid (PNU-100766) versus vancomycin in the treatment of hospitalized patients with nosocomial pneumonia: A randomized, double-blind, multicenter study. *Clin Infect Dis, 32*, 402–412.

Rybak, M. J., Bailey, E. M., Lamp, K. C., & Kaatz, G. W. (1992). Pharmacokinetics and bactericidal rates of daptomycin and vancomycin in intravenous drug abusers being treated for Gram-positive endocarditis and bacteremia. *Antimicrob Agents Chemother, 36*, 1109–1114.

Sadoyama, G., & Gontijo Filho, P. P. (2000). Risk factors for methicillin resistant and sensitive *Staphylococcus aureus* infection in a Brazilian university hospital. *Braz J Infect Dis, 4,* 135–143.

Sahm, D. F., Marsilio, M. K., & Piazza, G. (1999). Antimicrobial resistance in key bloodstream bacterial isolates: electronic surveillance with The Surveillance Network Database—USA. *Clin Infect Dis, 29,* 259–263.

Sakata, H. (2001). Isolation of methicillin-resistant *Staphylococcus aureus* from nasopharyngeal swabs on admission to a ward for pediatric patients: Comparison between 1992–1993 and 1997–1998. *Kansenshogaku Zasshi, 75,* 14–19.

Sambatakou, H., Giamarellos-Bourboulis, E. J., Grecka, P., Chryssouli, Z., & Giamarellou, H. (1998). In-vitro activity and killing effect of quinupristin/dalfopristin (RP59500) on nosocomial *Staphylococcus aureus* and interactions with rifampicin and ciprofloxacin against methicillin-resistant isolates. *J Antimicrob Chemother, 41,* 349–355.

Sanford, M. D., Widmer, A. F., Bale, M. J., Jones, R. N., & Wenzel, R. P. (1994). Efficient detection and long-term persistence of the carriage of methicillin-resistant *Staphylococcus aureus. Clin Infect Dis, 19,* 1123–1128.

Santos Sanches, I., Mato, R., de Lencastre, H., & Tomasz, A. (2000). Patterns of multidrug resistance among methicillin-resistant hospital isolates of coagulase-positive and coagulase-negative staphylococci collected in the international multicenter study RESIST in 1997 and 1998. CEM/NET Collaborators and the International Collaborators. *Microb Drug Resist, 6,* 199–211.

Scanvic, A., Denic, L., Gaillon, S., Giry, P., Andremont, A., & Lucet, J. C. (2001). Duration of colonization by methicillin-resistant *Staphylococcus aureus* after hospital discharge and risk factors for prolonged carriage. *Clin Infect Dis, 32,* 1393–1398.

Schentag, J. J., Hyatt, J. M., Carr, J. R., Paladino, J. A., Birmingham, M. C., Zimmer, G. S., & Cumbo, T. J. (1998). Genesis of methicillin-resistant *Staphylococcus aureus* (MRSA), how treatment of MRSA infections has selected for vancomycin-resistant *Enterococcus faecium*, and the importance of antibiotic management and infection control. *Clin Infect Dis, 26,* 1204–1214.

Schittek, B., Hipfel, R., Sauer, B., Bauer, J., Kalbacher, H., Stevanovic, S., Schirle, M., Schroeder, K., Blin, N., Meier, F., Rassner, G., & Garbe, C. (2001). Dermcidin: a novel human antibiotic peptide secreted by sweat glands. *Nat Immunol, 2,* 1133–1137.

Schmitz, F. J., Mackenzie, C. R., Hoffman, B., Verhoef, J., Finken-Eigen, M., Heinz, H. P., & Kohrer, K. (1997). Specific information concerning taxonomy, pathogenicity and methicillin resistance of staphylococci obtained by a multiplex PCR. *J Clin Microbiol, 46,* 773–778.

Schmitz, F. J., Krey, A., Sadurski, R., Verhoef, J., Milatovic, D., & Fluit, A. C. (2001). Resistance to tetracycline and distribution of tetracycline resistance genes in European *Staphylococcus aureus* isolates. *J Antimicrob Chemother, 47,* 239–240.

Shahin, R., Johnson, I. L., Jamieson, F., McGeer, A., Tolkin, J., & Ford-Jones, E. L. (1999). Methicillin-resistant *Staphylococcus aureus* carriage in a child care center following a case of disease. *Arch Pediatr Adolesc Med, 153,* 864–868.

Shinefield, H., Black, S., Fattom, A., Horwith, G., Rasgon, S., Ordonez, J., Yeoh, H., Law, D., Robbins, J. B., Schneerson, R., Muenz, L., & Naso, R. (2002). Use of a *Staphylococcus aureus* conjugate vaccine in patients receiving hemodialysis. *N Engl J Med, 346,* 491–496.

Shiomori, T., Yoshida, S., Miyamoto, H., & Makishima, K. (2000). Relationship of nasal carriage of *Staphylococcus aureus* to pathogenesis of perennial allergic rhinitis. *J Allergy Clin Immunol, 105,* 449–454.

Shopsin, B., Mathema, B., Zhao, X., Martinez, J., Kornblum, J., & Kreiswirth, B. N. (2000a). Resistance rather than virulence selects for the clonal spread of methicillin-resistant *Staphylococcus aureus*: implications for MRSA transmission. *Microb Drug Resist, 6,* 239–244.

Shopsin, B., Mathema, B., Martinez, J., Ha, E., Campo, M. L., Fierman, A., Krasinski, K., Kornblum, J., Alcabes, P., Waddington, M., Riehman, M., & Kreiswirth, B. N. (2000b). Prevalence of methicillin-resistant and methicillin-susceptible *Staphylococcus aureus* in the community. *J Infect Dis, 182*, 359–362.

Shuter, J., Hatcher, V. B., & Lowy, F. D. (1996). *Staphylococcus aureus* binding to human nasal mucin. *Infect Immun, 64*, 310–318.

Sievert, D. M., Boulton, M. L., Stoltman, G., Johnson, D., Stobierski, M. G., Downes, F. P., Somsel, P. A., Rudrik, J. T., Brown, W., Hafeez, W., Lundstrom, T., Flannagan, E., Johnson, R., Mitchell, J., Chang, S. (2002). *Staphylococcus aureus* resistant to vancomycin—United States, 2002 *MMWR, 51*, 565–567.

Simor, A. E., Ofner-Agostini, M., Bryce, E., Green, K., McGeer, A., Mulvey, M., & Paton, S. (2001). The evolution of methicillin-resistant *Staphylococcus aureus* in Canadian hospitals: 5 years of national surveillance. *CMAJ, 165*, 31–32.

Small, P. M., & Chambers, H. F. (1990). Vancomycin for *Staphylococcus aureus* endocarditis in intravenous drug users. *Antimicrob Agents Chemother, 34*, 1227–1231.

Soares, M. J., Tokumaru-Miyazaki, N. H., Noleto, A. L., & Figueiredo, A. M. (1997). Enterotoxin production by *Staphylococcus aureus* clones and detection of Brazilian epidemic MRSA clone (III: :B : A) among isolates from food handlers. *J Med Microbiol, 46*, 214–221.

Staples, A. M., Critchley, I. A., Thornsberry, C., Murfitt, K. S., & Sahm, D. F. (2000). Resistance to Oxacillin and other agents among *Staphylococcus aureus* in the United States, 40th Interscience Conference on Antimicrobial Agents and Chemotherapy (Toronto 2000), Abstract No. 161, p. 70.

Steinberg, J. P., Clark, C. C., & Hackman, B. O. (1996). Nosocomial and community-acquired *Staphylococcus aureus* bacteremias from 1980 to 1993: Impact of intravascular devices and methicillin resistance. *Clin Infect Dis, 23*, 255–259.

Stevens, D. L., Smith, L. G., Bruss, J. B., McConnell-Martin M. A., Duvall, S. E., Todd, W. M., & Hafkin, B. (2000). Randomized comparison of linezolid (PNU-100766) versus oxacillin-dicloxacillin for treatment of complicated skin and soft tissue infections. *Antimicrob Agents Chemother, 44*, 3408–3413.

Strauss, E. (2000). Fighting bacterial fire with bacterial fire. *Science, 290*, 2231–2233.

Suggs, A. H., Maranan, M. C., Boyle-Vavra, S., & Daum, R. S. (1999). Methicillin-resistant and borderline methicillin-resistant asymptomatic *Staphylococcus aureus* colonization in children without identifiable risk factors. *Pediatr Infect Dis J, 18*, 410–414.

Suh, K., Toye, B., Jessamine, P., Chan, F., & Ramotar, K. (1998). Epidemiology of methicillin-resistant *Staphylococcus aureus* in three Canadian tertiary-care centers. *Infect Contr Hosp Epidemiol, 19*, 395–400.

Suller, M. T. E., & Russell, A. D. (1999). Antibiotic and biocide resistance in methicillin-resistant *Staphylococcus aureus* and vancomycin-resistant enterococcus. *J Hosp Infect, 43*, 281–291.

Suller, M. T. E., & Russell, A. D. (2000). Triclosan and antibiotic resistance in *Staphylococcus aureus*. *J Antimicrob Chemother, 46*, 11–18.

Takahashi, N., Nishida, H., Kato, H., Imanishi, K., Sakata, Y., & Uchiyama, T. (1998). Exanthematous disease induced by toxic shock syndrome toxin 1 in the early neonatal period. *Lancet, 351*, 1614–1619.

Takahashi, N., Kato, H., Imanishi, K., Miwa, K., Yamanami, S., Nishida, H., & Uchiyama, T. (2000). Immunopathophysiological aspects of an emerging neonatal infectious disease induced by a bacterial superantigen. *J Clin Invest, 106*, 1409–1415.

Tam, A. C.-Y., & Yeung, C.-Y. (1988). The changing pattern of severe neonatal staphylococcal infection: A 10-year study. *Aust Pediatr J, 24*, 275–278.

Tang, Y. W., Waddington, M. G., Smith, D. H., Manahan, J. M., Kohner, P. C., Highsmith, L. M., Li, H., Cockerill, F. R., III, Thomson, R. L., Montgomery, S. O., & Persing, D. H. (2000). Comparison of protein A gene sequencing with pulsed-field gel electrophoresis and epidemiologic data for molecular typing of methicillin-resistant *Staphylococcus aureus*. *J Clin Microbiol, 38*, 1347–1353.

Teixeira, L. A., Resende, C. A., Ormonde, L. R., Rosenbaum, R., Figueiredo, A. M. S., de Lencastre, H., & Tomasz, A. (1995). Geographic spread of epidemic multi-resistant *Staphylococcus aureus* clone in Brazil. *J Clin Microbiol, 33*, 2400–2404.

Tenover, F. C., Arbeit, R. D., Goering, R. V., Michelson, P. A., Murray, B. E., Persing, D. H., & Swaminathan, B. (1995). Interpreting chromosomal DNA restriction patterns produced by pulsed-field gel electrophoresis: Criteria for bacterial strain typing. *J Clin Microbiol, 33*, 2233–2239.

Tenover, F. C., Biddle, J. W., & Lancaster, M. V. (2001). Increasing resistance to vancomycin and other glycopeptides in *Staphylococcus aureus*. *Emerging Infect Dis, 7*, 327–332.

Terpenning, M. S., Bradley, S. F., Wan, J. Y., Chenoweth, C. E., Jorgenson, K. A., & Kauffman, C. A. (1994). Colonization and infection with antibiotic-resistant bacteria in a long-term care facility. *J Am Geriatr Soc, 42*, 1062–1069.

Thompson, R. L., Cabezulo, I., & Wenzel, R. P. (1982). Epidemiology of nosocomial infections caused by methicillin-resistant *Staphylococcus aureus*. *Ann Intern Med, 97*, 309–317.

Tokue, Y., Shoji, S., Satoh, K., Watanabe, A., & Motomiya, M. (1992). Comparison of a polymerase chain reaction assay and conventional microbiologic method for detection of methicillin resistant *Staphylococcus aureus*. *Antimicrob Agents Chemother, 36*, 6–9.

Tomasz, A., Nachman, S., & Leaf, H. (1991). Stable classes of phenotypic expression in methicillin-resistant clinical isolates of staphylococci. *Antimicrob Agents Chemother, 35*, 124–129.

Tsiodras, S., Gold, H. S., Sakoulas, G., Eliopoulos, G. M., Wennersten, C., Venkataraman, L., Moellering, R. C., & Ferraro, M. J. (2001). Linezolid resistance in a clinical isolate of *Staphylococcus aureus*. *Lancet, 358*, 207–208.

Turnidge, J., & Grayson, M. L. (1993). Optimum treatment of staphylococcal infections. *Drugs, 45*, 353–366.

Udo, E. E., & Jacob, L. E. (2000). Characterization of methicillin-resistant *Staphylococcus aureus* from Kuwait hospitals with high-level fusidic acid resistance. *J Med Microbiol, 49*, 419–426.

Unal, S., Werner, K., DeGirolami, P., Barsanti, F., & Eliopoulos, G. (1994). Comparison of tests for detection of methicillin resistant *Staphylococcus aureus* in a clinical microbiology laboratory. *Antimicrob Agents Chemother, 38*, 345–347.

van Leeuwen, W. B., van Pelt, C., Luijendijk, A., Verbrugh, H. A., & Goessens, W. H. (1999). Rapid detection of methicillin resistance in *Staphylococcus aureus* isolates by the MRSA-screen latex agglutination test. *J Clin Microbiol, 37*, 3029–3030.

Vanuffel, P., & Cocito, C. (1996). Mechanism of action of Streptogramins and Macrolides. *Drugs, 51*(Suppl. 1), 21–30.

Verma, S., Joshi, S., Chitnis, V., Hemwani, N., & Chitnis, D. (2000). Growing problem of methicillin resistant staphylococci—Indian scenario. *Indian J Med Sci, 54*, 535–540.

Vincent, J. L., Bihari, D. J., Suter, P. M., Bruining, H. A., White, J., Nicolas-Chanoin, M.-H., Wolff, M., Spencer, R. C., & Hemmer, M. (1995). The prevalence of nosocomial infection in Intensive Care Units in Europe. *JAMA, 274*, 639–644.

von Eiff, C., Becker, C., Machka, K., Stammer, H., & Peters, G. (2001). Nasal carriage as a source of *Staphylococcus aureus* bacteremia. *N Engl J Med, 344*, 11–16.

Voss, A., Milatovic, D., Wallrauch-Schwarz, C., Rosdahl, V. T., & Bravenly, I. (1994). Methicillin-resistant *Staphylococcus aureus* in Europe. *Eur J Clin Microbiol Infect Dis, 13*, 50–55.

Wade, D., Silberring, J., Soliymani, R., Heikkinen, S., Kilpelainen, I., Lankinen, H., & Kuusela, P. (2000). Antibacterial activities of temporin A analogs. *FEBS Lett, 479*(1–2), 6–9.

Walker, J., Borrow, R., Goering, R. V., Egerton, S., Fox, A. J., & Oppenheim, B. A. (1999). Subtyping of methicillin-resistant *Staphylococcus aureus* isolates from the North-West of England: a comparison of standardised pulsed-field gel electrophoresis with bacteriophage typing including an inter-laboratory reproducibility study. *J Med Microbiol, 48*, 297–301.

Walsh, T. R., Bolmstrom, A., Qwarnstrom A., Ho, P., Wootton, M., Howe, R. A., MacGowan, A. P., & Diekema, D. (2001). Evaluation of current methods for detection of staphylococci with reduced susceptibility to glycopeptides. *J Clin Microbiol, 39*, 2439–2444.

Washio, M., Kiyohara, C., Arai, Y., Aoyagi, K., Okada, K., Fujisama, M., Maeda, M., & Ito, Y. (1998). Methicillin-resistant *Staphylococcus aureus* (MRSA) and *Pseudomonas aeruginosa* isolation from pharyngeal swab cultures among the Japanese elderly at admission to a geriatric hospital. *Public Health, 112*, 415–417.

Watanabe, H., Masaki, H., Asoh, N., Watanabe, K., Oishi, K., Furumoto, A., Kobayashi, S., Sato, A., & Nagatake, T. (2001). Emergence and spread of low-level mupirocin resistance in methicillin-resistant *Staphylococcus aureus* isolated from a community hospital in Japan. *J Hosp Infect, 47*, 294–300.

Wenzel, R. P., Nettleman, M. D., Jones, R. V., & Pfaller, M. A. (1991). Methicillin-resistant *Staphylococcus aureus*: Implications for the 1990's and effective control measures. *Am J Med, 91* (Suppl. 3B), 221S–226S.

Wenzel, R. P., Reagan, D. R., Bertino, J. S., Baron E. J., & Arias K. (1998). Methicillin-resistant *Staphylococcus aureus* outbreak: A consensus panel's definition and management guidelines. *Am J Infect Control, 26*, 102–110.

Werner, G., Cuny, C., Schmitz, F. J., & Witte, W. (2001). Methicillin-resistant, quinupristin–dalfopristin-resistant *Staphylococcus aureus* with reduced sensitivity to glycopeptides. *J Clin Microbiol, 39*, 3586–3590.

Wielders, C. L. C., Vriens, M. R., Brisse, S., de Graaf-Mittenburg, L. A. M., Troelsta, A., Fleer, A., Schmitz, F. J., Verhoef, J., & Fluit, A. C. (2001). Evidence for in-vivo transfer of mecA DNA between strains of *Staphylococcus aureus*. *Lancet, 357*, 1674–1675.

Wilson, D. R., Karchmer, A. W., Dajani, A. S., Taubert, K. A, Bayer, A., Kaye, D., Bisno, A. L., Ferrieri, P., Shulman, S. T., & Durack, D. T. (1995). Antibiotic treatment of adults with infective endocarditis due to streptococci, enterococci, staphylococci, and HACEK microorganisms. *JAMA, 274*, 1706–1713.

Wilson, P., Andrews, J. A., Charlesworth, R., Walesby, R., Singer, M., Farrell, D. J., & Robbins, M. (2003). Linezolid resistance in clinical isolates of *Staphylococcus aureus*. *J Antimicrob Chemother, 51*, 186–188.

Wongwanich, S., Tishyadhigama, P., Paisomboon, S., Ohta, T., & Hayashi, H. (2000). Epidemiological analysis of methicillin resistant *Staphylococcus aureus* in Thailand. *Southeast Asian J Trop Med Public Health, 31*, 72–76.

Wu, S., Piscitelli, C., de Lencastre, H., & Tomasz, A. (1996). Tracking the evolutionary origin or the methicillin resistance gene: Cloning and sequencing of a homologue of mecA from a methicillin susceptible strain of *Staphylococcus sciuri*. *Microb Drug Resist, 2*, 435–441.

York, M. K., Gibbs, L., Chehab, F., & Brooks, G. F. (1996). Comparison of PCR detection of mecA with standard susceptibility testing methods that determine methicillin resistance in coagulase-negative staphylococci. *J Clin Microbiol, 34*, 1023–1024.

Zarrouk, V., Bozdogan, B., Leclercq, R., Garry, L., Feger, C., Carbon, C., & Fantin, B. (2001). Activities of the combination of quinupristin–dalfopristin with rifampin in vitro and in experimental endocarditis due to *Staphylococcus aureus* strains with various phenotypes of resistance to macrolide-lincosamide-streptogramin antibiotics. *Antimicrob Agents Chemother, 45*, 1244–1248.

5

Vancomycin-Resistant Enterococci

Esteban C. Nannini and Barbara E. Murray

1. INTRODUCTION

The genus *Enterococcus* consists of Gram-positive, catalase negative, facultatively anaerobic organisms that are ovoid in shape and appear usually as short chains. These organisms were initially considered as streptococci, together with pyogenic, viridans, and lactic streptococci. However, enterococci are distinguished by their capability to grow at 10°C and 45°C, in sodium chloride concentrations of 6.5% and at pH 9.6, and to resist 60°C for 30 min (Sherman, 1937). In 1984, recognition of the low homology between nucleic acids of enterococci and those of streptococci led to the proposal of a new genus, *Enterococcus*, with inclusion of the species *E.* (*S.*) *faecalis*, *E.* (*S.*) *faecium*, and others (Schleifer & Kilpper-Bälz, 1984).

Enterococci are usual inhabitants of human and animal gastrointestinal tracts, and have also been found in vaginal and oral specimens. Most of the studies in healthy volunteers report that *E. faecalis* is more common and is found in higher numbers than *E. faecium* in feces, which may explain why *E. faecalis* outnumbers *E. faecium* as a cause of clinical infections. The presence of enterococci in the ecologic niche of the gastrointestinal tract and in wastewaters, also implies that this organism will be regularly exposed to different antibiotics.

The clinical manifestations of enterococci include causing an estimated 5–20% of the cases of infective endocarditis, which is now seen predominantly in older men, and can present with an acute or subacute course (Megran, 1992). Enterococcal bacteremia alone, however, is much more frequent than endocarditis. The source of the bacteremia without valve involvement is often the urinary tract, biliary tract, intra-abdominal or pelvic collections, intravascular catheters, and wound infections, situations in which the finding of polymicrobial bacteremia is not uncommon (Maki & Agger, 1988). Enterococci were reported as the third and the second most frequent agent recovered from community and nosocomial-acquired urinary tract infections (UTI), respectively (Bouza et al., 2001; Goldstein, 2000; Mathai et al., 2001). Enterococcal UTIs are more prevalent in the setting of structural abnormalities, instrumentation, or the presence of an indwelling bladder

Reemergence of Established Pathogens in the 21st Century
Edited by Fong and Drlica, Kluwer Academic/Plenum Publishers, New York, 2003

155

catheter. Intra-abdominal and pelvic infections, which typically originate from the patient's own endogenous flora, frequently involve enterococci. Although these infections often resolve with antibiotic therapy that does not specifically target enterococci, breakthrough infection and bacteremia caused by enterococci have been described. Other enterococcal infections include soft tissue infections (usually as part of mixed flora in diabetic foot infections, decubitus ulcers, burns, and post-abdominal surgical wounds) (Lewis & Zervos, 1990), sepsis and meningitis in neonates (Das & Gray, 1998), and more rarely nosocomial meningitis (Durand et al., 1993). Enterococci, overall, are considered an important nosocomial pathogen as reflected by the SCOPE program report from 49 U.S. hospitals, which found that enterococci were the third most common organism recovered from nosocomial bloodstream infections (Edmond et al., 1999). The proportion of noso-comial enterococci that are resistant to vancomycin has increased dramatically over the past 15 years, with 26.3% of intensive care units (ICUs) isolates collected between January and December 2000 being resistant to this agent (National Nosocomial Infection Surveillance [NNIS], 2001).

Historically, among infections caused by *Enterococcus* spp., *E. faecalis* was usually present in 80–90% of the cases, *E. faecium* in 5–20%, and the other species (e.g., *E. galli-narum, E. avium, E. casseliflavus,* and *E. raffinosus*) in 2–4% (Gordon et al., 1992; Lewis & Zervos, 1990; Maki & Agger, 1988; Moellering, 1992; Patterson et al., 1995). However, a change in the proportion of *Enterococcus* spp. recovered from clinical isolates has been observed, probably because of the increasing overall resistance to antibiotics among ente-rococci. For example, in a retrospective study from Nebraska, *E. faecalis* clinical isolates accounted for 83.9% of all the enterococci isolates in 1988–1989, while only 58.1% in 1994–1995; *E. faecium* isolates, on the other hand, showed a significant increase from 12.9% in 1988–1989 to 36.3% in 1994–1995 (Iwen et al., 1997), coincident with an increase in the percentage of vancomycin resistance from 0% to 22.2%. Another study (Vergis et al., 2001), which enrolled patients between 1995 and 1997 with clinically sig-nificant enterococcal bacteremia from four different states in the United States, found that of 398 enterococcal bacteremic episodes, 60% were caused by *E. faecalis* and 37% by *E. faecium*. These reports confirm a trend for an increase in *E. faecium* and likely reflect the prevalence of vancomycin-resistant (VR) enterococci (VRE) within specific areas.

One of the typical features of enterococci is the tolerance and/or resistance to differ-ent classes of antibiotics. The history of enterococci has been remarkable for the ability to develop or acquire resistance to antimicrobials (Table 5.1), which can be an inherent prop-erty of *Enterococcus* spp., secondary to a mutation in the existing DNA or secondary to acquisition of new DNA. Inherent resistance characteristics include resistance to semisyn-thetic penicillinase-resistant penicillins, cephalosporins, low levels of aminoglycosides, of clindamycin, and of quinupristin–dalfopristin (*E. faecalis*), and (in vivo) trimethoprim–sulfamethoxazole. Examples of acquired resistance include resistance to chloramphenicol, tetracycline, erythromycin, fluoroquinolones, high levels of clin-damycin, of aminoglycosides, and of penicillin (via penicillinase and non-penicillinase mechanism) (Murray, 1990). In addition to the inherent resistance to semisynthetic penicillinase-resistant penicillins and cephalosporins, enterococci display low-level resist-ance to penicillin, ampicillin, and ureidopenicillins, relative to streptococci, due to cell wall synthesis enzymes with low affinity for penicillin (so-called penicillin-binding pro-teins) (Fontana et al., 1983). Enterococci are inherently less susceptible to cell wall agents

Table 5.1
Reports of Drug Resistance Development in Clinical Isolates
of Enterococci (In Chronological Order)

Drug to which resistance was described	Enterococcal species	Reference
Streptomycin	Enterococci not identified to species level	Finland et al. (1950)
HLR to gentamicin	E. faecalis	Horodniceanu et al. (1979)
Penicillin (by β-lactamase production)	E. faecalis	Murray and Mederski-Samaroj (1983)
Vancomycin	E. faecium and E. faecalis	Uttley et al. (1988)
HLR to gentamicin	E. faecium	Eliopoulos et al. (1988)
Penicillin (by β-lactamase production)	E. faecium[a]	Coudron et al. (1992)
Quinupristin/dalfopristin	E. faecium	Collins et al. (1993)
Linezolid	E. faecium	Gonzales et al. (2001)

Note: HLR: high-level resistance.
[a] The only known β-lactamase positive *E. faecium* isolate reported.

and tolerant to the bactericidal activity of these agents (Handwerger & Tomasz, 1985; Krogstad & Pargwette, 1980). Penicillin resistance has been more prominent in *E. faecium* isolates, with high-level ampicillin resistance emerging in this species in recent years. The transfer of vancomycin and ampicillin resistance determinants from one *E. faecium* strain to another has been reported (Carias et al., 1998), and this might help explain the high occurrence of ampicillin resistance within VR *E. faecium* strains.

The rise in the incidence of multidrug-resistant enterococci and the occasional lack of effective therapy have made enterococcal infections an alarming and emerging infectious disease dilemma. Also of concern is the possibility of natural transmission of the vancomycin resistance traits from enterococci to other more pathogenic organisms, particularly *Staphylococcus aureus*, as was already attained in vitro and in an animal model (Noble et al., 1992), and more recently in two methicillin-resistant *S. aureus* (MRSA) isolates from patients (both *vanA*) (CDC, 2002a, 2002b).

2. MECHANISMS OF RESISTANCE TO VANCOMYCIN

As part of the synthesis of cell wall intermediates by vancomycin-susceptible (VS) enterococci (VSE), an intracellular ligase joins two D-alanine molecules to form D-alanyl-D-alanine (D-Ala-D-Ala). This dipeptide is then added to a tripeptide precursor, generating a pentapeptide precursor, which is transported through the cell membrane, transferred to the growing peptidoglycan chain by transglycosylation and subsequently cross-linked to the mature cell wall by transpeptidation. Glycopeptides can inhibit this process by binding with high affinity, in a non-covalent nature, to the C-terminal D-Ala-D-Ala of peptidoglycan precursors just after they cross the cell membrane. The relatively large molecules of vancomycin and teicoplanin effectively enclose the D-Ala-D-Ala terminal, inhibiting further enzyme-mediated peptidoglycan polymerization (Johnson et al., 1990). That is, these antibiotics form a complex with these cell wall precursors, blocking their incorporation into the bacterial cell wall (Reynolds, 1989).

Six types of glycopeptide resistance have been reported among enterococci, namely VanA, VanB, VanC, VanD, VanE, and VanG. The classification system is based on the specific ligase genes (e.g., *vanA, vanB*, etc.) carried by individual isolates. A related ligase gene, *vanF*, was identified in *Paenibacillus popilliae* (Rippere et al., 1998), and the associated glycopeptide resistance assigned the VanF designation. A phenotypic classification using the minimal inhibitory concentrations (MICs) of vancomycin and teicoplanin was initially used, but it lacks specificity. Genotypic classification is now preferred. Acquired glycopeptide resistance has been found most often in *E. faecium* and in *E. faecalis* (although with much higher frequency in the former) (Bingen et al., 1989; Green et al., 1991; Peset et al., 2000; Uttley et al., 1989), *Enterococcus durans* (Green et al., 1991; Robredo et al., 2000a), *Enterococcus mundtii* (Willey et al., 1993), *Enterococcus avium* (Descheemaeker et al., 2000), and *Enterococcus raffinosus* (Wilke et al., 1997); isolates of *Enterococcus hirae* (Robredo et al., 2000a) have also sporadically been found to carry vancomycin resistance genes.

Despite the different types of glycopeptide resistance described in enterococci, the common endpoint is the formation of a peptidoglycan precursor with less affinity for glycopeptides. VanA-, VanB-, and VanD-type of resistance produce a peptidoglycan precursor ending in the depsipeptide D-alanyl-D-lactate (D-Ala-D-Lac), while VanC and VanE isolates produce precursors terminating in the dipeptide D-alanyl-D-serine (D-Ala-D-Ser). The peptidoglycan precursors from VanG-type strains have not been described yet, and its ligase is the most dissimilar of the acquired ligases.

While resistance to vancomycin in enterococci is usually acquired, the motile species of enterococci, *E. gallinarum* and *E. casseliflavus/flavescens*, have been characterized as having intrinsic resistance to vancomycin (Navarro & Courvalin, 1994); these species carry the naturally occurring *vanC-1, vanC-2/vanC-3* genes that confer the VanC phenotype of glycopeptide resistance (although isolates of these species with the *vanA* or *vanB* cluster of genes have been reported [Dutka-Malen et al., 1994; Patel et al., 1997a]).

2.1. VanA

VanA type of resistance has been the most extensively explored. Typical VanA strains are highly resistant to vancomycin (MICs, ≥ 64 μg/ml) and teicoplanin (MICs, ≥ 16 μg/ml). The *vanA* gene cluster responsible for the development of glycopeptide resistance has generally been found on the transposon Tn*1546* or related elements (e.g., Tn*5482*) (Arthur et al., 1993; Handwerger & Skoble, 1995), which in turn have been found on transferable and nontransferable plasmids, as well as on the bacterial chromosome. Deletions, insertions, and mutations confer heterogeneity to the Tn*1546*-like elements (Brown et al., 2001; Willems et al., 1999; Woodford et al., 1998). The finding of identical Tn*1546* elements in different VR *E. faecium* strains from human and animal sources from the United States and Europe may indicate horizontal transfer of these genetic elements among these strains or from a common reservoir for glycopeptide resistance (Jensen et al., 1998a;

Robredo et al., 2000c). VanA type of resistance has been described primarily in *E. faecium* isolates but occasionally in *E. faecalis* strains and, more rarely, other species, again suggesting horizontal transmission.

The *vanA* gene cluster includes *vanR, vanS, vanH, vanA, vanX, vanY*, and *vanZ* (Figure 5.1). The three co-transcribed genes *vanHAX* are necessary and sufficient to confer resistance to glycopeptides (Arthur et al., 1992). These three genes encode a dehydrogenase (VanH), a ligase (VanA), and a D,D-dipeptidase (VanX). The dehydrogenase (VanH) reduces pyruvate into D-Lac, which is then used as a substrate by the ligase to synthesize the depsipeptide D-Ala-D-Lac (Arthur & Courvalin, 1993). D-Ala-D-Lac incorporation into cell wall precursors and further steps for cell wall assembly are generated by endogenous cell wall synthesis enzymes encoded by species-specific genes. Precursors of peptidoglycan ending in D-Ala-D-Lac instead of D-Ala-D-Ala have reduced affinity for glycopeptides and thus cell wall synthesis is not inhibited in the presence of vancomycin. The D,D-dipeptidase VanX appears to act on free dipeptides, resulting in the hydrolysis of D-Ala-D-Ala, thus reducing the formation of the normal D-Ala-D-Ala-containing precursor. Another gene that can contribute to the resistance machinery is *vanY*, which encodes a D,D-carboxypeptidase that cleaves the C-terminal D-Ala from late pentapeptide precursors (should any dipeptide escape the cleavage action of VanX and become incorporated into precursors), again reducing the formation of D-Ala-D-Ala-containing precursors (Arthur et al., 1998). *vanX* and, in some instances, *vanY* are important since the presence of D-Ala-D-Ala

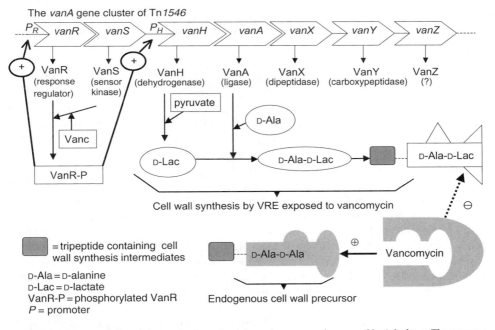

Figure 5.1. Representation of the mechanism of resistance to vancomycin among VanA isolates. The presence of vancomycin is sensed by VanS leading to phosphorylation of VanR (VanR-P), which upregulates the promoters P_R and P_H. The dehydrogenase VanH produces D-Lac from pyruvate, and then the ligase VanA forms the precursors ending in D-Ala-D-Lac. Vancomycin cannot attach to these precursors and cell wall synthesis continues in its presence.

precursors reduces the level of vancomycin resistance. VanZ increases the MICs of teicoplanin by an unknown mechanism, but its presence is not essential for VanA phenotype expression (Arthur et al., 1995).

The expression of the *vanA* cluster is regulated by a two-component regulatory system, composed of a membrane-associated sensor kinase (VanS) and a cytoplasmic regulator (VanR). VanS appears to sense the presence of glycopeptides in the medium by an unknown mechanism, leading to phosphorylation of a conserved histidine residue of the catalytic domain. The phosphoryl group is then transferred to the cytoplasmic response regulator (VanR), which causes increase in its affinity for the target promoters P_R (the promoter for the *vanRS* transcript) and P_H (the promoter for the *vanHAX* transcript) and results in transcriptional activation of the resistance genes and regulatory genes; this leads to increased transcription of *vanR* and accumulation of the phosphorylated (activated) cytoplasmic VanR, forming an amplification loop (Arthur & Quintiliani, 2001).

2.2. VanB

The VanB system of glycopeptide resistance imparts resistance to vancomycin but not, typically, to teicoplanin. The *vanB* gene cluster is homologous to much of the *vanA* gene cluster, and the counterparts are designated *vanH$_B$*, *vanX$_B$*, *vanY$_B$*, *vanR$_B$*, *vanS$_B$*, and *vanB*. The manner in which the VanA and VanB systems function is similar, although the *vanB* cluster contains a gene, *vanW*, not found in the *vanA* gene cluster. Another difference is that the VanB-type has no gene counterpart of the *vanZ* gene, found at one end of Tn*1546*.

The *vanB* cluster has been recognized primarily in *E. faecium* and *E. faecalis*; however, rare isolates of *E. casseliflavus* and *E. gallinarum* have been reported to carry these genes as well (Liassine et al., 1998). Occasionally, the *vanB* genes have been found in other organisms such as *Streptococcus gallolyticus* (Mevius et al., 1998), *Streptococcus bovis* (Poyart et al., 1997) (although misclassification between these two species has been reported [Devriese et al., 1998]), and anaerobes from human bowel flora such as *Eggerthella lenta* and *Clostridium innocuum* (Stinear et al., 2001).

The difference in susceptibility to teicoplanin between the VanA and VanB phenotype relates to differences in the two-component regulatory system (*vanS$_B$* and *vanR$_B$*). The presence of vancomycin results in activation of both VanA and VanB systems (Arthur et al., 1996) while teicoplanin does not activate the sensor kinase VanS$_B$, which differs from VanS$_A$ in the sensor domain (Evers & Courvalin, 1996). Thus, teicoplanin can induce the synthesis of VanA-related products while it does not induce the production of VanB-related proteins; however, teicoplanin-resistant mutants have been obtained from VanB-type enterococci when these organisms were plated onto teicoplanin-containing agar (Hayden et al., 1993). This phenomenon can be explained by the ability of teicoplanin to select mutants with alterations in VanS$_B$ (Arthur & Quintiliani, 2001), resulting in inducibility by teicoplanin, or in constitutive production of vancomycin-resistant proteins (i.e., loss of a requirement of an inducer). It was reported that a mutation of codon 221 in the *vanS$_B$* gene changes the VanS$_B$ function so that the presence of teicoplanin can trigger the cytoplasmic regulator (VanR$_B$), which in turn activates a promoter for transcription of the resistance genes (Lefort et al., 1999). Development of resistance to teicoplanin in a patient while on treatment with vancomycin (Hayden et al., 1993), as well as in vitro and in an animal model of experimental endocarditis treated with teicoplanin, has been reported (Aslangul et al., 1997). More recently, during a VanB-type VRE outbreak, a patient previously treated with teicoplanin was colonized with a VanB isolate resistant to teicoplanin (MIC, 32 μg/ml) that lacked the regulatory genes $vanR_B$ and $vanS_B$ and the promoter P_{YB} (Kawalec et al., 2001).

The *vanB* gene cluster was initially thought to be nontransferable, but a number of reports have found the gene cluster on chromosomally located transferable elements, as well as on transferable plasmids (Rice et al., 1998). The *vanB* gene cluster has also been found on the same plasmid as a gentamicin-resistance gene in a clinical *E. faecalis* isolate (Woodford et al., 1995).

2.3. VanC

The *vanC* genes have been found exclusively in the motile enterococci *E. gallinarum, E. casseliflavus*, and *E. flavescens* (the latter two are probably the same species), carrying the *vanC-1, vanC-2*, and *vanC-3* genes, respectively (Clark et al., 1998) (*vanC-2* and *vanC-3* genes are 98% identical [Navarro & Courvalin, 1994]). The VanC phenotype is characterized by, at most, low-level resistance to vancomycin while remaining susceptible to teicoplanin, although some strains test vancomycin susceptible. Of note, the National Committee for Clinical Laboratory Standards (NCCLS) breakpoints for vancomycin and enterococci are ≥32 μg/ml for resistant and ≤4 μg/ml for susceptible, while other groups consider an MIC of vancomycin of 8 μg/ml as resistant. Five genes, which are naturally occurring or inherent to these species, have been identified within the *vanC-1* cluster: *vanC-1*, which encodes a ligase that synthesizes the dipeptide D-Ala-D-Ser; *vanXY*, a D,D-dipeptidase-carboxypeptidase that hydrolyzes D-Ala-D-Ala; *vanT* (a homologue of *vanH* and *vanH_B*), encoding a serine racemase which provides D-Ser to be used by the VanC ligase; and *vanR-vanS* homologues which encode a two-component regulatory system (Arias et al., 2000). The presence of a system for the synthesis of D-Ala-D-Ala precursors, together with the *vanC* gene cluster which mediates the formation of D-Ala-D-Ser, may explain the variability in the vancomycin susceptibility of these species (Dutka-Malen et al., 1992); that is, isolates with higher production of the D-Ala-D-Ala precursors (high affinity for vancomycin) are predicted to have lower MICs of vancomycin (sometimes within the susceptible range: ≤4 μg/ml) than isolates that produce more D-Ala-D-Ser precursors (lower affinity for vancomycin).

2.4. VanD

The VanD-type of glycopeptide resistance was first reported in an *E. faecium* (BM4339) urinary isolate from a patient in a New York hospital in 1991 (Perichon et al., 1997). This isolate was constitutively resistant to moderate levels of vancomycin (MIC,

64 µg/ml) and lower levels of teicoplanin (MIC, 4 µg/ml). The deduced amino acid sequence of the VanD ligase has 69% identity with VanA and VanB and 43% identity with VanC. Three other strains have been identified in Boston, Massachusetts, with MICs of 128 and 4 µg/ml for vancomycin and teicoplanin, respectively (Ostrowsky et al., 1999). The *vanD* gene encodes a D-alanine : D-lactate ligase (Perichon et al., 1997) and the complete sequence of the *vanD* gene cluster was also found to encode a dehydrogenase (VanH$_D$) and a D,D-dipeptidase (VanX$_D$), which are highly similar to the corresponding proteins in VanA and VanB phenotypes. VanY$_D$ (a D,D-carboxypeptidase) has greater similarity to penicillin-binding proteins than to VanY$_A$ or VanY$_B$ (Casadewall & Courvalin, 1999). The original strain (*E. faecium* BM4339) was later found to be unable to synthesize D-Ala-D-Ala due to a mutation in its endogenous *ddl* ligase gene (Reynolds et al., 2001), which implies that the activity of the D,D-dipeptidase (VanX$_D$) and the D,D-carboxypeptidase (VanY$_D$) are not required for glycopeptide resistance and that vancomycin resistance is constitutively expressed. Two other *E. faecium* strains carrying this gene have since been reported (Boyd et al., 2000; Perichon et al., 2000). *vanD* appears to be located in the chromosome and, thus far, its transfer to other enterococci has not been reported.

2.5. VanE

The *vanE* glycopeptide resistance gene has been recently described in an *E. faecalis* strain (BM4405) (Fines et al., 1999). This isolate was noted to have some similarities to the intrinsic VanC-phenotype: low level resistance to vancomycin (MICs, 16 µg/ml), susceptibility to teicoplanin (MICs, 0.5 µg/ml), and the presence of serine racemase activity for the production of D-Ala-D-Ser precursors (Fines et al., 1999). Unlike VanC-type strains, *vanE* is not an inherent or a species-specific gene. The amino acid sequence of the VanE ligase has greater identity to VanC (55%) than to VanA (45%), VanD (44%), or VanB (43%). Another isolate of *E. faecalis* harboring the *vanE* gene has been reported recently in Canada (Van Caeseele et al., 2001).

2.6. VanF

The *vanF* gene has been found in *Paenibacillus* (formerly *Bacillus*) *popilliae* (a biopesticide used in the United States to suppress Japanese beetle population) strains collected in 1945 (Rippere et al., 1998). These strains were found to have a vancomycin resistance gene with approximate 77% and 69% nucleotide sequence identity to *vanA* and *vanB*, respectively. Later, the same group of investigators detected genes encoding other homologues of the *vanA* gene cluster (*vanY, vanZ, vanH*, and *vanX*) in a *P. popilliae* strain (Patel et al., 2000). The predicted amino acid sequences showed the following relatedness to those of the VanA-type of resistance: 61% identity for VanY$_F$, 21% for VanZ$_F$, 74% for VanH$_F$, 77% for VanF, and 79% for VanX$_F$. These findings are of more phylogenic than clinical interest because no human disease has been reported with this organism.

2.7. VanG

vanG is a vancomycin resistance gene found in an *E. faecalis* strain isolated from a hospitalized patient in Brisbane, Australia (McKessar et al., 2000). Three other isolates in the same institution had the same susceptibility pattern and were indistinguishable by pulsed-field gel electrophoresis (PFGE). These strains displayed moderate resistance to vancomycin (MICs, 12–16 μg/ml) and full susceptibility to teicoplanin (MICs, 0.5 μg/ml). The *vanG* cluster was found to encode the two-component regulatory proteins, $VanR_G$ and $VanS_G$; a ligase (VanG) with 39–47% similarity with other enterococcal ligases; a D,D-peptidase ($VanY_G$) and a racemase ($VanT_G$), but no VanX dipeptidase activity was detected (McKessar et al., 2000).

2.8. Vancomycin-Dependent Enterococci

The first vancomycin-dependent enterococcus (VDE) was described in 1993 in a urine sample from a patient heavily treated with vancomycin and who was known to be colonized with VRE (Fraimow et al., 1994). Its growth was observed only around a vancomycin disk and a disk containing the dipeptide D-Ala-D-Ala. Several reports of *E. faecalis* and *E. faecium* VDE isolated from multiple sites were reported thereafter (Dever et al., 1995; Green et al., 1995), including an outbreak in a bone marrow transplant (BMT) unit (Kirkpatrick et al., 1999). It has been shown that a mutation in the endogenous *ddl* gene of these VRE leads to the synthesis of an inactive D-Ala:D-Ala ligase, but, under vancomycin-inducing conditions, D-Ala-D-Lac precursors are produced from their *vanA* or *vanB* gene cluster, allowing the organisms to survive. When vancomycin is not present, its inducing effect ends and no more D-Ala-D-Lac precursors are produced; as the organism cannot make D-Ala-D-Ala, it cannot sustain growth. As expected, the growth of the VDE strain was supported when D-Ala-D-Ala was added to the plate (Fraimow et al., 1994). These VRE strains can revert to vancomycin-independent growth by restoring their normal activity of D-Ala : D-Ala ligase activity or by constitutively producing precursors ending in D-Ala-D-Lac (Van Bambeke et al., 1999); thus, the discontinuation of vancomycin may not be sufficient to adequately treat patients infected with VDE.

2.9. Origin of Vancomycin Resistance Genes

Several non-enterococcal bacteria harbor the *vanA* and *vanB* genes, including *Oerskovia turbata, Arcanobacterium haemolyticum* (Power et al., 1995), *S. bovis* (Poyart et al., 1997), *S. gallolyticus* (Mevius et al., 1998), and *Bacillus circulans* (Fontana et al., 1997). However, these appear to be sporadic examples, and there is no evidence to suggest that these non-enterococcal bacteria are the source or donor of *vanA/B* genes. Rather, they are occasional recipients. Some Gram-positive organisms are naturally resistant to vancomycin, such as *Leuconostoc* spp., *Lactobacillus* spp., and *Pediococcus* spp.; however, the D-Ala:D-Lac ligase and D-lactate dehydrogenase enzymes of these organisms are not closely related to VanA or VanB nor to VanH or $VanH_B$, respectively (Patel, 2000). *Erysipelothrix rhusiopathiae* is also vancomycin resistant, though *vanA* and *vanB* genes have not been detected in this organism (Facklam et al., 1989). *S. aureus* isolates with decreased susceptibility to vancomycin have been reported, although no *van*-like genes have been found.

As mentioned earlier, *E. gallinarum* carries the *vanC-1* gene and *E. casseliflavus* the *vanC-2* gene, which are responsible for the production of a D-Ala:D-Ser ligase. As the VanC enzymes have only a 37–39% amino acid sequence identity with those from the VanA/B phenotypes (Navarro & Courvalin, 1994), it is considered unlikely that the *vanC* genes are a recent origin of the high-level vancomycin-resistant genes *vanA* and *vanB*.

Some results suggest that the remote source of the vancomycin-resistant genes in VRE lies within glycopeptide-producing organisms. The D-Ala-D-Ala ligases from the glycopeptide-producing organisms, *Amycolatopsis orientalis* and *Streptomyces toyocaensis*, showed a high amino acid sequence similarity to the VanA and VanB ligases (Marshall et al., 1997), and contiguous genes from *A. orientalis* C329.2 and *S. toyocaensis* NRRL 15009 strains were found to encode products with striking homology to VanH and VanX of VRE (Marshall et al., 1998). No genes encoding the homologues of the two-component regulatory elements (VanR and VanS), the D,D-carboxy-peptidase VanY, or the unknown function proteins VanW or VanZ of VRE were found in the DNA flanking the *vanHAX*-like cluster in either organism. This, plus the relative lack of conservation of *vanS* and *vanR* homologues of the *vanA* and *vanB* gene clusters, in contrast to the *vanHAX* homologues, has led to the hypothesis that these genes were added to the *vanHAX* homologues from a different source. The G + C content of the glycopeptide resistance genes from *S. toyocaensis* and *A. orientalis* is much higher than that from the *vanA* and *vanB* gene clusters of VRE (65.5% and 63.6% vs. 44% and 49%, respectively) suggesting that, if the organisms are the origin, it is very remote. *vanHAX*-like gene clusters were found in other glycopeptide-producing organisms also (i.e., *A. orientalis* 18098, *A. orientalis* subsp. *lurida*, *A. coloradensis* subsp. *labeda*). It has been hypothesized that the presence of intermediate organisms between the glycopeptide-producing organisms and VRE could account for the dilution of the original G + C content (Marshall et al., 1998), presumably over thousands to millions of years. While important progress has been achieved in this area, the exact origin of the vancomycin resistance genes and how, when, and why these genes reached enterococci more so than other microorganisms, remain unanswered questions.

3. EPIDEMIOLOGY

The first report of VRE was from the United Kingdom in 1988, when 48 *E. faecium* and 7 *E. faecalis* strains recovered since 1986 were described (Uttley et al., 1988). In the same year, two VR *E. faecium* strains were recovered from the feces of two patients with acute leukemia in France (Leclercq et al., 1988). In 1989, a VanB *E. faecalis* clinical isolate recovered in 1987 was reported from St Louis, Missouri in the United States (Sahm et al., 1989). A dramatic spread of VRE, later identified as VanA *E. faecium*, was soon noted in New York hospitals, where the number of hospitals reporting VRE increased from

1 in 1989 to 38 in 1991 (Frieden et al., 1993). VRE isolates were subsequently reported in many European countries (Endtz et al., 1997; Kjerulf et al., 1996; Melhus & Tjernberg, 1996; Nourse et al., 2000) and from other continents including South America (Marin et al., 1998; Zanella et al., 1999), Australia (Bell et al., 1998), Africa (Budavari et al., 1997), and Asia (Chiew & Ling, 1998; Fujita et al., 1998), documenting a worldwide distribution.

3.1. The Scenario in Europe

Until 1997 about 30% of the total antibiotic usage in the European Union (EU) was directed to animal feeds in order to promote growth. Antibiotics used for that purpose were called feed savers or antimicrobial performance enhancers (van den Bogaard & Stobberingh, 2000). Most of these antimicrobials are active against Gram-positive organisms, and the most common agents used include avilamycin (an everninomycin), avoparcin (a glycopeptide), bacitracin (a polypeptide), flavomycin (a bambermycin), monesin (a polyether), tylosin and spiramycin (macrolides), and virginiamycin (a mixture of two streptogramins) (van den Bogaard & Stobberingh, 2000).

After the emergence of VRE as human pathogens, it was recognized that the glycopeptide avoparcin, commonly used as an animal growth enhancer in most of the EU-members countries, selects for VRE in the intestinal flora of animals (Bates et al., 1994). If VRE from food-producing animals were to reach the human intestinal flora, significant levels of colonization might result among healthy individuals outside the health-care environment. As examples, stool samples from 11 (28%) of 40 Belgian community volunteers not on antibiotics and without recent health-care contact were positive for VRE (Van der Auwera et al., 1996), and 50 (4.9%) of 1,026 employees from food processing companies in Switzerland were found to be VRE VanA-type carriers (Balzereit-Scheuerlein & Stephan, 2001).

Similar consequences have been described with enterococci resistant to erythromycin and quinupristin–dalfopristin isolated from fecal samples from pigs and healthy persons in The Netherlands, when animal feeds included related antibiotics like tylosin (macrolide) and virginiamycin (van den Bogaard et al., 1997b).

This apparent route of spread of resistant bacteria from the intestinal flora of food animals involves contamination of carcasses of slaughtered animals, followed by introduction into the intestinal tract of humans via the food chain (Bates et al., 1994). Supporting this chain of transmission, VanA-type VRE were found in 27.2% of food samples of chicken origin in Spain (Robredo et al., 2000a); an identical VRE strain by PFGE after *Sma*I digestion was isolated from a turkey farmer and from his turkeys in The Netherlands (van den Bogaard et al., 1997a); also in Spain, related genetic arrangements of the *vanA* gene cluster were detected in *E. faecium, E. faecalis, E. hirae*, and *E. durans* isolates from chicken and human stool samples (Robredo et al., 2000c). The same PFGE pattern was observed in VanA *E. faecium* strains from two poultry products and two humans samples (Robredo et al., 2000b).

After recognizing the selection pressure for VRE exerted by the use of avoparcin as an animal growth enhancer, its use was banned in EU countries. The avoparcin ban in Denmark in 1995 was followed by a decrease in the occurrence of VRE in broilers, from 72.7% in 1995 to 5.8% in 2000 (Aarestrup et al., 2001). However, the prevalence of VRE in pigs was only reduced after the use of the macrolide tylosin was also abandoned, suggesting that glycopeptide use was not the only cause for the persistence of VRE strains in animals. In Italy, a decreased rate of VRE contamination in meat products was observed, especially in poultry products, after avoparcin use was banned in 1997 (Grosso et al., 2000). More significantly, two years after the use of avoparcin in animal husbandry was discontinued, a significant decrease in the prevalence of VRE was observed in human volunteers from the same community in Germany (Klare et al., 1999).

Despite the widespread use of avoparcin in animal feeds, the prevalence of VRE in hospitalized patients in European countries has not reached the magnitude found in the United States. In a national surveillance study in Belgium hospitals (Vandamme et al., 1996) between January and April 1993, only 1.5% of the 472 isolates were identified as glycopeptide-resistant. Surveillance studies with rectal culture among 1,112 hospitalized patients in The Netherlands, between 1995 and 1998, yielded a 1.4% prevalence of VRE, most of which were *E. faecium* isolates with VanA-phenotype (van den Braak et al., 2000). More recently, from 4,208 clinical isolates of enterococci collected in 27 countries in Europe, VanA, VanB, and VanC accounted only for 0.4%, 0.1%, and 1.6% of the isolates (Schouten et al., 2000), although a higher prevalence was reported in three hospitals from Spain between January 1994 and April 1995, when 8% of enterococcal blood isolates were VRE (Balas et al., 1997). The transmission of VRE within hospitals in Europe also has been less dramatic than in the United States. One report from France (Bingen et al., 1991) found that all the VRE strains isolated within four wards in a children's hospital were different, a finding consistent with the existence of an important diverse reservoir in the community. However, healthy individuals from the community who are colonized with VRE can certainly introduce resistant strains and their resistance genes into health-care facilities (van den Bogaard & Stobberingh, 2000). Then, the hospital environment, which favors the resistant organism because of the high use of antibiotics, may facilitate selection and dissemination of resistant clones and/or resistance genes within it (Bates et al., 1994).

In summary, the epidemiology of VRE in Europe has emphasized the following: (1) the existence of a direct effect of antimicrobial growth promoters on the prevalence of VRE, not only in feces from food-producing animals but also in persons from the community; (2) that this effect may be reversible after stopping the use of the antibiotics as growth enhancers; and (3) the concept of transferring resistant organisms and/or resistance genes from animals to humans.

3.2. The Scenario in United States

In the United States, there was an initial strong correlation between ICU and VRE occurrence; however, this correlation diminished after 1995 and, in the following years, VRE extended to all size hospitals and also into long-term care facilities (LTCF) across the United States. A periodically updated report from the NNIS system of the Centers for Disease Control and Prevention (CDC) (accessible at: http://www.cdc.gov/ncidod/hip/SUR-VEILL/NNIS.HTM) found an overall rate of 26.3% of VRE among enterococci isolates in 2000. It was also found that, among enterococci causing nosocomial infections in ICU patients, a 40% and 31% increase in the vancomycin resistance rate was observed during the years 1999 and 2000, respectively, when compared with the mean rate of vancomycin resistance observed in the previous 5 years (NNIS, 2000, 2001).

Glycopeptides were never approved for use as antimicrobial growth enhancers to feed animals in the United States. However, the presence of VRE (*E. faecium*) in commercially prepared chicken feed (Schwalbe et al., 1999) and dry dog food (Dunne, 1996) has been reported, although the source of the organism was never discovered. Contrasting with European studies, no *vanA* or *vanB* genes were found in stool samples from 101 healthy volunteers without hospital exposure or in 52 animals (49 chickens and 3 turkeys) and 5 probiotic preparations from the community or environmental sources in the geographic area of Houston, Texas (Coque et al., 1996). Similarly, none of 21 healthy community volunteers had VRE isolated from stool samples in Baltimore, Maryland (Morris et al., 1995).

The first known isolate of VRE in the United States was identified in Missouri in 1987 (Sahm et al., 1989) and it was a VanB-type of glycopeptide-resistant *E. faecalis* (the genome of this strain, V583, has since been sequenced by The Institute for Genome Research [TIGR], accessible at http://www.tigr.org/tdb/mdb/mdbinprogress.html). Shortly thereafter, a number of the hospitals from the northeast and midwest United States began to recognize increasing number of cases of VRE infection or colonization. VanA- and VanB-type of glycopeptide resistance strains were initially reported as causing monoclonal outbreaks (Boyce et al., 1994; Frieden et al., 1993; Handwerger et al., 1993), but, subsequently, many hospitals found that their VRE were polyclonal, that is, they were different strains. (Montecalvo et al., 1994; Morris et al., 1995; Shay et al., 1995).

In the United States, the hospital is the main source of VRE, and the indiscriminate use of vancomycin in this setting is thought to be one of the culprits for the selection of these organisms. Vancomycin was licensed for use in the United States in 1958, although its use was not substantial until the 1980s. The total use of vancomycin (injectable and oral) in the United States experienced a dramatic increase from 2,000 kg/year in 1984, to 7,600 kg/year in 1989, and to 11,200 kg/year in 1996 (Kirst et al., 1998), most likely due to the increased occurrence of MRSA infections, prosthetic device-related infections, and *Clostridium difficile* colitis. Other antibiotics, including broad-spectrum cephalosporins and antianaerobic agents, have also been increasingly used in recent years. The use of these antimicrobials alter patients' bowel flora, rendering them more susceptible to colonization by VRE, which then may be transmitted to other patients or health-care workers (HCW). Colonized subjects will be discharged to LTCF or to the community, facilitating the spread of the vancomycin-resistant organisms to others who might be admitted to the health-care facility and be exposed to antibiotics at any time (McDonald et al., 1997).

3.3. Risk Factors

The key factors for the emergence of antibiotic resistance in general include mutations in bacterial genes, exchange of resistance genes among organisms, antibiotic selective pressure in health-care facilities and in the community, and finally, dissemination, sometimes globally, of resistant strains (clones). Antimicrobial drug resistance allows resistant bacteria to proliferate due to their specific advantage over sensitive strains in a setting where antibiotic selective pressure is present. Thus, settings where there is heavy use of antibiotics and in which spread of bacteria from person to person can easily occur tend to have a high rate of antibiotic resistance.

In the case of enterococci, asymptomatic gastrointestinal colonization by organisms with resistant traits is almost always the first step in the development of nosocomial enterococcal infection (Mundy et al., 2000). Suppression of gastrointestinal competitors by antibiotic pressure results in expansion of the enterococcal population, be it acquired or endogenous, carrying an advantageous resistant trait (Donskey et al., 2000a). As a result, persons with prolonged hospitalization and with chronic and more severe illnesses are more likely to have received multiple antibiotics courses as well as to have been exposed to the hospital's resistant organisms. Enterococcal bacteremia, for example, tends to occur in subjects with a serious underlying medical condition, who have undergone a recent major surgery, or have received antibiotics without antienterococcal activity (Maki & Agger, 1988; Pallares et al., 1993). Some authors have referred to enterococcal infections as markers for more serious underlying conditions. Risk factors associated with enterococcal bacteremia include malignant disease, use of urethral or intravascular catheter, recent surgery, major burn, multiple trauma, and prior antibiotic therapy (Maki & Agger, 1988; Shlaes et al., 1981; Wells & von Graevenitz, 1980).

When enterococcal species resistant to ampicillin, mainly *E. faecium*, emerged in the late 1980s (Grayson et al., 1991), several risk factors for its acquisition were described, such as duration of hospitalization, prior antimicrobial therapy (particularly imipenem, extended-spectrum cephalosporins, and metronidazole), nosocomial acquisition, and hospitalization on a surgery service (Chirurgi et al., 1992; McCarthy et al., 1994; Venditti et al., 1994). Similar associations had been noted previously in reports of an increased incidence of high-level gentamicin-resistant (HLGR) enterococci; in this case, the risk factors associated with HLGR were higher Acute Physiologic, Age, and Chronic Health Evaluation (APACHE) II score, prior antibiotic treatment and surgical procedures, prolonged hospitalization, chronic renal failure, ICU stay, and the presence of a urinary catheter (Axelrod & Talbot, 1989; Caballero-Granado et al., 1998; Viagappan & Holliman, 1999; Wells et al., 1992; Zervos et al., 1986). Not surprisingly, risk factors associated with the development of glycopeptide resistance in enterococci are comparable to the ones described above for ampicillin and HLGR strains. Some of the same risk factors were also previously reported for MRSA infections (Boyce, 1989).

Risk factors for VRE colonization and infection have been extensively evaluated, mostly as part of case-control, retrospective studies. Some of these studies have compared cases of VRE bacteremia with VSE bacteremia without specifying the enterococcal species (Lautenbach et al., 1999; Shay et al., 1995; Wells et al., 1995), while others made a comparison mostly between *E. faecium* (VRE) and *E. faecalis* (VSE) species (Lucas et al., 1998). Major differences between these studies also relate to the subjects selected for the control group. Some have used subjects with negative surveillance cultures for VRE (Boyce et al., 1994; Byers et al., 2001; Handwerger et al., 1993; Morris et al., 1995; Tokars et al., 1999); other studies used matched subjects without bacteremia (Edmond et al., 1995; Papanicolaou et al., 1996); and, finally, others included patients with vancomycin-susceptible infection within the same species as control subjects (*E. faecium* [Linden et al., 1996; Stosor et al., 1998; Tornieporth et al., 1996] and *E. faecalis* [Peset et al., 2000]).

Table 5.2 summarizes case–control studies assessing the risk factors for VRE colonization and VRE infection. The risk factors identified include prior treatment with antibiotics

Table 5.2
Case-Control Studies Analyzing Risk Factors for Vancomycin-Resistant Enterococci (VRE) Colonization and Infection

Hospital setting	Method of analysis	Cases	Ctrl	No. of cases	Risk factors	Reference
Outbr/ICU	Univariate	VREfm[a]	Neg SC	16	Prior treatment with oral vanc, IV aminoglycosides, and cephalosporins	Handwerger et al. (1993)
VanB outbr/MW	Univariate	VREfm[a]	Neg SC	37	Proximity to another VRE-positive patient, exposure to a nurse who cared for another case-patient	Boyce et al. (1994)
MW	Multivariate	VRE bact (95% Efm)	VSE bact[b]	46	Receipt of vanc, high APACHE II score, hematology malignancy or BMT	Shay et al. (1995)
Onc unit/ STC	Multivariate	VREfm[a]	Neg SC	75	Receipt of IV vanc and ciprofloxacin, high APACHE II score, and antimicrobial days	Morris et al. (1995)
VanA outbr/ Onc unit[c]	Univariate	VREfm bact	Matched without bact	11	Prior use of metronidazole, clindamycin, and imipenem, gastrointestinal colonization with VRE	Edmond et al. (1995)
Liver transplant service	Multivariate	VREfm bact	VSEfm bact	54	Length of hospitalization	Linden et al. (1996)
OLT recipients	Multivariate	VREfm infection	OLT recipient	32	Days in ICU and repeated exploratory laparotomy	Papanicolaou et al. (1996)
MW	Multivariate	VREfm[a]	Matched VSEfm[a]	145	Prior use of vanc and third-generation cephalosporins, length of hospitalization, and intra-hospital transfer	Tornieporth et al. (1996)
MW	Univariate	VREfm bact	VSEfm bact	53	Prior use of vanc and aminoglycosides, and presence of indwelling bladder catheter	Stosor et al. (1998)
MW	Multivariate	VRE bact (98% Efm)	VSE bact[b]	72	Receipt of vanc, renal insufficiency, antimicrobial days, and neutropenia	Lautenbach et al. (1999)
MW/LTCF	Multivariate	VREfm in SC	Neg SC	42	Antimicrobial days	Tokars et al. (1999)
VanA outbr	Multivariate	17 VRE bact (16 VREfc)	VSEfc bact	17	Receipt of glycopeptide, hemodialysis, use of steroids and chemotherapy, and prior surgery	Peset et al. (2000)

(continued)

Table 5.2

(continued)

Hospital setting	Method of analysis	Cases	Ctrl	No. of cases	Risk factors	Reference
MW	Multivariate	VRE isolates in SC	Neg SC	86	Prior treatment with metronidazole, proximity to a non-isolated VRE case, and history of major trauma	Byers et al. (2001)
MW	Multivariate	VRE bact (85% *Efm*)	VSE bact (89% *Efc*)	147	Previous vanc use, steroid use, and high APACHE II score	Vergis et al. (2001)

Notes
[a] Isolates from either colonization or infection.
[b] No identification to species were done.
[c] 10 of the 11 patients were neutropenic.
APACHE: acute physiologic, age, and chronic health evaluation; Bact: bacteremia; BMT: bone marrow transplant; Ctrl: control; *Efm: Enterococcus faecium; Efc: Enterococcus faecalis*; ICU: intensive care unit; IV: intravenous; LTCF: long-term care facility; MW: multiple wards; Neg: negative; Onc: oncology; OLT: orthotopic liver transplant; Outbr: outbreak; SC: surveillance cultures; STC: Shock-trauma center; Vanc: vancomycin; VRE: vancomycin-resistant enterococci; VSE: vancomycin-susceptible enterococci; VREfc: VR *E. faecalis*; VREfm: VR *E. faecium*; VSEfc: VS *E. faecalis*; VSEfm: VS *E. faecium*.

including oral or intravenous (IV) vancomycin, cephalosporins, ciprofloxacin, metronidazole, clindamycin, and imipenem; severity of the disease based on the APACHE II score; antimicrobial days; length of hospitalization or days in ICU; proximity to a VRE-infected or colonized case; exposure to a nurse who cared for another VRE case-patient; history of major trauma; gastrointestinal colonization with VRE; prior corticosteroid use; hemodialysis, previous chemotherapy or surgery; renal insufficiency and neutropenia; hematology malignancy, and BMT recipient; and repeated exploratory laparotomy in organ liver transplant recipients.

Some studies have debated the role of vancomycin, particularly when administered IV, versus other agents such as third-generation cephalosporins or antianaerobic agents as risks for VRE, and it is likely that each contributes, perhaps in different situations. A recent study (Fridkin et al., 2001) across the United States found that rates of vancomycin and third-generation cephalosporin use were independently associated with the prevalence of VRE in ICU. They also reported an association between the prevalence of VRE in non-ICU inpatients areas with the prevalence of VRE in ICUs.

A recent prospective study (Donskey et al., 2000a) has provided important insight into the effect of antibiotics on the colonization by VRE. Fifty-one VRE-colonized patients were followed for 7 months. The density of VRE in stool samples was evaluated during and after antibiotic therapy, comparing the effect of antibiotics with antianaerobic activity and those with minimal antianaerobic activity. The density of VRE colonization was very high (mean number of organisms, 7.8 ± 1.5 log per gram) in 33 patients during treatment with antianaerobic antibiotics, with subsequent reduction in the density of colonization after antibiotics were discontinued (of note, vancomycin was included in the antianaerobic group due to its activity against Gram-positive anaerobes). In a subgroup of patients who had not been on antianaerobic agents during the preceding week or more, the VRE density in stools increased a mean of 2.2 log per gram after an antianaerobic regimen (piperacillin–tazobactam, ampicillin–sulbactam, amoxicillin–clavulanate, cefoxitin, cefote-tan, imipenem–cilastatin, meropenem, metronidazole, clindamycin, alatrofloxacin, van-comycin, or ceftriaxone) was started as compared with a decrease of 0.6 log per gram in those who received antibiotics with minimal antianaerobic activity (ciprofloxacin, levo-floxacin, dicloxacillin, nafcillin, cephalexin, cefepime, aztreonam, gentamicin, or trimetho-prim–sulfamethoxazole). Interesting, the number of positive environmental cultures for VRE had a positive correlation with high VRE density in the stools (≥ 4 log per gram).

3.4. Mortality Associated with VRE

When morbidity and mortality rates are compared for enterococcal infections, differ-ences in the host and the infecting bacterial species have to be considered. *E. faecalis* has long been able to produce infection in non-hospitalized healthy individuals, specifically community-acquired native valve endocarditis. *E. faecium*, on the other hand, more often infects debilitated, sometimes immunocompromised patients, who have been hospitalized for prolonged time and have been previously exposed to broad-spectrum antibiotic, having an overall high mortality rate reflecting the severity of the underlying disease. Indeed, the presence of *E. faecium* is considered a marker of poor prognosis. Two studies (Noskin et al., 1995a; Suppola et al., 1998) assessing the differences between bacteremic patients due to *E. faecium* and *E. faecalis* found that nosocomial acquisition, cancer, neutropenia, renal insufficiency, current corticosteroid therapy, and previous treatment with antibiotics (aminoglycosides, vancomycin, metronidazole, clindamycin, and cephalosporins) were significantly more frequently observed in patients in the *E. faecium* group than in the *E. faecalis* group. None of these studies found significant difference in the crude mortality and in the enterococcal-attributed mortality rate between the two groups after adjustment was done for underlying illness severity.

Several studies have tried to measure the mortality associated with VRE infections (Table 5.3), one of which reported a 67% attributable mortality rate in subjects with VRE bacteremia compared with only 30% in a matched group without bacteremia (Edmond et al., 1996), indicating the clinical significance and the need for therapy of enterococcal bacteremia. Other studies compared VRE-infected subjects with VSE-infected ones with-out identification to species (Lautenbach et al., 1999; Shay et al., 1995; Stroud et al., 1996; Wells et al., 1995), which carries the risk of comparing patients infected with *E. faecium* versus patients infected with *E. faecalis*, because the former will account for most of the VRE and the later for most of the VSE strains. Comparing patients infected with different species may confound the estimation of mortality attributable to vancomycin resistance. The acquisition of resistance traits (vancomycin, in this case) by any microorganism is not known to be associated with augmented virulence properties, although this possibility has not been well studied.

Three other studies have compared the mortality rate of patients with enterococcal bacteremia, including patients having bacteremia with a vancomycin-susceptible strain of the same enterococcal species (*E. faecium*) in the control group (Garbutt et al., 2000; Linden et al., 1996; Stosor et al., 1998). In two of these studies patients with what were considered clinically significant *E. faecium* bacteremia were enrolled from multiple wards

Table 5.3

Epidemiological Studies of Mortality Associated with Vancomycin-Resistant Enterococcal
Bacteremia

Cases and controls	Crude mortality (%)			Attributable mortality (%)			Outcome/Comments	Reference dates	Study
	VRE	Ctrl	*P* value	VRE	VSE	*P* value			
27 VRE (89% *Efm*) vs. 27 matched subjects without bact	67	30	0.01	37	—	—	Higher mortality rate for VRE bact than matched controls without bact	Edmond et al. (1996)	1993–1995
46 VRE (95% *Efm*) vs. 46 VSE[a]	33	6	0.004	N/A	N/A	—	Vancomycin resistance was not associated with mortality when adjusted for disease severity	Shay et al. (1995)	1992–1993
54 VRE (*Efm*) vs. 48 VSE (*Efm*)	57	35	0.04	46	25	0.04	Higher attributable mortality in the VRE group	Linden et al. (1996)	1991–1994
21 VRE (*Efm*) vs. 32 VSE (*Efm*)	76	41	0.009	38	9	0.01	Higher attributable mortality in the VRE group	Stosor et al. (1998)	1992–1995
72 VRE (98% *Efm*) vs. 188 VSE[a]	20	41	<0.001	N/A	N/A	—	Vancomycin resistance was not an independent predictor of mortality	Lautenbach et al. (1999)	1991–1995
46 VRE (*Efm*) vs. 23 VSE (*Efm*)	48	30	0.17	N/A	N/A	—	Vancomycin resistance was not an independent predictor of mortality	Garbutt et al. (2000)	1995–1997
17 VRE (94% *Efc*) vs. 169 VSE (76% *Efc*, 19% *Efm*, 5% other species)	23	12	0.254	N/A	N/A	—	Type of resistance did not affect mortality rate. Inappropriate antimicrobial treatment was a risk factor only in univariate analysis	Peset et al. (2000)	1994–1996
147 VRE (85% *Efm*) vs. 251 VSE (89% *Efc*)	64	36	<0.001	N/A	N/A	—	Higher mortality in the VRE group. Effective treatment was associated with better survival	Vergis et al. (2001)	1995–1997

[a] No identification to species level was done.
N/A: not available.
For abbreviations see Table 5.2.

while the third included only patients with severe liver disease from the liver transplant
service (Linden et al., 1996). Two of the studies concluded that the presence of vancomycin
resistance was an independent predictor of mortality. The first one (Linden et al., 1996)
included 102 patients with severe liver disease, the majority of whom were receiving immuno-
suppressive therapy; active antienterococcal antibiotics were given to 22 of 51 patients
and to 42 of 46 patients in the VRE and VSE group, respectively. The in-hospital death rate
and the enterococcal-associated mortality were significantly higher in the VRE (57% and
46%) than the VSE group (35% and 25%) ($p = 0.04$ for both variables). Vancomycin resistance, shock, and liver failure were associated with an increased risk of death. The second

study (Stosor et al., 1998) evaluated 53 patients from multiple wards. Based on the information provided, it is difficult to assess treatment efficacy, but active agents were given more frequently in the VSE group. Again, the crude mortality rate and mortality attributed to the bacteremic episode were significantly higher in the VRE group (76% and 41%) than in the VSE group (38% and 9%) ($p = 0.009$ and $p = 0.01$, respectively). The third and more recent study failed to demonstrate any association between resistance to vancomycin and mortality (Garbutt et al., 2000) in 69 bacteremic patients, of which more than half were in an ICU. Disease severity and shock were significant independent predictors of death, but the association with vancomycin resistance did not reach significance. This study was performed a few years later than the other two studies, and the failure of vancomycin resistance to predict mortality may reflect the availability and use of more active agents against VRE. Supporting these findings, a recent prospective multicenter study (Vergis et al., 2001) compared 147 patients with VRE bacteremia (85% were *E. faecium* and 15% *E. faecalis* strains) versus 251 patients with VSE bacteremia (11% were *E. faecium* and 89% *E. faecalis* strains), finding that hematologic malignancy, vancomycin resistance and high APACHE II score were significantly associated with mortality rate; however, for the subgroup of 208 patients with monomicrobial enterococcal bacteremia, the use of effective treatment was associated with better survival regardless of the presence of vancomycin resistance. Accordingly, in a case-control study of patients with enterococcal bacteremia, the 30-day mortality rate was independently associated with inappropriate therapy (Caballero-Granado et al., 2001), and in another recently published report, mortality and length of hospital stay were higher in the VRE group (69% were *E. faecium* strains) than in the VSE group (83% were *E. faecalis* strains) but again, only 18.9% of the subjects in the VRE group received appropriate therapy compared with 75% of those in the VSE group (Lodise et al., 2002).

Common sense conclusions to the questions about VRE-associated mortality are probably now supported by scientific data. One of these is that, if serious infections are not treated adequately, increased direct mortality associated with the VRE infection will likely be observed.

3.5. VRE and *Clostridium difficile*

There are several epidemiological similarities between VRE and *C. difficile*. Many risk factors have been described as associated with both conditions, including length of hospitalization, broad-spectrum antimicrobial exposure, severity of the underlying disease, and contamination of inanimate objects within the environment and HCWs' hands (Bignardi, 1998; Clabots et al., 1992; Gerding, 1997; Johnson & Gerding, 1998; Kim et al., 1981). In the case of VRE colonization, the presence of diarrhea has also been associated with greater environmental contamination (Boyce et al., 1994) and probable increased spread of VRE.

Another point of convergence between these two entities is the finding that *C. difficile* associated-diarrhea by itself was recognized as the only statistically significant risk factor for VRE bacteremia in a small group of VRE-colonized patients with acute leukemia (Roghmann et al., 1997). The immunosuppression of the host, probably the effect of the

C. difficile on the intestinal lining, and the prior antibiotic exposure (especially antianaerobic drugs), may all have played a role in facilitating the bacteremia in these patients.

In other studies examining the association between these two pathogens, VRE (excluding two *E. gallinarum* strains) was found in 13.9% of the stool samples sent for *C. difficile* analysis and in 29.6% of those positive for *C. difficile* cytotoxin assay; 61.6% of the samples positive for VRE were also *C. difficile*-toxin positive (Rafferty et al., 1997). In a more recent study, VRE was found in 19.8% of stool specimens submitted for *C. difficile* toxin assay and in 41.4% of the stool samples that were positive for *C. difficile* toxin (Leber et al., 2001), perhaps as a reflection of the nationwide increase in VRE. Hospital surveillance studies for VRE colonization in specimens submitted for *C. difficile* toxin assay or in those positive for *C. difficile* toxin may represent an opportunity to assess nosocomial VRE prevalence or to increase its detection, and was felt to be cost-effective in at least one hospital setting (Leber et al., 2001). However, some VRE-positive patients will be missed with this approach. Overall, more studies are needed to establish recommendations in this regard.

3.6. Transmission

Early reports of outbreaks of VRE typically represented clonal dissemination of a single *E. faecium* strain, which frequently could be reduced or eliminated through infection control measures (Boyce et al., 1994; Karanfil et al., 1992; Rubin et al., 1992). It was suggested that it was easier for an isolate carrying the resistant trait to spread than for resistance to evolve in different strains at the same time (Murray, 1994). In contrast, later outbreaks have tended to involve different strains of enterococci, with VanA as well as VanB isolates, and to be associated with difficulty in eradicating VRE from the hospital setting (Frieden et al., 1993; Montecalvo et al., 1994; Morris et al., 1995; Shay et al., 1995). However, even after VRE becomes endemic in a hospital setting, monoclonal spread of resistant strains can still occur (Kim et al., 1999), and may even displace other endemic VRE strains (Fridkin et al., 1998).

Intra- and inter-hospital dissemination of enterococcal isolates have been previously observed with gentamicin-resistant *E. faecalis* (Zervos et al., 1987), penicillin-resistant *E. faecium* (Grayson et al., 1991; Miranda et al., 1991) and β-lactamase producing *E. faecalis* strains (Murray et al., 1991; Seetulsingh et al., 1996). Inter-hospital spread of VRE was also confirmed by detecting the same VRE strain by PFGE in 13 hospitals from Cleveland, Ohio (Donskey et al., 1999b), another VRE strain in 7 hospitals from San Antonio, Texas (Moreno et al., 1995), and another in 12 LTCF and in two acute care facilities from Sioux City, Iowa (Trick et al., 1999).

HCWs, the environment, and VRE-colonized patients play a role as reservoirs and agents of transmission in the nosocomial and inter-hospital dissemination of VRE. The actual proportion of VRE-colonized patients may act as an intensification factor within a certain health-care setting. One study found that the proportion of VRE-positive subjects, known as "colonization pressure," was the most important factor for VRE acquisition in an ICU (Bonten et al., 1998). Person to person transmission via the carriage by HCW's hands was implicated as the route of enterococcal transmission more than 15 years ago (Coudron et al., 1984; Zervos et al., 1987). More recently, surveillance studies have recovered VRE from HCWs' hands from 0% to 41%, including studies using different culture techniques and after having hands washed with antiseptic soap (Bonilla et al., 1997; Boyce et al., 1995; Shay et al., 1995; Wells et al., 1995). Results from experimental studies have demonstrated that both longer contact with the cleansing agent and the use of antiseptics instead of bland soap are associated with more effective decontamination of VRE colonized hands (Hayden, 2000). The use of gloves reduces the contamination of hands from Gram-negative rods or enterococci after patient contact (Olsen et al., 1993), and its use is recommended when entering a room of a VRE-colonized patient (CDC, 1995). However, among 17 HCWs whose gloves were culture positive for a patient's VRE strain after patient-care contact, 5 still had the same strain when their hands were cultured (Tenorio et al., 2001), stressing even more the importance of the recommendation for handwashing after glove removal. Notably, HCWs' hands can become colonized with a patient's VRE strain, even if they did not experience direct contact with the colonized patient (Tenorio et al., 2001), presumably from environmental contamination.

Further evidence of the role of transmission of VRE within the hospital environment, during a monoclonal outbreak caused by a VanB-type of VRE, the major risk factors for acquisition of the outbreak strain were the proximity to a VRE-positive patient and the exposure to a nurse who cared for a colonized patient (Boyce et al., 1994). A surveillance study (Bonten et al., 1996) in an ICU reported that in 85% of the patients the same VRE strain was found in another patient at the same time. In the same report, 38% of the VRE-colonized patients had the same strain isolated from upper body sites, such as oropharynx, arm, trachea, and stomach, and the number of VRE-positive body sites was directly correlated with the proportion of VRE-positive environmental cultures such as blood-pressure cuffs, drawsheets, bedrails, enteral feed, counter tops, and urine containers (Bonten et al., 1996).

The ability of enterococci (including VRE) to survive in different milieu, for instance, on hospital fabrics and plastics (Neely & Maley, 2000) or on countertops, telephone handpieces, stethoscopes, and fingertips (Noskin et al., 1995b), helps explain their relatively common recovery from environmental surfaces in rooms of VRE-positive patients, where the frequency of positive samples for VRE has ranged between 7% and 37% (Karanfil et al., 1992; Livornese et al., 1992; Slaughter et al., 1996); room contamination was noted to be exacerbated in colonized patients with diarrhea (Boyce et al., 1994).

Using data from a prior study that measured the efficacy of barrier precautions in preventing the nosocomial dissemination of VRE (Slaughter et al., 1996), a group of investigators recently applied the Ross–Macdonald model of vector-borne disease transmission to the spread of VRE in ICU (Austin et al., 1999), where the "vectors" (HCWs) were spreading VRE isolates between the susceptible "hosts" (ICU patients). The basic reproductive number (R_0), which plays a central role in this equation, defines the number of secondary colonized cases generated by the index VRE-positive case. The impact of new VRE-positive admissions on the endemic prevalence will also depend on the R_0 factor. Therefore, if the number of patients that are newly colonized from each VRE-colonized patient admitted is high, the number of patients persistently colonized in the ICU will subsequently increase. The measures that could diminish the R_0 in the most significant way were judged to be handwashing and staff cohorting. Reducing antibiotic use was also useful, although the effect would be less evident with a high R_0 value. This mathematical model may help to define the degree of control measures required to prevent the nosocomial spread of VRE.

3.7. The Role of Long-Term Care Facilities (LTCFs)

LTCFs have been viewed as important reservoirs of resistant organisms, contributing substantially to the overall burden of antimicrobial resistance (Goodall & Tompkins, 1994). LTCFs residents are frequently colonized or infected with multidrug-resistant pathogens at the time of hospital admission, a situation that is occasionally followed by hospital outbreaks, as was well described in the 1970s with MRSA (O'Toole et al., 1970) and multidrug-resistant *Klebsiella pneumoniae* (Gerding et al., 1979). As in the hospital setting, spread of a single strain was identified in an early VRE outbreak in LTCFs and multiple strains have been implicated in later years. For example, a prevalence study of patients colonized with VRE while residing in health-care facilities (4 acute and 26 LTCFs) from the Siouxland region showed that 4 different genotypes determined by PFGE accounted for the 40 VRE isolates in 1997, 10 genotypes for the 25 isolates in 1998, and in 1999, 7 genotypes were found among the 10 isolates recovered (Ostrowsky et al., 2001).

Different rates of prevalence of VRE among LTCFs residents have been reported. This disparity may be in part due to different methods for collection and screening used in each study, a probable geographic variation, and the setting in which the study was performed (i.e., VRE outbreak or surveillance study). For example, a high colonization rate with VRE was reported in LTCFs from Ann Arbor, Michigan, with the concomitant presence of important environmental and HCWs contamination (Bonilla et al., 1997); during a prospective surveillance study, only one of 92 LTCFs residents admitted to an inpatient acute geriatrics service was positive for VRE, between June and July 2000 in Buffalo, New York (Mylotte et al., 2001); and in another prevalence survey, a 1.7% prevalence of VRE colonization within LTCFs from Sioux City, Iowa in 1997 was observed (Trick et al., 1999). Of note, a prospective study of 36 patients colonized with VR *E. faecium* in LTCFs found that the majority of them were free of VRE colonization at a median of 67 days, although receipt of an antimicrobial agent was associated with a significant delay in VRE clearance (Brennen et al., 1998).

3.8. Prevention and Control Measures

Several factors should be taken into account when considering the infection control recommendations for preventing nosocomial VRE dissemination.

1. The nosocomial incidence of VRE is, in some ways, linked to that of MRSA. A high occurrence rate of MRSA infections will lead to an increased use of vancomycin, which in turn may select for VRE strains within the hospital (Herwaldt, 1999). Therefore, control of MRSA transmission may be an important measure for VRE prevention.

2. The morbidity and mortality associated with VRE infection is certainly influenced by the population under consideration (Hayden, 2000), and more aggressive VRE-control programs might be warranted in settings such as transplant centers and ICUs.

3. The natural history of an uncontrolled monoclonal outbreak has been shown to progress to polyclonal endemicity (Kim et al., 1999), and VRE will be more difficult to control in institutions where it is highly endemic, despite infection control measures. Thus, early recognition of VRE is important for subsequent control.

4. Adequate staff education and reduction of antibiotic pressure should be included in all the steps of measures to control nosocomial transmission of VRE.

In 1995, the Hospital Infection Control Practices Advisory Committee (HICPAC) published recommendations for preventing the spread of vancomycin resistance (CDC, 1995). These recommendations focused primarily on the prudent use of vancomycin; educational programs; the role of the microbiology laboratory in the detection, reporting, and control of VRE; and finally, on the specific measures for preventing and controlling nosocomial spread of VRE. The HICPAC had previously recommended that once VRE has been detected in a hospital, all enterococcal isolates should be screened for vancomycin resistance (CDC, 1994).

3.8.1. Appropriate Use of Vancomycin and Other Antibiotics

The HICPAC recommended that the use of vancomycin should be discouraged in a number of situations (Table 5.4). However, despite these recommendations, the use of vancomycin has continued to increase even though its use is often deemed to be inappropriate. The effect of vancomycin restriction on the prevalence of VRE has been difficult to assess because of the use of other antibiotics and accompanying infection control measures. Studies showing some degree of beneficial effect as well as no changes in the VRE prevalence after decreased oral and IV vancomycin use have been described (Austin et al., 1999; Morris et al., 1995; Quale et al., 1996).

Table 5.4

Situations in which the Use of Vancomycin should be Discouraged (HICPAC Recommendations)

Routine surgical prophylaxis, unless the patient has a life-threatening β-lactam allergy.

Empiric therapy for febrile neutropenic patient, unless evidence exists for Gram-positive infection in hospitals where the prevalence of methicillin-resistant *S. aureus* (MRSA) is substantial

Treatment of single positive blood culture for coagulase-negative staphylococci if other blood cultures taken during the same time

Continued empiric use in patients whose cultures are negative for β-lactam resistant Gram-positive organisms

Prophylaxis for intravascular catheters placement

Selective decontamination of the digestive tract

Eradication of MRSA colonization

Primary treatment of antibiotic-associated colitis

Routine prophylaxis in low-birthweight infants and patients on continuous ambulatory peritoneal dialysis or hemodialysis

Treatment of β-lactam susceptible Gram-positive microorganisms in patients with renal failure (often considered because of dosing convenience)

Topical application or irrigation use

Certainly, the use of other antibiotics may affect the incidence of VRE in a certain hospital. In a mouse model of intestinal colonization with VRE, the use of ceftriaxone and ticarcillin–clavulanate administered concomitantly with an oral inoculum of a VanB *E. faecium* isolate was associated a high-level establishment of VRE colonization, while a group of mice that received piperacillin–tazobactam showed a level similar to those in the control group (Donskey et al., 2000b). However, in the same mouse model, when VRE colonization was already established, the use of vancomycin or antibiotics with potent antianaerobic effect, including piperacillin–tazobactam, produced higher density of VRE in stools than the administration of antibiotics lacking antianaerobic activity (ceftriaxone, cefepime, ciprofloxacin, and aztreonam) (Donskey et al., 1999a). In humans, it was reported that the use of third-generation cephalosporins for empiric therapy in febrile neutropenic patients was associated with an increased prevalence of VRE as compared to a period when piperacillin–tazobactam was the agent of choice (Bradley et al., 1999). While these preliminary data suggest that the use of antibiotics with better antienterococcal activity might be associated with a lower risk for VRE acquisition or establishment of colonization, a more recent prospective study (Donskey et al., 2000a) found that high-density VRE colonization was more frequently seen with the use of antianaerobic agents (including piperacillin–tazobactam) than with the use of those without antianaerobic activity, supporting the hypothesis that suppression of intestinal anaerobes may be an important factor for VRE overgrowth in the gut.

3.8.2. Implementation of Infection Control Measures

The HICPAC recommendations regarding preventing and controlling nosocomial transmission of VRE include a first step of notification of HCW about the institution's policies regarding VRE infected or colonized patients, as well as establishing a system for monitoring appropriate procedures and outcome measures. VRE-infected or colonized patients should be placed in private rooms or in the same room as other patients who have VRE. The recommended isolation precautions for persons who will enter the room of a VRE-infected or colonized patient include wearing clean, nonsterile gloves, and a clean nonsterile gown if any contact with the patient or the room's environment is anticipated or if the patient has diarrhea, fecal incontinence, an ileostomy or colostomy, or a wound drainage not contained by a dressing. It is also recommended that gloves be removed before leaving the patient's rooms, hands washed with antiseptic soap or waterless antiseptic agent, and care taken after glove and gown removal and handwashing to avoid contact with potentially contaminated surfaces (e.g., door knob). In addition, inanimate items as stethoscopes, sphygmomanometers, or rectal thermometers, should be dedicated to a single patient or a cohort of patients with VRE.

Roommates of patients found to be VRE-positive for the first time should be screened for VRE with stool culture or rectal swab to rule out cross-transmission, and further screening of patients should be done at the discretion of the infection-control staff. Since VRE can persist as part of the colonizing flora in the intestinal tract, perhaps indefinitely, any decision regarding discontinuation of isolation precautions should be made only after very careful consideration. At least three consecutive negative VRE cultures, one week apart, from rectal swab, perianal area, axilla or umbilicus, wound, Foley catheter, colostomy sites if present, or any known positive site, have been recommended as a criterion before removing a patient from isolation precautions. Even when a patient is deemed as VRE free, the possibility of relapse should be considered. One recent report (Baden et al., 2001) found that out of 21 patients previously considered cleared or VRE free (after having at least three negative stool and index site cultures during a period of $\geq$3 weeks), five were found to be colonized with VRE after weekly cultures for 5 weeks using a broth-enrichment technique. These five patients were more likely to have received antimicrobial agents with Gram-negative and antianaerobic activity within the prior month than the other 16 patients. Two of the five isolates were genotypically related to the patient's historical strain. Thus, standard methods for declaring patients free of VRE are inadequate. When the patient becomes ill and receives broad-spectrum antibiotics, VRE relapse might be considered. In this situation, the burden of organisms might increase enough to be detected by standard cultures techniques, allowing more efficient transmission and, in the appropriate setting, place the patient at risk for bloodstream infections. When previously known VRE colonized patients are readmitted, isolation precautions should resume, and an effective system should be established to let the medical staff know about the VRE colonization status of the patient.

The HICPAC provides other measures to be taken in hospitals where VRE is endemic or in situations where the incidence continues to rise despite implementation of the measures described. Areas with a high rate of VRE (i.e., ICU) can serve as a reservoir as well as a place for propagation within the hospital, so the following control efforts should focus on those areas.

1. Minimize HCWs contact between VRE-positive and other patients through staff cohorting.
2. Perform surveillance cultures and/or personnel examination (especially when chronic skin and nails problems are present) to detect VRE-carriers among HCWs who, in the case of a high prevalence rate, may need to be removed from the care of VRE-negative patients.
3. Ensure adequate procedures for cleaning and disinfection of environmental objects, including environmental cultures for verification of VRE eradication after the cleaning of a VRE-positive room. If environmental cultures are positive after using conventional cleaning, one may consider using the "bucket method," which leaves quaternary ammonium compound drenching over all surfaces for 10 min before being dried with a clean towel. This method resulted in 100% efficacy with a single application (Byers et al., 1998).

Isolation of VRE-colonized or infected patients coupled with the use of surveillance cultures was successful at decreasing the prevalence of VRE from 2.2% in 1997 to 0.5% in 1999 among 30 acute and LTCF in the Siouxland region (Ostrowsky et al., 2001). Other measures, such as assignment of colonized patients to geographic cohorts, education of patients, cohorting of nursing staff, and assessment of patients on antibiotics by an Infectious Diseases specialist also appeared effective in reducing the incidence of VRE bacteremia and VRE colonization in an adult oncology unit where VRE was endemic (Montecalvo et al., 1999). Another study (Lai et al., 1998) found that similar infection control measures applied for about 3 years (although the use of vancomycin was restricted only during the last year of the study) in an ICU setting could decrease but not eradicate the rate of VRE in the hospital. Other simple measures, such as switching from oral and rectal thermometers to tympanic ones, have been associated with reduction not only of VRE but also of *C. difficile* infections (Brooks et al., 1998).

3.9. Treatment of VRE-Colonized Patients

Since gastrointestinal VRE colonization is a risk factor for VRE bacteremia and since it has been considered that most of the bacteremic episodes of VRE arise from an endogenous source, several antimicrobial agents have been evaluated to achieve gastrointestinal VRE decolonization, or at least to significantly reduce the degree of colonization. Agents effective in decreasing the density of VRE in stools should also help to diminish the spread of VRE within health-care facilities, and would probably reduce the overall risk of infection with these resistant organisms.

Reports from small, non-controlled studies using oral doxycycline and rifampin (Dembry et al., 1996), novobiocin and tetracycline (Montecalvo et al., 1995), oral bacitracin (Chia et al., 1995; O'Donovan et al., 1994) showed variable results. A recent prospective study of a 2-week course of oral bacitracin and doxycycline found no difference in the colonization rate after the intervention was stopped (Weinstein et al., 1999). Another prospective study evaluated ramoplanin, a non-absorbable glycolipodepsipeptide, whose activity is not affected by the presence of glycopeptide resistance in enterococci (Reynolds & Somner, 1990). At the end of a 1-week course of ramoplanin, more than 75% of the subjects were free of VRE; however, no difference in VRE colonization rate between the two dosage groups of ramoplanin and the placebo group was found 2 weeks after stopping the antibiotic (Wong et al., 2001). These studies showed that, with the intra-luminal presence of active agents against VRE, temporary suppression of VRE in stools (or at least its reduction below the level of detection of the screening test) is achievable. Patients colonized with VRE experiencing situations where the risk of bloodstream infections is considered high, such as intense chemotherapy with subsequent neutropenia and/or mucositis or patients with *C. difficile* colitis, might receive some benefits from this therapeutic approach. There is currently an ongoing phase III trial evaluating the administration of ramoplanin to patients at high risk for VRE bacteremia during the entire period of neutropenia or hospitalization.

4. TREATMENT OF VRE INFECTIONS

4.1. General Considerations

The choice of antibiotic(s) for treatment of infections caused by VRE is determined by several factors including the species involved, the seriousness of the infection, the phenotype and level of glycopeptide resistance of the infecting strain, and the presence of resistance to other agents. The immune status of the host may also influence the aggressiveness of the therapeutic approach.

4.1.1. Enterococcal Species

Effective therapy for VRE has been limited because *E. faecium* isolates are seldom susceptible to β-lactams, and nosocomial strains are also typically resistant to other antimicrobial agents. In the case of VRE infections caused by *E. faecalis*, ampicillin or penicillin is the drug of choice because the rate of ampicillin resistance among *E. faecalis* strains is very low (Edmond et al., 1999; Jones et al., 1997; Vergis et al., 2001).

Laboratory tests showing that the infecting VRE strain is motile indicate the presence of the VanC species *E. gallinarum* or *E. casseliflavus/flavescens*. These strains account only for 1–3% of the enterococcal bacteremia episodes, they have low-level resistance to vancomycin (MICs, 2–16 μg/ml), and their treatment should include ampicillin or penicillin, with or without gentamicin depending on the need for bactericidal combination. The use of vancomycin should be avoided because failures have been reported (Reid et al., 2001).

4.1.2. Type of Glycopeptide Resistance

Strains carrying the *vanB* gene cluster remain susceptible to teicoplanin because the VanS$_B$ membrane-bound kinase senses the presence of vancomycin but not teicoplanin. Teicoplanin in combination with gentamicin was effective in the treatment of rabbits with experimental endocarditis caused by VanB-type *E. faecalis* strains; however, resistance to teicoplanin was observed when this agent was used alone (Aslangul et al., 1997; Lefort et al., 1999). Unfortunately, this problem has also been reported in clinical practice. Emergence of resistance to teicoplanin was demonstrated in a patient with VanB-type *E. faecium* bacteremia while on treatment with this agent (Hayden et al., 1993), and in another patient with prosthetic valve endocarditis due to VanB *E. faecium* after a 4-month course of treatment with teicoplanin (Furlong & Rakowski, 1997). Therefore, if teicoplanin is to be used for VanB-type strains, it should be given in combination with an aminoglycoside and with close follow-up to detect in vivo development of resistance.

Against a VanE-type enterococcus, which usually displays MICs of vancomycin of 16 μg/ml and of teicoplanin of 0.5 μg/ml, teicoplanin and high-dose vancomycin (resulting in a peak of 38.3 ± 5.2 μg/ml and a trough of 15.0 ± 8.3 μg/ml) successfully decreased the mean vegetation counts in an experimental rabbit model of endocarditis (Lafaurie et al., 2001). However, unless clinical efficacy is demonstrated, a judicious approach would avoid the use of glycopeptides, particularly vancomycin, against this still unusual type of VRE.

4.1.3. Necessity of Bactericidal Therapy

Clinical scenarios where bactericidal activity is usually required for enterococcal infections include endocarditis and possibly meningitis and bacteremia in neutropenic patients. The primary mean of achieving bactericidal activity against enterococci has been by the synergistic effect between cell wall active agents and aminoglycosides (Watanakunakorn & Bakie, 1973), if the organism is not highly resistant to the latter. Greater clinical efficacy was observed in the treatment of enterococcal endocarditis when a bactericidal combination was utilized (Geraci & Martin, 1954; Herzstein et al., 1984), and this combination has been considered the treatment of choice of this entity since then. Fortunately, most infections in non-immunocompromised subjects, (intra-abdominal, soft tissue, and UTIs) are caused by relatively susceptible enterococci and can often be treated with ampicillin, amoxicillin, or penicillin alone (or with glycopeptides, if the patient is allergic to β-lactams), or with nitrofurantoin or fluoroquinolones in the case of lower UTIs (Lefort et al., 2000a).

When serious infections are to be treated and no regimen is able to achieve bactericidal activity, other interventions should be sought more aggressively, such as foreign body removal, local debridement, and surgical drainage; in some cases, valve replacement may be needed. The importance of these measures in the treatment of VRE infections was highlighted by a retrospective study of 28 VRE infected patients (Lai, 1996). Many of these patients had resolution of symptoms without specific antimicrobial therapy against VRE, but with line removal in catheter-related bacteremia, debridement in patients with soft tissue infections, surgical drainage in patients with pelvic abscesses, and Foley catheter removal in UTIs.

4.2. Therapeutic Options (Table 5.5)

4.2.1. Lower UTIs

In hospital settings where VRE are endemic, finding VRE strains in urine samples is not uncommon, although in the majority of the cases these VRE isolates appear to

Table 5.5
Therapeutic Options for VRE

	Advantages	Disadvantages
Nitrofurantoin	High concentration in urine. Useful in cystitis	Should be avoided in patients with renal insufficiency and when upper UTI is suspected
Fosfomycin tromethamine salt	Probably useful for cystitis	More clinical data needed for *E. faecium*
High-dose ampicillin (20–30 g/day)	Only if the MIC of the isolate is ≥64 µg/ml	Few anecdotal reports. May need to be combined with aminoglycosides
Teicoplanin (not available in the USA)	Only for VanB strains	Risk of development in vivo resistance; use in combination with gentamicin or streptomycin (if HLR-G or HLR-S not present) may reduce risk of resistance
Quinupristin–dalfopristin	FDA approved for use in VR *E. faecium* infections	Usually requires a central line for administration. Myalgias and/or arthralgias are present in about 10% of patients. May interact with drugs metabolized through the cytochrome P450 3A4 enzyme pathway. Not active against *E. faecalis*
Oxazolididones (linezolid)	100% oral bioavailability. FDA approved for use in VR *E. faecium* infections	Reversible myelosuppression (particularly thrombocytopenia) is of concern, especially after 2 weeks of therapy (weekly complete blood count recommended)

Notes: FDA: Food and Drug Administration; UTI: urinary tract infection; HLR-G: high-level resistance to gentamicin; HLR-S: high-level resistance to streptomycin; MIC: minimal inhibitory concentration.

correspond to urine colonization. The actual rate of UTI in urine cultures positive for VRE was found to be only 13% (Wong et al., 2000). In the management of lower UTIs, agents that are concentrated at high levels in the urine, such as nitrofurantoin and fosfomycin, are reasonable choice; however, when the clinical picture is more compatible with pyelonephritis, then the use of these agents should be avoided and antibiotics that attain higher systemic levels should be used.

Nitrofurantoin has maintained good in vitro activity against vancomycin-susceptible and VRE strains (Zhanel et al., 2001) and, in individuals with normal renal function, adequate urinary levels are achieved after its oral administration. In the presence of renal insufficiency, the use of this drug should be avoided. Nitrofurantoin does not attain good concentration in prostatic tissue; however, its combination with rifampin for 6 weeks was reported to be successful to treat a liver transplant recipient patient with VR *E. faecium* prostatitis (Taylor et al., 1998).

Fosfomycin tromethamine salt has also been used as an oral agent for the treatment of uncomplicated UTI because of its broad spectrum of antimicrobial activity with documented clinical efficacy for *E. faecalis* UTIs. In an in vitro study, this drug inhibited 94–97% of various VanA, VanB, and VanC isolates (including *E. faecalis, E. faecium, E. gallinarum,* and *E. casseliflavus* isolates) with MIC_{90} values in the intermediate range of susceptibility (32–64 µg/ml) (Allerberger & Klare, 1999). Because the oral administration of 3 g of fosfomycin achieves a urinary concentration greater than 128 µg/ml in subjects with normal creatinine clearance (Patel et al., 1997b), this agent is a reasonable choice for the treatment of uncomplicated UTI caused by VRE, although clinical trials including infections caused by *E. faecium* strains have not been reported.

4.2.2. Diverse Agents and Combinations in Vitro and in Animal Models

Several diverse drug combinations against VRE have been examined in vitro and in animal model experiments; however, these combinations have not been tested in humans, and due to the availability of new agents described below, may not be needed. For instance, the combination of imipenem and ampicillin was more effective than either agent alone in a model of experimental endocarditis caused by a VR *E. faecium* (Brandt et al., 1996); ceftriaxone, vancomycin, and gentamicin, given in combination, achieved in vitro bactericidal effect and in vivo efficacy in a rabbit model of endocarditis against a highly β-lactam-resistant VR *E. faecium*, although resistance to the synergistic effect was seen after 5 days of treatment (Caron et al., 1995). Initial in vitro experiments combining ampicillin and vancomycin against highly β-lactam resistant VRE showed a positive interaction (Leclercq et al., 1991), but only for some strains. The later fluoroquinolones have better in vitro activity against Gram-positive organisms than the older agents; however, some have not been studied against enterococcal infections in humans and the development of some of the more active compounds (i.e., clinafloxacin) has been stopped due to diverse adverse events.

4.2.3. Approved Agents for VRE Infections

Since 1999, two drugs have received approval from the Food and Drug Administration (FDA) for the treatment infections cause by VR *E. faecium*. The first one was quinupristin–dalfopristin in September 1999 and, a few months later, linezolid, in April 2000.

4.2.3a. Quinupristin–Dalfopristin. This is an injectable agent composed of two streptogramin antibiotics (quinupristin, a streptogramin B, and dalfopristin, a streptogramin A) mixed in a 30/70 ratio. The two streptogramins bind to different sites of the bacterial ribosomes, leading to a synergistic inhibition of bacterial protein synthesis. Dalfopristin binding causes conformational changes in the ribosome that increase the affinity of quinupristin, which can result in irreversible protein synthesis inhibition accounting for its bactericidal effect against some Gram-positive organisms. Particularly against *E. faecium* strains, quinupristin–dalfopristin displayed in vitro bacteriostatic to modest bactericidal activity, which was dependent on the inoculum growth phase, the medium, the erythromycin susceptibility pattern (constitutive expression of the *erm* gene common to most clinical VRE isolates eliminates the bactericidal activity of quinupristin–dalfopristin) and the incubation time (Caron et al., 1997). *E. faecalis*, on the other hand, is naturally resistant to quinupristin–dalfopristin due to an efflux mechanism (Singh et al., 2002), and superinfection with this species has been reported in patients receiving this agent (Chow et al., 1997; Moellering et al., 1999). Quinupristin–dalfopristin against VR *E. faecium* infections was evaluated in two open labeled non-randomized clinical trials. One included 396 seriously ill patients with various infections (Moellering et al., 1999), and another one evaluated 23 patients, most of whom had bacteremia (Winston et al., 2000). In these two studies, favorable bacteriological outcome was observed in more than 70% of the patients, except in 48% of those with bacteremia of unknown origin and 75% of those with endocarditis (only four subjects were evaluable). IV plus intraventricular quinupristin–dalfopristin has been successfully used in some reports of shunt-related meningitis (Nachman et al., 1995; Williamson et al., 2002). The most common side effects are venous adverse events (46% when the agent is given through peripheral veins), arthralgias (9.1%), and myalgias (6.6%) (the discontinuation rate due to adverse events was about 8%) (Moellering et al., 1999).

Resistance to quinupristin–dalfopristin in VR *E. faecium* human isolates has been uncommon in the United States, where 98.9% of the strains were inhibited by ≤ 2 µg/ml (Eliopoulos et al., 1998), as well as in France (Bozdogan & Leclercq, 1999). A much higher rate (17%) was found in chicken carcasses (McDonald et al., 2001), which is probably related to the widespread administration of virginiamycin (another mixture of two streptogramins with cross-resistance to quinupristin–dalfopristin) to feed farm animals in the United States and in the EU. In a clinical trial, molecular typing of VRE was used to demonstrate emergence of resistance (4- to 8-fold increase in baseline MIC) to quinupristin–dalfopristin in originally susceptible strains while on therapy in 1.2% of the cases (Moellering et al., 1999).

Resistance to streptogramin B compounds in enterococci is often related to the presence of erythromycin ribosomal methylation (*erm*) or virginiamycin factor B hydrolase (*vgb*) genes. The Erm(B) methylase, commonly found in enterococci, adds one or two methyl groups to the 23S rRNA moiety, decreasing the binding site affinity for erythromycin as well as for the newer macrolides, lincosamides, and streptogramin B compounds (Roberts et al., 1999), therefore named MLS_B phenotype resistance; *erm*(B) can be inducible or constitutively expressed. Dalfopristin is not affected by this resistant mechanism, and quinupristin–dalfopristin shows an in vitro inhibitory bacteriostatic activity comparable with that of MLS_B-susceptible *E. faecium* strains (Fantin et al., 1997). In the rabbit endocarditis model, quinupristin–dalfopristin was significantly more effective in reducing the bacterial titers in vegetations of an erythromycin-susceptible *E. faecium* strain than of an MLS_B-inducible strain, although probably due in part to a different degree of diffusion within the vegetation of the two streptogramins (Fantin et al., 1997). Overall, the bactericidal activity of quinupristin–dalfopristin appears to be reduced in the presence of the MLS_B phenotype. The other gene involved in streptogramin B resistance, the *vgb* gene, has been rarely identified in streptogramin-resistant *E. faecium* strains (Jensen et al., 1998b). Streptogramin A compounds (i.e., dalfopristin) can be inactivated by acetyltransferases encoded by the genes *vat*(D) (previously *satA*) and *vat*(E) (previously *satG*). Both genes have been frequently found in streptogramin-resistant *E. faecium* strains from animals and individuals of some Western European countries (Haroche et al., 2000; Jensen et al., 1998b; Soltani et al., 2000). When quinupristin–dalfopristin was tested in vitro against different *E. faecium* constructs using recombinant plasmids carrying the *erm*(B), *vat*(D), and *vgb* genes, at least two of these genes had to be present to increase the quinupristin–dalfopristin MIC above 4 µg/ml (Bozdogan & Leclercq, 1999).

4.2.3b. Linezolid.   The oxazolidinones are a new class of agents discovered in the 1980s, among which linezolid has attained FDA approval for the treatment of infections caused by VR *E. faecium* infections. These compounds have a unique mechanism of action by inhibition of protein synthesis at an early stage. They bind to the bacterial 23S ribosomal RNA of the 50S subunit preventing the formation of a functional 70S initiation complex, thus, hindering the binding of the mRNA to the ribosome at the initiation of the translation (Shinabarger et al., 1997). In a rat model of endocarditis caused by a VanA *E. faecium* strain, linezolid showed a bacteriostatic activity (Patel et al., 2001). Published studies in humans have reported microbiological cure in 67% of patients with multiple pre-existing conditions (recent major surgical procedure or orthotopic liver transplantation) and diverse VRE infections (bacteremia, peritonitis, intra-abdominal abscess and wound infection) treated with linezolid (Chien et al., 2000). In another study, patients with different VRE infections were randomized to receive two doses of linezolid (600 or 200 mg IV every 12 hr), finding a non-statistically significant better response in the higher dose group, with 67% and 52% of cure rate, respectively (Hartman et al., 2000). The compassionate-use program of linezolid reported 55 patients with VRE infections attaining a cure rate of 87.5% in soft tissue infections, 90.9% in primary bacteremia, 91.7% in abdominal or pelvic infections, and 100% for catheter-related bacteremia (Leach et al., 2000). Other reports on the efficacy of linezolid for VRE infections include a post-BMT patient with septic thrombophlebitis and persistent bacteremia (McNeil et al., 2000), and a patient with congenital cyanotic heart disease with tricuspid valve endocarditis (and probable aortic involvement) (Babcock et al., 2001). Linezolid has been successfully used in a few case reports of meningitis caused by VRE (Hachem et al., 2001; Shaikh et al., 2001; Steinmetz et al., 2001; Zeana et al., 2001). In one, the linezolid cerebrospinal fluid concentration was 74% of that achieved in plasma, 7 hr after the administered dose (600 mg IV) (Zeana et al., 2001). Side effects associated with linezolid have been predominantly gastrointestinal (nausea, vomiting, diarrhea), headache, taste alteration, and hematological; when given for more than 2 weeks, an increased incidence of reversible myelosuppression (in particular thrombocytopenia) has been reported.

Resistance to linezolid was initially thought to be a rare event, although serial passages in linezolid resulted in derivatives with high MICs and mutations in the 23S rRNA gene region (Prystowsky et al., 2001). Recently, clinical *E. faecium* isolates resistant to glycopeptides and linezolid have been reported (Gonzales et al., 2001). The reported isolates have generally come from immunosuppressed patients with prolonged linezolid exposure (21–40 days) and complicated infections with high bacterial inocula (i.e., liver abscesses, empyema). It is likely that resistance to linezolid will be increasingly seen in clinical practice sooner than previously expected. A linezolid-resistant VRE strain has recently produced nosocomial spread in a transplantation unit at the Mayo Clinic in Rochester, Minnesota (Herrero et al., 2002).

4.2.4. Other Options and Anecdotal Reports

One of the possible options for the treatment of VRE infections is the administration of high-dose ampicillin (20–24 g per day) when the ampicillin MIC of the VRE strain is less than 64 μg/ml (MICs ≥16 μg/ml is regarded as resistant on NCCLS recommendations) because, with this high dose, serum concentrations of ampicillin that are several times the MIC can be achieved (Murray, 1997). If the organism does not show HLR, an aminoglycoside should be added; this regimen was actually successful in some reports (Dodge et al., 1997).

Another agent used to treat patients with serious VRE infections was chloramphenicol, but its efficacy has not been tested in controlled trials. One retrospective study evaluated 51 patients with VRE bacteremia treated with chloramphenicol, showing a 61% and 79% rate of clinical and microbiological response, respectively, although no effect on mortality was observed (Lautenbach et al., 1998). Interesting, and probably because of its good CNS penetration, a pediatric case of ventricular shunt-associated meningitis caused by VR *E. faecium* was successfully treated with 3 weeks of IV chloramphenicol and new shunt placement at the end of therapy (Perez Mato et al., 1999). Some other agents, alone or in combination, have occasionally succeeded in the therapy of VRE infections, such as tetracycline in a neutropenic patient with persistent VRE bacteremia (Howe et al., 1997) (although there was no mention about the timing of resolution of neutropenia), the combination of novobiocin and doxycycline in three patients with VRE bacteremia (Montecalvo et al., 1995), and chloramphenicol plus minocycline in a patient with prosthetic valve endocarditis without valve replacement (Safdar et al., 2002).

4.3. Agents in Development

Daptomycin is a lipopeptide antibiotic with activity against Gram-positive pathogens that was initially in development in the mid-1980s. This agent requires the presence of calcium, and it is recommended that this cation be added to the media when susceptibilities to this compound are being tested. Daptomycin produces disruption of the bacterial membranes affecting lipoteichoic acid synthesis, as studied in *E. hirae* (Canepari et al., 1990), although recent investigations have questioned this mechanism of action in *S. aureus* (Laganas & Silverman, 2001). The main adverse event noted in early animal studies and in phase I and phase II trials in humans was myopathy, especially in the twice-daily dosing schedule and at the highest administered dose. Subsequent studies have focused on its once-daily administration, at a dose of 4 mg/kg for complicated skin and soft tissue infection and pneumonia, with which they were able to maintain the efficacy and to increase the safety of the compound (Tally & DeBruin, 2000). Recent trials are using a once-daily dose of 6 mg/kg for more severe diseases.

Oritavancin (LY333328) is a new semi-synthetic glycopeptide, structurally related to vancomycin and teicoplanin, and a derivative of the parent compound LY264826. While its exact mechanism of action remains unclear, it is thought to be similar to that of the other glycopeptides. The activity of this agent against VRE strains may derive from its ability to bind to bacterial membrane and dimerize (Allen et al., 1997). Oritavancin displayed MIC_{90} values of 0.5 and 1.0 μg/ml, and 1.0 and 2.0 μg/ml for VS and VR *E. faecium*, and VS and VR *E. faecalis*, respectively (Schwalbe et al., 1996). Of note, the MICs and the minimal bactericidal concentrations (MBCs) were consistently 2- to 4-fold higher for VRE strains than for VSE ones. Another study also showed decreased bactericidal activity of oritavancin against VanA and VanB strains, although a synergistic effect was noted when this drug was combined with gentamicin (Lefort et al., 2000b). In the rabbit model of endocarditis, oritavancin displayed only modest response against an *E. faecalis* strain (JH2-2) and two transconjugants strains with VanA and VanB phenotype (Lefort et al., 2000b; Saleh-Mghir et al., 1999), which was attributed to the high protein binding propensity of this drug in rabbit sera and the heterogeneous diffusion into the vegetations. Rather worrisome is the observation that in half of the rabbits infected with the VanA strain, strains with MICs 4–10 times higher than the parental strain were recovered from the vegetations, while no such mutants were found in animals infected with the VanB, the VS *E. faecalis* strain, or when oritavancin was given in combination with gentamicin (Lefort et al., 2000b). Moderate level resistance to oritavancin (MICs, ≤16 μg/ml) was previously observed in VR *E. faecalis* strains with higher production of D-Ala-D-Lac precursors, with expression of the *vanZ* gene, or with mutations in the $vanS_B$ sensor gene of the *vanB* cluster conferring cross-resistance to teicoplanin and oritavancin (Arthur et al., 1999). These data suggest that, even though oritavancin has in vitro activity against VRE, development of resistance in vivo may not be an uncommon finding. Oritavancin entered phase III clinical trials in the United States in January 2001.

Another active agent against VRE in development is tigecycline (GAR-936), a glycylcycline, which is a derivative of minocycline. In an in vitro protein synthesis system using *E. coli* isolates, glycylcyclines displayed protein synthesis inhibition, even against strains carrying the *tet*(M) gene, which encodes a cytoplasmatic protein that blocks the action of tetracyclines, doxycycline, and minocycline at the ribosomal level (TetM-protected ribosomes) (Rasmussen et al., 1994). This agent showed an MIC_{90} of 0.12 μ/ml and 0.25 μg/ml for VS and VR *E. faecalis* strains, respectively, and 0.12 μg/ml for both VS and VR *E. faecium* strains; the MIC_{90} against minocycline-resistant enterococci was ≤0.25 μg/ml (Gales & Jones, 2000). Tigecycline was effective in a rat model of experimental endocarditis against both VS and VR *E. faecalis* strains (Murphy et al., 2000), and in a mice peritonitis model against several VRE and VSE strains, as well as against tetracycline- and minocycline-resistant and -susceptible *E. faecalis* and *E. faecium* strains (Nannini et al., 2001). This agent is currently in phase III trials.

5. CONCLUSION

The incidence of nosocomial infections caused by VRE has consistently increased during the past decade across all types of health-care facilities, especially in the United States. More rigorous infection control measures and reduction in the use of antimicrobials for the treatment of human infections and/or new preventative modalities will likely be necessary to decrease the development of drug resistance in enterococci, as well as in other microorganisms. Restriction of the use of antibiotics as animal growth enhancers in the EU has resulted in decreased transmission of these organisms (and their resistant genes) from animals to humans. This interchange between animals and humans has become even more worrisome after a recent description of an *E. faecium* outbreak causing severe hemorrhagic disease in pigs and 40 local farmers (12 of them died) in a region of China (Lu et al., 2002). Newer therapeutic agents have been developed and used with relative effectiveness (although without a bactericidal activity) for the treatment of VRE infections, but the propensity of enterococci to develop resistance suggest that VRE will continue to be a therapeutic and infection control challenge for the immediate future.

References

Aarestrup, F. M., Seyfarth, A. M., Emborg, H. D., Pedersen, K., Hendriksen, R. S., & Bager, F. (2001). Effect of abolishment of the use of antimicrobial agents for growth promotion on occurrence of antimicrobial resistance in fecal enterococci from food animals in Denmark. *Antimicrob Agents Chemother 45*, 2054–2059.
Allen, N. E., LeTourneau, D. L., & Hobbs, J. N., Jr. (1997). The role of hydrophobic side chains as determinants of antibacterial activity of semisynthetic glycopeptide antibiotics. *J Antibiot (Tokyo) 50*, 677–684.
Allerberger, F., & Klare, I. (1999). In-vitro activity of fosfomycin against vancomycin-resistant enterococci. *J Antimicrob Chemother 43*, 211–217.
Arias, C. A., Courvalin, P., & Reynolds, P. E. (2000). *vanC* cluster of vancomycin-resistant *Enterococcus gallinarum* BM4174. *Antimicrob Agents Chemother 44*, 1660–1666.
Arthur, M., & Courvalin, P. (1993). Genetics and mechanisms of glycopeptide resistance in enterococci. *Antimicrob Agents Chemother 37*, 1563–1571.
Arthur, M., Depardieu, F., Cabanie, L., Reynolds, P., & Courvalin, P. (1998). Requirement of the VanY and VanX D,D-peptidases for glycopeptide resistance in enterococci. *Mol Microbiol 30*, 819–830.
Arthur, M., Depardieu, F., Molinas, C., Reynolds, P., & Courvalin, P. (1995). The *vanZ* gene of Tn*1546* from *Enterococcus faecium* BM4147 confers resistance to teicoplanin. *Gene 154*, 87–92.
Arthur, M., Depardieu, F., Reynolds, P., & Courvalin, P. (1996). Quantitative analysis of the metabolism of soluble cytoplasmic peptidoglycan precursors of glycopeptide-resistant enterococci. *Mol Microbiol 21*, 33–44.
Arthur, M., Depardieu, F., Reynolds, P., & Courvalin, P. (1999). Moderate-level resistance to glycopeptide LY333328 mediated by genes of the *vanA* and *vanB* clusters in enterococci. *Antimicrob Agents Chemother 43*, 1875–1880.
Arthur, M., Molinas, C., & Courvalin, P. (1992). The VanS-VanR two-component regulatory system controls synthesis of depsipeptide peptidoglycan precursors in *Enterococcus faecium* BM4147. *J Bacteriol 174*, 2582–2591.

Arthur, M., Molinas, C., Depardieu, F., & Courvalin, P. (1993). Characterization of Tn*1546*, a Tn*3*-related transposon conferring glycopeptide resistance by synthesis of depsipeptide peptidoglycan precursors in *Enterococcus faecium* BM4147. *J Bacteriol 175*, 117–127.

Arthur, M., & Quintiliani, R., Jr. (2001). Regulation of VanA- and VanB-type glycopeptide resistance in enterococci. *Antimicrob Agents Chemother 45*, 375–381.

Aslangul, E., Baptista, M., Fantin, B., Depardieu, F., Arthur, M., Courvalin, P., & Carbon, C. (1997). Selection of glycopeptide-resistant mutants of VanB-type *Enterococcus faecalis* BM4281 in vitro and in experimental endocarditis. *J Infect Dis 175*, 598–605.

Austin, D. J., Bonten, M. J., Weinstein, R. A., Slaughter, S., & Anderson, R. M. (1999). Vancomycin-resistant enterococci in intensive-care hospital settings: Transmission dynamics, persistence, and the impact of infection control programs. *Proc Natl Acad Sci USA 96*, 6908–6913.

Axelrod, P., & Talbot, G. H. (1989). Risk factors for acquisition of gentamicin-resistant enterococci. A multivariate analysis. *Arch Intern Med 149*, 1397–1401.

Babcock, H. M., Ritchie, D. J., Christiansen, E., Starlin, R., Little, R., & Stanley, S. (2001). Successful treatment of vancomycin-resistant *Enterococcus* endocarditis with oral linezolid. *Clin Infect Dis 32*, 1373–1375.

Baden, L. R., Thiemke, W., Skolnik, A., Chambers, R., Strymish, J., Gold, H. S., Moellering, Jr, R. C., & Eliopoulos, G. M. (2001). Prolonged colonization with vancomycin-resistant *Enterococcus faecium* in long-term care patients and the significance of clearance. *Clin Infect Dis 33*, 1654–1660.

Balas, D., Perea, B., Wilhelmi, I., Romanyk, J., Alos, J. I., & Gomez-Garces, J. L. (1997). Prevalence of antimicrobial resistance in enterococci isolated from blood in Madrid (1994–1995). *Enferm Infecc Microbiol Clin 15*, 22–23.

Balzereit-Scheuerlein, F., & Stephan, R. (2001). Prevalence of colonisation and resistance patterns of vancomycin-resistant enterococci in healthy, non-hospitalised persons in Switzerland. *Swiss Med Wkly 131*, 280–282.

Bates, J., Jordens, J. Z., & Griffiths, D. T. (1994). Farm animals as a putative reservoir for vancomycin-resistant enterococcal infection in man. *J Antimicrob Chemother 34*, 507–514.

Bell, J., Turnidge, J., Coombs, G., & O'Brien, F. (1998). Emergence and epidemiology of vancomycin-resistant enterococci in Australia. *Commun Dis Intell 22*, 249–252.

Bignardi, G. E. (1998). Risk factors for Clostridium difficile infection. *J Hosp Infect 40*, 1–15.

Bingen, E., Lambert-Zechovsky, N., Mariani-Kurkdjian, P., Cezard, J. P., & Navarro, J. (1989). Bacteremia caused by a vancomycin-resistant *Enterococcus*. *Pediatr Infect Dis J 8*, 475–476.

Bingen, E. H., Denamur, E., Lambert-Zechovsky, N. Y., & Elion, J. (1991). Evidence for the genetic unrelatedness of nosocomial vancomycin-resistant *Enterococcus faecium* strains in a pediatric hospital. *J Clin Microbiol 29*, 1888–1892.

Bonilla, H. F., Zervos, M. A., Lyons, M. J., Bradley, S. F., Hedderwick, S. A., Ramsey, M. A., Paul, L. K., & Kauffman, C. A. (1997). Colonization with vancomycin-resistant *Enterococcus faecium*: Comparison of a long-term-care unit with an acute-care hospital. *Infect Control Hosp Epidemiol 18*, 333–339.

Bonten, M. J., Hayden, M. K., Nathan, C., van Voorhis, J., Matushek, M., Slaughter, S., Rice, T., & Weinstein, R. A. (1996). Epidemiology of colonisation of patients and environment with vancomycin-resistant enterococci. *Lancet 348*, 1615–1619.

Bonten, M. J., Slaughter, S., Ambergen, A. W., Hayden, M. K., van Voorhis, J., Nathan, C., & Weinstein, R. A. (1998). The role of "colonization pressure" in the spread of vancomycin-resistant enterococci: An important infection control variable. *Arch Intern Med 158*, 1127–1132.

Bouza, E., San Juan, R., Munoz, P., Voss, A., & Kluytmans, J. (2001). A European perspective on nosocomial urinary tract infections I. Report on the microbiology workload, etiology and antimicrobial susceptibility (ESGNI-003 study). European Study Group on Nosocomial Infections. *Clin Microbiol Infect 7*, 523–531.

Boyce, J. M. (1989). Methicillin-resistant *Staphylococcus aureus*. Detection, epidemiology, and control measures. *Infect Dis Clin North Am 3*, 901–913.

Boyce, J. M., Mermel, L. A., Zervos, M. J., Rice, L. B., Potter-Bynoe, G., Giorgio, C., & Medeiros, A. A. (1995). Controlling vancomycin-resistant enterococci [see comments] [erratum appears in *Infect Control Hosp Epidemiol* 1996 Apr;*17*(4), 211]. *Infect Control Hosp Epidemiol 16*, 634–637.

Boyce, J. M., Opal, S. M., Chow, J. W., Zervos, M. J., Potter-Bynoe, G., Sherman, C. B., Romulo, R. L., Fortna, S., & Medeiros, A. A. (1994). Outbreak of multidrug-resistant *Enterococcus faecium* with transferable vanB class vancomycin resistance. *J Clin Microbiol 32*, 1148–1153.

Boyd, D. A., Conly, J., Dedier, H., Peters, G., Robertson, L., Slater, E., & Mulvey, M. R. (2000). Molecular characterization of the *vanD* gene cluster and a novel insertion element in a vancomycin-resistant *Enterococcus* isolated in Canada. *J Clin Microbiol 38*, 2392–2394.

Bozdogan, B., & Leclercq, R. (1999). Effects of genes encoding resistance to streptogramins A and B on the activity of quinupristin-dalfopristin against *Enterococcus faecium*. *Antimicrob Agents Chemother 43*, 2720–2725.

Bradley, S. J., Wilson, A. L., Allen, M. C., Sher, H. A., Goldstone, A. H., & Scott, G. M. (1999). The control of hyperendemic glycopeptide-resistant *Enterococcus* spp. on a haematology unit by changing antibiotic usage. *J Antimicrob Chemother 43*, 261–266.

Brandt, C. M., Rouse, M. S., Laue, N. W., Stratton, C. W., Wilson, W. R., & Steckelberg, J. M. (1996). Effective treatment of multidrug-resistant enterococcal experimental endocarditis with combinations of cell wall-active agents. *J Infect Dis 173*, 909–913.

Brennen, C., Wagener, M. M., & Muder, R. R. (1998). Vancomycin-resistant *Enterococcus faecium* in a long-term care facility. *J Am Geriatr Soc 46*, 157–160.

Brooks, S., Khan, A., Stoica, D., Griffith, J., Friedeman, L., Mukherji, R., Hameed, R., & Schupf, N. (1998). Reduction in vancomycin-resistant *Enterococcus* and *Clostridium difficile* infections following change to tympanic thermometers. *Infect Control Hosp Epidemiol 19*, 333–336.

Brown, A. R., Townsley, A. C., & Amyes, S. G. (2001). Diversity of Tn*1546* elements in clinical isolates of glycopeptide-resistant enterococci from Scottish hospitals. *Antimicrob Agents Chemother 45*, 1309–1311.

Budavari, S. M., Saunders, G. L., Liebowitz, L. D., Khoosal, M., & Crewe-Brown, H. H. (1997). Emergence of vancomycin-resistant enterococci in South Africa. *S Afr Med J 87*, 1557.

Byers, K. E., Anglim, A. M., Anneski, C. J., Germanson, T. P., Gold, H. S., Durbin, L. J., Simonton, B. M., & Farr, B. M. (2001). A hospital epidemic of vancomycin-resistant *Enterococcus*: Risk factors and control. *Infect Control Hosp Epidemiol 22*, 140–147.

Byers, K. E., Durbin, L. J., Simonton, B. M., Anglim, A. M., Adal, K. A., & Farr, B. M. (1998). Disinfection of hospital rooms contaminated with vancomycin-resistant *Enterococcus faecium*. *Infect Control Hosp Epidemiol 19*, 261–264.

Caballero-Granado, F. J., Becerril, B., Cuberos, L., Bernabeu, M., Cisneros, J. M., & Pachon, J. (2001). Attributable mortality rate and duration of hospital stay associated with enterococcal bacteremia. *Clin Infect Dis 32*, 587–594.

Caballero-Granado, F. J., Cisneros, J. M., Luque, R., Torres-Tortosa, M., Gamboa, F., Diez, F., Villanueva, J. L., Perez-Cano, R., Pasquau, J., Merino, D., Menchero, A., Mora, D., Lopez-Ruz, M. A., & Vergara, A. (1998). Comparative study of bacteremias caused by *Enterococcus* spp. with and without high-level resistance to gentamicin. The grupo Andaluz para el estudio de las enfermedades infecciosas. *J Clin Microbiol 36*, 520–525.

Canepari, P., Boaretti, M., del Mar Lleo, M., & Satta, G. (1990). Lipoteichoic acid as a new target for activity of antibiotics: Mode of action of daptomycin (LY146032). *Antimicrob Agents Chemother 34*, 1220–1226.

Carias, L. L., Rudin, S. D., Donskey, C. J., & Rice, L. B. (1998). Genetic linkage and cotransfer of a novel, *vanB*-containing transposon (Tn*5382*) and a low-affinity penicillin-binding protein 5 gene in a clinical vancomycin-resistant *Enterococcus faecium* isolate. *J Bacteriol 180*, 4426–4434.

Caron, F., Gold, H. S., Wennersten, C. B., Farris, M. G., Moellering, R. C., Jr., & Eliopoulos, G. M. (1997). Influence of erythromycin resistance, inoculum growth phase, and incubation time on assessment of the bactericidal activity of RP 59500 (quinupristin-dalfopristin) against vancomycin-resistant *Enterococcus faecium. Antimicrob Agents Chemother 41*, 2749–2753.

Caron, F., Pestel, M., Kitzis, M. D., Lemeland, J. F., Humbert, G., & Gutmann, L. (1995). Comparison of different beta-lactam-glycopeptide-gentamicin combinations for an experimental endocarditis caused by a highly beta-lactam-resistant and highly glycopeptide-resistant isolate of *Enterococcus faecium. J Infect Dis 171*, 106–112.

Casadewall, B., & Courvalin, P. (1999). Characterization of the *vanD* glycopeptide resistance gene cluster from *Enterococcus faecium* BM4339. *J Bacteriol 181*, 3644–3648.

CDC. (1994). Preventing the Spread of Vancomycin Resistance—A Report from the Hospital Infection Control Practices Advisory Committee prepared by the Subcommittee on Prevention and Control of Antimicrobial-Resistant Microorganisms in Hospitals; comment period and public meeting—CDC. Notice. *Federal Register 59*, 25758–25763.

CDC. (2002a). *Staphylococcus aureus* resistant to vancomycin—United States, 2002. *MMWR 51*, 565–567.

CDC. (2002b). Vancomycin-resistant *Staphylococcus aureus*—Pennsylvania, 2002. *MMWR 51*, 902.

CDC. (1995). Recommendations for preventing the spread of vancomycin resistance. Recommendations of the Hospital Infection Control Practices Advisory Committee (HICPAC). *MMWR 44*, 1–13.

Chia, J. K., Nakata, M. M., Park, S. S., Lewis, R. P., & McKee, B. (1995). Use of bacitracin therapy for infection due to vancomycin-resistant *Enterococcus faecium. Clin Infect Dis 21*, 1520.

Chien, J. W., Kucia, M. L., & Salata, R. A. (2000). Use of linezolid, an oxazolidinone, in the treatment of multidrug-resistant Gram-positive bacterial infections. *Clin Infect Dis 30*, 146–151.

Chiew, Y. F., & Ling, M. L. (1998). Two cases of vancomycin-resistant enterococci from Singapore. *J Infect 36*, 133–134.

Chirurgi, V. A., Oster, S. E., Goldberg, A. A., & McCabe, R. E. (1992). Nosocomial acquisition of beta-lactamase—negative, ampicillin-resistant *Enterococcus. Arch Intern Med 152*, 1457–1461.

Chow, J. W., Davidson, A., Sanford, E., 3rd, & Zervos, M. J. (1997). Superinfection with *Enterococcus faecalis* during quinupristin/dalfopristin therapy. *Clin Infect Dis 24*, 91–92.

Clabots, C. R., Johnson, S., Olson, M. M., Peterson, L. R., & Gerding, D. N. (1992). Acquisition of *Clostridium difficile* by hospitalized patients: Evidence for colonized new admissions as a source of infection. *J Infect Dis 166*, 561–567.

Clark, N. C., Teixeira, L. M., Facklam, R. R., & Tenover, F. C. (1998). Detection and differentiation of *vanC-1, vanC-2*, and *vanC-3* glycopeptide resistance genes in enterococci. *J Clin Microbiol 36*, 2294–2297.

Collins, L. A., Malanoski, G. J., Eliopoulos, G. M., Wennersten, C. B., Ferraro, M. J., & Moellering, R. C., Jr. (1993). In vitro activity of RP59500, an injectable streptogramin antibiotic, against vancomycin-resistant Gram-positive organisms. *Antimicrob Agents Chemother 37*, 598–601.

Coque, T. M., Tomayko, J. F., Ricke, S. C., Okhyusen, P. C., & Murray, B. E. (1996). Vancomycin-resistant enterococci from nosocomial, community, and animal sources in the United States. *Antimicrob Agents Chemother 40*, 2605–2609.

Coudron, P. E., Markowitz, S. M., & Wong, E. S. (1992). Isolation of a beta-lactamase-producing, aminoglycoside-resistant strain of *Enterococcus faecium. Antimicrob Agents Chemother 36*, 1125–1126.

Coudron, P. E., Mayhall, C. G., Facklam, R. R., Spadora, A. C., Lamb, V. A., Lybrand, M. R., & Dalton, H. P. (1984). *Streptococcus faecium* outbreak in a neonatal intensive care unit. *J Clin Microbiol 20*, 1044–1048.

Das, I., & Gray, J. (1998). Enterococcal bacteremia in children: A review of seventy-five episodes in a pediatric hospital. *Pediatr Infect Dis J 17*, 1154–1158.

Dembry, L. M., Uzokwe, K., & Zervos, M. J. (1996). Control of endemic glycopeptide-resistant ente-
    rococci. *Infect Control Hosp Epidemiol 17*, 286–292.
Descheemaeker, P., Ieven, M., Chapelle, S., Lammens, C., Hauchecorne, M., Wijdooghe, M.,
    Vandamme, P., & Goossens, H. (2000). Prevalence and molecular epidemiology of glycopeptide-
    resistant enterococci in Belgian renal dialysis units. *J Infect Dis 181*, 235–241.
Dever, L. L., Smith, S. M., Handwerger, S., & Eng, R. H. (1995). Vancomycin-dependent *Enterococcus
    faecium* isolated from stool following oral vancomycin therapy. *J Clin Microbiol 33*, 2770–2773.
Devriese, L. A., Vandamme, P., Pot, B., Vanrobaeys, M., Kersters, K., & Haesebrouck, F. (1998).
    Differentiation between *Streptococcus gallolyticus* strains of human clinical and veterinary origins
    and *Streptococcus bovis* strains from the intestinal tracts of ruminants. *J Clin Microbiol 36*,
    3520–3523.
Dodge, R. A., Daly, J. S., Davaro, R., & Glew, R. H. (1997). High-dose ampicillin plus streptomycin
    for treatment of a patient with severe infection due to multiresistant enterococci. *Clin Infect Dis
    25*, 1269–1270.
Donskey, C. J., Chowdhry, T. K., Hecker, M. T., Hoyen, C. K., Hanrahan, J. A., Hujer, A. M., Hutton-
    Thomas, R. A., Whalen, C. C., Bonomo, R. A., & Rice, L. B. (2000a). Effect of antibiotic therapy
    on the density of vancomycin-resistant enterococci in the stool of colonized patients [see com-
    ments]. *N Engl J Med 343*, 1925–1932.
Donskey, C. J., Hanrahan, J. A., Hutton, R. A., & Rice, L. B. (1999a). Effect of parenteral antibiotic
    administration on persistence of vancomycin-resistant *Enterococcus faecium* in the mouse gas-
    trointestinal tract. *J Infect Dis 180*, 384–390.
Donskey, C. J., Hanrahan, J. A., Hutton, R. A., & Rice, L. B. (2000b). Effect of parenteral antibiotic
    administration on the establishment of colonization with vancomycin-resistant *Enterococcus fae-
    cium* in the mouse gastrointestinal tract. *J Infect Dis 181*, 1830–1833.
Donskey, C. J., Schreiber, J. R., Jacobs, M. R., Shekar, R., Salata, R. A., Gordon, S., Whalen, C. C.,
    Smith, F., & Rice, L. B. (1999b). A polyclonal outbreak of predominantly VanB vancomycin-
    resistant enterococci in northeast Ohio. Northeast Ohio vancomycin-resistant *Enterococcus* sur-
    veillance program. *Clin Infect Dis 29*, 573–579.
Dunne, W. M. (1996). Watch out where the huskies go. *ASM News 62*, 283.
Durand, M. L., Calderwood, S. B., Weber, D. J., Miller, S. I., Southwick, F. S., Caviness, V. S., Jr., &
    Swartz, M. N. (1993). Acute bacterial meningitis in adults. A review of 493 episodes. *N Engl J
    Med 328*, 21–28.
Dutka-Malen, S., Blaimont, B., Wauters, G., & Courvalin, P. (1994). Emergence of high-level resist-
    ance to glycopeptides in *Enterococcus gallinarum* and *Enterococcus casseliflavus*. *Antimicrob
    Agents Chemother 38*, 1675–1677.
Dutka-Malen, S., Molinas, C., Arthur, M., & Courvalin, P. (1992). Sequence of the *vanC* gene of
    Enterococcus gallinarum BM4174 encoding a D-alanine: D-alanine ligase-related protein neces-
    sary for vancomycin resistance. *Gene 112*, 53–58.
Edmond, M. B., Ober, J. F., Dawson, J. D., Weinbaum, D. L., & Wenzel, R. P. (1996). Vancomycin-
    resistant enterococcal bacteremia: Natural history and attributable mortality. *Clin Infect Dis 23*,
    1234–1239.
Edmond, M. B., Ober, J. F., Weinbaum, D. L., Pfaller, M. A., Hwang, T., Sanford, M. D., &
    Wenzel, R. P. (1995). Vancomycin-resistant *Enterococcus faecium* bacteremia: Risk factors for
    infection. *Clin Infect Dis 20*, 1126–1133.
Edmond, M. B., Wallace, S. E., McClish, D. K., Pfaller, M. A., Jones, R. N., & Wenzel, R. P. (1999).
    Nosocomial bloodstream infections in United States hospitals: A three-year analysis. *Clin Infect
    Dis 29*, 239–244.
Eliopoulos, G. M., Wennersten, C., Zighelboim-Daum, S., Reiszner, E., Goldmann, D., &
    Moellering, R. C., Jr. (1988). High-level resistance to gentamicin in clinical isolates of
    Streptococcus (Enterococcus) faecium. *Antimicrob Agents Chemother 32*, 1528–1532.

Eliopoulos, G. M., Wennersten, C. B., Gold, H. S., Schulin, T., Souli, M., Farris, M. G., Cerwinka, S., Nadler, H. L., Dowzicky, M., Talbot, G. H., & Moellering, R. C., Jr. (1998). Characterization of vancomycin-resistant *Enterococcus faecium* isolates from the United States and their susceptibility in vitro to dalfopristin-quinupristin. *Antimicrob Agents Chemother 42*, 1088–1092.

Endtz, H. P., van den Braak, N., van Belkum, A., Kluytmans, J. A., Koeleman, J. G., Spanjaard, L., Voss, A., Weersink, A. J., Vandenbroucke-Grauls, C. M., Buiting, A. G., van Duin, A., & Verbrugh, H. A. (1997). Fecal carriage of vancomycin-resistant enterococci in hospitalized patients and those living in the community in The Netherlands. *J Clin Microbiol 35*, 3026–3031.

Evers, S., & Courvalin, P. (1996). Regulation of VanB-type vancomycin resistance gene expression by the VanS(B)-VanR (B) two-component regulatory system in *Enterococcus faecalis* V583. *J Bacteriol 178*, 1302–1309.

Facklam, R., Hollis, D., & Collins, M. D. (1989). Identification of Gram-positive coccal and coccobacillary vancomycin-resistant bacteria. *J Clin Microbiol 27*, 724–730.

Fantin, B., Leclercq, R., Garry, L., & Carbon, C. (1997). Influence of inducible cross-resistance to macrolides, lincosamides, and streptogramin B-type antibiotics in *Enterococcus faecium* on activity of quinupristin-dalfopristin in vitro and in rabbits with experimental endocarditis. *Antimicrob Agents Chemother 41*, 931–935.

Fines, M., Perichon, B., Reynolds, P., Sahm, D. F., & Courvalin, P. (1999). VanE, a new type of acquired glycopeptide resistance in *Enterococcus faecalis* BM4405. *Antimicrob Agents Chemother 43*, 2161–2164.

Finland, M., Wilcox, C., & Frank, P. F. (1950). In vitro sensitivity of human pathogens strains of streptococci to seven antibiotics. *Am J Clin Pathol 20*, 208–217.

Fontana, R., Cerini, R., Longoni, P., Grossato, A., & Canepari, P. (1983). Identification of a streptococcal penicillin-binding protein that reacts very slowly with penicillin. *J Bacteriol 155*, 1343–1350.

Fontana, R., Ligozzi, M., Pedrotti, C., Padovani, E. M., & Cornaglia, G. (1997). Vancomycin-resistant *Bacillus circulans* carrying the *vanA* gene responsible for vancomycin resistance in enterococci. *Eur J Clin Microbiol Infect Dis 16*, 473–474.

Fraimow, H. S., Jungkind, D. L., Lander, D. W., Delso, D. R., & Dean, J. L. (1994). Urinary tract infection with an *Enterococcus faecalis* isolate that requires vancomycin for growth. *Ann Intern Med 121*, 22–26.

Fridkin, S. K., Edwards, J. R., Courval, J. M., Hill, H., Tenover, F. C., Lawton, R., Gaynes, R. P., & McGowan, J. E., Jr. (2001). The effect of vancomycin and third-generation cephalosporins on prevalence of vancomycin-resistant enterococci in 126 U.S. adult intensive care units. *Ann Intern Med 135*, 175–183.

Fridkin, S. K., Yokoe, D. S., Whitney, C. G., Onderdonk, A., & Hooper, D. C. (1998). Epidemiology of a dominant clonal strain of vancomycin-resistant *Enterococcus faecium* at separate hospitals in Boston, Massachusetts. *J Clin Microbiol 36*, 965–970.

Frieden, T. R., Munsiff, S. S., Low, D. E., Willey, B. M., Williams, G., Faur, Y., Eisner, W., Warren, S., & Kreiswirth, B. (1993). Emergence of vancomycin-resistant enterococci in New York City. *Lancet 342*, 76–79.

Fujita, N., Yoshimura, M., Komori, T., Tanimoto, K., & Ike, Y. (1998). First report of the isolation of high-level vancomycin-resistant *Enterococcus faecium* from a patient in Japan. *Antimicrob Agents Chemother 42*, 2150.

Furlong, W. B., & Rakowski, T. A. (1997). Therapy with RP 59500 (quinupristin/dalfopristin) for prosthetic valve endocarditis due to enterococci with VanA/VanB resistance patterns. *Clin Infect Dis 25*, 163–164.

Gales, A. C., & Jones, R. N. (2000). Antimicrobial activity and spectrum of the new glycylcycline, GAR-936 tested against 1,203 recent clinical bacterial isolates. *Diagn Microbiol Infect Dis 36*, 19–36.

Garbutt, J. M., Ventrapragada, M., Littenberg, B., & Mundy, L. M. (2000). Association between resistance to vancomycin and death in cases of *Enterococcus faecium* bacteremia. *Clin Infect Dis 30*, 466–472.

Geraci, J. E., & Martin, W. J. (1954). Antibiotic therapy of bacterial endocarditis. VI. Subacute enterococcal endocarditis: Clinical, pathologic and therapeutic consideration of 33 cases. *Circulation 10*, 173–194.

Gerding, D. N. (1997). Is there a relationship between vancomycin-resistant enterococcal infection and *Clostridium difficile* infection? *Clin Infect Dis 25*(Suppl 2), S206–210.

Gerding, D. N., Buxton, A. E., Hughes, R. A., Cleary, P. P., Arbaczawski, J., & Stamm, W. E. (1979). Nosocomial multiply resistant Klebsiella pneumoniae: Epidemiology of an outbreak of apparent index case origin. *Antimicrob Agents Chemother 15*, 608–615.

Goldstein, F. W. (2000). Antibiotic susceptibility of bacterial strains isolated from patients with community-acquired urinary tract infections in France. Multicentre Study Group. *Eur J Clin Microbiol Infect Dis 19*, 112–117.

Gonzales, R. D., Schreckenberger, P. C., Graham, M. B., Kelkar, S., DenBesten, K., & Quinn, J. P. (2001). Infections due to vancomycin-resistant *Enterococcus faecium* resistant to linezolid. *Lancet 357*, 1179.

Goodall, B., & Tompkins, D. S. (1994). Methicillin resistant staphylococcal infection. Nursing homes act as reservoir. [letter; comment]. *BMJ 308*, 58.

Gordon, S., Swenson, J. M., Hill, B. C., Pigott, N. E., Facklam, R. R., Cooksey, R. C., Thornsberry, C., Jarvis, W. R., & Tenover, F. C. (1992). Antimicrobial susceptibility patterns of common and unusual species of enterococci causing infections in the United States. Enterococcal Study Group. *J Clin Microbiol 30*, 2373–2378.

Grayson, M. L., Eliopoulos, G. M., Wennersten, C. B., Ruoff, K. L., De Girolami, P. C., Ferraro, M. J., & Moellering, R. C. (1991). Increasing resistance to beta-lactam antibiotics among clinical isolates of *Enterococcus faecium*: A 22-year review at one institution. *Antimicrob Agents Chemother 35*, 2180–2184.

Green, M., Barbadora, K., & Michaels, M. (1991). Recovery of vancomycin-resistant Gram-positive cocci from pediatric liver transplant recipients. *J Clin Microbiol 29*, 2503–2506.

Green, M., Shlaes, J. H., Barbadora, K., & Shlaes, D. M. (1995). Bacteremia due to vancomycin-dependent *Enterococcus faecium*. *Clin Infect Dis 20*, 712–714.

Grosso, M. D., Caprioli, A., Chinzari, P., Fontana, M. C., Pezzotti, G., Manfrin, A., Giannatale, E. D., Goffredo, E., & Pantosti, A. (2000). Detection and characterization of vancomycin-resistant enterococci in farm animals and raw meat products in Italy. *Microb Drug Resist 6*, 313–318.

Hachem, R., Afif, C., Gokaslan, Z., & Raad, I. (2001). Successful treatment of vancomycin-resistant *Enterococcus meningitis* with linezolid. *Eur J Clin Microbiol Infect Dis 20*, 432–434.

Handwerger, S., Raucher, B., Altarac, D., Monka, J., Marchione, S., Singh, K. V., Murray, B. E., Wolff, J., & Walters, B. (1993). Nosocomial outbreak due to *Enterococcus faecium* highly resistant to vancomycin, penicillin, and gentamicin. *Clin Infect Dis 16*, 750–755.

Handwerger, S., & Skoble, J. (1995). Identification of chromosomal mobile element conferring high-level vancomycin resistance in *Enterococcus faecium*. *Antimicrob Agents Chemother 39*, 2446–2453.

Handwerger, S., & Tomasz, A. (1985). Antibiotic tolerance among clinical isolates of bacteria. *Rev Infect Dis 7*, 368–386.

Haroche, J., Allignet, J., Aubert, S., Van Den Bogaard, A. E., & El Solh, N. (2000). *satG*, conferring resistance to streptogramin A, is widely distributed in *Enterococcus faecium* strains but not in staphylococci. *Antimicrob Agents Chemother 44*, 190–191.

Hartman, C. S., Leach, T. S., Kaja, R. W., Schaser, R. J., Todd, W. M., & Hafkin, B. (2000, September 17–20). Linezolid in the treatment of vancomycin-resistant *Enterococcus*: A dose comparative, multicenter phase III trial. *Proceedings of 40th Interscience Conference on Antimicrobial Agents and Chemotherapy (Abstract No. 2235), Toronto, Canada. Washington, DC: American Society for Microbiology.*

Hayden, M. K. (2000). Insights into the epidemiology and control of infection with vancomycin-resistant enterococci. *Clin Infect Dis 31*, 1058–1065.

Hayden, M. K., Trenholme, G. M., Schultz, J. E., & Sahm, D. F. (1993). In vivo development of teicoplanin resistance in a VanB *Enterococcus faecium* isolate. *J Infect Dis 167*, 1224–1227.

Herrero, I. A., Issa, N. C., & Patel, R. (2002). Nosocomial spread of linezolid-resistant, vancomycin-resistant *Enterococcus faecium*. *N Engl J Med 346*, 867–869.

Herwaldt, L. A. (1999). Control of methicillin-resistant *Staphylococcus aureus* in the hospital setting. *Am J Med 106*, 11S–18S; discussion 48S–52S.

Herzstein, J., Ryan, J. L., Mangi, R. J., Greco, T. P., & Andriole, V. T. (1984). Optimal therapy for enterococcal endocarditis. *Am J Med 76*, 186–191.

Horodniceanu, T., Bougueleret, L., El-Solh, N., Bieth, G., & Delbos, F. (1979). High-level, plasmid-borne resistance to gentamicin in *Streptococcus faecalis* subsp. *zymogenes*. *Antimicrob Agents Chemother 16*, 686–689.

Howe, R. A., Robson, M., Oakhill, A., Cornish, J. M., & Millar, M. R. (1997). Successful use of tetracycline as therapy of an immunocompromised patient with septicaemia caused by a vancomycin-resistant *Enterococcus*. *J Antimicrob Chemother 40*, 144–145.

Iwen, P. C., Kelly, D. M., Linder, J., Hinrichs, S. H., Dominguez, E. A., Rupp, M. E., & Patil, K. D. (1997). Change in prevalence and antibiotic resistance of *Enterococcus* species isolated from blood cultures over an 8-year period. *Antimicrob Agents Chemother 41*, 494–495.

Jensen, L. B., Ahrens, P., Dons, L., Jones, R. N., Hammerum, A. M., & Aarestrup, F. M. (1998a). Molecular analysis of Tn*1546* in *Enterococcus faecium* isolated from animals and humans. *J Clin Microbiol 36*, 437–442.

Jensen, L. B., Hammerum, A. M., Aerestrup, F. M., van den Bogaard, A. E., & Stobberingh, E. E. (1998b). Occurrence of *satA* and *vgb* genes in streptogramin-resistant *Enterococcus faecium* isolates of animal and human origins in the Netherlands. *Antimicrob Agents Chemother 42*, 3330–3331.

Johnson, A. P., Uttley, A. H., Woodford, N., & George, R. C. (1990). Resistance to vancomycin and teicoplanin: An emerging clinical problem. *Clin Microbiol Rev 3*, 280–291.

Johnson, S., & Gerding, D. N. (1998). *Clostridium difficile*—Associated diarrhea. *Clin Infect Dis 26*, 1027–1034; quiz 1035–1026.

Jones, R. N., Marshall, S. A., Pfaller, M. A., Wilke, W. W., Hollis, R. J., Erwin, M. E., Edmond, M. B., & Wenzel, R. P. (1997). Nosocomial enterococcal blood stream infections in the SCOPE Program: Antimicrobial resistance, species occurrence, molecular testing results, and laboratory testing accuracy. SCOPE Hospital Study Group. *Diagn Microbiol Infect Dis 29*, 95–102.

Karanfil, L. V., Murphy, M., Josephson, A., Gaynes, R., Mandel, L., Hill, B. C., & Swenson, J. M. (1992). A cluster of vancomycin-resistant *Enterococcus faecium* in an intensive care unit. *Infect Control Hosp Epidemiol 13*, 195–200.

Kawalec, M., Gniadkowski, M., Kedzierska, J., Skotnicki, A., Fiett, J., & Hryniewicz, W. (2001). Selection of a teicoplanin-resistant *Enterococcus faecium* mutant during an outbreak caused by vancomycin-resistant enterococci with the VanB phenotype. *J Clin Microbiol 39*, 4274–4282.

Kim, K. H., Fekety, R., Batts, D. H., Brown, D., Cudmore, M., Silva, J., Jr., & Waters, D. (1981). Isolation of *Clostridium difficile* from the environment and contacts of patients with antibiotic-associated colitis. *J Infect Dis 143*, 42–50.

Kim, W. J., Weinstein, R. A., & Hayden, M. K. (1999). The changing molecular epidemiology and establishment of endemicity of vancomycin resistance in enterococci at one hospital over a 6-year period. *J Infect Dis 179*, 163–171.

Kirkpatrick, B. D., Harrington, S. M., Smith, D., Marcellus, D., Miller, C., Dick, J., Karanfil, L., & Perl, T. M. (1999). An outbreak of vancomycin-dependent *Enterococcus faecium* in a bone marrow transplant unit. *Clin Infect Dis 29*, 1268–1273.

Kirst, H. A., Thompson, D. G., & Nicas, T. I. (1998). Historical yearly usage of vancomycin. *Antimicrob Agents Chemother 42*, 1303–1304.

Kjerulf, A., Pallesen, L., & Westh, H. (1996). Vancomycin-resistant enterococci at a large university hospital in Denmark. *APMIS 104*, 475–479.

Klare, I., Badstubner, D., Konstabel, C., Bohme, G., Claus, H., & Witte, W. (1999). Decreased incidence of VanA-type vancomycin-resistant enterococci isolated from poultry meat and from fecal samples of humans in the community after discontinuation of avoparcin usage in animal husbandry. *Microb Drug Resist 5*, 45–52.

Krogstad, D. J., & Pargwette, A. R. (1980). Defective killing of enterococci: A common property of antimicrobial agents acting on the cell wall. *Antimicrob Agents Chemother 17*, 965–968.

Lafaurie, M., Perichon, B., Lefort, A., Carbon, C., Courvalin, P., & Fantin, B. (2001). Consequences of VanE-type resistance on efficacy of glycopeptides in vitro and in experimental endocarditis due to *Enterococcus faecalis. Antimicrob Agents Chemother 45*, 2826–2830.

Laganas, V., & Silverman, J. A. (2001, December 16–19). Inhibition of lipoteichoic acid biosynthesis is not the target of daptomycin in *Staphylococcus aureus*. *Proceedings of 41st Interscience Conference on Antimicrobial Agents and Chemotherapy (Abstract No. C1-1802). Chicago, IL. Washington, DC: American Society for Microbiology*.

Lai, K. K. (1996). Treatment of vancomycin-resistant *Enterococcus faecium* infections. *Arch Intern Med 156*, 2579–2584.

Lai, K. K., Kelley, A. L., Melvin, Z. S., Belliveau, P. P., & Fontecchio, S. A. (1998). Failure to eradicate vancomycin-resistant enterococci in a university hospital and the cost of barrier precautions. *Infect Control Hosp Epidemiol 19*, 647–652.

Lautenbach, E., Bilker, W. B., & Brennan, P. J. (1999). Enterococcal bacteremia: Risk factors for vancomycin resistance and predictors of mortality. *Infect Control Hosp Epidemiol 20*, 318–323.

Lautenbach, E., Schuster, M. G., Bilker, W. B., & Brennan, P. J. (1998). The role of chloramphenicol in the treatment of bloodstream infection due to vancomycin-resistant *Enterococcus*. *Clin Infect Dis 27*, 1259–1265.

Leach, T. S., Schaser, R. J., Hempsall, K. A., & Todd, W. M. (2000). Clinical efficacy of linezolid for infections caused by vancomycin-resistant enterococci (VRE) in a compassionate-use program (abstract no. 66). *Clin Infect Dis 31*, 224.

Leber, A. L., Hindler, J. F., Kato, E. O., Bruckner, D. A., & Pegues, D. A. (2001). Laboratory-based surveillance for vancomycin-resistant enterococci: Utility of screening stool specimens submitted for *Clostridium difficile* toxin assay. *Infect Control Hosp Epidemiol 22*, 160–164.

Leclercq, R., Bingen, E., Su, Q. H., Lambert-Zechovski, N., Courvalin, P., & Duval, J. (1991). Effects of combinations of beta-lactams, daptomycin, gentamicin, and glycopeptides against glycopeptide-resistant enterococci. *Antimicrob Agents Chemother 35*, 92–98.

Leclercq, R., Derlot, E., Duval, J., & Courvalin, P. (1988). Plasmid-mediated resistance to vancomycin and teicoplanin in *Enterococcus faecium*. *N Engl J Med 319*, 157–161.

Lefort, A., Baptista, M., Fantin, B., Depardieu, F., Arthur, M., Carbon, C., & Courvalin, P. (1999). Two-step acquisition of resistance to the teicoplanin-gentamicin combination by VanB-type *Enterococcus faecalis* in vitro and in experimental endocarditis. *Antimicrob Agents Chemother 43*, 476–482.

Lefort, A., Mainardi, J. L., Tod, M., & Lortholary, O. (2000a). Antienterococcal antibiotics. *Med Clin North Am 84*, 1471–1495.

Lefort, A., Saleh-Mghir, A., Garry, L., Carbon, C., & Fantin, B. (2000b). Activity of LY333328 combined with gentamicin in vitro and in rabbit experimental endocarditis due to vancomycin-susceptible or -resistant *Enterococcus faecalis*. *Antimicrob Agents Chemother 44*, 3017–3021.

Lewis, C. M., & Zervos, M. J. (1990). Clinical manifestations of enterococcal infection. *Eur J Clin Microbiol Infect Dis 9*, 111–117.

Liassine, N., Frei, R., Jan, I., & Auckenthaler, R. (1998). Characterization of glycopeptide-resistant enterococci from a Swiss hospital. *J Clin Microbiol 36*, 1853–1858.

Linden, P. K., Pasculle, A. W., Manez, R., Kramer, D. J., Fung, J. J., Pinna, A. D., & Kusne, S. (1996). Differences in outcomes for patients with bacteremia due to vancomycin-resistant *Enterococcus faecium* or vancomycin-susceptible *E. faecium*. *Clin Infect Dis 22*, 663–670.

Livornese, L. L., Dias, S., Samel, C., Romanowski, B., Taylor, S., May, P., Pitsakis, P., Woods, G., Kaye, D., & Levison, M. E. (1992). Hospital-acquired infection with vancomycin-resistant *Enterococcus faecium* transmitted by electronic thermometers. *Ann Intern Med 117*, 112–116.

Lodise, T. P., McKinnon, P. S., Tam, V. H., & Rybak, M. J. (2002). Clinical outcomes for patients with bacteremia caused by vancomycin-resistant *Enterococcus* in a level 1 trauma center. *Clin Infect Dis 34*, 922–929.

Lu, H. Z., Weng, X. H., Li, H., Yin, Y. K., Pang, M. Y., & Tang, Y. W. (2002). Enterococcus faecium-related outbreak with molecular evidence of transmission from pigs to humans. *J Clin Microbiol 40*, 913–917.

Lucas, G. M., Lechtzin, N., Puryear, D. W., Yau, L. L., Flexner, C. W., & Moore, R. D. (1998). Vancomycin-resistant and vancomycin-susceptible enterococcal bacteremia: Comparison of clinical features and outcomes. *Clin Infect Dis 26*, 1127–1133.

Maki, D. G., & Agger, W. A. (1988). Enterococcal bacteremia: Clinical features, the risk of endocarditis, and management. *Medicine (Baltimore), 67*, 248–269.

Marin, M. E., Mera, J. R., Arduino, R. C., Correa, A. P., Coque, T. M., Stamboulian, D., & Murray, B. E. (1998). First report of vancomycin-resistant *Enterococcus faecium* isolated in Argentina. *Clin Infect Dis 26*, 235–236.

Marshall, C. G., Broadhead, G., Leskiw, B. K., & Wright, G. D. (1997). D-Ala-D-Ala ligases from glycopeptide antibiotic-producing organisms are highly homologous to the enterococcal vancomycin-resistance ligases VanA and VanB. *Proc Natl Acad Sci USA 94*, 6480–6483.

Marshall, C. G., Lessard, I. A., Park, I., & Wright, G. D. (1998). Glycopeptide antibiotic resistance genes in glycopeptide-producing organisms. *Antimicrob Agents Chemother 42*, 2215–2220.

Mathai, D., Jones, R. N., & Pfaller, M. A. (2001). Epidemiology and frequency of resistance among pathogens causing urinary tract infections in 1,510 hospitalized patients: A report from the SENTRY Antimicrobial Surveillance Program (North America). *Diagn Microbiol Infect Dis 40*, 129–136.

McCarthy, A. E., Victor, G., Ramotar, K., & Toye, B. (1994). Risk factors for acquiring ampicillin-resistant enterococci and clinical outcomes at a Canadian tertiary-care hospital. *J Clin Microbiol 32*, 2671–2676.

McDonald, L. C., Kuehnert, M. J., Tenover, F. C., & Jarvis, W. R. (1997). Vancomycin-resistant enterococci outside the health-care setting: Prevalence, sources, and public health implications. *Emerg Infect Dis 3*, 311–317.

McDonald, L. C., Rossiter, S., Mackinson, C., Wang, Y. Y., Johnson, S., Sullivan, M., Sokolow, R., DeBess, E., Gilbert, L., Benson, J. A., Hill, B., & Angulo, F. J. (2001). Quinupristin-dalfopristin-resistant *Enterococcus faecium* on chicken and in human stool specimens. *N Engl J Med 345*, 1155–1160.

McKessar, S. J., Berry, A. M., Bell, J. M., Turnidge, J. D., & Paton, J. C. (2000). Genetic characterization of *vanG*, a novel vancomycin resistance locus of *Enterococcus faecalis*. *Antimicrob Agents Chemother 44*, 3224–3228.

McNeil, S. A., Clark, N. M., Chandrasekar, P. H., & Kauffman, C. A. (2000). Successful treatment of vancomycin-resistant *Enterococcus faecium* bacteremia with linezolid after failure of treatment with synercid (quinupristin/dalfopristin). *Clin Infect Dis 30*, 403–404.

Megran, D. W. (1992). Enterococcal endocarditis. *Clin Infect Dis 15*, 63–71.

Melhus, A., & Tjernberg, I. (1996). First documented isolation of vancomycin-resistant *Enterococcus faecium* in Sweden. *Scand J Infect Dis 28*, 191–193.

Mevius, D., Devriese, L., Butaye, P., Vandamme, P., Verschure, M., & Veldman, K. (1998). Isolation of glycopeptide resistant *Streptococcus gallolyticus* strains with *vanA, vanB*, and both *vanA* and *vanB* genotypes from faecal samples of veal calves in The Netherlands. *J Antimicrob Chemother* *42*, 275–276.

Miranda, A. G., Singh, K. V., & Murray, B. E. (1991). DNA fingerprinting of *Enterococcus faecium* by pulsed-field gel electrophoresis may be a useful epidemiologic tool. *J Clin Microbiol 29*, 2752–2757.

Moellering, R. C., Jr. (1992). Emergence of *Enterococcus* as a significant pathogen. *Clin Infect Dis 14*, 1173–1176.

Moellering, R. C., Linden, P. K., Reinhardt, J., Blumberg, E. A., Bompart, F., & Talbot, G. H. (1999). The efficacy and safety of quinupristin/dalfopristin for the treatment of infections caused by vancomycin-resistant *Enterococcus faecium*. Synercid emergency-use study group. *J Antimicrob Chemother 44*, 251–261.

Montecalvo, M. A., Horowitz, H., Gedris, C., Carbonaro, C., Tenover, F. C., Issah, A., Cook, P., & Wormser, G. P. (1994). Outbreak of vancomycin-, ampicillin-, and aminoglycoside-resistant *Enterococcus faecium* bacteremia in an adult oncology unit. *Antimicrob Agents Chemother 38*, 1363–1367.

Montecalvo, M. A., Horowitz, H., Wormser, G. P., Seiter, K., & Carbonaro, C. A. (1995). Effect of novobiocin-containing antimicrobial regimens on infection and colonization with vancomycin-resistant *Enterococcus faecium*. *Antimicrob Agents Chemother 39*, 794.

Montecalvo, M. A., Jarvis, W. R., Uman, J., Shay, D. K., Petrullo, C., Rodney, K., Gedris, C., Horowitz, H. W., & Wormser, G. P. (1999). Infection-control measures reduce transmission of vancomycin-resistant enterococci in an endemic setting. *Ann Intern Med 131*, 269–272.

Moreno, F., Grota, P., Crisp, C., Magnon, K., Melcher, G. P., Jorgensen, J. H., & Patterson, J. E. (1995). Clinical and molecular epidemiology of vancomycin-resistant *Enterococcus faecium* during its emergence in a city in southern Texas. *Clin Infect Dis 21*, 1234–1237.

Morris, J. G., Jr., Shay, D. K., Hebden, J. N., McCarter, R. J., Jr., Perdue, B. E., Jarvis, W., Johnson, J. A., Dowling, T. C., Polish, L. B., & Schwalbe, R. S. (1995). Enterococci resistant to multiple antimicrobial agents, including vancomycin. Establishment of endemicity in a university medical center. *Ann Intern Med 123*, 250–259.

Mundy, L. M., Sahm, D. F., & Gilmore, M. (2000). Relationships between enterococcal virulence and antimicrobial resistance. *Clin Microbiol Rev 13*, 513–522.

Murphy, T. M., Deitz, J. M., Petersen, P. J., Mikels, S. M., & Weiss, W. J. (2000). Therapeutic efficacy of GAR-936, a novel glycylcycline, in a rat model of experimental endocarditis. *Antimicrob Agents Chemother 44*, 3022–3027.

Murray, B. E. (1990). The life and times of the *Enterococcus*. *Clin Microbiol Rev 3*, 46–65.

Murray, B. E. (1994). Can antibiotic resistance be controlled? [letter; comment]. *N Engl J Med 330*, 1229–1230.

Murray, B. E. (1997). Vancomycin-resistant enterococci. *Am J Med 102*, 284–293.

Murray, B. E., & Mederski-Samaroj, B. (1983). Transferable beta-lactamase. A new mechanism for in vitro penicillin resistance in *Streptococcus faecalis*. *J Clin Invest 72*, 1168–1171.

Murray, B. E., Singh, K. V., Markowitz, S. M., Lopardo, H. A., Patterson, J. E., Zervos, M. J., Rubeglio, E., Eliopoulos, G. M., Rice, L. B., & Goldstein, F. W. (1991). Evidence for clonal spread of a single strain of beta-lactamase-producing *Enterococcus (Streptococcus) faecalis* to six hospitals in five states. *J Infect Dis 163*, 780–785.

Mylotte, J. M., Goodnough, S., & Tayara, A. (2001). Antibiotic-resistant organisms among long-term care facility residents on admission to an inpatient geriatrics unit: Retrospective and prospective surveillance. *Am J Infect Control 29*, 139–144.

Nachman, S. A., Verma, R., & Egnor, M. (1995). Vancomycin-resistant Enterococcus faecium shunt infection in an infant: An antibiotic cure. *Microb Drug Resist 1*, 95–96.

Nannini, E. C., Singh, K. V., & Murray, B. E. (2001, December 16–19). Efficacy of GAR-936, a novel glycylcycline, against enterococci in a mouse peritonitis model. *Proceedings of*

41st Interscience Conference on Antimicrobial Agents and Chemotherapy (Abstract No. B-1651). Chicago, IL. Washington, DC: American Society for Microbiology.

Navarro, F., & Courvalin, P. (1994). Analysis of genes encoding D-alanine-D-alanine ligase-related enzymes in *Enterococcus casseliflavus* and *Enterococcus flavescens*. *Antimicrob Agents Chemother 38*, 1788–1793.

Neely, A. N., & Maley, M. P. (2000). Survival of enterococci and staphylococci on hospital fabrics and plastic. [see comments]. *J Clin Microbiol 38*, 724–726.

NNIS. (2000). National Nosocomial Infections Surveillance (NNIS) system report, data summary from January 1992–April 2000, issued June 2000. *Am J Infect Control 28*, 429–448.

NNIS. (2001). National Nosocomial Infections Surveillance (NNIS) System Report, Data Summary from January 1992–June 2001, issued August 2001. *Am J Infect Control 29*, 404–421.

Noble, W. C., Virani, Z., & Cree, R. G. (1992). Co-transfer of vancomycin and other resistance genes from *Enterococcus faecalis* NCTC 12201 to *Staphylococcus aureus*. *FEMS Microbiol Lett 72*, 195–198.

Noskin, G. A., Peterson, L. R., & Warren, J. R. (1995a). *Enterococcus faecium* and *Enterococcus faecalis* bacteremia: Acquisition and outcome. *Clin Infect Dis 20*, 296–301.

Noskin, G. A., Stosor, V., Cooper, I., & Peterson, L. R. (1995b). Recovery of vancomycin-resistant enterococci on fingertips and environmental surfaces [see comments]. *Infect Control Hosp Epidemiol 16*, 577–581.

Nourse, C., Byrne, C., Kaufmann, M., Keane, C. T., Fenelon, L., Smyth, E. G., Hone, R., & Butler, K. (2000). VRE in the Republic of Ireland: Clinical significance, characteristics and molecular similarity of isolates. *J Hosp Infect 44*, 288–293.

O'Donovan, C. A., Fan-Havard, P., Tecson-Tumang, F. T., Smith, S. M., & Eng, R. H. (1994). Enteric eradication of vancomycin-resistant *Enterococcus faecium* with oral bacitracin. *Diagn Microbiol Infect Dis 18*, 105–109.

Olsen, R. J., Lynch, P., Coyle, M. B., Cummings, J., Bokete, T., & Stamm, W. E. (1993). Examination gloves as barriers to hand contamination in clinical practice. *JAMA 270*, 350–353.

Ostrowsky, B. E., Clark, N. C., Thauvin-Eliopoulos, C., Venkataraman, L., Samore, M. H., Tenover, F. C., Eliopoulos, G. M., Moellering, R. C., Jr., & Gold, H. S. (1999). A cluster of VanD vancomycin-resistant *Enterococcus faecium*: Molecular characterization and clinical epidemiology. *J Infect Dis 180*, 1177–1185.

Ostrowsky, B. E., Trick, W. E., Sohn, A. H., Quirk, S. B., Holt, S., Carson, L. A., Hill, B. C., Arduino, M. J., Kuehnert, M. J., & Jarvis, W. R. (2001). Control of vancomycin-resistant *Enterococcus* in health care facilities in a region. *N Engl J Med 344*, 1427–1433.

O'Toole, R. D., Drew, W. L., Dahlgren, B. J., & Beaty, H. N. (1970). An outbreak of methicillin-resistant *Staphylococcus aureus* infection. Observations in hospital and nursing home. *JAMA 213*, 257–263.

Pallares, R., Pujol, M., Pena, C., Ariza, J., Martin, R., & Gudiol, F. (1993). Cephalosporins as risk factor for nosocomial *Enterococcus faecalis* bacteremia. A matched case-control study. *Arch Intern Med 153*, 1581–1586.

Papanicolaou, G. A., Meyers, B. R., Meyers, J., Mendelson, M. H., Lou, W., Emre, S., Sheiner, P., & Miller, C. (1996). Nosocomial infections with vancomycin-resistant *Enterococcus faecium* in liver transplant recipients: Risk factors for acquisition and mortality. *Clin Infect Dis 23*, 760–766.

Patel, R. (2000). Enterococcal-type glycopeptide resistance genes in non-enterococcal organisms. *FEMS Microbiol Lett 185*, 1–7.

Patel, R., Piper, K., Cockerill, F. R., 3rd, Steckelberg, J. M., & Yousten, A. A. (2000). The biopesticide *Paenibacillus popilliae* has a vancomycin resistance gene cluster homologous to the enterococcal *vanA* vancomycin resistance gene cluster. *Antimicrob Agents Chemother 44*, 705–709.

Patel, R., Rouse, M. S., Piper, K. E., & Steckelberg, J. M. (2001). Linezolid therapy of vancomycin-resistant *Enterococcus faecium* experimental endocarditis. *Antimicrob Agents Chemother 45*, 621–623.

Patel, R., Uhl, J. R., Kohner, P., Hopkins, M. K., & Cockerill, F. R., 3rd. (1997a). Multiplex PCR detection of *vanA, vanB, vanC-1*, and *vanC-2/3* genes in enterococci. *J Clin Microbiol 35*, 703–707.

Patel, S. S., Balfour, J. A., & Bryson, H. M. (1997b). Fosfomycin tromethamine. A review of its antibacterial activity, pharmacokinetic properties and therapeutic efficacy as a single-dose oral treatment for acute uncomplicated lower urinary tract infections. *Drugs 53*, 637–656.

Patterson, J. E., Sweeney, A. H., Simms, M., Carley, N., Mangi, R., Sabetta, J., & Lyons, R. W. (1995). An analysis of 110 serious enterococcal infections. Epidemiology, antibiotic susceptibility, and outcome. *Medicine (Baltimore), 74*, 191–200.

Perez Mato, S., Robinson, S., & Begue, R. E. (1999). Vancomycin-resistant *Enterococcus faecium* meningitis successfully treated with chloramphenicol. *Pediatr Infect Dis J 18*, 483–484.

Perichon, B., Casadewall, B., Reynolds, P., & Courvalin, P. (2000). Glycopeptide-resistant *Enterococcus faecium* BM4416 is a VanD-type strain with an impaired D-Alanine:D-Alanine ligase. *Antimicrob Agents Chemother 44*, 1346–1348.

Perichon, B., Reynolds, P., & Courvalin, P. (1997). VanD-type glycopeptide-resistant *Enterococcus faecium* BM4339. *Antimicrob Agents Chemother 41*, 2016–2018.

Peset, V., Tallon, P., Sola, C., Sanchez, E., Sarrion, A., Perez-Belles, C., Vindel, A., Canton, E., & Gobernado, M. (2000). Epidemiological, microbiological, clinical, and prognostic factors of bacteremia caused by high-level vancomycin-resistant *Enterococcus* species. *Eur J Clin Microbiol Infect Dis 19*, 742–749.

Power, E. G., Abdulla, Y. H., Talsania, H. G., Spice, W., Aathithan, S., & French, G. L. (1995). *vanA* genes in vancomycin-resistant clinical isolates of *Oerskovia turbata* and *Arcanobacterium* (*Corynebacterium*) *haemolyticum*. *J Antimicrob Chemother 36*, 595–606.

Poyart, C., Pierre, C., Quesne, G., Pron, B., Berche, P., & Trieu-Cuot, P. (1997). Emergence of vancomycin resistance in the genus *Streptococcus*: Characterization of a *vanB* transferable determinant in *Streptococcus bovis*. *Antimicrob Agents Chemother 41*, 24–29.

Prystowsky, J., Siddiqui, F., Chosay, J., Shinabarger, D. L., Millichap, J., Peterson, L. R., & Noskin, G. A. (2001). Resistance to linezolid: Characterization of mutations in rRNA and comparison of their occurrences in vancomycin-resistant enterococci. *Antimicrob Agents Chemother 45*, 2154–2156.

Quale, J., Landman, D., Saurina, G., Atwood, E., DiTore, V., & Patel, K. (1996). Manipulation of a hospital antimicrobial formulary to control an outbreak of vancomycin-resistant enterococci. *Clin Infect Dis 23*, 1020–1025.

Rafferty, M. E., McCormick, M. I., Bopp, L. H., Baltch, A. L., George, M., Smith, R. P., Rheal, C., Ritz, W., & Schoonmaker, D. (1997). Vancomycin-resistant enterococci in stool specimens submitted for *Clostridium difficile* cytotoxin assay. *Infect Control Hosp Epidemiol 18*, 342–344.

Rasmussen, B. A., Gluzman, Y., & Tally, F. P. (1994). Inhibition of protein synthesis occurring on tetracycline-resistant, TetM-protected ribosomes by a novel class of tetracyclines, the glycylcyclines. *Antimicrob Agents Chemother 38*, 1658–1660.

Reid, K. C., Cockerill, I. F., & Patel, R. (2001). Clinical and epidemiological features of *Enterococcus casseliflavus/flavescens* and *Enterococcus gallinarum* bacteremia: A report of 20 cases. *Clin Infect Dis 32*, 1540–1546.

Reynolds, P. E. (1989). Structure, biochemistry and mechanism of action of glycopeptide antibiotics. *Eur J Clin Microbiol Infect Dis 8*, 943–950.

Reynolds, P. E., Ambur, O. H., Casadewall, B., & Courvalin, P. (2001). The VanYD D,D-carboxypeptidase of *Enterococcus faecium* BM4339 is a penicillin-binding protein. *Microbiol 147*, 2571–2578.

Reynolds, P. E., & Somner, E. A. (1990). Comparison of the target sites and mechanisms of action of glycopeptide and lipoglycodepsipeptide antibiotics. *Drugs Exp Clin Res 16*, 385–389.

Rice, L. B., Carias, L. L., Donskey, C. L., & Rudin, S. D. (1998). Transferable, plasmid-mediated VanB-type glycopeptide resistance in *Enterococcus faecium*. *Antimicrob Agents Chemother 42*, 963–964.

Rippere, K., Patel, R., Uhl, J. R., Piper, K. E., Steckelberg, J. M., Kline, B. C., Cockerill, F. R., 3rd, and Yousten, A. A. (1998). DNA sequence resembling *vanA* and *vanB* in the vancomycin-resistant biopesticide *Bacillus popilliae. J Infect Dis 178*, 584–588.

Roberts, M. C., Sutcliffe, J., Courvalin, P., Jensen, L. B., Rood, J., & Seppala, H. (1999). Nomenclature for macrolide and macrolide-lincosamide-streptogramin B resistance determinants. *Antimicrob Agents Chemother 43*, 2823–2830.

Robredo, B., Singh, K. V., Baquero, F., Murray, B. E., & Torres, C. (2000a). Vancomycin-resistant enterococci isolated from animals and food. *Int J Food Microbiol 54*, 197–204.

Robredo, B., Singh, K. V., Torres, C., & Murray, B. E. (2000b). Streptogramin resistance and shared pulsed-field gel electrophoresis patterns in vanA-containing *Enterococcus faecium* and *Enterococcus hirae* isolated from humans and animals in Spain. *Microb Drug Resist 6*, 305–311.

Robredo, B., Torres, C., Singh, K. V., & Murray, B. E. (2000c). Molecular analysis of Tn*1546* in *vanA*-containing *Enterococcus* spp. isolated from humans and poultry. *Antimicrob Agents Chemother 44*, 2588–2589.

Roghmann, M. C., McCarter, R. J., Jr., Brewrink, J., Cross, A. S., & Morris, J. G., Jr. (1997). *Clostridium difficile* infection is a risk factor for bacteremia due to vancomycin-resistant entero-cocci (VRE) in VRE-colonized patients with acute leukemia. *Clin Infect Dis 25*, 1056–1059.

Rubin, L. G., Tucci, V., Cercenado, E., Eliopoulos, G., & Isenberg, H. D. (1992). Vancomycin-resistant *Enterococcus faecium* in hospitalized children. *Infect Control Hosp Epidemiol 13*, 700–705.

Safdar, A., Bryan, C. S., Stinson, S., & Saunders, D. E. (2002). Prosthetic valve endocarditis due to vancomycin-resistant Enterococcus faecium: Treatment with chloramphenicol plus minocycline. *Clin Infect Dis 34*, E61–63.

Sahm, D. F., Kissinger, J., Gilmore, M. S., Murray, P. R., Mulder, R., Solliday, J., & Clarke, B. (1989). In vitro susceptibility studies of vancomycin-resistant *Enterococcus faecalis. Antimicrob Agents Chemother 33*, 1588–1591.

Saleh-Mghir, A., Lefort, A., Petegnief, Y., Dautrey, S., Vallois, J. M., Le Guludec, D., Carbon, C., & Fantin, B. (1999). Activity and diffusion of LY333328 in experimental endocarditis due to vancomycin-resistant *Enterococcus faecalis. Antimicrob Agents Chemother 43*, 115–120.

Schleifer, K. H., & Kilpper-Bälz, R. (1984). Transfer of *Streptococcus faecalis* and *Strepto-coccus faecium* to the genus *Enterococcus* nom. rev. as *Enterococcus faecalis* comb. nov. and *Enterococcus faecium* comb. nov. *Int J Syst Bacteriol 34*, 31–34.

Schouten, M. A., Hoogkamp-Korstanje, J. A., Meis, J. F., & Voss, A. (2000). Prevalence of vancomycin-resistant enterococci in Europe. *Eur J Clin Microbiol Infect Dis 19*, 816–822.

Schwalbe, R. S., McIntosh, A. C., Qaiyumi, S., Johnson, J. A., Johnson, R. J., Furness, K. M., Holloway, W. J., & Steele-Moore, L. (1996). In vitro activity of LY333328, an investigational gly-copeptide antibiotic, against enterococci and staphylococci. *Antimicrob Agents Chemother 40*, 2416–2419.

Schwalbe, R. S., McIntosh, A. C., Qaiyumi, S., Johnson, J. A., & Morris, J. G., Jr. (1999). Isolation of vancomycin-resistant enterococci from animal feed in USA. *Lancet 353*, 722.

Seetulsingh, P. S., Tomayko, J. F., Coudron, P. E., Markowitz, S. M., Skinner, C., Singh, K. V., & Murray, B. E. (1996). Chromosomal DNA restriction endonuclease digestion patterns of beta-lactamase-producing *Enterococcus faecalis* isolates collected from a single hospital over a 7-year period. *J Clin Microbiol 34*, 1892–1896.

Shaikh, Z. H., Peloquin, C. A., & Ericsson, C. D. (2001). Successful treatment of vancomycin-resistant *Enterococcus faecium* meningitis with linezolid: Case report and literature review. *Scand J Infect Dis 33*, 375–379.

Shay, D. K., Maloney, S. A., Montecalvo, M., Banerjee, S., Wormser, G. P., Arduino, M. J., Bland, L. A., & Jarvis, W. R. (1995). Epidemiology and mortality risk of vancomycin-resistant enterococcal bloodstream infections. *J Infect Dis 172*, 993–1000.

Sherman, J. M. (1937). The streptococci. *Bacteriol Rev 1*, 3–97.

Shinabarger, D. L., Marotti, K. R., Murray, R. W., Lin, A. H., Melchior, E. P., Swaney, S. M., Dunyak, D. S., Demyan, W. F., & Buysse, J. M. (1997). Mechanism of action of oxazolidinones: Effects of linezolid and eperezolid on translation reactions. *Antimicrob Agents Chemother 41*, 2132–2136.

Shlaes, D. M., Levy, J., & Wolinsky, E. (1981). Enterococcal bacteremia without endocarditis. *Arch Intern Med 141*, 578–581.

Singh, K. V., Weinstock, G. M., & Murray, B. E. (2002). An *Enterococcus faecalis* ABC homologue (Lsa) is required for the resistance of this species to clindamycin and quinupristin-dalfopristin. *Antimicrob Agents Chemother 46*, 1845–1850.

Slaughter, S., Hayden, M. K., Nathan, C., Hu, T. C., Rice, T., Van Voorhis, J., Matushek, M., Franklin, C., & Weinstein, R. A. (1996). A comparison of the effect of universal use of gloves and gowns with that of glove use alone on acquisition of vancomycin-resistant enterococci in a medical intensive care unit. *Ann Intern Med 125*, 448–456.

Soltani, M., Beighton, D., Philpott-Howard, J., & Woodford, N. (2000). Mechanisms of resistance to quinupristin-dalfopristin among isolates of *Enterococcus faecium* from animals, raw meat, and hospital patients in Western Europe. *Antimicrob Agents Chemother 44*, 433–436.

Steinmetz, M. P., Vogelbaum, M. A., De Georgia, M. A., Andrefsky, J. C., & Isada, C. (2001). Successful treatment of vancomycin-resistant enterococcus meningitis with linezolid: Case report and review of the literature. *Crit Care Med 29*, 2383–2385.

Stinear, T. P., Olden, D. C., Johnson, P. D., Davies, J. K., & Grayson, M. L. (2001). Enterococcal *vanB* resistance locus in anaerobic bacteria in human faeces. *Lancet 357*, 855–856.

Stosor, V., Peterson, L. R., Postelnick, M., & Noskin, G. A. (1998). *Enterococcus faecium* bacteremia: Does vancomycin resistance make a difference? *Arch Intern Med 158*, 522–527.

Stroud, L., Edwards, J., Danzing, L., Culver, D., & Gaynes, R. (1996). Risk factors for mortality associated with enterococcal bloodstream infections. *Infect Control Hosp Epidemiol 17*, 576–580.

Suppola, J. P., Kuikka, A., Vaara, M., & Valtonen, V. V. (1998). Comparison of risk factors and outcome in patients with *Enterococcus faecalis* vs *Enterococcus faecium* bacteraemia. *Scand J Infect Dis 30*, 153–157.

Tally, F. P., & DeBruin, M. F. (2000). Development of daptomycin for Gram-positive infections. *J Antimicrob Chemother 46*, 523–526.

Taylor, S. E., Paterson, D. L., & Yu, V. L. (1998). Treatment options for chronic prostatitis due to vancomycin-resistant *Enterococcus faecium*. *Eur J Clin Microbiol Infect Dis 17*, 798–800.

Tenorio, A. R., Badri, S. M., Sahgal, N. B., Hota, B., Matushek, M., Hayden, M. K., Trenholme, G. M., & Weinstein, R. A. (2001). Effectiveness of gloves in the prevention of hand carriage of vancomycin-resistant enterococcus species by health care workers after patient care. *Clin Infect Dis 32*, 826–829.

Tokars, J. I., Satake, S., Rimland, D., Carson, L., Miller, E. R., Killum, E., Sinkowitz-Cochran, R. L., Arduino, M. J., Tenover, F. C., Marston, B., & Jarvis, W. R. (1999). The prevalence of colonization with vancomycin-resistant *Enterococcus* at a Veterans' Affairs institution. *Infect Control Hosp Epidemiol 20*, 171–175.

Tornieporth, N. G., Roberts, R. B., John, J., Hafner, A., & Riley, L. W. (1996). Risk factors associated with vancomycin-resistant *Enterococcus faecium* infection or colonization in 145 matched case patients and control patients. *Clin Infect Dis 23*, 767–772.

Trick, W. E., Kuehnert, M. J., Quirk, S. B., Arduino, M. J., Aguero, S. M., Carson, L. A., Hill, B. C., Banerjee, S. N., & Jarvis, W. R. (1999). Regional dissemination of vancomycin-resistant enterococci resulting from interfacility transfer of colonized patients. *J Infect Dis 180*, 391–396.

Uttley, A. H., Collins, C. H., Naidoo, J., & George, R. C. (1988). Vancomycin-resistant enterococci. *Lancet 1*, 57–58.

Uttley, A. H., George, R. C., Naidoo, J., Woodford, N., Johnson, A. P., Collins, C. H., Morrison, D., Gilfillan, A. J., Fitch, L. E., & Heptonstall, J. (1989). High-level vancomycin-resistant enterococci causing hospital infections. *Epidemiol Infect 103*, 173–181.

Van Bambeke, F., Chauvel, M., Reynolds, P. E., Fraimow, H. S., & Courvalin, P. (1999). Vancomycin-dependent *Enterococcus faecalis* clinical isolates and revertant mutants. *Antimicrob Agents Chemother 43*, 41–47.

Van Caeseele, P., Giercke, S., Wylie, J., Boyd, D., Mulvey, M., Amin, S., & Ofner-Agostini, M. (2001). Identification of the first vancomycin-resistant *Enterococcus faecalis* harbouring *vanE* in Canada. *Can Commun Dis Rep 27*, 101–104.

van den Bogaard, A. E., Jensen, L. B., & Stobberingh, E. E. (1997a). Vancomycin-resistant enterococci in turkeys and farmers. *N Engl J Med 337*, 1558–1559.

van den Bogaard, A. E., Mertens, P., London, N. H., & Stobberingh, E. E. (1997b). High prevalence of colonization with vancomycin- and pristinamycin-resistant enterococci in healthy humans and pigs in The Netherlands: Is the addition of antibiotics to animal feeds to blame? *J Antimicrob Chemother 40*, 454–456.

van den Bogaard, A. E., & Stobberingh, E. E. (2000). Epidemiology of resistance to antibiotics. Links between animals and humans. *Int J Antimicrob Agents 14*, 327–335.

van den Braak, N., Ott, A., van Belkum, A., Kluytmans, J. A., Koeleman, J. G., Spanjaard, L., Voss, A., Weersink, A. J., Vandenbroucke-Grauls, C. M., Buiting, A. G., Verbrugh, H. A., & Endtz, H. P. (2000). Prevalence and determinants of fecal colonization with vancomycin-resistant *Enterococcus* in hospitalized patients in The Netherlands. *Infect Control Hosp Epidemiol 21*, 520–524.

Van der Auwera, P., Pensart, N., Korten, V., Murray, B. E., & Leclercq, R. (1996). Influence of oral glycopeptides on the fecal flora of human volunteers: Selection of highly glycopeptide-resistant enterococci. *J Infect Dis 173*, 1129–1136.

Vandamme, P., Vercauteren, E., Lammens, C., Pensart, N., Ieven, M., Pot, B., Leclercq, R., & Goossens, H. (1996). Survey of enterococcal susceptibility patterns in Belgium. *J Clin Microbiol 34*, 2572–2576.

Venditti, M., Fimiani, C., Baiocchi, P., Santini, C., Tarasi, A., Capone, A., Di Rosa, R., & Micozzi, A. (1994). Infections by ampicillin-resistant enterococci: A case-control study. *J Chemother 6*, 121–126.

Vergis, E. N., Hayden, M. K., Chow, J. W., Snydman, D. R., Zervos, M. J., Linden, P. K., Wagener, M. M., Schmitt, B., & Muder, R. R. (2001). Determinants of vancomycin resistance and mortality rates in enterococcal bacteremia: A prospective multicenter study. *Ann Intern Med 135*, 484–492.

Viagappan, M., & Holliman, R. E. (1999). Risk factors for acquisition of gentamicin-resistant enterococcal infection: A case-controlled study. *Postgrad Med J 75*, 342–345.

Watanakunakorn, C., & Bakie, C. (1973). Synergism of vancomycin-gentamicin and vancomycin-streptomycin against enterococci. *Antimicrob Agents Chemother 4*, 120–124.

Weinstein, M. R., Dedier, H., Brunton, J., Campbell, I., & Conly, J. M. (1999). Lack of efficacy of oral bacitracin plus doxycycline for the eradication of stool colonization with vancomycin-resistant *Enterococcus faecium*. *Clin Infect Dis 29*, 361–366.

Wells, C. L., Juni, B. A., Cameron, S. B., Mason, K. R., Dunn, D. L., Ferrieri, P., & Rhame, F. S. (1995). Stool carriage, clinical isolation, and mortality during an outbreak of vancomycin-resistant enterococci in hospitalized medical and/or surgical patients. *Clin Infect Dis 21*, 45–50.

Wells, L. D., & von Graevenitz, A. (1980). Clinical significance of enterococci in blood cultures from adult patients. *Infection 8*, 147–151.

Wells, V. D., Wong, E. S., Murray, B. E., Coudron, P. E., Williams, D. S., & Markowitz, S. M. (1992). Infections due to beta-lactamase-producing, high-level gentamicin-resistant *Enterococcus faecalis*. *Ann Intern Med 116*, 285–292.

Wilke, W. W., Marshall, S. A., Coffman, S. L., Pfaller, M. A., Edmund, M. B., Wenzel, R. P., & Jones, R. N. (1997). Vancomycin-resistant *Enterococcus raffinosus*: Molecular epidemiology, species identification error, and frequency of occurrence in a national resistance surveillance program. *Diagn Microbiol Infect Dis 29*, 43–49.

Willems, R. J., Top, J., van den Braak, N., van Belkum, A., Mevius, D. J., Hendriks, G., van Santen-Verheuvel, M., & van Embden, J. D. (1999). Molecular diversity and evolutionary relationships of Tn*1546*-like elements in enterococci from humans and animals. *Antimicrob Agents Chemother 43*, 483–491.

Willey, B. M., Kreiswirth, B. N., Simor, A. E., Faur, Y., Patel, M., Williams, G., & Low, D. E. (1993). Identification and characterization of multiple species of vancomycin-resistant enterococci, including an evaluation of Vitek software version 7.1. *J Clin Microbiol 31*, 2777–2779.

Williamson, J. C., Glazier, S. S., & Peacock, J. E., Jr. (2002). Successful treatment of ventriculostomy-related meningitis caused by vancomycin-resistant Enterococcus with intravenous and intraventricular quinupristin/dalfopristin. *Clin Neurol Neurosurg 104*, 54–56.

Winston, D. J., Emmanouilides, C., Kroeber, A., Hindler, J., Bruckner, D. A., Territo, M. C., & Busuttil, R. W. (2000). Quinupristin/Dalfopristin therapy for infections due to vancomycin-resistant *Enterococcus faecium*. *Clin Infect Dis 30*, 790–797.

Wong, A. H., Wenzel, R. P., & Edmond, M. B. (2000). Epidemiology of bacteriuria caused by vancomycin-resistant enterococci—A retrospective study. *Am J Infect Control 28*, 277–281.

Wong, M. T., Kauffman, C. A., Standiford, H. C., Linden, P., Fort, G., Fuchs, H. J., Porter, S. B., & Wenzel, R. P. (2001). Effective suppression of vancomycin-resistant *Enterococcus* species in asymptomatic gastrointestinal carriers by a novel glycolipodepsipeptide, ramoplanin. *Clin Infect Dis 33*, 1476–1482.

Woodford, N., Adebiyi, A. M., Palepou, M. F., & Cookson, B. D. (1998). Diversity of VanA glycopeptide resistance elements in enterococci from humans and nonhuman sources. *Antimicrob Agents Chemother 42*, 502–508.

Woodford, N., Jones, B. L., Baccus, Z., Ludlam, H. A., & Brown, D. F. (1995). Linkage of vancomycin and high-level gentamicin resistance genes on the same plasmid in a clinical isolate of *Enterococcus faecalis*. *J Antimicrob Chemother 35*, 179–184.

Zanella, R. C., Valdetaro, F., Lovgren, M., Tyrrel, G. J., Bokermann, S., Almeida, S. C., Vieira, V. S., & Brandileone, M. C. (1999). First confirmed case of a vancomycin-resistant *Enterococcus faecium* with VanA phenotype from Brazil: Isolation from a meningitis case in Sao Paulo. *Microb Drug Resist 5*, 159–162.

Zeana, C., Kubin, C. J., Della-Latta, P., & Hammer, S. M. (2001). Vancomycin-resistant *Enterococcus faecium* meningitis successfully managed with linezolid: Case report and review of the literature. *Clin Infect Dis 33*, 477–482.

Zervos, M. J., Dembinski, S., Mikesell, T., & Schaberg, D. R. (1986). High-level resistance to gentamicin in *Streptococcus faecalis*: Risk factors and evidence for exogenous acquisition of infection. *J Infect Dis 153*, 1075–1083.

Zervos, M. J., Kauffman, C. A., Therasse, P. M., Bergman, A. G., Mikesell, T. S., & Schaberg, D. R. (1987). Nosocomial infection by gentamicin-resistant *Streptococcus faecalis*. An epidemiologic study. *Ann Intern Med 106*, 687–691.

Zhanel, G. G., Hoban, D. J., & Karlowsky, J. A. (2001). Nitrofurantoin is active against vancomycin-resistant enterococci. *Antimicrob Agents Chemother 45*, 324–326.

6

Multi-Resistant *Enterobacteriaceae* in Hospital Practice

Maria I. Morosini, Rafael Cantón, and José L. Martínez

1. INTRODUCTION

Antibiotics were so succesful in the treatment of infections that in the 1980s a point was reached where the battle against infection was thought to be won. Health programs could be devoted to other more important topics, such as cancer or cardiovascular diseases. Unfortunately, this optimistic view was far from being accurate, as bacteria have evolved to be resistant to antibiotics. Infections are still the main health problem, according to the World Health Organization (2000). Infections by multidrug resistant *Enterobacteriaceae* have been highlighted as particularly problematic for hospital practice (Dennesen et al., 1998). We want to stress here that recurrent infections might compromise several hospital practices such as immunosuppression for organ transplantation, major surgery, anticancer therapy, intubation and catetherization, with therapeutic failures occurring, not as a consequence of the therapeutic protocol, but as a consequence of infection. The problem is more relevant when the microorganisms that produce the infections are resistant to antibiotics, because in this case they are barely treatable (Neu, 1992). Antibiotic resistance can be an intrinsic property of some bacterial species or it can be acquired as the consequence of selection during antibiotic treatment. Clear examples of the first situation is the lack of susceptibility of Gram-negative bacteria to macrolides and the decreased susceptibility of some non-fermenters (*Pseudomonas aeruginosa*, *Burkholderia cepacia*, *Stenotrophomonas maltophilia*, ...) to several antibiotic families (Quinn, 1998). Although not be discussed in depth in this chapter, intrinsic antibiotic resistance is a major problem at hospitals. Most intrinsically resistant bacterial species have an environmental origin and are only capable of producing infection in people having a previous basal pathology (Alonso et al., 2001). Nevertheless, these microbes are refractory to treatment. Indeed, antibiotic treatment is a risk factor for infections by intrinsically resistant nosocomial pathogens such as those cited previously. For this reason these organisms are important to infections suffered by hospitalized patients (Quinn, 1998).

Reemergence of Established Pathogens in the 21st Century
Edited by Fong and Drlica, Kluwer Academic/Plenum Publishers, New York, 2003

In the case of *Enterobacteriaceae* previously susceptible populations have been replaced by multidrug-resistant populations through the acquisition of antibiotic resistance genotypes. Acquired antibiotic resistance can arise from two different genetic mechanisms. One is mutation (Martinez & Baquero, 2000). To produce an effect on the bacterial cell, the antibiotic needs to traverse different cellular envelopes, in some cases to undergo modification by bacterial enzymes, to avoid the effect of detoxification mechanisms (antibiotic inactivating enzymes and efflux pumps, see below), and ultimately inhibit its target. Mutations that prevent the entry of the antibiotic, modify its target, or activate bacterial detoxification mechanisms may produce an antibiotic resistance phenotype. The other way by which an antibiotic resistance phenotype can be acquired is by the horizontal transfer of antibiotic resistance genes (Davies, 1997). Horizontal gene transfer is so frequent among bacteria that the concept of "common bacterial genome" has been coined to denote the plethora of elements that contibute to gene transfer among bacterial populations.

2. MOLECULAR BASIS OF ANTIBIOTIC RESISTANCE IN *ENTEROBACTERIACEAE*

In this section, we discuss two aspects of the molecular mechanisms that allow the emergence and dissemination of antibiotic resistant *Enterobacteriaceae*. One is the basis for the transfer of antibiotic resistance determinants among different bacteria. The second is the basis for resistance to antibiotics with the greatest impact on clinical practice (quinolone resistance, β-lactam resistance, and multidrug resistance).

2.1. Horizontal Gene Tranfer

Whereas conjugative transposons have a very important role in gene transfer in Gram-positive bacteria, gene transfer in Gram-negative bacteria is mainly due to plasmid transfer (Gomez-Lus, 1998). Antibiotic resistance plasmids are ubiquitously distributed among bacterial populations, contributing to the wide distribution and further evolution of antibiotic resistance genes. Of major concern are the plasmids encoding extended spectrum β-lactamases (ESBLs, see below), aminoglycoside inactivating enzymes (Shaw et al., 1993), or tetracycline resistance genes (Mendez et al., 1980). Almost all ESBLs are encoded by conjugative, multi-resistant plasmids that belong to a limited number of incompatibility groups (Jacoby & Sutton, 1991). The presence of antibiotic resistance genes in these transmissible elements undoubtedly facilitates the interspecies transmission of resistance genes in settings such as Intensive Care Units (ICUs) and other hospital facilities where antibiotic pressure is omnipresent.

Antibiotic resistance plasmids have evolved by sequentially acquiring antibiotic resistance genes (Davies, 1997), and now multidrug resistance plasmids are the rule rather than the exception in *Enterobacteriaceae*. Moreover, transfer of multidrug resistance plasmids is frequent both within the same species and among different bacterial species. In this respect, epidemics of multidrug-resistant organisms can be due to the dissemination of a single virulent clone containing a multidrug-resistant plasmid or to the dissemination of a multidrug-resistance plasmid among different clones of the same species or even among different bacterial species (Martínez-Suárez et al., 1987). A situation has been observed in which the same β-lactamase is present in different plasmids and in different strains of the same species producing an "epidemic outbreak" that is atributable to neither the plasmid nor to a specific bacterial clone but rather to the β-lactamase itself (Coque et al., 2002).

The origin of antibiotic resistance plasmids was revealed in the seminal work in the 1980s of Datta and Hughes. They demonstrated that bacterial isolates from the pre-antibiotic era contained plasmids similar to those isolated recently, both in terms of plasmid number and incomptibility groups. However, the plasmids isolated after antibiotic usage contained antibiotic resistance genes that were absent from those isolated in the pre-antibiotic era (Datta & Hughes, 1983; Hughes & Datta, 1983). These data indicate that antibiotic resistance plasmids have evolved through the acquisisiton of antibiotic resistance genes (from antibiotic producers (Davies, 1997) and from other bacteria (Alonso et al., 2001)) plus further selection by antibiotic pressure. It is widely recognized that antibiotic resistance plasmids can evolve by acquisition of genes directly from the chromosome (F plasmids), by the insertion of transposons, which can subsequently jump to the chromosome when the plasmid enters in a new host and by the insertion of integrons (Hall & Collis, 1995; Rowe-Magnus & Mazel, 1999). A recent 30-year retrospective analysis of IncFI plasmids from multidrug epidemic clones of *Salmonella enterica typhimurium* has shown that IncFI plasmids are evolving through sequential acquisition of integrons carrying various arrays of antibiotic resistance genes (Carattoli et al., 2001).

Integrons turn out to be the primary systems for the capture of antibiotic resistance genes in Gram-negative bacteria (Hall & Collis, 1995; Rowe-Magnus & Mazel, 1999). Integrons (Figure 6.1) are formed by gene cassettes located downstream of a recombinase-encoding conserved sequence that includes a strong promoter. This organization allows the formation of large arrays of gene cassettes that can be transferred as a whole between different replicons (Hall & Collis, 1995; Rowe-Magnus & Mazel, 1999). Integrons contaning antibiotic resistance genes are now known to reside in chromosomes of the

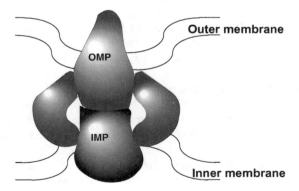

Figure 6.1. Structure of MDR efflux pumps from Gram-negative bacteria. Most multidrug efflux pumps so far characterized in *Enterobacteriaceae* are composed by three proteins. An inner membrane protein (IM), an outer membrane protein (OM), and a peroplasmic protein that helps in the formation of the chanel required for the efflux of the antibiotics coupled to the entrance of protons.

Enterobacteriaceae as well as within multidrug resistance plasmids (Martínez-Freijó et al., 1998; White et al., 2001). For example, many ESBLs, such as VEB-1, GES-1, and IBC-1, are located in class 1 integrons that carry other resistance gene cassettes in addition to the bla_{ESBL} gene (Giakkoupi et al., 2000; Poirel et al., 1999, 2000). These integrons are located on conjugative multi-resistance plasmids and in some cases within transposable elements, which greatly favors the spread of resistance. In fact, it has been recently suggested that the prevalence of integrons in the genomes of *Enterobacteriaceae* is increasing (Schmitz et al., 2001), probably as a result of antibiotic treatment.

The main problem with antibiotic resistance plasmids is their ability to transfer several different antibiotic resistance determinants at once. Thus, treatment with one antibiotic selectively enriches bacteria that are multidrug resistant. This phenomenon casts doubts on the utility of antibiotic cycling and antibiotic restriction as discussed below.

2.2. Mechanisms of Resistance

2.2.1. Quinolone Resistance

Quinolones interact with two related bacterial targets that are essential for bacterial DNA replication, the class II topoisomerases DNA gyrase and topoisomerase IV (Berger et al., 1996; Peng & Marians, 1993). Both enzymes are tetramers, composed of two GyrA and GyrB subunits in the case of gyrase and two ParC and ParE subunits in the case of topoisomerase IV. GyrA is homologous to ParC and GyrB is homologous to ParE.

Fluoroquinolone resistance can be mediated by (1) mutations in encoding for the target enzymes (2) reducing intracellular accumulation due to (a) efflux of the antibiotic which is actively removed from the bacterial cells by energy-dependent efflux pumps (see below) or (b) mutations that affect expression of porins or lipopolysaccharide (Hooper, 1999; Piddock, 1999). Until recently, all quinolone resistance mechanisms described were chromosomally mediated, but now plasmid-mediated resistance, transferable to other *Enterobacteriaceae* has been described in a *Klebsiella pneumoniae* isolate (Martínez-Martínez et al., 1998).

The primary target of fluoroquinolones in Gram-negative bacteria is DNA gyrase, which is more sensitive to quinolones than topoisomerase IV (Drlica & Zhao, 1997; Hooper, 1999; Piddock, 1999). Thus, first step quinolone resistance mutations occur in *gyrA*, the coding gene of GyrA subunit. Mutations in the subunits of topoisomerase IV may generate no significant resistance phenotype except in the presence of mutations in the primary target enzyme (Zhao et al., 1997). The N-termini of both GyrA and ParC exhibit extensive homology, and amino acid substitutions in these segments are associated with quinolone resistance (Nakamura, 1997). They define a so-called quinolone resistance-determining region (QRDR). In *Escherichia coli*, the GyrA QRDR spans amino acids 51 to 106 (Friedman et al., 2001), with hotspot-alterations at serine 83 and aspartate 87 associated with clinical resistance (Piddock, 1999). This association has been observed in other enteric microorganisms (Chu et al., 1998; Nishino et al., 1997; Weigel et al., 1998). Other resistance *loci* have been described, although less frequently than at positions 83 and 87.

The presence of two targets for quinolone interaction within bacterial cells allows stepwise mutations in both enzymes, and the development of high-level fluoroquinolone resistance. Once one or two substitutions within the QRDR of GyrA have accumulated (Conrad et al., 1994; Vila et al., 1994), subsequent substitutions in the QRDR of ParC lead to a further increase in resistance. Among clinical isolates, low level resistance (Ciprofloxacin MIC <2 mg/L) are due to a single *gyrA* mutation (Ser-83-Leu), and high-level resistant isolates (Ciprofloxacin MIC >4 mg/L) often arises from one or two *gyrA* mutations plus a mutation affecting *parC* (Piddock, 1999). In addition, clinical strains often have impaired drug accumulation due to mutations that allow overproduction of the *acrAB* efflux-pump system (Oethinger et al., 2000). A study of *gyrA* mutations associated with fluoroquinolone resistance has been performed in eight species of *Enterobacteriaceae* (Weigel et al., 1998). Among the interesting conclusions are: (1) overall QRDR amino acid sequences are highly conserved among the studied species (2) amino acid changes were conserved in the QRDRs of *Citrobacter freundii*, *Klebsiella oxytoca* and *Enterobacter aerogenes* (Ser-83 to Thr), and *Providencia stuartii* (Val-69 to Ile and Asp-87 to Glu), and (3) substitutions at Gly-81, Ser-83, and/or Asp-87 were found in all clinical strains with Ciprofloxacin MICs higher than 2 mg/L. *E. coli* was the only species that required double mutations in *gyrA* to express high-level fluoroquinolone resistance. Among the other tested species, some isolates that displayed high-level fluoroquinolone resistance with only a GyrA substitution at Ser-83 or Thr-83. Quinolone-resistant clinical isolates of *Serratia marcescens* exhibited the greatest diversity in amino acid substitutions: Gly-81-Cys, Ser-83-Ile or Arg, and Asp-87-Asn without double mutations in any of the isolates.

Molecular analysis of mutations producing antibiotic resistance is an important tool for defining antibiotic/bacteria interactions and further search of novel antibiotic targets. It can also be an important method for rapid detection of antibiotic resistant bacteria based in molecular tools. These methods are increasingly being used for detecting antiviral resistances, and have been recently suggested for detecting rifampin resistance in *Mycobacterium tuberculosis* using DNA extracted directly from sputum (El Hajj et al., 2001).

2.2.2. *Extended Spectrum β-lactamases (ESBLs)*

Resistance to β-lactam antibiotics in Gram-negative bacteria may be due to (1) reduced permeation of the compound into the cell, (2) altered susceptibility of the target penicillin-binding proteins (PBPs), and (3) enzymatic inactivation due to the hydrolytic activity of β-lactamases. Production of β-lactamases is the most significant cause of resistance in Gram-negative bacilli, particularly among *Enterobacteriaceae* (Livermore, 1995). Although the first β-lactamase was described in 1940, 20 years passed until the appearance of TEM-1, the first plasmid-mediated-β-lactamase found in an *E. coli* clinical isolate (Abraham & Chain, 1940; Datta & Kontomichalou, 1965). Since then, an uninterrupted race has taken place between the development of new β-lactam compounds and the appearance of new β-lactamases capable of inactivating the compounds. Many different factors have contributed to this phenomenon: (1) the presence of resistance determinants (*bla* genes) on plasmids or other mobile genetic elements, (2) the plasticity of the enzyme molecule that allows different and co-existing mutations to expand the spectrum of substrates hydrolyzed without loss of the main catalytic features, (3) the clonal spread of bacterial host, and (4) the dissemination of genetic determinants in environments especially prone to resistance development, for example, hospital settings. Due to these characteristics, a scenario for the emergence of "a myriad of novel β-lactamases" that was advanced many years ago (Bush, 1989) came true. At present, more than 150 ESBLs have been described.

Despite differences in their spectrum of activity, ESBLs hydrolyze all β-lactams with the exception of cephamycins and carbapenems. Lower hydrolytic activity is observed with oxacephems (moxalactam) and the so-called fourth generation cephalosporins, cefpirome, and cefepime. Clavulanic-acid, sulbactam, and tazobactam exert, with different affinities, a generalized inhibitory activity towards these enzymes.

β-lactamases have been classified in a variety of ways. The most useful are the Ambler and the Bush classifications (Table 6.1). Ambler's molecular classification comprises four classes, form A to D, and considers the sequence of key unchanged residues despite mutations in other more variable positions. (Ambler, 1980). Bush's functional scheme (Bush et al., 1995) correlates structure and function with molecular classes of β-lactamases. ESBLs can be defined as enzymes that belong to the functional group 2be (Bush's classification) and structural class A (Ambler's classification). ESBLs are mainly derived from plasmid-encoded TEM and SHV β-lactamases. Point mutations in the structural *bla* genes result in the expansion of their hydrolytic spectrum to third- and fourth-generation cephalosporins and monobactams. However, they concomitantly produce an increased susceptibility to older β-lactams and β-lactamase inhibitors, because substitutions

Table 6.1
Functional and Molecular Classification Schemes of β-Lactamases[a]

Functional group	Subgroup	Molecular class	Inhibition by clavulanic-acid	β-lactamase characteristics
1		C	No	Chromosomally or plasmid-mediated cephalosporinases in Gram-negatives. Broad-spectrum of β-lactam resistance, except carbapenems.
2		A, D	Yes/diminished	
	2a	A	Yes	Includes staphylococcal and enterococcal penicinallases.
	2b	A	Yes	Broad spectrum TEM-1, TEM-2 and SHV-1.
	2be	A	Yes	Extended-spectrum β-lactamases (ESBLs), *K. oxytoca* K1. Resistance to oximino β-lactams and monobactams.
	2br	A	No/diminished	Inhibitor-resistance TEM (IRTs) and inhibitor-resistant SHV-derivatives.
	2c	A	Yes	Carbenicillin-hydrolyzing enzymes.
	2d	D	Diminished	Cloxacillin-hydrolyzing enzymes.
	2e	A	Yes	Cephalosporinases from *Proteus vulgaris*, *Bacteroides fragilis* CepA.
	2f	A	Yes	Carbapenem-hydrolyzing enzymes with active site-serine.
3	3a, 3b, 3c	B	No	Metallo-enzymes. Susceptibility to monobactams. Resistance to the rest of β-lactams including carbapenems.
4		Unknown		Miscellaneous group. Heterogeneous and unsequenced enzymes.

[a] Table is adapted from Bush et al. (1995) and Medeiros (1997).

that enlarge the active site cavity of the enzyme allow the introduction of compounds with bulky radicals that simultaneously displace the β-lactam ring from the active-site serine-70 and decrease its catalytic efficiency (Bush, 1997; Knox, 1995; Medeiros, 1997). Nevertheless, only certain residues are able to change without compromising the integrity of the enzyme molecule. Those residues constitute hotspots that are commonly substituted in different enzyme-variants. For example, TEM-ESBLs derive from TEM-1 and TEM-2 with 1 to 5 amino acid substitutions (and their combinations) in a region that accounts less than 2% of the protein sequence. That is enough to dramatically enlarge their β-lactam hydrolytic attributes.

The susceptibility levels of ESBLs-producing bacteria also depend on the amount of enzyme produced. To compensate for weakening the catalytic capacity of the ESBLs, enzyme production needs to be increased to reach clinically relevant resistance levels. This may arise from the presence of more active promoters, such as those found in TEM-2, in many TEM-ESBL derivatives, and in SHV-2a (Sougakoff et al., 1989; Tzouvelekis & Bonomo, 1999). They can be due to the presence of an insertion sequence in the promoter region, as in bla_{TEM-6} which has an insertion of 116 bp related to IS1 in its promoter (Goussard et al., 1991). Enzyme production can also increase from the presence of multiple copies of the *bla* gene in the encoding plasmid. Other mechanisms, such as impaired outer membrane permeability due to the loss of porins and/or the simultaneous presence of other β-lactamases, can also contribute to resistance. In this regard, co-existence of an ESBL with a parent enzyme in the same isolate frequently increases resistance levels among clinical isolates (Bradford et al., 1994; Medeiros, 1997).

A feasible scheme for the stepwise broadening of the spectrum of ESBLs can be summarized by saying that antibiotic pressure favors the selection of substitutions with favorable catalytic properties, even very tiny ones. It has been demonstrated that a variant population, despite extremely small phenotypic differences from the parental type, is selected at a narrow range of antibiotic concentrations (Baquero et al., 1998). Subsequent replacements rendering more complex and efficient enzyme derivatives may be fixed by selective antibiotic concentrations and/or fluctuating antibiotic selective pressure (Blázquez et al., 2000). In fact it has been found that detrimental mutations are compensated by other mutations suppressing the enzyme instability created and/or by mutations strengthening the transcription of the *bla* promoter. The balance between neutral, favorable, and detrimental changes (in the presence of selective antibiotic pressure) may modulate the stability of the enzyme structure and should ultimately be responsible for the establishment or loss of the new variants. The presence of ESBLs in easily spreading clonal isolates and/or in mobile genetic carriers completes the scenario for wide dispersion, particularly in hospitals.

SHV-derived ESBLs have evolved from the SHV-1 enzyme, which seems itself to have derived from a chromosomal β-lactamase of *Klebsiella pneumoniae* (Tzouvelekis & Bonomo, 1999). These variants have spread to many enteric bacilli (*E. coli, K. oxytoca, Enterobacter* spp., *Serratia marcescens, Citrobacter diversus, Proteus mirabilis, Salmonella enterica*), although *K. pneumoniae* still remains the most common bacterial host (Tzouvelekis & Bonomo, 1999). SHV-ESBLs are more efficient than their TEM counterparts in hydrolyzing broad-spectrum β-lactams (Tzouvelekis & Bonomo, 1999). However, fewer changed residues are described if compared with those in TEM derivatives, making the number of SHV-ESBLs fewer than TEM-ESBLs.

CTX-M-ESBLs constitute a group of class A ESBLs having an enhanced ability to hydrolyze cefotaxime. The low ability to hydrolyze ceftazidime has in most cases irrelevant impact on clinical resistance. A remarkable feature of these enzymes is that they are better inhibited by tazobactam than by clavulanic-acid and sulbactam. This group, encoded by transferable plasmids, has been described in many enteric isolates, although they have preferentially been found in *Salmonella typhimurium* and *E. coli*. A controversy has arisen concerning the possible ancestors of these enzymes. A significant degree of homology (over 75%) exists between CTX-Ms and certain chromosomally encoded class A cephalosporinases from *K. oxytoca, C. diversus*, and *P. vulgaris*. However a significant homology has recently been found between this group and the chromosomal AmpC of *Kluyvera ascorbata* (Bradford, 2001). The epidemiology of these enzymes is rather peculiar. They are almost all isolated from localized outbreaks in South America (Argentina, Brazil), Japan, and Eastern Europe mainly involving *Salmonella typhimurium* isolates expressing different CTX-M types (Bradford, 2001). Another focus has been recently reported in Spain comprising *E. coli* and *Salmonella virchow* isolates harboring CTX-M-9. Another variant, CTX-M-10 has also been recently described in Spain in a clinical *E. coli* isolate (Oliver et al., 2001).

Although most ESBLs are TEM or SHV derivatives, there are many ESBLs that comprise a heterogeneous group that, although belonging to class A, are unrelated to TEM, SHV or other well categorized family of enzymes (Table 6.2). Most have been recently isolated from quite dispersed geographical areas and do not share significant common features. These novel ESBLs could still be in an early phase of dissemination and evolution like that already observed for TEM and SHV β-lactamases. An increasing number in the types of β-lactamases is potentially dangerous.

Three other groups of β-lactamases, although not comprising ESBLs *sensu stricto* are briefly mentioned below.

2.2.2a. Inhibitor-Resistant TEM-β-Lactamases (IRTs).   It was initially thought that the main mechanisms of resistance to combinations of β-lactams/β-lactamase inhibitors was

Table 6.2
Characteristics of Novel, Unrelated ESBLs[a]

Enzyme (pI)	Species	Preferred substrate
PER-1 (5.4)	*S. typhimurium*	Ceftazidime
PER-2 (5.4)	*S. typhimurium*	Ceftazidime
FEC-1 (8.2)	*E. coli*	Cefotaxime
SFO-1 (7.3)	*E. cloacae*	Cefotaxime
VEB-1 (5.35)	*E. coli*	Ceftazidime, aztreonam
GES-1 (5.8)	*K. pneumoniae*	Ceftazidime
TLA-1 (9.0)	*E. coli*	Cefotaxime, ceftazidime, aztreonam
BES-1 (7.5)	*S. marcescens*	Cefotaxime, ceftazidime, aztreonam
IBC-1 (6.9)[b]	*E. cloacae*	Cefotaxime, ceftazidime, aztreonam

[a] Data from Bradford (2001).
[b] Giakkoupi et al. (2000).

overproduction of TEM-1 β-lactamase (Martínez et al., 1987; Reguera et al., 1991) encoded by multi-copy plasmids (Martínez et al., 1989). However, IRTs rapidly emerged in bacterial populations. These enzymes have been found in many enterobacterial genera such as *E. coli, K. pneumoniae, K. oxytoca, Proteus mirabilis*, and *C. freundii*. They confer resistance to the combinations of clavulanic-acid/β-lactams and sulbactam/β-lactams. Significantly, they retain a considerable degree of susceptibility to tazobactam and to piperacillin–tazobactam. IRTs do not hydrolyze broad-spectrum β-lactams. Only four mutations in the *bla* structural gene lead to the inhibitor-resistant phenotype. Other, less frequent mutations have also been described in these derivatives in which more than one amino acid substitution can be found (Bradford, 2001; Bush, 1999). SHV-10, the first naturally occurring inhibitor-resistant SHV variant described, was found in a clinical *E. coli* isolate that was probably selected by amoxicillin–clavulanate treatment. Three amino acid substitutions are present in this enzyme: Gly238→Ser, Glu240→Lys, and Ser130→Gly. Despite the presence of the combination Gly238/Glu240 substitution, SHV-10 does not display an extended-spectrum of hydrolysis. Apparently it is suppressed by the dominant effect of the substitution at position 130 (Gly for Ser) (Prinarakis, 1997; Tzouvelekis & Bonomo, 1999).

The co-existence of ESBLs and IRT mutations in the same enzyme variant, like those found in TEM-50 and TEM-68, may be of concern as it strongly reduces therapeutic options due to the complexity of the resulting resistance phenotype (Bradford, 2001). A new ESBL, named SHV-26, was found in a clinical isolate of *K. pneumoniae* with reduced susceptibility to clavulanate. It could be the first among the SHV enzymes to combine a mutation responsible for a broad hydrolytic spectrum with one that reduces susceptibility to a β-lactamase inhibitor (Chang et al., 2001).

2.2.2b. Plasmid-Mediated AmpC β-Lactamases. The presence of an *ampC* gene on a plasmid was first reported in 1988 with the description of the MIR-1 enzyme (Papanicolau et al., 1990). Subsequently, many plasmid-encoded AmpC β-lactamases have been found among the *Enterobacteriaceae* (Philippon et al., 2002). Substrate and inhibition patterns of these enzymes resemble their chromosomal counterparts. Certain species such as *K. pneumoniae*, which produce low levels of chromosomal β-lactamase, and *Salmonella*, which does not produce it at all, are among the bacterial hosts of these enzymes (Bush, 1999). In addition, the AmpC-type DHA-1 found in a *Salmonella enteritidis* isolate is inducible by virtue of the simultaneous presence of *ampR* in the encoding plasmid (Barnaud et al., 1998). Most of these enzymes evolved into two groups. One group clusters around CMY-2. The corresponding enzymes are very similar and show a close relationship to the chromosomal AmpC β-lactamase of *C. freundii*. The other group centers around CMY-1. This group is heterogeneous and is not so closely related to chromosomal AmpC cephalosporinases.

2.2.2c. Carbapenem-Hydrolyzing Enzymes (Carbapenemases). Until the appearance of class A carbapenemases, imipenem and other carbapenems escaped the hydrolyzing activity of the most serine β-lactamases. At present four enzymes of this type have been described, NMC-A and IMI-1 from *E. cloacae*, Sme-1 from *S. marcescens*, and KPC-1 from *K. pneumoniae* (Livermore, 1995; Yigit et al., 2001). NMC-A, IMI-1, and Sme are chromosomally encoded and are resistant to the inhibition by clavulanic acid, whereas

KPC-1 is plasmid-mediated and susceptible to the inhibition by clavulanic-acid. Despite the low prevalence of this group of enzymes they must not be ignored because they have emerged in different geographical areas and they have appeared in multiple isolates at the same hospital (Bush, 1999). A plasmid-mediated class B metallo-β-lactamase, IMP-1 was initially found in *S. marcescens* and *P. aeruginosa* clinical isolates from Japan (Osano et al., 1994). The same or very similar alleles were subsequently identified in *K. pneumoniae* and *C. freundii* isolates among others. In all cases, the bla_{IMP-1} gene has been plasmid-transferred. IMP-1 has a notable extended-spectrum of β-lactam hydrolysis, with the exception of aztreonam. It is poorly inhibited by available inhibitors. Apart from its plasmid codification, this enzyme is located on a mobile gene cassette inserted into a class 1 integron (Laraki et al., 1999).

Amino acid sequences of TEM, SHV, and OXA derived ESBLs and IRTs can be found at the web site www.lahey.org/studies/webt.htm

2.3. Multidrug Efflux Pumps

As previously stated, some bacteria are intrinsically resistant to certain antibiotic families. This intrinsic resistance is due to an interplay between the impermeability of the cellular envelopes and the activity of pumps that extrude a wide range of compounds, including antibiotics. In fact, even for bacteria considered as susceptible, elimination of efflux pumps makes them more susceptible to antibiotics. Most multidrug (MDR) efflux pumps analyzed in Gram-negative bacteria (Nikaido, 1998; Poole, 2000) are composed of three elements: an inner membrane protein, an outer membrane protein, and a membrane fusion protein located in the periplasm that facilitates the interaction between the two channels (Figure 6.2). Less well studied are efflux pumps belonging to the ABC family of drug transporters which are similar to those present in Gram-positive bacteria and mammals. An example of this pump type is MacAB (Kobayashi et al., 2001), which is involved in intrinsic resistance to macrolides in *E. coli*.

The expression of MDR pumps is exquisitely downregulated, but mutants capable of overexpressing them are readily selected by antibiotic pressure both in vitro and in vivo

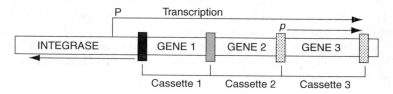

Figure 6.2. Structure of an integron. Integrons are genetic elements, elements that mediate the acquisition and spread of genes in bacterial populations through recombination. Integrons are formed by a integrase gene, an adjacent recombination site (black box), followed by several cassettes, each one including one gene and one 59 bp. element (dotted boxes) that favors recombination. Transcription of the genes arrangement is controlled by a strong promoter (P) located within the integrase gene. In some cases, the gene cassettes also have specific promoters (*p*). This structure favors the formation of large arrays of genes (sometimes more than one hundred) which are transferred as single elements among bacterial populations.

(Nikaido, 1998; Poole, 2000). Those mutants have an increased resistance to antibiotics belonging to several different structural families. Thus, treatment with one antibiotic might select mutants that resist not only the selecting agent but also unselected antibiotics. Some MDR pumps can also accomodate antiseptics and detergents. Consequently, routine cleaning procedures might eventually select MDR mutants in bacterial populations (Moken et al., 1997).

The increase in MICs of MDR mutants is frequently tiny. Thus these bacteria may not be classified as antibiotic resistant mutants accordingly to NCCLS rules. However, overexpression of MDR pumps is needed, at least in some cases, to reach a full antibiotic resistant phenotype, usually in association with other mechanisms of resistance. An example of this is the association of mutations in topoisomerases and overproduction of the MDR pump *acrAB* that is frequently encountered in quinolone resistant clinical isolates of *E. coli* (Mazzariol et al., 2000). Another is the finding that antibiotic efflux (mainly of quinolones) is frequent among clinical isolates of *Enterobacteriaceae* (Berlanga et al., 2000; Everett et al., 1996; Giraud et al., 2000; Ishii et al., 1991). It is important to emphasize that MDR pumps have been found in all microorganisms so far analyzed (Saier et al., 1998). In fact, *E. coli* contains several MDR pumps in its genome (Sulavik et al., 2001), with *acrAB-tolC* (Okusu et al., 1996) being the most relevant one. Biochemical and genetic analyses support the idea that MDR pumps are present in the genomes of all *Enterobacteriaceae* species.

3. EPIDEMIOLOGY AND EXTENSION OF THE PROBLEM

Despite geographical variations, an increase in the frequency of use of antimicrobials have been observed in most countries (Guillemot, 1999). Overuse, and the misuse of antimicrobials, has been considered responsible for the escalation of antimicrobial resistance (Gaynes & Monnet, 1997). Several surveillance programs have demonstrated an increase of resistance among *Enterobacteriaceae* and the importance of antibiotic-resistant *Enterobacteriaceae* isolates for both hospital and community-acquired infections (Fridkin et al., 1999; Gaynes & Monnet, 1997). Of particular concern is the increased prevalence of resistant *Enterobacteriaceae* isolates in ICUs, since patients infected with these organisms have a poor prognosis (Fridkin & Gaynes, 1999; Kollef, 2001). In a recent multicenter study performed in ICUs from 118 European hospitals, the *Enterobacteriaceae* represented nearly 60% of all isolates associated with nosocomial infections, and they were frequently resistant to third-generation cephalosporins. Moreover, these isolates were frequently resistant to aminoglycosides and fluoroquinolones (Hanberger et al., 1999). These trends have also been observed in the United States during the last decade (Fridkin & Gaynes, 1999). *E. coli, Enterobacter* spp., and *K. pneumoniae* isolates are among the eight most common pathogens associated with nosocomial infections in ICU patients, and they represent 20% of all isolates. These organisms are usually resistant to antimicrobials commonly used to treat infections. The National Nosocomial Infections Surveillance System (NNIS) demonstrated that at least 3% of *E. coli*, 10% of *K. pneumoniae*, and 35% of *Enterobacter* spp. isolates recovered from patients at ICUs were resistant to third generation cephalosporins. These figures are clearly higher than those obtained when all isolates recovered from nosocomial infections were analyzed (NNIS, 1999).

3.1. Extended-Spectrum β-Lactamase Producing Isolates

A recent review of β-lactam resistance phenotypes among different species of *Enterobacteriaceae* recovered from different geographic areas of the world showed important variations of ESBL phenotypes depending on location (Winokour et al., 2001). *K. pneumoniae* had the highest prevalence of isolates expressing this phenotype, being greatest in Latin America (45.5%), followed by the Western Pacific region (24.6%), Europe (22.6%), the United States (7.6%), and Canada (4.9%). A careful review of previous studies shows an increased trend of ceftazidime resistance in *K. pneumoniae* isolates, particularly those performed in the ICU setting (Hanberger et al., 2001). In some studies from European countries, ceftazidime resistance rose to nearly 35% (Livermore & Yuan, 1996). This prevalence is even much higher in certain areas, such as Turkey, where ceftazidime and other third generation cephalosporin resistance increased to 75% in *K. pneumoniae* ICU isolates (Aksaray et al., 2000). In the United States, resistance to ceftazidime also increased during the 1990s; however, the percentage of these isolates is much lower than that obtained in Turkey.

The clinical relevance of ESBL-producing *K. pneumoniae* isolates has been clearly demonstrated (Bush, 2001). Although identical resistance genes have been found in different isolates and plasmid dissemination has been documented (Arlet et al., 1994; Asensio et al., 2000; Essack et al., 2001; Gniadkowski et al., 1998a, 1998b; Wiener et al., 1999), the spread of an epidemic strain remains the most commonly reported mechanism of ESBL dissemination (Yuan et al., 1998). Most outbreaks are limited to high-risk patient-care areas (Asensio et al., 2000; Philippon et al., 1994), but they have also involved outpatients such as those from nursing homes (Wiener et al., 1999). The spread of ESBL-producing *K. pneumoniae* strains from one hospital to another has been demonstrated (Arlet et al., 1994; Bradford et al., 1994; Fiett et al., 2000; Gniadkowski et al., 1998a, 1998b; Philippon et al., 1994). Less common is dissemination between countries (Philippon et al., 1994; Shannon et al., 1998).

ESBL outbreaks usually involve a large number of hospitalized patients, which make these situations difficult to resolve unless third-generation cephalosporin restriction and barrier precautions are implemented (Meyer et al., 1993). Despite this fact and the suspicion that the increase of ESBL-producing *K. pneumoniae* isolates could be due to the spread of particular clones, recent work revealed a high heterogeneity of clonal types associated with ESBL production (Coque et al., 2002; Essack et al., 2001). These observations revealed the importance of horizontal transmission of ESBL genetic determinants, probably accelerated by the inclusion of these elements on integrons and transposable elements in addition to plasmid structures. Despite these findings, we cannot exclude the idea that the concurrent detection of different ESBL variants in multiple geographic locations may also result from convergent gene evolution of widely spread, broad-spectrum non-ESBL enzymes. Moreover, the evolution of the resistant determinants due to the accumulation of point mutations has been demonstrated, which advances the understanding of the co-emergence of ESBL-producing isolates. This possibility has been discussed with SHV-type ESBL (Chang et al., 2001), but it can also be applied to TEM-type ESBL enzymes.

The rapid dissemination of ESBL-producing organisms may be facilitated by the fact that these organisms are also resistant to non-β-lactam antibiotics, including aminoglycosides, tetracyclines, chloramphenicol, trimethoprim, and sulphonamides (Fernández-Rodríguez et al., 1992; Jacoby & Sutton, 1991; Nordmann, 1998; Philippon et al., 1994; Yuan et al., 1998). This multi-resistance phenotype is generally plasmid-encoded and thus co-transferred with the third-generation cephalosporin resistance. Moreover, fluoroquinolone resistance has also increased among ESBL-producing strains (Paterson et al., 2000; Winokour et al., 2001). Since quinolone resistance is not plasmid-encoded (see above), a genetic linkage between ESBLs and quinolone resistance does not exist, although an epidemiological linkage does.

ESBL-producing *E. coli* is an emerging problem, although in general it appears at a lower frequency than ESBL-producing *K. pneumoniae* (Winokour et al., 2001). However, in some European countries, such as Spain, a rapid spread of certain CTX-M enzymes (Coque et al., 2001) have increased its prevalence. This family emerged in South America and Europe in 1989 at nearly the same time (Tzouvelekis et al., 2000), and its dissemination might be accelerated since they are encoded in transposable elements (Oliver, personal communication). An interesting feature of this group of enzymes is their close relationship with chromosomal β-lactamases found in environmental bacteria such as *Kluyvera ascorbata* and *Kluyvera criocrescens* (Oliver et al., 2000).

A dangerous possibility is that the prevalence of ESBL-producing bacteria may be underestimated mainly due to the utilization of breakpoints that are too high and inaccurate susceptibility testing methods (Thomson, 2001). Moreover, ESBL genes can be harbored in AmpC β-lactamase-producing *Enterobacteriaceae* and *P. aeruginosa*, which makes it difficult to detect ESBLs by routine susceptibility testing methods (Cantón et al., 2001). In fact, outbreaks due to AmpC β-lactamase-producing isolates (mainly *Enterobacter aerogenes*) harboring ESBL enzymes have been described (De Gheldre et al., 2001; Galdbart et al., 2000). In addition, many clinical laboratories, as well as the wider medical community, are not fully aware of the importance of ESBL-producing organisms (Bush, 2001; Thomson, 2001). This situation may facilitate the dissemination of ESBLs, since awareness is needed to set up barrier precautions and adequate antibiotic policies.

3.1.1. AmpC Hyperproducing Enterobacter

High-level AmpC-related resistance has recently become predominat, particularly in ICU settings (Fridkin & Gaynes, 1999). Third-generation cephalosporins-resistant *E. cloacae, E. aerogenes, C. freundii, M. morganii*, and *S. marcesecens* are commonly involved in nosocomial infections. In a recent report, 36% of *Enterobacter* spp. isolates from ICU infections were resistant to broad-spectrum cephalosporins (NNIS report, 1999). The emergence of this resistance correlates with exposure to these antimicrobials (Kaye et al., 2001). Approximately 20% of patients under prescription with broad-spectrum cephalosporins develop resistance. This percentage is significantly higher among patients with bacteriemia than among patients with wound, tissue, or urine infections.

E. cloacae is the most frequently reported *Enterobacter* species recovered from nosocomial infections. However, in certain geographic areas, *E. aerogenes* has recently emerged. This situation is favoured by the production of an ESBL (TEM-24) in addition to the inducible AmpC β-lactamase (De Gheldre et al., 2001; Galdbart et al., 2000). The prevalence of ceftazidime and cefotaxime resistance in *E. cloacae* has reached 70% in Turkey and 50% countries like Portugal and Russia (Hanberger et al., 2001). In the United States, this resistance is slightly lower (nearly 35%) (Fridkin et al., 1999), but it is currently increasing (Hanberger et al., 2001). Despite these alarmingly high resistance values, implementing antibiotic intervention policies and barrier precautions can still reduce these trends (Struelens et al., 1999). Reduction may be due to the cessation of the emergence of AmpC hyperproducing clones from AmpC inducible clones, perhaps because AmpC hyperproduction results in higher biological cost (Morosini et al., 2000). Unfortunately, non-β-lactam resistance is increasing among Ceftazidime-resistant *E. cloacae* isolates (Fluit et al., 2001), which may facilitate co-selection processes.

3.1.2. Carbapenem Resistance

Carbapenemases have been detected rarely in *Enterobacteriaceae*. Nevertheless, they have been recognized in Group 1 β-lactamase-producing isolates (Table 6.1), mainly in *E. cloacae* and *S. marcescens*, and to a lesser extent in *C. freundii*. They have also been recognized in *K. pneumoniae*. Although these enzymes are thought not to be widely distributed among *Enterobacteriaceae* isolates, some geographic areas, such as Japan, seem to be hot spots for carbapenemase-producing isolates (Livermore & Woodford, 2000). As previously stated, the genes encoding them are located in transferable elements, including plasmids and transposons (Ito et al., 1995; Yigit et al., 2001). That is expected to accelerate their transmission under carbapenem selective pressure. They have also been linked to integron structures (Bennet, 1999), which can stabilize their presence in bacterial populations. Despite these observations, the most prevalent carbapenem resistance mechanisms among *Enterobacteriaceae* are those associated with decreased outer-membrane permeability and hyperproduction of Group 1 (Cornaglia et al., 1995) or plasmid-mediated AmpC (Bradford et al., 1997) β-lactamases. The former has been described in *E. cloacae* whereas the latter in *K. pneumoniae*. It is important to note that in both cases, isolates were resistant to carbapenems and also to third-generation cephalosporins.

Recent analyses of resistance trends have shown that carbapenem resistance in *Enterobacteriacae* is much lower than that observed in *P. aeruginosa*. Imipenem resistance in *Enterobacter* spp. from ICU studies is normally below 5% (Hanberger et al., 2001). The corresponding figure for *K. pneumoniae* is lower than 3%, and it is very unusual in *E. coli*. However, some multicenter studies from Turkey (Aksaray et al., 2000) demonstrated imipenem resistance in more that 5% of *K. pneumoniae* and more than 10% in *Enterobacter* spp. isolates.

3.2. Quinolone Resistance and Multi-Resistance in *Enterobacteriaceae*

Fluorinated quinolones are particularly active against enteric bacteria. However, widespread use of these antibiotics has resulted in an increasing incidence of resistance among *Enterobacteriaceae*. The concomitant use of certain members of this class in veterinary medicine has played a significant role in selecting resistance strains that could pass to the food chain and thereby to create a serious public health problem (Everett et al., 1996). Although the ICARE surveillance program failed to show high resistance to ciprofloxacin in *E. coli* isolates (1.4% in ICU isolates) (NNIS, 1999), other programs such as the SENTRY Antimicrobial Surveillance Program showed higher resistance values. For example, in Europe, 9.5% of the *E. coli* isolates during 1997 and 1998 were resistant to ciprofloxacin. This value increased to 11% during 1999, mainly due to the situation in Southern European ICUs (Hanberger et al., 2001). An alarmingly high (19%) ciprofloxacin resistance in *E. coli* was seen in ICUs in Turkey (Aksaray et al., 2000). The ciprofloxacin resistance prevalence was lower in *K. pneumoniae* (7%) during 1997 and 1998, but it also dramatically increased during 1999 (24%). In *Enterobacter* spp. the situation was similar, as 20% of these isolates were resistant to fluoroquinolones. Single-step mutation to low level resistance to fluoroquinolones occurs at a frequency of $\leq 10^{-10}$ for many bacterial species at drug concentrations up to ten times the MIC (Hooper, 1999). The relevance of this resistance would not be, at first sight, of clinical importance for susceptible organisms but higher resistance levels can be readily selected by serial exposure of these isolates to increasing drug concentrations (Hooper, 2000). High-level resistance may be also shared with structurally unrelated compounds due to overexpression of efflux pumps (see above). Two main aspects related to resistance in clinical setting deserve consideration: emergence of resistant mutants during antibiotic treatment and superinfection by previously selected antibiotic resistant mutants. Emergence of resistance has been particularly observed in *P. aeruginosa*. This bacterial species is more likely than others to develop quinolone resistance because it has a high mutation rate and a low therapeutic ratio of the antibiotic is common in many systemic infections (Le Thomas et al., 2001). Emergence of resistance in other bacterial species, including enteric microorganisms during or after fluoroquinolone prescription, has been reported (Garau et al., 1999; Truong et al., 1995). Quinolone-resistant *E. coli* strains have been isolated from outpatients with urinary tract infections, from neutropenic patients after prophylaxis or in the community as the consequence of fecal contamination (Van Kraaij, 1998; Wagenlehner, 2000). Superinfection, although infrequent, is more likely to occur in those genera where quinolone activity is suboptimal due to intrinsic microbial features like *P. aeruginosa*, other Gram-negative bacilli, *Streptococcus* spp., *Enterococcus* spp., and yeasts, among others (Zervos et al., 1988).

Development of resistance and emergence of quinolone resistant mutants are expected to depend markedly on the dual target recognition of these drugs. The frequency at which resistance would develop should be lower if concentrations could be obtained at which both targets were inhibited (a double mutation will be required for resistance). The C-8 methoxy fluoroquinolones show promise in this regard (Lu et al., 1999; Zhao et al., 1997).

As stated above, of particular concern is the fact that a high percent of ciprofloxacin resistant *Enterobacteriaceae* are also resistant to third-generation cephalosporins (Fluit et al., 2001). During 1997 and 1998, nearly 50% and 70% of ciprofloxacin-resistant *Enterobacter* spp. and *K. pneumoniae* isolates, respectively, were also resistant to ceftazidime. This association is particularly noticeable with ESBL producing isolates: one third of ESBL-producing *K. pneumoniae* recovered in the United States were resistant to ciprofloxacin. This value was even higher in the Western Pacific area, reaching 44% (Winokour et al., 2001). A similar situation has been detected in *E. coli* and *P. mirabilis* harboring ESBLs. Moreover, resistance to other antimicrobials in ESBL producing strains was also high (Figure 6.3), a situation that can facilitate the spread of these isolates. Cross-resistance in *E. cloacae* is also high for other antibiotics. For example, nearly 30% of ceftazidime-resistant isolates are also resistant to gentamicin (Fluit et al., 2001). Aminoglycoside resistance due to

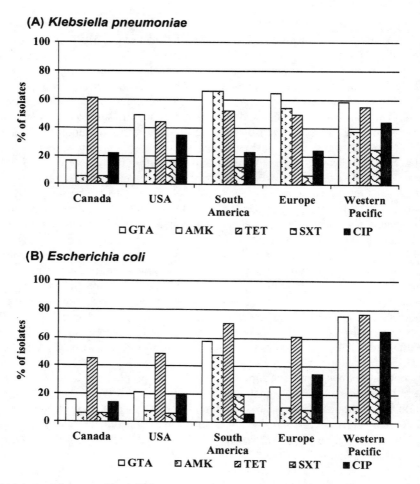

Figure 6.3. Co-resistance in *K. pneumoniae* (A) and *E. coli* (B) isolates from SENTRY Antimicrobial Surveillance Programm (1998) from different geographic areas that expressed an ESBL clinical phenotype (data from Winokour, 2001). GTA: gentamycin; AMK: amikacin; TET: tetracycline; SXT: trimethoprim-sulfamethoxazole; CIP: ciprofloxacin. A high prevalence of resistance to different antibiotics not belonging to the β-lactam family was found among ESBL producing *K. pneumoniae* and *E. coli* isolates in all cases, although some difference in prevalence were observed among different countries. These resistances may facilitate ESBL producing isolates to disseminate (clonal dissemination). With the exception of quinolone resistance, the other resistance genes are normally encoded in the same plasmid that harbored the ESBL gene which also facilitate the spread of plasmids harboring ESBL (plasmid dissemination).

the production of the aminoglycoside modifying enzyme AAC(6′)-I is also higher in *E. aerogenes* isolates, particularly in those strains producing TEM-24 ESBL (Galdbart et al., 2000).

The increase of *Enterobacteriacae* with cross-resistance to aminoglycoside and other antimicrobials, including ceftazidime, cotrimoxazole, and ciprofloxacin, has been recognized in ICUs. In a recent study, the incidence of ciprofloxacin-resistant *E. cloacae* and *E. coli* isolates increased in a hematology unit in the Netherlands from <0.5% to 20.7%

and <0.5% to 64%, respectively, from 1996 to 1999. In addition, clonal spread of single genotypes was documented (Van Belkum et al., 2001).

4. INTENSIVE CARE UNITS AS THE EPICENTER OF THE PROBLEM

Current health care trends underscore the importance of bacterial resistance in noso-comial infections in the ICUs (Fridkin & Gaynes 1999; Fridkin et al., 1999; Kollef, 2001). Patients who received care in ICUs are at increased risk for nosocomial infections, and treatment of these infections has become difficult, if not impossible, due to the emergence of antimicrobial resistance in pathogens (Kollef, 2001). Some of the clearest data relating antibiotic use and resistance have come from studies of ICU populations. Reports com-paring antimicrobial/organism combinations noted significantly higher resistance rates in ICU patients than in other hospital or out-patient groups (Archival et al., 1997). Data from the Intensive Care Antimicrobial Resistance Epidemiology (ICARE) Project in the United States showed that for each of the antimicrobial groups used at higher rates in ICU areas there was a corresponding higher prevalence of the respective resistant pathogen among ICU patients compared with non-ICU in-patients (Fridkin et al., 1999). This trend was clearly observed with Gram-negative organisms, including *Enterobacteriaceae* isolates.

Although the increasing incidence of resistance in ICU has been clearly stated, as is the relationship between antimicrobial use and the rise in nosocomial infections (Swartz, 1994), the association of these resistant organisms with increased mortality has not been so clearly documented. However, several investigations have demonstrated a strong asso-ciation between inadequate antibiotic treatment and in-hospital mortality of patients with ICU nosocomial infection (Kollef & Fraser, 2001). A recently reported 5-year analysis in a single institution demonstrated the relationship between antimicrobial consumption and low susceptibility for nosocomial pathogens (White et al., 2000). This observation was sig-nificantly pronounced in the ICUs but significant relationship was often not apparent when the entire hospital was considered.

It is clear that the antimicrobial use in the ICU environment is higher than in the com-munity or other hospitalization areas, which easily facilitates the selection of resistant bac-teria. In addition, there is a tendency to employ homogeneous antibiotic prescribing with a limited number of antibiotic classes in the ICU setting. Levy (1997) has defined the con-cept of "selection density," which when applied to ICUs may explain the emergence of resistant bacteria in these units. The selection density is the total amount of antibiotic used per individual per geographic area. This value is higher in the ICUs than other hospital-ization areas facilitating the selection of resistant bacteria. Moreover, cross-transmission of antimicrobial-resistant pathogens is facilitated by the special architectural characteris-tics of these units, the nature of critical care, and the commonly compromised situation of patient host defenses (Fridkin & Gaynes, 1999). In this scenario, patients become rapidly colonized by resistant bacteria and easily develop infections by these organisms. Therefore, the ICUs serve as incubators of resistant pathogens.

The objective of antibiotic treatment in humans is to exert a deleterious action against bacterial pathogens. However, when these drugs are administered to a given patient, there is also an antibacterial effect exerted on the "normal bacterial flora" that often contributes to patient colonization by resistant bacteria (Hooker & Di Piro, 1988). We have to recall here that several infections in ICUs are due to bacteria such as *E. coli* that belong to the "normal bacterial flora" of healthy individuals. In this respect, selection of antibiotic resistance in the normal bacterial flora could have a major impact on the development of antibiotic resistance among enterobacterial isolates involved in infections in ICUs. Moreover, selective decontamination processes used in ICUs to reduce bacterial flora might select antibiotic-resistant bacteria, in some cases due to overexpression of multidrug efflux pumps. In fact, it has been shown that these decontamination procedures promote patient colonization with resistant bacteria, mainly with enteric Gram-negative organisms (Bonten & Weistein, 1996).

5. FUTURE DIRECTIONS

The correct treatment of infections to avoid the emergence and further spread of antibiotic-resistant microorganisms requires appropriate treatment strategies and the use of novel compounds for bacteria that are already antibiotic resistant. Hygiene, prophylaxis, good management of infection, and the establishment of adequate surveillance networks on a global scale are required to avoid, as much as possible the replacement of susceptible populations by multidrug-resistant bacteria.

5.1. Prevention

Obviously, the best strategy for the treatment of an infection is to avoid the infection itself. Hygiene and prophylaxis are the best ways for avoiding the spread of epidemic clones of pathogenic bacteria. Vaccination has been very useful for preventing or even eradicating infections. For the moment, however, vaccination has not helped in the prevention of *Enterobacteriaceae* infections. The different approaches for obtaining *Enterobacteriacea* vaccines (Levine & Noriega, 1995) include intact, dead cells, living attenuated vaccines (Hoiseth & Stocker, 1981), polysaccharide (Conlan et al., 2000), virulence determinants (Mason et al., 1998), or even DNA vaccines (Alves et al., 2000). Some of these approaches are under development; thus the possibility for obtaining a useful *Enterobacteriaceae* vaccine is still open.

In the case of the hospital environment, careful protocols must be implemented to avoid not only infection but cross-contamination between patients or between patients and hospital workers who are carriers of pathogens. Hospitals are overcrowded habitats in which people are already sick and thus more susceptible to infection, even by non-professional pathogens (opportunistic pathogens). Hospitals are also "antibiotic-rich" environments. Thus, hospitals are optimal ecosystems for the evolution (by mutation and acquisition of antibiotic resistance determinants) and rapid dissemination of pathogenic bacteria. Prevention must then include protocols for avoiding and detecting bacterial contamination, for the early detection of infection, for the isolation of potential epidemic *foci* before an epidemic outbreak occurs, and for the surveillance of epidemic clones (or eventually multidrug resistance plasmids) in the in-hospital bacterial populations. Prevention must also include the best strategies for antibiotic treatment to reduce as much as possible the selection of antibiotic resistant *Enterobacteriaceae*, that can replace susceptible populations and afterwards disseminate in the environment.

Approaches to minimize the emergence of antibiotic resistance should thus be directed to the implementation of straight epidemiological surveillance for prompt detection of community- and nosocomial-resistant strains; the use of adequate dosing regimens (appropriate therapeutic index) against well-known susceptible strains; use of combination drug therapy (minimizing the emergence of resistant mutants for each compound) cycling with other structurally unrelated agents, and use of new antibiotics with chemical and pharmacokinetically improved properties.

5.2. Management

Management of infections requires effective protocols for the treatment of each individual patient. These protocols must incorporate the pharmacological and pharmacokinetic properties of the antibiotics. If drug concentration at the site of infection exceeds the MIC of first-step resistance mutants of the pathogen, no selection of these mutants will occur (favorable therapeutic index). A concept that deserves to be mentioned here is the mutant prevention concentration (MPC, antibiotic concentration that blocks the growth of mutants) because, when determined for a given pair antimicrobial drug-pathogen, it could help to define a dosing regimen that would require the cells to develop at least two concurrent resistant mutations for growth (Zhao & Drlica, 2001). When serum drug concentration exceeds the MPC threshold, restriction or even prevention of selection of resistant mutants would be likely. In contrast, the growth and persistence of first-step mutants is favored by the use of inadequately low doses of the drug (normally used to clear infections) or by deficient delivery of the compound to the site of infection. Such doses contribute to subsequent step-wise development of mutants due to repetitive exposure to the drug, eventually giving rise to high-level resistant variants (Zhao & Drlica, 2001; Zhou et al., 2000).

The management of the infected patient must take in account not only the treatment required for suppresion of the disease, but also the effect that this treatment might have for the community. Infection is a worldwide health problem, since an antibiotic resistant clone selected in one patient as the consequence of an inappropriate treatment regime can be transferred to new patients. In this respect, a global strategy for the management of infections must be implemented in order to reduce the problem of antibiotic resistance among bacterial populations. Many surveillance programs (Verhoef et al., 1999), like SENTRY, WHONET, ENARE, ... have been implemented to improve the guidelines for empiric treatment in the community in hospitals. It is hoped that this will reduce the emergence of antibiotic resistant bacteria in hospital, slow the spread, and provide fast information on local and worldwide changes in resistance patterns in order to improve the guidelines for antibiotic treatment. To that goal, data must be collected and distributed among clinicians at all levels, from hospitals to worldwide networks. Also the implementation of accurate policies of antibiotic usage are required for reducing the emergence and dissemination of antibiotic resistant *Enterobacteriaceae*.

5.2.1. Antibiotic Policies

A close association between a history of antimicrobial use and the emergence of antimicrobial resistance both in Gram-positive and Gram-negative bacteria has been demonstrated. Likewise, improvements in susceptibility recovery have been observed when antibiotic use is controlled, and improvement in antibiotic use decreases or delays the emergence and spread of resistance (Monroe & Polk, 2000), particularly in hospital practice (Gould, 1999; Kollef, 2001; Shlaes et al., 1997). It seems that some changes on the antimicrobial politics might lead to a decrease in the infections due to Gram-negative bacteria (De Man et al., 2000; Gerding et al., 1991; Giamarellou & Antoniadou, 1997; Gruson et al., 2000; Kollef et al., 1997, 2000; Mebis et al., 1998; Rahal et al., 1998; Rice et al., 1996; Saez-Llorens et al., 2000; Urban et al., 2000; Van der Zwet et al., 1999). In contrast, other experiences have demonstrated no substantial changes in antibiotic susceptibility profiles over time (Domíngez et al., 2000) or even an increase in the recovery of multi-resistant organisms (Rahal et al., 1998). These different effects may be related to the strategy used (see below) and the environment where these antibiotic policies were implemented.

Several recent studies have shown the benefit of applying antibiotic use strategies for reducing bacterial resistance and infections in hospital settings, particularly in ICUs. Due to rapid dissemination of resistant bacteria and/or resistance determinants, these strategies should also be implemented in the community (John & Rice, 2000; Osterbland et al., 2000). In that sense, it has been well demonstrated that patients in long-term care units are commonly colonized by multi-resistant organisms, including *Enterobacteriaceae* (Wiener et al., 1999). These patients represent a major route for the introduction or reintroduction of resistant bacteria to the intensive-care environment (Nicolle, 2001).

Antibiotic usage strategies include limiting unnecessary antibiotic administration and optimization of antimicrobial effectiveness (Table 6.3). However, an avoidance of risk factors associated with the acquisition and horizontal transmission of antibiotic-resistant bacterial infections is commonly needed to curb the increase or resistance. As a result, antibiotic policy programs usually superimpose different strategies, and for this reason the

Table 6.3
General Strategies for Reducing the Emergence of Antibiotic Resistance

---

1. *Limit unnecessary antibiotic administration*
   Develop educational programs
   Create an antibiotic use quality improvement team
   Consultation to infectious diseases specialist
   Computer-guided prescribing
   Implementation of antibiotic guidelines (automated protocols and guidelines)
   Antibiotic restriction use
   Antibiotic stop order
   Prior authorization for antibiotic use
2. *Optimize antimicrobial effectiveness*
   Antibiotic cycling and scheduled antibiotic changes
   Use of combination therapy
   Use of narrow spectrum and older antibiotic
   Use of antimicrobials with low selecting action
   Promotion of antimicrobial heterogeneity use

---

outcomes of such programs are difficult to assess owing to the complex variables involved. Herein we will review some of the antibiotic policies currently in use at hospitals.

5.2.1a. Automated use of Protocols and Guidelines and Prior Consultation with an Infectious Diseases Specialist. The implementation of antibiotic guidelines has been widely recommended to improve antibiotic use (Yates, 1999). This effort should be locally adapted, even to specific areas of hospitals, since antibiotic susceptibility profiles vary among different units and wards. Moreover, to improve the effectiveness of these protocols they should be defined with the active participation of practicing clinicians (Onion & Bartzokas, 1998). In some institutions, an infection team should authorize the prescribed antibiotic. This approach does not negatively affect patients' recovery, and it has decreased nosocomial infections and colonization with multi-resistant bacteria (Frank et al., 1997). Such strategies can benefit from automated, computer-based decisions (Evans et al., 1994), and are associated with more stable antibiotic susceptibility patterns for Gram-negative bacteria (Burke, 1998; Pestonik et al., 1996).

Automated and non-automated interventions combined with prior consultation with an infectious disease specialist can be successfully used to reduce unnecessary antibiotic use, which can reduce bacterial resistance profiles. Infected patients treated by an infectious diseases specialist are less likely to receive inadequate antimicrobial treatment, less likely to receive broad-spectrum antibiotics, and less likely to suffer from infections due to antibiotic-resistant bacteria (Byl et al., 1999). For these reasons, consultation with an infectious disease specialist has also been used to improve hospital susceptibility profiles. This strategy has been successfully implemented, reducing resistance in Gram-negative enteric bacilli (Saez-Llorens et al., 2000).

5.2.1b. Antibiotic Restriction. This method is generally implemented to reduce antimicrobial cost, but it can also influence antimicrobial resistance. Modification of the formulary is a general practice when an outbreak is detected. Restrictions have been successfully used to reduce specific outbreaks, particularly with multi-resistant *Enterobacteriaceae*. Interestingly, restriction policies are also beneficial for resistant organism not responsible for the outbreak. For example, White et al. (1997) showed that restricted antibiotic used in the management of resistant *Acinetobacter* achieved a significant decrease in the antibiotic resistance of *Enterobacteriaceae*. A common fear associated with this strategy is that antibiotic restriction gives successful results initially, but prolonged restrictions may provoke the appearance of new resistant bacteria to non-restricted antibiotics (Meyer et al., 1993; Rahal et al., 1998). For this reason, the complete control of all prescribed antibiotics has been advocated.

In a 30-year-old milestone study, the complete cessation of all antibiotic prescribing was necessary to control an outbreak of multi-resistant *Klebsiella* infection in a neurosurgical unit (Price & Sleigh, 1970). More recently, restriction of cephalosporin showed reduction of multi-resistant Gram-negative bacilli (Ballow & Schentag, 1992; Jones, 1992). Table 6.4 shows some recent experiences by summarizing the design, indicators, and major findings of shifting from intensively prescribed antimicrobials, mostly third generation cephalosporins, to another class of broad-spectrum antimicrobials, such as a penicillin-β-lactamase inhibitor combination, a fluoroquinolone, or a fourth generation cephalosporin.

The relationship between antibiotic use and resistance is more evident when resistance is due to mutations selected during therapy that result in clinical failure (Fish et al., 1995).

Table 6.4
Modification of Antimicrobial Use

Resistant pathogen	Intervention	Outcome	Reference
ESBL producing *K. pneumoniae*	Ceftazidime restriction and piperacillin–tazobactam inclusion in the formulary with educational programs and patient surveillance	Reduction of ESBL-producing *K. pneumoniae* (75%), decreased consumption of ceftazidime with no increase in piperacillin–tazobactam	Rice et al. (1996)
Multi-resistant Gram-negative bacteria	Restrictive use of broad-spectrum antibiotics, particularly cephalosporins and quinolones. Educational programs and control of risk factors	Reduction in antimicrobial resistance, decreased consumption of restricted antibiotics with no increase in non-restricted antibiotics	Giamarellou and Antoniadou (1997)
Ceftazidime-resistant inducible *Enterobacteriaceae*	Ceftazidime replaced by cefepime-amikacin	Reduction (80–100%) of resistant *Enterobacter* spp. and *Citrobacter* spp.	Mebis et al. (1998)
Ceftazidime and ciprofloxacin resistant *E. aerogenes*	Ceftazidime and ciprofloxacin replaced by cefepime	Reduction (75%) of resistant *Enterobacteriaceae*, including *E. aerogenes*	Struelens et al. (1998)
ESBL producing *K. pneumoniae*	Restrictive use of cephalosporins	Reduction of ESBL producing *K. pneumoniae* infections	Peña et al. (1998)
ESBL producing *K. pneumoniae*	Cephalosporin restriction	Reduction of multi-resistant Gram-negative bacteria, including ESBL-producing *K. pneumoniae*. Increased use of imipenem and parallel increment of imipenem resistant *P. aeruginosa*	Rahal et al. (1998)
Gentamicin resistant *K. pneumoniae*	Replacing gentamicin by amikacin	Disappearance of the gentamicin resistant *K. pneumoniae* outbreak	Van der Zwet et al. (1999)
ESBL producing *K. pneumoniae*	Replacing gentamicin and ceftazidime by amikacin and meropenem	Disappearance of the ESBL outbreak	Asensio et al. (2000)
ESBL (TEM-26) producing *K. pneumoniae*	Cephalosporin restriction	Reduction of ESBL (TEM-26) producing *K. pneumoniae*. Emergence of new ESBL	Urban et al. (2000)

Third generation cephalosporin resistance in ESBL and Bush group-1 β-lactamase producing *E. coli, K. pneumoniae*, and *Enterobacter* spp. arise from mutations. ESBL producing organisms have been controlled by restricting the use of third generation cephalosporins and implementing carbapenem or piperacillin–tazobactam therapy (Meyer et al., 1993; Rice et al., 1996). In a recent study, it has been demonstrated that class restriction applied to cephalosporins increased susceptibility among *K. pneumoniae* isolates due to the replacement of ESBL producers by non-ESBL producers (Urban et al., 2000). Paterson et al. (2001) also controlled an outbreak due to ESBL-producing *E. coli* in a liver transplantation unit by a combination of contact isolation, hand hygiene, and gut decontamination with an orally administered fluoroquinolone. However, these approaches should be taken with caution, since fluoroquinolone resistance is increasing in ESBL producing isolates (Winokour et al., 2001), and the receipt of fluoroquinolone is a risk factor for the acquisition of fluoroquinolone-resistant Gram-negative organisms (Richard et al., 2001).

Due to the usual linkage of aminoglycoside modifying resistance determinants in plasmids harboring bla_{ESBLs}, restriction of cephalosporins should be coupled with restriction of aminoglycosides to clearly diminish infections due to ESBL producers and the reservoir for these isolates (Toltzis et al.,1998). In that sense, restriction of an affected aminoglycoside and substitution by an unaffected one may be useful to resolve outbreak situations (Asensio et al., 2000; Van der Zwet, 1999).

Resistance to third-generation-cephalosporins due to hyperproduction of Bush group-1 β-lactamases in *Enterobacter cloacae* has also been demonstrated in relation to the use of several antimicrobials, including ceftazidime (Ballow & Schentag, 1992). Enforcement of third-generation cephalosporin-usage restriction led to a decrease in resistance to *E. cloacae* (Banberger & Dahl, 1992). Moreover, the replacement of ceftazidime by cefepime plus amikacin decreased an endemic presence of ceftazidime-resistant inducible *Enterobacteriaceae* from a hematology ward (Mebis et al., 1998). A similar effect has also been observed with non β-lactam antibiotics, generally fluoroquinolones (Kollef et al., 1997; Struelens et al., 1998).

Restriction policies reduce antimicrobial heterogeneity and make a displacement of treatments to non-restricted antimicrobials. Thus, an unintended consequence of these programs is the increase in bacterial resistance to the new antimicrobials. This has been very well documented when cephalosporins have been restricted and an increase in carbapenem use was noted concomitantly with the emergence of infections due to imipenem-resistant *P. aeruginosa* and *Acinetobacter baumanii* (Meyer et al., 1993; Rahal et al., 1998). Thus, the effect of limiting usage of one antibiotic or antibiotic family may increase the use of another agent and resistance to this might then emerge. This phenomenon has been termed "squeezing the balloon" (Burke, 1998).

5.2.1c. Antibiotic Cycling. Antibiotic cycling is characterized by the withdrawal of a specific antibiotic from use during a predefined period and its reintroduction at a later time (Table 6.5). The main goal of cycling is to allow resistance rates for specific antibiotics to decrease or at least to remain stable (Kollef, 2001). Theoretically, this strategy periodically removes from the environment specific antimicrobials that could induce or select resistance. Antibiotic cycling is based on two assumptions: (1) antibiotic selection is the major force promoting the emergence of resistance determinants (McGowan & Gerding, 1996); (2) acquisition of an antibiotic resistant phenotype has a physiological cost for bacteria

Table 6.5

Antibiotic Cycling Experiences Involving Gram-Negative Bacilli

Resistant pathogen	Intervention	Outcome	Reference
Gram-negatives resistant to ceftazidime	Scheduled change to ciprofloxacin for empirical treatment of Gram-negative infections	Reduction (78%) of Gram-negatives resistant to ceftazidime and ICU infections associated with these isolates	Kollef et al. (1997)
Gram-negatives resistant to gentamicin	Cycling of gentamicin and amikacin using time cycles of 12–52 month over 10 years	Reduction of Gram-negatives resistant to gentamicin and ICU infections associated with these isolates	Gerding (2000)
Gram-negatives resistant to ceftazidime	Scheduled change to ciprofloxacin (6 months) followed by cefepime (6 months) for empirical treatment of Gram-negatives infections	Reduction of inadequate empirical antibiotic treatments	Kollef and Fraser (2001)
Multidrug resistant Gram-negatives and vancomycin resistant enterococci	Cycling of four antibiotic regimens (4–6 months) over 19 months among neutropenic patients	No increase of bacterial resistance but increment of enterococcal infections	Domínguez et al. (2000)
Gram-negatives resistant to ceftazidime and ciprofloxacin	Restricted use of ceftazidime and ciprofloxacin and cycling of empirical treatments on the basis of monthly review of bacterial susceptibility profiles	Reduction of infections due to resistant Gram-negatives and reduction of inadequate empirical antibiotic treatments	Gruson et al. (2000)

(Andersson & Levin, 1999), so that in the absence of antibiotic selective pressure, the susceptible bacterial populations will overgrow the resistant ones. Rotational usage practices are likely to be most appropriate against Gram-negative bacilli because of the wide variety of available agents for cycling (Gerding, 2000).

Evidence suggesting that cycling of antimicrobial therapy is useful in limiting resistance is inconclusive. A prospective, nonrandomized observational trial cycling antimicrobials (4–6 months) in a hematology-oncology unit demonstrated that Gram-negative susceptibility profiles showed no increase in resistance (Domínguez et al., 2000). In contrast, cycling of aminoglycosides and scheduled changes with fluoroquinolones and β-lactams reduced the occurrence of infections due to resistant bacteria (Gerding, 2000; Gruson et al., 2000; Kollef, 2001; Kollef et al., 1997). Moreover, the replacement of a first-choice aminoglycoside by another which had never been used in the institution may resolve outbreaks situations (Van der Zwet et al., 1999), but it may have worse results when reintroduced (Gerding et al., 1991). These varying results may be due to differences in methodological cycling strategies. Not all antibiotic-cycling strategies may elicit the disappearance or emergence of resistant determinants in all species at all times. At present, few rotation schemes have been suggested (McGowan & Tenover, 1997), and it is not clear how many antibiotics should be needed in the cycling process, how long the prescribing cycling period should be, and how long one needs to observe and evaluate the results. Recent studies in intensive care units recommended that rotation strategies should be adapted in parallel to continuous antimicrobial surveillance of resistant bacteria (Gruson et al., 2000). This surveillance includes re-evaluations of all treatments with antibiotics at day 3 and day 10 of the program to check the appropriateness of the initial therapy and the influence of the antibiotics on the microbial ecology (more or less antibiotic resistant bacteria, prevalence of microorganisms involved in infection, ...) at the ICUs.

Although the antibiotic cycling approach was designed to reduce the emergence of bacterial resistance and potentially restore the effectiveness of withdrawn antimicrobials (Sanders & Sanders, 1997), some fears concerning the efficacy of this approach have recently arisen. Limitations have been theoretically related with practical utility and the persistence of resistance genes (John & Rice, 2000; McGowan, 2000). The genetic mechanism involved in acquiring antimicrobial resistance may favor stability of resistance genes even in the absence of antibiotic pressure. In fact, it has been observed that the bacterial fitness cost associated with resistance may decline with compensatory mutations, which can be maintained in the absence of the antibiotic (Björkman & Andersson, 2000). On the other hand, the ability of a given antibiotic to select resistant strains is complex. It depends on its intrinsic lethal activity, if any, the ability of the organisms to mutate target genes while maintaining their functionality (Martínez & Baquero, 2000), the proximity to other species that possess transferable resistant determinants, and the ability to tolerate and express acquired resistance determinants (Bonhoeffer et al., 1997).

It has been recently postulated that the persistence of antimicrobial resistance determinants in the environment after the reduction of specific antimicrobial selective pressure can be governed by at least three general rules: (1) resistance determinants will have a shorter half-life if their expression is disadvantageous for survival in an antibiotic-free medium; (2) resistance will have shorter half-lives if they confer a disadvantage in the presence of a new antibiotic pressure during the cycling period; and (3) resistance phenotypes that are inducible may be more persistent than those that are expressed constitutively

(John & Rice, 2000). In addition, concomitant presence of various resistance determinants in a common genetic structure leading to co-selection processes may enhance the persistence of resistance determinants. In Gram-negative bacteria, sequential antimicrobial exposure may promote the evolution of plasmids towards multidrug resistance simply by adding gene cassettes (either alone or forming part of novel integrons) to the plasmid structure. Once that occurs, selection with one antibiotic or another will maintain the resistance to all agents represented on the multidrug-resistance element (Alonso et al., 2001; Chiew et al., 1998).

The problem with ESBLs illustrates the possibility of cycling failure. Ceftazidime restriction in a single institution with a late-detected outbreak of ESBL-producing *K. pneumoniae* isolates decreased the presence of these isolates, but the reintroduction of this antibiotic resulted in their re-emergence (Meyer et al., 1993; Rahal et al., 1998). More recently, total restriction of all cephalosporin class antibiotics in the same institution increased susceptibility among ESBL-producing isolates, but new variants of ESBL arose, indicating the possibility that other antimicrobials, different from cephalosporins, participated in the selection process (Urban et al., 2000). In addition, the co-selection processes might be common for ESBL isolates, as ESBL producers can be resistant to several other classes of antibiotics, including aminoglycosides, tetracyclines, and trimethoprim-sulphamethoxazole and, more recently, fluoroquinolones (Jacoby & Sutton, 1991; Winokur et al., 2001).

In cycling strategies it is important to monitor the susceptibility patterns of the isolates, not only in clinical samples but also in patients microflora and even in the environment, to adapt cycling strategies to susceptibility patterns, and to identify possible reservoirs of resistant bacteria that may be responsible for rotation failure (Gerding, 2000). The environmental gene pool may contribute to the persistence of a resistance determinant that may arise with antibiotic changes. This situation has been observed in ESBL-producing *Enterobacteriaceae*, as these isolates can be introduced and reintroduced from long-term care facility patients when they are hospitalized (Nicolle, 2001; Wiener et al., 1999). Moreover, the presence of bla_{ESBL} in environmental isolates and the possibility of transmission to nosocomial pathogens may enhance the persistence of these isolates.

5.2.1d. Use of Narrow Spectrum and Older Antibiotics.   As previously stated, the avoidance of broad-spectrum antibiotics (i.e., cephalosporins, carbapanems, and quinolones) may reduce bacterial resistance to antimicrobials. In parallel, the use of narrow spectrum and older antibiotics, particularly in empiric and prophylaxis protocols, are promoted to reduce the selection of the broad spectrum resistant bacteria. In an recent report, De Man et al. (2000) modified the empiric antibiotic regimens in a neonatal ICU to remove the selective pressure that favored resistant bacteria. They demonstrated that restriction of a combination of amoxicillin–cefotaxime for early-onset septicemia and the use of a regimen consisting of older antibiotics, penicillin–tobramycin, reduced infections due to *E. cloacae*: the risk for colonization with bacteria resistant to the empirical therapy was 18 times lower. Moreover, the colonization pattern with resistant bacteria may decrease with "classical" regimens, as they normally have little or no impact on the normal flora (Höiby, 2000).

5.2.1e. Use of Combination Antibiotic Therapy.   The use of combination antibiotic therapy is generally recommended in empiric treatment in neutropenic patients. Combination regimens increase the pathogen coverage and have the potential to reduce the emergence of bacterial resistance and to reverse resistance trends. Mathematical models favor combination regimes as the best method of preventing both the emergence and clonal spread of resistance (Lipsitch & Levin, 1997). It has also been stated that combination therapy may reduce the "mutant selection window" if the normalized pharmacokinetic profiles of the antimicrobials superimpose at the concentrations that inhibit growth (Zhao & Drlica, 2001). Decreasing antibiotic resistance of *Enterobacteriaceae* by introducing antibiotic combination therapy was observed in neutropenic febrile patients (Mebis et al., 1998). Similar results were reported when ceftazidime use was discontinued and substituted by piperacillin plus an aminoglycoside, reducing by 25% the ceftazidime resistance prevalence in *E. cloacae* (Ballow & Schentag, 1992). Moreover, the use of combination therapy demonstrated in ICU patients a reduction of ventilator-associated pneumonia by multiresistant Gram-negative bacteria (Trouillet et al., 1998).

5.2.1f. Use of Antimicrobials with Low Selecting Action. This strategy has been used mainly to avoid the selection of *Enterobacteriaceae* or *P. aeruginosa* resistant to third-generation cephalosporins due to Bush group-1 β-lactamase production. Cefepime, a fourth-generation cephalosporin with a low selective window, has been used alone and in combination with aminoglycosides to avoid the selection of β-lactamase hyperproducer populations of *Enterobacter* spp. and *Cifrobacter freundii* (Mebis et al., 1998; Struelens et al., 1998).

5.2.1g. Utilization of Antimicrobial Heterogeneity. Recently, antimicrobial heterogeneity has been advocated as the best practice for reducing the emergence of antimicrobial resistance (Kollef & Fraser, 2001). This strategy can be viewed as the use of a variety of antibiotics rather than one a few number of agents for any specific clinical indication. This approach is new and has been specifically designed against Gram-negative bacteria in ICU setting (Kollef & Fraser, 2001). Theoretically, the selection density for a given antibiotic is lower than that obtained with restrictive policies, because the number of patients being treated by a single antibiotic type is lower than in classical antibiotic treatment protocols. If the selection density is lower, the probability for selecting antibiotic resistance mutants will be then lower, because the number of bacteria "at risk" (under antibiotic selective pressure) will also be lower.

6. NEW AGENTS ON THE HORIZON

Several antibiotics are currently used for the treatment of infection by *Enterobacteriaceae*. However, all belong to few structural families. Thus, resistance to one antibiotic frequently reduces susceptibility to other members of the same family. Novel antibiotics belonging to different structural families are needed in to fight antibiotic-resistant bacteria. Some novel families of antibiotics may be launched by 2005. Knowledge derived from the sequencing of whole microbial genomes, combinatorial chemistry, rational design by computerized molecular modelling of crystal structures of potential targets, new methods for screening natural compounds, and widely used methods of high throughput screening are potentially useful tools for obtaining new antibiotics (Tan et al., 2000). In the meantime, new antibiotics from the known structural families have been marketed or are close to be approved for use.

Among the new antibiotics, we can cite fluoroquinolones (Fix et al., 2000) such as gemifloxacin (Lowe & Lamb, 2000), moxafloxacin and gatifloxacin (Perry et al., 1999), tetracyclines such as glycylcycline (Johnson & Jones, 1996; Sum et al., 1998), and β-lactams, particularly those belonging to the carbapenem family that are unaffected by ESBLs. Carbapenems under development include two prodrugs that are active after oral administration (Miyazaki et al., 2001; Weiss et al., 1999). New families under development include antimicrobial cationic peptides, analogues of host defense peptides (Hancock & Lehrer, 1998). These peptides can be useful for the treatment of infections by *Enterobacteriaceae* because they prevent the initiation of systemic inflammatory reactions as well as killing the bacteria.

Finally, we want to mention inhibitors of antibiotic resistance mechanisms. These inhibitors can restore the susceptibility of bacteria to old antibiotics. Well known examples are β-lactamase inhibitors (Maiti et al., 1998). These agents have been extremely useful for the treatment of infections by β-lactamase-producing Gram-negative bacteria. Among these compounds are novel inhibitors of class C β-lactamases, such as boronic acids (Weston et al., 1998). These novel inhibitors have a very different chemical structure from previous β-lactamase inhibitors that are β-lactams, so that it is unlikely that they will induce the expression of β-lactamases. Inhibitors of MDR efflux pumps are also under development (Lomovskaya et al., 2001). Efflux pump inhibitors might have an added value for the treatment of infections, because MDR pumps contribute both to intrinsic and acquired resistance of bacterial populations. For example, the intrinsic resistance to macrolides displayed by Gram-negative bacteria is partly due to the activity of MDR efflux pumps. It is conceivable that MDR inhibitors, in combination with macrolides, could be active against Gram-negative bacteria. This opens the possibility of using antibiotics in combination with appropriate inhibitors for the treatment of infection by bacteria previously classified as intrinsically resistant to such drugs.

References

Abraham, E. P., & Chain, E. (1940). An enzyme from bacteria able to destroy penicillin. *Nature, 146*, 837.

Aksaray, S., Dokuzo-Guz, B., Guvener, E., Yucesoy, M., Yulug, N., Kocagoz, S., Unal, S., Cetin, S., Calangu, S., Gunaydin, M., Leblebicioglu, H., Esen, S., Bayar, B., Willke, A., Findik, D., Tuncer, I., Baysal, B., Gunseren, F., & Mamikoglu, L. (2000). Surveillance of antimicrobial resistance among Gram-negative isolates from intensive care units in a hight hospital in Turkey. *J Antimicrob Chemother, 45*, 695–699.

Alonso, A., Sanchez, P., & Martinez, J. L. (2001). Environmental selection of antibiotic resistance genes. *Environ Microbiol, 3*, 1–9.

Alves, A. M., Lasaro, M. O., Almeida, D. F., & Ferreira, L. C. (2000). DNA immunisation against the CFA/I fimbriae of enterotoxigenic *Escherichia coli* (ETEC). *Vaccine, 19*, 788–795.

Ambler, R. P. (1980). The structure of β-lactamases. *Phil Trans R Soc Lond Biol, 289*, 321–331.

Andersson, D. I., & Levin, B. R. (1999). The biological cost of antibiotic resistance. *Curr Opin Microbiol, 2*, 489–493.

Archival, L., Phillips, L., Monnet, D., McGowan, J. E. J., Tenover, F., & Gaynes, R. (1997). Antimicrobial resistance in isolates from inpatients and outpatients in the United States: Increasing importance of the intensive care unit. *Clin Infect Dis, 24*, 211–215.

Arlet, G., Rouveau, M., Casin, I., Bouvet, P. J. M., Lagrange, P. H., & Philippon, P. (1994). Molecular epidemiology of *Klebsiella pneumoniae* strains that produce SHV-4 β-lactamase and which were isolated in 14 French hospitals. *J Clin Microbiol, 32*, 2553–2558.

Asensio, A., Oliver, A., González-Diego, P., Baquero, F., Pérez-Díaz, J. C., Ros, P., Cobo, J., Palacios, M., Lasheras, D., & Cantón, R. (2000). Outbreak of a multiresistant *Klebsiella pneumoniae* strain in an intensive care unit: Antibiotic use as risk factor for colonization and infection. *Clin Infect Dis, 30*, 55–60.

Ballow, C. H., & Schentag, J. J. (1992). Trends in antibiotic utilization and bacterial resistance. Report of the National Nosocomial Resistance Surveillance Group. *Diagn Microbiol Infect Dis, 15*, 37S–42S.

Banberger, D. M., & Dahl, S. L. (1992). Impact of voluntary *vs* enforced compliance of third-generation cephalosporin use in a teaching hospital. *Arch Intern Med, 152*, 554–557.

Baquero, F., Negri, M. C., Morosini, M. I., & Blázquez, J. (1998). Antibiotic-selective environments. *Clin Infect Dis, 27*, S5–S11.

Barnaud, G., Arlet, G., Verdet, C. H., Gaillot, O., Lagrange, P. H., & Philippon, A. (1998). *Salmonella enteritidis*: AmpC plasmid-mediated inducible β-lactamase (DHA-1) with an *ampR* gene from *Morganella morganii*. *Antimicrob Agents Chemother, 42*, 2352–2358.

Bennet, P. M. (1999). Integrons and gene cassetes: A genetic construction kit for bacteria. *J Antimicrob Chemother, 43*, 1–4.

Berger, J. M., Gamblin, S. J., Harrison, S. C., & Wang, J. C. (1996). Structure and mechanism of DNA topoisomerase II. *Nature, 379*, 225–232.

Berlanga, M., Vazquez, J. L., Hernandez-Borrell, J., Montero, M. T., & Viñas, M. (2000). Evidence of an efflux pump in *Serratia marcescens*. *Microb Drug Resist Mech E Dis, 6*, 111–117.

Björkman, J., & Andersson, D. I. (2000). The cost of antibiotic resistance from a bacterial perspective. *Drug Resist Updat, 3*, 237–245.

Blázquez, J., Morosini, M. I., Negri, M. C., & Baquero, F. (2000). Selection of naturally occurring extended-spectrum TEM β-lactamase variants by fluctuating β-lactam pressure. *Antimicrob Agents Chemother, 44*, 2182–2184.

Bonhoeffer, S., Lipsitch, M., & Levin, B. R. (1997). Evaluating treatment protocols to prevent antibiotic resistance. *Proc Natl Acad Sci, USA, 94*, 12106–12111.

Bonten, M. J. M., & Weinstein, R. A. (1996). The role of colonization in the pathogenesis of nosocomial infections. *Infect Control Hosp Epidemiol, 17*, 193–200.

Bradford, P. A. (2001). Extended-spectrum β-lactamases in the 21st century: Characterization, epidemiology, and detection of this important resistance threat. *Clin Microbiol Rev, 14*, 933–951.

Bradford, P. A., Cherubin, C. E., Idemyor, V., Rasmussen, B. A., & Bush, K. (1994). Multiply resistant *Klebsiella pneumoniae* from two Chicago hospitals: Identification of the extended-spectrum β-lactamase TEM-12 and TEM-10 ceftazidime-hydrolyzing β-lactamases in a single isolate. *Antimicrob Agents Chemother, 38*, 761–766.

Bradford, P. A., Urban, C., Mariano, N., Projam, S. J., Rahal, J. J., & Bush, K. (1997). Imipenem resistance in *Klebsiella pneumoniae* is associated with the combination of ACT-1, a plasmid-mediated AmpC β-lactamase, and the loss of outer membrane protein. *Antimicrob Agents Chemother, 41*, 563–569.

Burke, J. P. (1998). Antibiotic-resistance—squeezing the balloon? *JAMA, 280*, 1270–1271.

Bush, K. (1989). Characterization of β-lactamases. *Antimicrob Agents Chemother, 33*, 259–263.

Bush, K. (1997). The evolution of beta-lactamases. *Ciba Found Symp, 207*, 152–163.

Bush, K. (1999). β-lactamases of increasing clinical importance. *Curr Pharmaceut Des, 5*, 839–845.

Bush, K. (2001). New beta-lactamases in Gram-negative bacteria: Diversity and impact on the selection of antimicrobial therapy. *Clin Infect Dis, 32*, 1085–1089.

Bush, K., Jacoby, G. A., & Medeiros, A. A. (1995). A functional classification scheme for β-lactamases and its correlation with molecular structure. *Antimicrob Agents Chemother, 39*, 1211–1233.

Byl, B., Clevenbergh, P., Jacobs, F., Struelens, M. J., Zech, F., Kentos, A., & Thys, J. P. (1999). Impact of infectious disease specialist and microbiological data on the appropriateness of antimicrobial therapy for bacteriemia. *Clin Infect Dis, 29*, 60–66.

Cantón, R., Pérez-Vázquez, M. P., Oliver, A., Coque, T. M., Loza, E., Ponz, F., & Baquero, F. (2001). Validation of the VITEK2 and the Advance Expert System with a Collection of *Enterobacteriaceae* harboring Extended Spectrum or Inhibitor Resistant β-lactamases. *Diagn Microbiol Infect Dis, 41*, 65–70.

Carattoli, A., Villa, L., Pezzella, C., Bordi, E., & Visca, P. (2001). Expanding drug resistance through integron acquisition by Inc*FI* plasmids of *Salmonella Enterica Typhimurium. Emerg Infect Dis, 7*, 444–447.

Chang, Y., Siu, L. K., Fung, C. P., Huang, M. H., & Ho, M. (2001). Diversity of SHV and TEM β-lactamases in *Klebsiella pneumoniae*: Gene evolution in northern Taiwan and two novel β-lactamases SHV-25 and SHV-26. *Antimicrob Agents Chemother, 45*, 2407–2413.

Chiew, Y. F., Yeo, S. F., Hall, L. M. C., & Livermore, D. (1998). Can susceptibility to an antimicrobial be restored by halting its use? The case of streptomycin versus *Enterobacteriaceae*. *J Antimicrob Chemother, 41*, 247–251.

Chu, Y. W., Houang, E. T. S., & Cheng, A. F. B. (1998). Novel combination of mutations in the DNA gyrase and topoisomerase IV genes in laboratory-grown fluoroquinolone-resistant *Shigella flexneri* mutants. *Antimicrob Agents Chemother, 42*, 3051–3052.

Conlan, J. W., Kuo-Lee, R., Webb, A., Cox, A. D., & Perry, M. B. (2000). Oral immunization of mice with a glycoconjugate vaccine containing the O157 antigen of *Escherichia coli* O157:H7 admixed with cholera toxin fails to elicit protection against subsequent colonization by the pathogen. *Can J Microbiol, 46*, 283–290.

Conrad, S. M., Oethinger, M., Kaifel, K., Klotz, G., Marre, R., & Kern, W. V. (1994). *gyrA* mutations in high-level fluoroquinolone-resistant *Escherichia coli* clinical isolates. *J Antimicrob Chemother, 38*, 443–455.

Coque, T. M., Valera, M. C., Oliver, A., Morosini, M. I., & Cantón, R. (2001). Shifting epidemiology of extended-spectrum beta-lactamases (ESBL) in a Spanish hospital (1988–2000): From SHV to CTXM derivel ESBL. In Programs and abstracts 41st Interscience Conference on Antimicrobial Agents and Chemotherapy. American Society for Microbiology.

Coque, T. M., Oliver, A., Pérez-Díaz, J. C., Baquero, F., & Cantón, R. (2002). Genes Encoding TEM-4, SHV-2, and CTX-M-10 Extended Spectrum β-Lactamases are Carried by Multiple *Klebsiella pneumoniae* Clones in a Single Hospital (Madrid, 1989–2000). *Antimicrob Agents Chemother, 46*, 500–510.

Cornaglia, G., Roussel, K., Satta, G., & Fontana, R. (1995). Relative importances of outer membrane permeability and group 1 β-lactamase as determinants of meropenem and imipenem activities against *Enterobacter cloacae*. *Antimicrob Agents Chemother, 39*, 350–355.

Datta, N., & Kontomichalou, P. (1965). Penicillinase synthesis controlled by infectious R factors in *Enterobacteriaceae*. *Nature, 208*, 239–241.

Datta, N., & Hughes, V. M. (1983). Plasmids of the same *Inc* groups in *Enterobacteria* before and after the medical use of antibiotics. *Nature, 306*, 616–617.

Davies, J. E. (1997). Origins, acquisition and dissemination of antibiotic resistance determinants. *Ciba Found Symp, 207*, 15–27.

De Gheldre, Y., Struelens, M. J., Glupczynski, Y., De Mol, P., Maes, N., Nonhoff, C., Chetoui, H., Sion, C., Ronveaux, O., Vaneechoutte, M., & le Groupement Pour Le Dépistage, L'Etude et la Prevencion de Infections Hospitalières (GDEPIH-GOSPIZ). (2001). National epidemiologic surveys of *Enterobacter aerogenes* in Belgian hospitals from 1996 to 1998. *J Clin Microbiol, 39,* 889–896.

De Man, P., Verhoeven, B. A., Verbrugh, H. A., Vos, M. C., & van den Anker, J. N. (2000). An antibiotic policy to prevent emergence of resistant bacilli. *Lancet, 355,* 973–978.

Dennesen, P. J., Bonten, M. J., & Weinstein, R. A. (1998). Multiresistant bacteria as a hospital epidemic problem. *Ann Med, 30,* 176–185.

Domínguez, E. A., Smith, T. L., Reed, E., Sanders, C. C., & Sanders, W. E., Jr. (2000). A pilot study of antibiotic cycling in a hematology-oncology unit. *Infect Control Hosp Epidemiol, 21,* S4–S8.

Drlica, K., & Zhao, X. L. (1997). DNA gyrase, topoisomerase IV, and the 4-quinolones. *Microbiol Mol Biol Rev, 61,* 377–392.

Drusano, G. L. (2000). Fluoroquinolone pharmacodynamics: Prospective determination of the relationships between exposure and outcome. *J Chemother, 12,* S21–S26.

El-Hajj, H. H., Marras, S. A., Tyagi, S., Kramer, F. R., & Alland, D. (2001). Detection of rifampin resistance in Mycobacterium tuberculosis in a single tube with molecular beacons. *J Clin Microbiol, 39,* 4131–4137.

Essack, E. S., Hall, L. M. C., Pillay, D. G., McFadyen, M. L., & Livermore, D. M. (2001). Complexity and diversity of *Klebsiella pneumoniae* strains with extended-spectrum β-lactamases isolated in 1994 and 1996 at a teaching hospital in Durban, South Africa. *Antimicrob Agents Chemother, 45,* 88–95.

Evans, R. S., Classen, D. C., Pestonik, S. L., Lundsgaarde, H. P., & Burke, J. P. (1994). Improving antibiotic selection using computer decision support. *Arch Intern Med, 154,* 878–884.

Everett, M. J., Jin, Y. F., Ricci, V., & Piddock, L. J. V. (1996). Contributions of individual mechanisms to fluoroquinolone resistance in 36 *Escherichia coli* strains isolated from humans and animals. *Antimicrob Agents Chemother, 40,* 2380–2386.

Fernández-Rodríguez, A., Cantón, R., Pérez-Díaz, J. C., Martínez-Beltrán, J., Picazo, J. J., & Baquero, F. (1992). Aminoglycoside-modifying enzymes in clinical isolates harboring extended-spectrum β-lactamases. *Antimicrob Agents Chemother, 36,* 2536–2538.

Fiett, J., Palucha, A., Miaczynska, B., Stankiewicz, M., Przondo-Mordaska, H., Hryniewicz, W., & Gniadkowski, M. (2000). A novel complex mutant β-lactamase, TEM-68, identified in a *Klebsiella pneumoniae* isolate from an outbreak of extended spectrum β-lactamase-producing Klebsiellae. *Antimicrob Agents Chemother, 44,* 1499–1505.

Fish, D. N., Piscitelli, S. C., & Danziger, L. H. (1995). Development of resistance during antimicrobial therapy: A review of antibiotic classes and patient characteristics in 173 studies. *Pharmacotherapy, 15,* 279–291.

Fix, A. M., Pfaller, M. A., Biedenbach, D. J., Beach, M. L., & Jones, R. N. (2001). Comparative antimicrobial spectrum and activity of BMS284756 (T-3811, a desfluoroquinolone) tested against 656 *Enterobacteriaceae*, including preliminary *in vitro* susceptibility test comparisons and development. *Int J Antimicrob Agents, 18,* 141–145.

Fluit, A. C., Schmitz, F. J., Verhoef, J., & European SENTRY participants. (2001). Multi-resistance to antimicrobial agents for the ten most frequently isolated bacterial pathogens. *In J Antimicrob Agents, 18,* 147–160.

Frank, M. O., Batteiger, B. E., Sorensen, S. J., Hartstein, A. I., Carr, J. A., McComb, J. S., Clark, C. D., Abel, S. R., Mikuta, J. M., & Jones, R. B. (1997). Decreased in expenditures and selected nosocomial infections following implementation of an antimicrobial-prescribing improved program. *Clin Perform Quality Health Care, 5,* 180–188.

Fridkin, S. K., & Gaynes, R. P. (1999). Antimicrobial resistance in intensive care units. *Clin Chest Med, 20,* 303–315.

Fridkin, S. K., Steward, C. D., Edwards, J. R., Pryor, E. R., McGowan, J. E., Jr, Archivald, L. K., Gaynes, R. P., & Tenover, F. C. (1999). Surveillance of antimicrobial use and resistance in US hospitals: Project ICARE phase 2: project intensive care antimicrobial resistance epidemiology (ICARE) hospitals. *Clin Infect Dis, 29*, 245–252.

Friedman, S. M., Lu, T., & Drlica, K. (2001). Mutation in DNA gyrase A gene of *Escherichia coli* that expands the quinolone resistance-determining region. *Antimicrob Agents Chemother, 45*, 2378–2380.

Galdbart, J. O., Lémann, F., Ainouz, D., Féron, P., Lambert-Zechovsky, N., & Branger, C. (2000). TEM-24 extended-spectrum β-lactamase-producing *Enterobacter aerogenes*: Long-term clonal dissemination in French hospitals. *Clin Microbiol Infect, 6*, 316–323.

Garau, J., Xercavins, M., Rodríguez-Caballeira, M., Gómez-Vera, J. R., Coll, I., Vidal, D., Llovet, T., & Ruiz-Bremon. A. (1999). Emergence and dissemination of quinolone-resistant *Escherichia coli* in the community. *Antimicrob Agents Chemother, 43*, 2736–2741.

Gaynes, R., & Monnet, D. (1997). The contribution of antibiotic use on the frequency of antibiotic resistance in hospitals. *Ciba Found Symp, 207*, 47–60.

Gerding, D. N. (2000). Antimicrobial cycling: Lessons learned from aminoglycoside experience. *Infect Control Hosp Epidemiol, 21*, S12–S17.

Gerding, D. N., Larson, T. A., Hughes, R. A., Weiler, M., Shanholtzer, C., & Peterson, L. R. (1991). Aminoglycoside resistance and aminoglycoside usage: Ten years of experience in one hospital. *Antimicrob Agents Chemother, 35*, 1284–1290.

Giakkoupi, P., Tzouvelekis, L. S., Tsakris, A., Loukova, V., Sofianou, D., & Tzelepi, E. (2000). IBC-1, a novel integron-associated class A β-lactamase with extended-spectrum properties produced by an *Enterobacter cloacae* clinical strain. *Antimicrob Agents Chemother, 44*, 2247–2253.

Giamarellou, H., & Antoniadou, A. (1997). The effect of monitoring of antibiotic use on decreasing antibiotic resistance in the hospital. *Ciba Found Symp, 207*, 76–86.

Giraud, E., Cloeckaert, A., Kerboeuf, D., & Chaslus-Dancla, E. (2000). Evidence for active efflux as the primary mechanism of resistance to ciprofloxacin in Salmonella enterica serovar typhimurium. *Antimicrob Agents Chemother, 44*, 1223–1228.

Gniadkowski, M., Palucha, A., Grzesiowsk, P., & Hryniewicz, W. (1998a). Outbreak of ceftazidime-resistant *Klebsiella pneumoniae* in Warsaw, Poland: Clonal spread of the TEM-47 extended spectrum β-lactamase (ESBL)-producing strain and transfer of a plasmid carrying the SHV-5 like ESBL-encoding gene. *Antimicrob Agents Chemother, 42*, 3079–3085.

Gniadkowski, M., Schneider, I., Jungwirth, R., Hryniewicz, W., & Bauernfeind, A. (1998b). Ceftazidime-resistant *Enterobacteriaceae* isolates from three Polish hospitals: Identification of three novel TEM- and SHV-5 type extended spectrum β-lactamase-producing *Klebsiellae*. *Antimicrob Agents Chemother, 42*, 514–520.

Gomez-Lus, R. (1998). Evolution of bacterial resistance to antibiotics during the last three decades. *Int Microbiol, 1*, 279–284.

Gould, I. (1999). A review of the role of antibiotic policies in the control of antibiotic resistance. *J Antimicrob Chemother, 43*, 459–465.

Goussard, S., Sougakoff, W., Mabilat, C., Bauernfeind, A., & Courvalin, P. (1991). An IS*1*-like element is responsible for high-level synthesis of extended-spectrum β-lactamase TEM-6 in *Enterobacteriaceae*. *J Gen Microbiol, 137*, 2681–2687.

Gruson, D., Hilbert, G., Vargas, F., Valentino, R., Bebear, C., Allery, A., Bebear, C., Gbikpi-Benisson, G., & Cardinaus, J. P. (2000). Rotation and restricted use of antibiotics in a medical intensive care unit. Impact on the incidence of ventilator associated pneumonia caused by antibiotic-resistant Gram-negative bacteria. *Am J Respir Crit Care Med, 162*, 837–843.

Guillemot, D. (1999). Antibiotic use in humans and bacterial resistance. *Curr Opin Microbiol, 2*, 494–498.

Hall, R. M., & Collis, C. M. (1995). Mobile gene cassettes and integrons: Capture and spread of genes by site-specific recombination. *Mol Microbiol, 15*, 593–600.

Hancock, R. E., & Lehrer, R. (1998). Cationic peptides: A new source of antibiotics. *Trends Biotechnol, 16*, 82–88.

Hanberger, H., García-Rodriguez, J. A., Gobernado, M., Groossens, H., Nilsson, L. E., & Struelens, M. J. (1999). Antibiotic susceptibility among aerobic Gram-negative bacilli in intensive care units in 5 European countries. *JAMA, 281*, 67–71.

Hanberger, H., Diekema, D., Fluit, A., Jones, R., Struelens, M., Spencer, M., & Wolff, M. (2001). Surveillance of antibiotic resistance in European ICUs. *J Hosp Infect, 48*, 161–176.

Heisig, P. (1996). Genetic evidence for a role of *parC* mutations in development of high-level fluoroquinolone resistance in *Escherichia coli*. *Antimicrob Agents Chemother, 40*, 879–885.

Höiby, N. (2000). Ecological antibiotic policy. *J Antimicrob Chemother, 46*, 59–62.

Hoiseth, S. K., & Stocker, B. A. (1981). Aromatic-dependent *Salmonella typhimurium* are non-virulent and effective as live vaccines. *Nature, 291*, 238–239.

Hooker, K. D., & Di Piro, J. T. (1988). Effect of antimicrobial therapy on bowel flora. *Clin Pharm, 7*, 878–888.

Hooper, D. C. (1999). Mechanisms of fluoroquinolone resistance. *Drug Resist Updates, 2*, 38–55.

Hooper, D. C. (2000). New uses for new and old quinolones and the challenge of resistance. *Clin Infect Dis, 30*, 243–254.

Hooper, D. C. (2001). Mechanisms of action of antimicrobials: Focus on fluoroquinolones. *Clin Infect Dis, 32*, S9–S15.

Hughes, V. M., & Datta, N. (1983). Conjugative plasmids in bacteria of the "pre-antibiotic" era. *Nature, 302*, 725–726.

Ishii, H., Sato, K., Hoshino, K., Sato, M., Yamaguchi, A., Sawai, T., & Osada, Y. (1991). Active efflux of ofloxacin by a highly quinolone-resistant strain of *Proteus vulgaris*. *J Antimicrob Chemother, 28*, 827–836.

Ito, H., Arakawa, Y., Ohsuka, S., Wacharotayanku, R., Kato, N., & Ohta, M. (1995). Plasmid-mediated dissemination of metallo β-lactamase gen bla_{IMP} among clinically isolated strains of *Serratia marcescens*. *Antimicrob Agents Chemother, 39*, 824–829.

Jacoby, G. A., & Sutton, L. (1991). Properties of plasmids responsible for production of extended-spectrum β-lactamases. *Antimicrob Agents Chemother, 35*, 164–169.

John, J. F., & Rice, L. B. (2000). The microbial genetics of antibiotic cycling. *Infect Control Hosp Epidemiol, 21*, S22–S31.

Johnson, D. M., & Jones, R. N. (1996). Two investigational glycylcyclines, DMG-DMDOT and DMG-MINO. Antimicrobial activity studies against Gram-positive species. *Diagn Microbiol Infect Dis, 24*, 53–57.

Jones, R. N. (1992). The current and future impact of antimicrobial resistance among nosocomial bacterial pathogens. *Diagn Microbiol Infect Dis, 15*, 3S–10S.

Kaye, K. S., Cosgrove, S., Harris, A., Eliopoulos, G. M., & Carmeli, Y. (2001). Risk factors for emergence of resistance to broad spectrum cephalosporin among *Enterobacter* spp. *Antimicrob Agents Chemother, 45*, 2628–2630.

Knox, J. R. (1995). Extended-spectrum and inhibitor-resistant TEM-type β-lactamases: Mutations, specificity and three-dimensional structure. *Antimicrob Agents Chemother, 39*, 2593–2601.

Kobayashi, N., Nishino, K., & Yamaguchi, A. (2001) Novel macrolide-specific ABC-type efflux transporter in *Escherichia coli*. *J Bacteriol, 183*, 5639–5644.

Kollef, M. H. (2001). Is there a role for antibiotic cycling in the intensive care unit? *Crit Care Med, 29*, N135–N142.

Kollef, M. H., & Fraser, V. J. (2001). Antibiotic resistance in the intensive care unit. *Ann In Med, 134*, 298–314.

Kollef, M. H., Vlasnik, J., Sharpless, L., Pasque, C., Murphy, D., & Fraser, V. (1997). Schedule rotation of antibiotic classes. A strategy to decrease the incidence of ventilator associated pneumonia due to antibiotic-resistant Gram-negative bacteria. *Am J Respir Crit Care Med, 156*, 1040–1048.

Kollef, M. H., Ward, S., Sherman, G., Prentice, D., Schaiff, R., Huey, W., & Fraser, V. (2000). Inadequate treatment of nosocomial infections is associated with certain empiric antibiotic choice. *Crit Care Med, 28*, 3456–3464.

Laraki, N., Galleni, M., Thamm, I., Riccio, M. L., Amicosante, G., Frère, J. M., & Rossolini, G. M. (1999). Structure of In31, a *bla* $_{IMP}$-containing *Pseudomonas aeruginosa* integron phyletically related to In5, which carries an unusual array of gene cassettes. *Antimicrob Agents Chemother, 43*, 890–901.

Le Thomas, I., Coutdic, G., Clermont, O., Brahimi, N., Plesiat, P., & Bingen, E. (2001). *In vivo* selection of a target/efflux double mutant of *Pseudomonas aeruginosa* by ciprofloxacin therapy. *J Antimicrob Chemother, 48*, 553–555.

Levine, M. M., & Noriega, F. (1995). A review of the current status of enteric vaccines. *P N G Med J, 38*, 325–331.

Levy, S. B. (1997). Antibiotic resistance: An ecological imbalance. *Ciba Found Symp, 207*, 1–9.

Lipsitch, M., & Levin, B. R. (1997). The population dynamics of antimicrobial chemotherapy. *Antimicrob Agents Chemother, 41*, 363–373.

Livermore, D. M. (1995). β-lactamases in laboratory and clinical resistance. *Clin Microbiol Rev, 8*, 557–584.

Livermore, D. M., & Yuan, M. (1996). Antibiotic resistance and production of extended-spectrum β-lactamases amongst *Klebsiella* spp. from intensive care units in Europe. *J Antimicrob Chemother, 38*, 409–424.

Livermore, D. M., & Woodford, N. (2000). Carbapenemases: A problem in waiting? *Curr Opin Microbiol, 3*, 489–495.

Lomovskaya, O., Warren, M. S., Lee, A., Galazzo, J., Fronko, R., Lee, M., Blais, J., Cho, D., Chamberland, S., Renau, T., Leger, R., Hecker, S., Watkins, W., Hoshino, K., Ishida, H., & Lee, V. J. (2001). Identification and characterization of inhibitors of multidrug resistance efflux pumps in *Pseudomonas aeruginosa*: Novel agents for combination therapy. *Antimicrob Agents Chemother, 45*, 105–116.

Lowe, M. N., & Lamb, H. M. (2000). Gemifloxacin. *Drugs, 59*, 1137–1147.

Lu, T., Zhao, X., & Drlica, K. (1999). Gatifloxacin activity against quinolone-resistant gyrase: Allele-specific enhancement of bacteriostatic bactericidal activities by the C-8-methoxy group. *Antimicrob Agents Chemother, 43*, 2969–2974.

Maiti, S. N., Phillips, O. A., Micetich, R. G., & Livermore, D. M. (1998). Beta-lactamase inhibitors: Agents to overcome bacterial resistance. *Curr Med Chem, 5*, 441–456.

Martínez, J. L., & Baquero, F. (2000). Mutation frequencies and antibiotic resistance. *Antimicrob Agents Chemother, 44*, 1771–1777.

Martínez, J. L., Cercenado, E., Rodríguez-Creixems, M., Vicente-Pérez, M. F., Delgado-Iribarren, A., & Baquero, F. (1987). Resistance to beta-lactam/clavulanate. *Lancet, 8573*, 1473.

Martínez, J. L., Vicente, M. F., Delgado-Iribarren, A., Pérez-díaz, J. C., & Baquero, F. (1989). Small plasmids are involved in amoxycillin-clavulanate resistance in *Escherichia coli. Antimicrob Agents Chemother, 33*, 595.

Martínez-Freijó, P., Fluit, A. C., Schmitz, F. J., Grek, V. S. C., Verhoef, J., & Jones, M. E. (1998). Class 1 integrons in Gram-negative isolates from different European hospitals and associations with decreased susceptibility to multiple antibiotic compounds. *J Antimicrob Chemother, 42*, 689–696.

Martínez-Martínez, L., Pascual, A., & Jacoby, G. A. (1998). Quinolone resistance from a transferable plasmid. *Lancet, 351*, 797–799.

Martínez-Suárez, J., Martínez, J. L., López de Goicoechea, M. J., Pérez-Díaz, J. C., Baquero, F., Meseguer, M., & Baquero, F. (1987). Acquisition of antibiotic resistance plasmids *in vivo* by extraintestinal *Salmonella* spp. *J Antimicrob Chemother, 20*, 452–453.

Mason, H. S., Haq, T. A., Clements, J. D., & Arntzen, C. J. (1998). Edible vaccine protects mice against *Escherichia coli* heat-labile enterotoxin (LT): Potatoes expressing a synthetic LT-B gene. *Vaccine, 16*, 1336–1343.

Mazzariol, A., Tokue, Y., Kanegawa, T. M., Cornaglia, G., & Nikaido, H. (2000). High-level fluoroquinolone-resistant clinical isolates of *Escherichia coli* overproduce multidrug efflux protein AcrA. *Antimicrob Agents Chemother, 44*, 3441–3443.

McGowan, J. E., Jr. (2000). Strategies for study of the role of cycling on antimicrobial use and resistance. *Infect Control Hosp Epidemiol, 21,* S36–S43.

McGowan, J. E., Jr., & Gerding, D. N. (1996). Does antibiotic restriction prevent resistance? *New Horiz, 4,* 370–376.

McGowan, J. E., & Tenover, F. C. (1997). Control of antimicrobial resistance in the health care system. *Infect Dis Clin North Am, 11,* 297–311.

Mebis, J., Goossens, H., Bryneel, P., Sion, J. P., Meeus, I., van Droogenbroeck, J., Schroyens, W., & Berneman, Z. N. (1998). Decreasing antibiotic resistance of *Enterobacteriaceae* by introducing a new antibiotic combination therapy by neutropenic fever patients. *Leukemia, 12,* 1627–1629.

Medeiros, A. A. (1997). Evolution and dissemination of β-lactamases accelerated by generations of β-lactam antibiotics. *Clin Infect Dis, 24,* S19–S45.

Mendez, B., Tachibana, C., & Levy, S. B. (1980). Heterogeneity of tetracycline resistance determinants. *Plasmid, 3,* 99–108.

Meyer, K. S., Urban, C., Eagan, J. A., Berger, B. J., & Rahal, J. J. (1993). Nosocomial outbreak of *Klebsiella* infection resistant to late-generation cephalosporins. *Ann Intern Med, 119,* 353–358.

Miyazaki, S., Hosoyama, T., Furuya, N., Ishii, Y., Matsumoto, T., Ohno, A., Tateda, K., & Yamaguchi, K. (2001). *In vitro* and *in vivo* antibacterial activities of L-084, a novel oral carbapenem, against causative organisms of respiratory tract infections. *Antimicrob Agents Chemother, 82,* 203–207.

Moken, M. C., McMurry, L. M., & Levy, S. B. (1997). Selection of multiple-antibiotic-resistant (Mar) mutants of *Escherichia coli* by using the disinfectant pine oil: Roles of the *mar* and *acrAB* loci. *Antimicrob Agents Chemother, 41,* 2770–2772.

Monroe, S., & Polk, R. (2000). Antibimicrobial use and bacterial resistance. *Curr Opin Microbiol, 3,* 496–501.

Morosini, M. I., Ayala, J. A., Baquero, F., Martínez, J. L., & Blazquez, J. (2000). Biological cost of AmpC production for *Salmonella enterica* serotype Typhimurium. *Antimicrob Agents Chemother, 44,* 3137–3143.

Nakamura, S. (1997). Mechanisms of quinolone resistance. *J Infect Chemother, 3,* 128–138.

Neu, H. C. (1992). The crisis in antibiotic resistance. *Science, 257,* 1064–1073.

Nicolle, L. E. (2001). Preventing infections in non-hospital settings: Long-term care. *Emerg Infect Dis, 7,* 205–207.

Nikaido, H. (1998). Multiple antibiotic resistance and efflux. *Curr Opin Microbiol, 1,* 516–523.

Nishino, Y., Deguchi, T., Yasuda, M., Kawamura, T., Nakano, M., Kanematsu, E., Ozeki, S., & Kawada, Y. (1997). Mutations in the *gyrA* and *parC* genes associated with fluoroquinolone resistance in clinical isolates of *Citrobacter freundii*. *FEMS Microbiol Lett, 154,* 409–414.

NNIS. (1999). Intensive Care Antimicrobial Resistance Epidemiology (ICARE) surveillance report, data summary from January 1996 through December 1997: A report from the National Nosocomial Infections Surveillance (NNIS) System. *Am J Infect Control, 27,* 279–284.

Nordmann, P. (1998). Trends in β-lactam resistance among *Enterobacteriaceae*. *Clin Infect Dis, 27,* S1000–S1006.

Oethinger, M., Kern, W. V., Jellen-Ritter, A. S., McMurry, L. M., & Levy, S. B. (2000). Ineffectiveness of topoisomerase mutations in mediating clinically significant fluoroquinolone resistance in *Escherichia coli* in the absence of the AcrAB efflux pump. *Antimicrob Agents Chemother, 44,* 10–13.

Okusu, H., Ma, D., & Nikaido, H. (1996). AcrAB efflux pump plays a major role in the antibiotic resistance phenotype of *Escherichia coli* multiple-antibiotic-resistance (Mar) mutants. *J Bacteriol, 178,* 306–308.

Oliver, A., Pérez-Díaz, J. C., Coque, T. M., Baquero, F., & Cantón, R. (2000). Nucleotide sequence and characterization of a novel cetotaxime-hydrolyzing beta-lactamase (CTX-M-10) isolated in Spain. *Antimicrob Agents Chemother, 44,* 2549–2553.

Onion, C. W., & Bartzokas, C. A. (1998). Changing attitudes to infection management in primary care: A controlled trial of active versus passive guideline implementation. *Farm Pract, 15*, 99–104.

Osano, E., Arakawa, Y., Wacharotayankum, R., Ohta, M., Horii, T., Ito, H., Yoshimura, F., & Kato, N. (1994). Molecular characterization of an enterobacterial metallo-β-lactamase found in a clinical isolate of *Serratia marcescens* that shows imipenem resistance. *Antimicrob Agents Chemother, 38*, 71–78.

Osterblad, M., Hakanen, A., Manninen, R., Leistevuo, T., Peltonen, R., Meurman, O., Huovinen, P., & Kotilainen, P. (2000). A between-species comparison of antimicrobial resistance in enterobacteria in fecal flora. *Antimicrob Agents Chemother, 44*, 1479–1484.

Papanicolaou, G. A., Medeiros, A. A., & Jacoby, G. A. (1990). Novel-plasmid mediated β-lactamase (MIR-1) conferring resistance to oxyimino- and α-methoxy β-lactams in clinical isolates of *Klebsiella pneumoniae*. *Antimicrob Agents Chemother, 34*, 2200–2209.

Paterson, D. L., Mulazimoglu, L., Casellas, J. M., Ko, W. C., Goosens, H., Von Gottberg, A., Mohapatra, S., Trenholme, G. M., Klugman, K. P., McCormack, J. G., & Yu, V. L. (2000). Epidemiology of ciprofloxacin resistance and its relationship to extended-spectrum beta-lactamase production in *Klebsiella pneumoniae* isolates causing bacteremia. *Clin Infect Dis, 30*, 473–478.

Paterson, D. L., Singh, N., Rihs, J. D., Squier, C., Rihs, B. L., & Muder, R. R. (2001). Control of an outbreak of infection due to extended-spectrum ESBL producing *E. coli* in a liver transplantation unit. *Clin Infect Dis, 33*, 126–128.

Peng, H., & Marians, K. J. (1993). *Escherichia coli* topoisomerase IV. Purification, characterization, subunit structure, and subunit interactions. *J Biol Chem, 268*, 24481–24490.

Peña, C., Pujol, M., Ardanuy, C., Ricart, A., Pallares, R., Linares, J., Ariza, J., & Gudiol, F. (1998). Epidemiology and successful control of a large outbreak due to *Klebsiella pneumoniae* producing extended-spectrum β-lactamases. *Antimicrob Agents Chemother, 42*, 53–58.

Perry, C. M., Barman Balfour, J. A., & Lamb, H. M. (1999). Gatifloxacin. *Drugs, 58*, 683–696.

Pestotnik, S. L., Classen, D. C., Evans, R. S., & Burke, J. P. (1996). Implementing antibiotic practice guidelines through computer-assisted decision support: Clinical and financial outcomes. *Ann Intern Med, 12*, 884–890.

Philippon, A., Arlet, G., & Lagrange, P. H. (1994). Origin and impact of plasmid-mediated of extended spectrum β-lactamases. *Eur J Clin Microbiol Infect Dis, 13*, S17–S29.

Philippon, A., Arlet, G., & Jacoby, G. A. (2002). Plasmid-determined AmpC-type β-lactamases. *Antimicrob Agents Chemother, 46*, 1–11.

Piddock, L. J. V. (1999). Mechanisms of fluoroquinolone resistance: An update 1994–1998. *Drugs, 58*, S11–S18.

Poirel, L., Naas, T., Guibert, M., Chaibi, E. B., Labia, R., & Nordmann, P. (1999). Molecular and biochemical characterization of VEB-1, a novel class A extended-spectrum β-lactamase encoded by an *Escherichia coli* integron gene. *Antimicrob Agents Chemother, 43*, 573–581.

Poirel, L., Le Thomas, I., Naas, T., Karim, A., & Nordmann, P. (2000). Biochemical sequence analysis of GES-1, a novel class A extended-spectrum β-lactamase, and the class 1 Integron In52 from *Klebsiella pneumoniae*. *Antimicrob Agents Chemother, 44*, 622–632.

Poole, K. (2000). Efflux-mediated resistance to fluoroquinolones in Gram-negative bacteria. *Antimicrob Agents Chemother, 44*, 2233–2241.

Price, D. J. E., & Sleigh, J. D. (1970). Control infection due to *Klebsiella aerogenes* in a neurosurgical unit by withdrawal of all antibiotics. *Lancet, 7685*, 1213–1215.

Prinarakis, E. E., Miriagou, V., Tzelepi, E., Gazouli, M., & Tzouvelekis, L. S. (1997). Emergence of an inhibitor-resistant β-lactamase (SHV-10) derived from an SHV-5 variant. *Antimicrob Agents Chemother, 41*, 838–840.

Quinn, J. P. (1998). Clinical problems posed by multiresistant nonfermenting Gram-negative pathogens. *Clin Infect Dis, 27*, S117–S124.

Rahal, J. J., Urban, C., Horn, D., Freeman, K., Segal-Maurer, S., Maurer, J., Mariano, N., Marks, S., Burns, J. M., Dominick, D., & Lim, M. (1998). Class restriction of cephalosporin use to control total cephalosporin resistance in nosocomial *Klebsiella*. *JAMA, 280,* 1233–1237.

Reguera, J. A., Baquero, F., Pérez-Díaz, J. C., & Martínez, J. L. (1991). Factors determining resistance to β-lactam combined with β-lactamase inhibitors in *Escherichia coli*. *J Antimicrob Chemother, 27,* 569–575.

Rice, L. B., Eckstein, E. C., DeVente, J., & Shlaes, D. M. (1996). Ceftazidime-resistant *Klebsiella pneumoniae* isolates recovered at the Cleveland Department of Veteran Affairs Medical Center. *Clin Infect Dis, 23,* 118–124.

Richard, P., Delangle, M. H., Raffi, F., Espaze, E., & Richet, H. (2001). Impact of fluoroquinolone administration on the emergence of fluoroquinolone-resistant Gram-negative bacilli from gastrointestinal flora. *Clin Infect Dis, 32,* 162–166.

Rowe-Magnus, D. A., & Mazel, D. (1999). Resistance gene capture. *Curr Opin Microbiol, 2,* 483–488.

Saez-Llorens, X., Castrejon de Wong, M. M., Castano, E., De Suman, O., De Moros, D., & De Atencio, I. (2000). Impact of an antibiotic restriction policy on a hospital expenditures and bacterial susceptibility: A lesson from a pediatric institution in a developing country. *Ped Infect Dis J, 19,* 200–206.

Saier, M. H., Paulsen, I. T., Sliwinski, M. K., Pao, S. S., Skurray, R. A., & Nikaido, H. (1998). Evolutionary origins of multidrug and drug-specific efflux pumps in bacteria. *FASEB J, 12,* 265–274.

Sanders, W. E., Jr., & Sanders, C. C. (1997). Circumventing antibiotic resistance in specialized hospital units. *Clin Microbiol Infect, 3,* 272–273.

Schmitz, F. J., Hafner, D., Geisel, R., Follmann, P., Kirschke, C., Verhoef, J., Kohrer, K., & Fluit, A. C. (2001). Increased prevalence of class I integrons in *Escherichia coli, Klebsiella* species, and *Enterobacter* species isolates over a 7-year period in a German university hospital. *J Clin Microbiol, 39,* 3724–3726.

Shannon, K., Stapleton, P., Xiang, X., Johnson, A., Beattie, H., El Bakri, F., Cookson, B., & French, G. (1998). Extended-spectrum β-lactamase-producing *Klebsiella pneumoniae* strains causing nosocomial outbreaks of infection in the United Kingdom. *J Clin Microbiol, 36,* 3105–3110.

Shaw, K. J., Rather, P. N., Hare, R. S., & Miller, G. H. (1993). Molecular genetics of aminoglycoside resistance genes and familial relationships of the aminoglycoside-modifying enzymes. *Microbiol Rev, 57,* 138–163.

Shlaes, D. M., Gerding, D. N., John, J. F., Jr., Craig, W. A., Bornstein, D. L., Duncan, R. A., Eckman, M. R., Farrer, W. E., Greene, W. H., Lorian, V., Levy, S., McGowan, J. E., Jr., Paul, S. M., Ruskin, J., Tenover, F. C., & Watanakunakorn, C. (1997). Society for Healthcare Epidemiology of America and Infectious Diseases Society of America Joint Committee on the Prevention of Antimicrobial Resistance: Guidelines for the prevention of antimicrobial resistance in hospitals. *Infect Control Hosp Epidemiol, 18,* 275–291.

Sougakoff, W., Petit, A., Goussard, S., Sirot, D., Buré, A., & Courvalin, P. (1989). Characterization of the plasmid genes *bla* $_{T-4}$ and *bla* $_{T-5}$ which encode the broad-spectrum β-lactamases. *Gene, 78,* 339–348.

Struelens, M. J., Bly, B., Govaerts, D., De Gheldre, Y., Jacibs, E., Thys, J. P., Lievin, V., & Vincent, J. L. (1998). Modification of antibiotic policy associated with decrease in antibiotic-resistant Gram-negative bacilli in intensive care units. (Abstract K12). In Programs and abstracts 38th Interscience Conference on Antimicrobial Agents and Chemotherapy. American Society for Microbiolgy, p. 502.

Struelens, M. J., Byl, B., & Vincent, J. L. (1999). Antibiotic policy: A tool for controlling resistance of hospital pathogens. *Clin Microbiol Infect, 5,* S19–S24.

Sulavik, M. C., Houseweart, C., Cramer, C., Jiwani, N., Murgolo, N., Greene, J., DiDomenico, B., Shaw, K. J., Miller, G. H., Hare, R., & Shimer, G. (2001). Antibiotic susceptibility profiles of

Escherichia coli strains lacking multidrug efflux pump genes. *Antimicrob Agents Chemother, 45,* 1126–1136.

Sum, P. E., Sum, F. W., & Projan, S. J. (1998). Recent developments in tetracycline antibiotics. *Curr Pharm Des, 4,* 119–132.

Swartz, M. N. (1994). Hospital-acquired infections: Diseases with increasingly limited therapies. *Proc Natl Acad Sci USA, 91,* 2420–2427.

Tan, Y. T., Tillett, D. J., & McKay, I. A. (2000). Molecular strategies for overcoming antibiotic resistance in bacteria. *Mol Med Today, 6,* 309–314.

Thomson, K. S. (2001). Controversies about extended-spectrum and AmpC beta-lactamases. *Emerg Infect Dis, 7,* 333–336.

Toltzis, P., Yamashita, T., Vilt, L., Green, M., Morrissey, A., Spinner-Block, S., & Blumer, J. (1998). Antibiotic restriction does not alter endemic colonization with resistant Gram-negative rods in a pediatric intensive care unit. *Crit Care Med, 26,* 1893–1899.

Trouillet, J. L., Chastre, J., Vuagnat, A., Joly-Guillou, M. L., Combaux, D., Dombret, M. C., & Gibert, C. (1998). Ventilator-associated pneumonia caused by potentially drug-resistant bacteria. *Am J Respir Crit Care Med, 157,* 531–539.

Truong, Q. C., Quabdesselam, S., Hooper, D. C., Moreau, N. J., & Soussy, C. J. (1995). Sequential mutations of *gyrA* in *Escherichia coli* associated with quinolone therapy. *J Antimicrob Chemother, 36,* 1055–1059.

Tzouvelekis, L. S., & Bonomo, R. A. (1999). SHV-type β-lactamases. *Curr Pharmaceut Des, 5,* 847–864.

Tzouvelekis, L. S., Tzelepi, E., Tassios, P. T., & Legakis, N. J. (2000). CTX-M-Type β-lactamases: An emerging group of extended-spectrum enzymes. *Int J Antimicrob Agents, 14,* 137–142.

Urban, C., Mariano, N., Rahman, N., Queena, A., Montenegro, D., Bush, K., & Rahal, J. J. (2000). Detection of multirresistant ceftazidime-susceptible *Klebsiella pneumoniae* isolates lacking TEM-26 after class restriction of cephalosporins. *Microb Drug Resist, 6,* 297–303.

Van Belkum, A., Goessens, W., van Der Schee, C., Lemmens-Den Toom, N., Vos, M. C., Cornelissen, J., Lugtenburg, E., de Marie, S., Verbrugh, H., Lowenberg, B., & Endtz, H. (2001). Rapid emergence of ciprofloxacin-resistant *Enterobacteriaceae* containing multiple gentamicin resistance-associated integrons in a Dutch hospital. *Emerging Infect Dis, 7,* 862–871.

Van der Zwet, W. C., Parlevliet, G. A., Savelkoul, P. H., Stoof, J., Kaiser, A. M., Koeleman, J. G., & Vandenbroucke-Grauls, C. M. (1999). Nosocomial outbreak of gentamicin-resistant *Klebsiella pneumoniae* in a neonatal intensive care unit controlled by change in antibiotic policy. *J Hosp Infect, 42,* 295–302.

Van Kraaij, M. G., Dekker, A. W., Peters, E., Fluit, A., Verdonck, L. F., & Rozenberg-Arska, M. (1998). Emergence and infectious complications of ciprofloxacin-resistant *Escherichia coli* in haematological cancer patients. *Eur J Clin Microbiol Infect Dis, 17,* 591–592.

Verhoef, J., Acar, J. F., Gupta, R., & Jones, R. (1999). Surveillance of resistance against antimicrobial agents. *Int J Antimicrob Agents, 12,* 77–79.

Vila, J., Ruiz, J., Marco, F., Barcelo, A., Goñi, P., Giralt, E., & Jimenez de Anta, T. (1994). Association between double mutation in *gyrA* gene of ciprofloxacin-resistant clinical isolates of *Escherichia coli* and MICs. *Antimicrob Agents Chemother, 38,* 2477–2479.

Wagenlehner, F., Stower-Hoffmann, J., Schneider-Brachert, W., Naber, K. G., & Lehn, N. (2000). Influence of prophylactic single dose of ciprofloxacin on the level of resistance of *Escherichia coli* to fluoroquinolones in urology. *Int J Antimicrob Agents, 15,* 207–211.

Weigel, L. M., Steward, C. D., & Tenover, F. (1998). *gyrA* mutations associated with fluoroquinolone resistance in eight species of *Enterobacteriaceae*. *Antimicrob Agents Chemother, 42,* 2661–2667.

Weiss, W. J., Mikels, S. M., Petersen, P. J., Jacobus, N. V., Bitha, P., Lin, Y. I., & Testa, R. T. (1999). In vivo activities of peptidic prodrugs of novel aminomethyl tetrahydrofuranyl-1 beta-methylcarbapenems. *Antimicrob Agents Chemother, 43,* 460–464.

Weston, G. S., Blazquez, J., Baquero, F., & Shoichet, B. K. (1998). Structure-based enhancement of boronic acid-based inhibitors of AmpC beta-lactamase. *J Med Chem, 41*, 4577–4586.

White, A. C., Jr., Atmar, R. L., Wilson, J., Cate, T. R., Stager, C. E., & Greenberg, S. B. (1997). Effects of requiring prior authorization for selected antimicrobials expenditures, susceptibility, and clinical outcomes. *Clin Infect Dis, 25*, 230–239.

White, P. A., McIver, C. J., & Rawlinson, W. D. (2001). Integrons and gen cassetes in the *Enterobacteriaceae*. *Antimicrob Agents Chemother, 45*, 2658–2661.

White, R. L., Friedrich, L. V., Mihm, L. B., & Bosso, J. A. (2000). Assessment of the relationship between antimicrobial usage and susceptibility: Differences between hospitals and specific patient-care areas. *Clin Infect Dis, 31*, 16–23.

Wiener, J., Quinn, J. P., Bradford, P. A., Goering, R. V., Nathan, C., Bush, K., & Weinstein, R. A. (1999). Multiple antibiotic-resistant *Klebsiella* and *Escherichia coli* in nursing homes. *JAMA, 281*, 517–523.

Winokour, P. L., Cantón, R., Casellas, J. M., & Legakis, N. (2001). Variations in the prevalence of strains expressing an extended-spectrum β-lactamase phenotype and characterization of isolates from Europe, the Americas, and the Western Pacific region. *Clin Infect Dis, 32*, S94–S103.

World Health Organization. (2000). Overcoming antibiotic resistance. World Health Organization Report in Infectious Diseases 2000.

Yates, R. R. (1999). New intervention strategies for reducing antibiotic resistance. *Chest, 115*, 24S–27S.

Yigit, H., Queenan, A. M., Anderson, G. J., Domenech-Sánchez, A., Biddle, J. W., Steward, C. H. D., Alberti, S., Bush, K., & Tenover, F. (2001). Novel carbapenem-hydrolyzing β-lactamase, KPC-1, from a carbapenem-resistant strain of *Klebsiella pneumoniae*. *Antimicrob Agents Chemother, 45*, 1151–1161.

Yuan, M., Aucken, H., Hall, L. M. C., Pitt, T. L., & Livermore, D. M. (1998). Epidemiological typing of *Klebsiellae* with extended-spectrum β-lactamases from European intensive care units. *J Antimicrob Chemother, 41*, 527–539.

Zervos, M. J., Bacon, A. E., Patterson, J. E., Schaberg, D. R., & Kauffman, C. A. (1988). Enterococcal superinfection in patients treated with ciprofloxacin. *J Antimicrob Chemother, 21*, 113–115.

Zhao, X., Xu, C., Domagala, J., & Drlica, K. (1997). DNA topoisomerase targets of the fluoro-quinolones: A strategy for avoiding bacterial resistance. *Proc Natl Acad Sci USA, 94*, 13991–13996.

Zhao, X., & Drlica, K. (2001). Restricting the selection of antibiotic-resistant mutants: A general strategy derived from fluoroquinolone studies. *Clin Infect Dis, 33*, S147–S156.

Zhou, J., Dong, Y., Zhao, X., Lee, S., Amin, A., Ramaswamy, S., Domagala, J., Musser, J. M., & Drlica, K. (2000). Selection of antibiotic-resistant bacterial mutants: Allelic diversity among fluoroquinolone-resistant mutations. *J Infect Dis, 182*, 517–525.

7

Multidrug-Resistant Tuberculosis (MDRTB)

Philip Spradling and Renee Ridzon

1. OVERVIEW

1.1. History

Drug-resistant tuberculosis (TB), in the clinically relevant sense, is a man-made phenom-enon, the history of which dates back to the advent of antituberculosis chemotherapy. Soon after its introduction, Pyle (1947) described resistance to streptomycin, the probable exis-tence of a heterogeneous population of organisms in persons harboring large numbers of *Mycobacterium tuberculosis* bacilli (some of which were naturally resistant), and the potential for a single drug to exert a selective and promoting effect on these resistant populations. The hypothesis of innately resistant variants was confirmed in 1952, when Lederberg and Lederberg demonstrated that resistance of the tubercle bacillus to anti-microbial agents was not created by the action of a drug upon a particular organism, but a process whereby pre-existing resistant variants within a population of organisms were effectively selected for survival. In 1955, Cavalli-Sforza and Lederberg confirmed the spontaneous origin of streptomycin-resistant variants by the use of repetitive subcultures in liquid medium. Concurrent observations attested to the occurrence of isoniazid resist-ance shortly after its introduction. Middlebrook (1952) demonstrated that the incidence of isoniazid-resistant variants of *M. tuberculosis* was even greater than with streptomycin, and that these resistant strains had little or no catalase activity (Middlebrook, 1954).

From a clinical standpoint, bacillary population size and the ability to multiply were identified as two critical prerequisites for the emergence of bacterial resistance. Studies of resected pulmonary tissue from patients without prior chemotherapy permitted estimations of bacillary populations within various tuberculous lesions. Canetti (1965) estimated populations in cavities and hard casseous foci to be on the order of 10^7–10^9 and 10^2–10^4 organisms, respectively. By demonstrating that streptomycin resistance occurred more fre-quently during treatment of cavitary versus non-cavitary TB, Howard et al. (1949) and Howlett et al. (1949) showed a fundamental link between antimicrobial resistance and

Reemergence of Established Pathogens in the 21st Century
Edited by Fong and Drlica, Kluwer Academic/Plenum Publishers, New York, 2003

large initial bacillary populations. Expanding upon the work of Pyle, Crofton and Mitchison (1948) described the clinical manifestations of the process of selection and subsequent growth of resistant variants, during which large numbers of drug-susceptible bacilli are destroyed by a single drug, while drug-resistant bacilli are not, resulting in the permissive proliferation of drug-resistant variants (Crofton & Mitchison, 1948; Mitchison, 1950). Upon replication, these drug-resistant variants constitute a greater proportion of the population of infecting organisms. This phenomenon became known as the "fall and rise" phenomenon, and remains a practical means of detecting by sputum microscopy, the presence of drug resistance and incipient treatment failure after an apparent initial response.

Over the following years, as new antituberculosis drugs were developed, descriptions of resistance to individual agents, and cross-resistance among agents from particular drug classes, generally ensued (Canetti, 1962; Middlebrook, 1954; Mitchison, 1965, 1984; Wehrli, 1988; Yeager et al., 1952). Though all drugs used against TB were shown capable of inducing resistance by selection of pre-existing resistant variants, the rapidity and extent to which this occurs with the use of individual agents varied. Canetti (1965) found that the capacity of a single antituberculosis agent to augment the selection of resistant variants was dependent upon attainable drug concentrations of the agent in vivo, and a consequence of the drug's ability to more fully eradicate drug-susceptible portions of the microbial population. Later, David (1970) showed that the frequency of spontaneously resistant variants in a sample of wild-type mycobacteria should be 3.5×10^{-6} for isoniazid, 3.8×10^{-6} for streptomycin, 3.1×10^{-8} for rifampin, and 0.5×10^{-4} for ethambutol. Based on these frequencies, the probability of a naturally occurring bacillus that is resistant to isoniazid and rifampin would be the product of frequencies, or roughly 1 in 10^{14}.

It was evident, then, that successful treatment of TB and the prevention of drug resistance hinged upon the use of multiple chemotherapeutic agents, particularly in the early phases of treatment when bacterial populations were large enough to contain significant numbers of naturally occurring drug-resistant variants. As a result, two phases in the chemotherapy for TB were described; the initial phase, when numbers of organisms are high, and the second, "continuation," phase, when smaller numbers of organisms require a prolonged chemotherapeutic approach to ensure eradication (Canetti, 1962). This strategy continues to be the guiding principle of modern antituberculosis therapy.

More recently, some molecular determinants for resistance to the two most powerful antituberculosis drugs, isoniazid and rifampin, have been elucidated. Zhang et al. (1992) demonstrated the restoration of isoniazid susceptibility after transfer of the katG gene into isoniazid-resistant M. tuberculosis, providing strong evidence to support that the lack of catalase-peroxidase is in part associated with isoniazid resistance. Mutations in the gene encoding for the InhA protein have also been associated with isoniazid resistance (Rouse et al., 1995). Rifampin-resistant M. tuberculosis has been shown to have mutations in the region of the rpoB gene, a gene that is able to confer rifampin resistance (Telenti et al., 1993).

1.2. Definition

Although the term multidrug-resistant TB (MDRTB) has been used to described resistance to any two or more antituberculosis drugs, the more recently accepted definition is resistance to at least isoniazid and rifampin. This designation is not arbitrary, because no two other antituberculosis drugs have as profound an impact on the success of TB treatment than do these two agents. Initially synthesized in 1912, and used first in clinical trials in 1951, isoniazid remains one of the most important compounds used to treat TB disease and latent *M. tuberculosis* infection (LTBI). It is bactericidal against *M. tuberculosis*, well absorbed from the gastrointestinal tract, and penetrates well into all body fluids and cavities, producing concentrations similar to those found in serum.

Rifampin, derived from a class of compounds initially isolated from forest soil and produced by the fungus *Amycolatopsis mediterranei*, is also bactericidal, relatively nontoxic, and easily administered. In their description of rifampin as the most potent of antituberculosis agents in terms of sputum culture conversion, Dickinson and Mitchison (1981) ascribed the "sterilizing" effect of rifampin to its ability to affect dormant *M. tuberculosis* organisms that are metabolically active for only short periods of time.

The importance of rifampin to multiple drug regimens for the treatment of TB cannot be overemphasized. As a result of its powerful bactericidal effect and sterilizing capacity, the inclusion of rifampin in antituberculosis regimens allows for a much shorter course of treatment. This is principally the consequence of the drug's effect on shortening the duration of the continuation phase of treatment, when relatively small numbers of slow-growing organisms persist in tuberculous lesions. Multiple large clinical trials conducted in the 1970s and 1980s demonstrated that use of rifampin (with pyrazinamide) in multidrug regimens could shorten the duration of treatment from 18 to 24 months to 6 to 9 months (Algerian Working Group/British Medical Research Council Cooperative Study, 1984; British Thoracic and Tuberculosis Association, 1975; British Thoracic Association, 1982; Hong Kong Chest Service/British Medical Research Council, 1987; Snider et al., 1984).

The terms "primary" and "acquired" resistance (among others) have been used to differentiate between cases of drug-resistant TB that either have (acquired) or have not (primary) received previous treatment. Such terms, however, may inappropriately suggest the exact causative nature of drug resistance in a patient, which in many cases may not be possible to assess. Patients may be erroneously labeled as having "primary" drug resistance if they do not disclose previous treatment for TB. Conversely, patients who fail treatment (and therefore labeled with acquired resistance) may do so because their strain was initially resistant and not because it acquired resistance during the course of treatment. In the most recent global survey of antituberculosis drug resistance, the World Health Organization (WHO) and the International Union Against Tuberculosis and Lung Disease (IUATLD) recommend the terms "drug resistance among new cases" (for cases with less than 1 month of antituberculosis treatment in the past) and "resistance among previously treated cases" (cases with at least 1 month of treatment in the past), instead of primary resistance and acquired resistance (WHO, 2000a). Previously treated cases are often referred to as "retreatment" cases.

1.3. Public Health Importance

Without the benefit of use of the two most powerful antituberculosis drugs, treatment of TB cases resistant to both isoniazid and rifampin represents a highly formidable clinical challenge. The loss of susceptibility to isoniazid and rifampin greatly diminishes the chances of cure, increases the cost and morbidity of treatment, and can dramatically increase mortality, particularly among immunocompromised patients. In the larger context of public health, diminished rates of cure mean that patients with MDRTB may have an increased propensity to transmit drug-resistant *M. tuberculosis* isolates to other persons. Unlike regimens for the treatment of drug-susceptible TB, which have been established as the result of extensive clinical trials conducted over several decades, treatment regimens for MDRTB are not clearly defined. Therefore, treatment of patients with MDRTB requires significant expertise and the use of largely empiric regimens (guided by specialized drug susceptibility to the so-called second line antituberculosis agents) of comparatively untested clinical utility.

In 1994, WHO, IUATLD, and several partners initiated the Global Project on Antituberculosis Drug Resistance Surveillance, also referred to as the "Global Project." Since then, two reports on the prevalence and trends in the global epidemiology of MDRTB have been published, and will be more fully discussed in subsequent portions of this chapter (WHO, 1997, 2000). Both reports have highlighted the ubiquitous nature of drug resistance, and have illustrated that MDRTB is a worldwide phenomenon.

In addition to a review of the epidemiology of MDRTB, which is to follow, this chapter will review the pathophysiology, transmission, diagnosis, treatment, and prevention of MDRTB. An additional section will focus on the impact of human immunodeficiency virus (HIV) infection on the epidemiology, transmission, and treatment of MDRTB.

2. EPIDEMIOLOGY

2.1. Domestic

With the cooperation of state and local health departments, the Centers for Disease Control and Prevention (CDC) has collected data on the number of reported TB cases for the purpose of national surveillance since 1953. Before 1993, however, no national data were systematically collected with regard to drug susceptibility test results of incident TB cases. Prior to that, a number of nationwide surveys of selected hospitals and health departments throughout the United States were conducted to ascertain the degree of drug-resistant TB. Kent (1993) reviewed several surveys conducted by the CDC since the early 1960s of drug resistance among new cases of TB. All the surveys were conducted on non-random samples of hospital, state, and city laboratories over three time periods. These surveys allow some analyses in trends of antituberculosis drug resistance, although none was done in the same location or carried out in the same manner. In the first survey, from 1961 to 1968, involving 22 hospitals and sanatoria, the rate of resistance to a single drug was 3.5% and 1.0% to two or more drugs, and the rate of resistance did not rise over the 8-year period of the survey (Doster et al., 1976). A second survey, covering March 1975 through September 1982, involved 20 city and state laboratories and reported rates of resistance to a single and two or more drugs of 6.9% and 2.3%, respectively (CDC, 1983). As with the first survey, younger age groups had significantly higher rates of primary drug resistance, although overall rates of resistance declined over the survey period. Resistance to rifampin, in use since 1972, was rare (<0.01%). A third survey, for the period March 1982 through March 1986, involved 31 health departments and reported a rate of drug resistance among new cases of 9% (Snider et al., 1991). Despite the higher reported rate of resistance than the second survey, methodological differences between the second and third surveys were such that the latter report likely did not represent a true increase in the rate of primary drug resistance. Resistance to rifampin reported in the third survey remained rare (0.6%) and actually declined over the period of the survey. Of note, this survey reported a rate of resistance to both isoniazid and rifampin of 0.5%. Overall, these three surveys, despite absolute differences in the rates of primary drug resistance, suggested that nationwide rates remained stable or declined during the periods of survey.

In contrast, a number of regional surveys reported higher rates of drug resistance among new TB cases and higher overall rates of MDRTB. A survey conducted at a California hospital for the period 1969 through 1984 reported rates of drug resistance among new cases of 23% and among retreatment cases of 59%, and noted overall rates of MDRTB as high as 12% as early as 1972 (Ben-Dov & Mason, 1987). Stottmeier (1976) described the emergence of rifampin resistance in Massachusetts soon after its introduction in antituberculosis regimens, noting that most of the rifampin-resistant isolates were also resistant to other antituberculosis drugs and illustrating the potential for transmission of rifampin-resistant bacilli. In a survey of pediatric patients in New York City, new TB cases with isolates resistant to isoniazid and which were MDRTB were 9.7% and 6.7%, respectively, both of which exceeded rates of adults in the region at that time (Steiner et al., 1970). Although national surveys reported relatively low rates of drug resistance (and MDR) throughout the 1970s and 1980s, it was apparent that in some urbanized regions of the country and among certain age groups, the prevalence of drug resistance and MDR was higher. Moreover, the appearance of drug resistance among new TB cases and younger age groups demonstrated that recent transmission of drug-resistant *M. tuberculosis* isolates from inadequately treated patients was occurring, a phenomenon that would later assume much greater importance in the late 1980s and early 1990s during several large institutional outbreaks of MDRTB. From a national perspective, however, the continuation of drug resistance surveys did not appear warranted. In 1986, given resource constraints and competing priorities, the CDC discontinued surveillance of antituberculosis drug resistance (Snider et al., 1991).

In 1990, after the CDC, in collaboration with state and local health departments, investigated outbreaks of drug-resistant TB in two hospitals, one in Miami (Beck-Sague et al., 1992) and one in New York City (Edlin et al., 1992), interest in ongoing drug resistance surveillance intensified. The first comprehensive nationwide survey of antituberculosis drug resistance was conducted for the first quarter of 1991 and included all incident culture-positive TB cases in the United States with drug susceptibility test results (Bloch et al., 1994). Resistance to one or more drugs was found in 14.2% of cases and resistance to isoniazid and/or rifampin was 9.5%. MDRTB was found in 3.5% of cases, existing in 35 counties in 13 states. New York City accounted for 61.4% of the nation's MDRTB cases, with the relative risk of MDRTB much higher among racial and ethnic minorities than among White patients. In another survey of drug resistance among TB patients in New York City, rates of MDRTB were 15% and 14% for the first quarters of 1991 and 1992, respectively (Driver et al., 1994). Patients with MDRTB were as likely to be U.S. born as to be foreign-born, although more likely to be younger.

Responding to this growing public health crisis, the National MDRTB Task Force rec-ommended in 1992 that drug susceptibility testing be performed on initial *M. tuberculosis* isolates from each TB patient and that the results be reported to CDC. In 1993, CDC inten-sified TB surveillance with an expanded version of a Report of a Verified Case of TB (RVCT) form intended for use by state and local health departments. Additional data col-lected through the use of the RVCT included results of drug susceptibility testing, treat-ment used, HIV testing, occupation, history of substance abuse, homelessness, residence in a correctional or long-term care facility, and additional data related to outcomes of anti-tuberculosis therapy (CDC, 1994).

Subsequent to the implementation of expanded TB surveillance, Moore et al. (1997) described the results of the first 4 years (1993–1996) of national surveillance for drug resistance among all reported TB case patients in the United States. Overall resistance to isoniazid and rifampin was 2.2%; rates of MDRTB were significantly higher for patients with a prior episode of TB, but rates were similar for U.S. and foreign-born cases. MDRTB cases occurred in 41 states; 38% of cases of MDRTB were reported from New York City. Although the proportion of MDRTB cases in the United States decreased from the previ-ous survey, the decline was largely attributed to the fall in the number of MDRTB cases in New York City.

The CDC continues to monitor the rates of MDRTB annually. From 1993 through 2000, the number of MDRTB cases in the United States among cases declined from 485 to 141. Over this period, however, the proportion of MDRTB in foreign-born persons in the United States has substantially increased. Of the 485 cases in 1993, 30.9% occurred in foreign-born persons, while in 2000, the proportion had increased to 71.6% of all MDRTB cases in the United States (CDC, 2001).

2.2. International

Unlike recent trends in the U.S. and other established market economies, reports of MDRTB have been increasing rapidly in many different areas of the world, and represent an unprecedented public health threat. Initially, efforts to ascertain the extent of antituber-culosis drug resistance were hampered by problems with laboratory quality and epidemio-logical methods, particularly in less affluent countries. In a review of 63 surveys of resistance to antituberculosis drugs that were performed between 1985 and 1994, the rates of resistance were compared between isolates from patients with (retreatment) and with-out (new) previous treatment (Cohn et al., 1997). Among isolates from new TB cases, rates of resistance were as follows: isoniazid (median, 4.1%), streptomycin (median, 3.5%), rifampin (median, 0.2%), and ethambutol (median, 0.1%). For retreatment cases, however, rates of resistance were much higher, and the median rate of resistance to isoniazid was 10.6%, to streptomycin, 4.9%, to rifampin, 2.4%, and to ethambutol, 1.8%. In this review, the rates of MDRTB among new cases ranged from 0 to 10.8% (median, 0.5%); however, among retreatment cases, the rates were startling: Nepal (48.0%), Gujarat, India (33.8%), New York City (30.1%), Bolivia (15.3%), and Korea (14.5%).

As a result, the WHO and IUATLD established the global project on antituberculosis drug resistance surveillance in 1994. The aim of the project was to determine the levels of resistance to isoniazid, rifampin, ethambutol, and streptomycin in nationally representative populations using standardized methods, and a network of supranational reference laboratories was established to provide quality assurance through validation of susceptibility data. Emphasis was placed on sampling methods to ensure representativeness and on differentiating new from retreatment TB cases, so that the quality of national TB programs (NTP) and the degree of transmission of drug-resistant *M. tuberculosis* could be determined. In this schema, the degree of drug resistance among new TB cases was a measure of the degree of transmission of drug-resistant *M. tuberculosis*, whereas the degree of resistance among retreatment cases was an indicator of the extent to which patients with TB were appropriately treated. Two rounds of the global survey were completed by 2000, the first covering 1994–1996 (Pablos-Mendez et al., 1998) and the second, 1996–1999 (Espinal et al., 2001a, 2001b). Seventy-two countries or regions within countries were included in at least one of the surveys, and isolates from over 118,000 patients were tested. Twenty-eight areas participated in both surveys, thus allowing trends in drug resistance to be determined. For the two surveys combined, the data covered geographic areas representing 33% of the world population. The results of the surveys showed that while drug-resistant TB cases constituted a relatively small proportion of all cases worldwide, the problem of drug resistance was present in every country surveyed (Cegielski et al., 2002).

In the second survey, for new TB cases, the median resistance to any of the four first-line antituberculosis drugs (isoniazid, rifampin, ethambutol, or streptomycin) drugs was 11%, with a range of 1.7–37%. Resistance to isoniazid and streptomycin predominated, while rates of resistance to rifampin and ethambutol were much lower. The median prevalence of MDRTB was 1%, with a range of 0–14.1%. Seven geographic areas had particularly high levels of MDRTB (>5%) among new cases; four of these sites (Estonia, Latvia, and Ivanovo and Tomsk Oblasts of the Russian Federation) were in the former Soviet Union. Eight sites, all in Western Europe, had no detectable MDRTB (WHO, 2002). Figure 7.1 shows the prevalence of MDRTB and any other drug resistance among new TB for 1996–1999.

With regard to new cases, 28 sites provided data for at least 2 years between 1994 and 1999. In a few middle-income countries (Estonia and Peru), as well as in three high-income, low-incidence countries (Denmark, Germany, and New Zealand), there was a significant rise in the rates of isoniazid and streptomycin resistance, while the rates of resistance to rifampin and ethambutol remained stable. Most notably, rates of MDRTB did not increase in any of these geographic areas. In contrast, rates of MDRTB among new cases are alarming in the former Soviet Union regions surveyed, ranging from 4.0% to 14.4% among new TB cases. Whether these focal surveys reflect the whole picture of MDRTB in the former Soviet Union, however, is unclear. Additional surveys are vitally needed in other areas of the former Soviet Union to gain a more representative perspective of the problem (Cegielski et al., 2002).

Among retreatment cases in the global surveys, resistance to isoniazid and streptomycin were highest; the duration of treatment showed a dose-response effect. Prior treatment of greater than 12 months duration had a stronger impact on the prevalence of MDRTB than did prior treatment ranging from 6 to 12 months. Among the 58 countries or regions surveyed, the prevalence of isoniazid resistance was again the highest, but resistance to rifampin was second, unlike the situation among new cases. For MDRTB, the prevalence ranged from 0% to 48.2%, with a median of 9.1%. Among retreatment cases

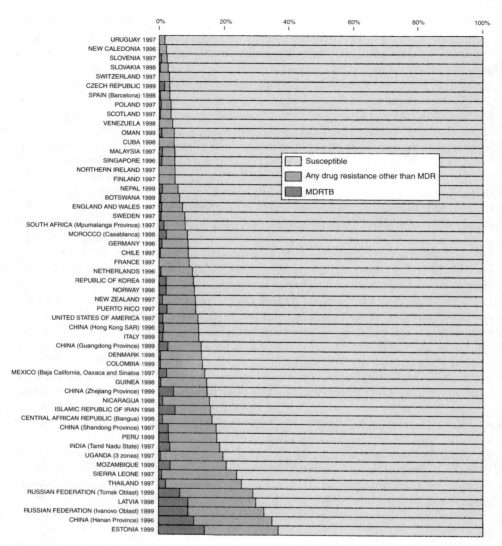

Figure 7.1. Prevalence of multidrug-resistant tuberculosis (MDRTB) and any other drug resistance among new TB cases, 1996–1999 (source, with permission of the publisher: World Health Organization. (2000). Antituberculosis drug resistance in the world, report no. 2: Prevalence and trends. Geneva, Switzerland [WHO/CDS/TB/2000.278]).

from countries or regions surveyed at least twice, Korea reported significant decreases in MDRTB; Estonia reported an increase in the prevalence of MDRTB, from 19.2% in 1994 to 37.8% in 1998. In other countries twice surveyed, the prevalence of MDRTB among retreatment cases remained stable or fell slightly (WHO, 2000). Figure 7.2 displays the prevalence of MDRTB and any other drug resistance among retreatment TB cases for

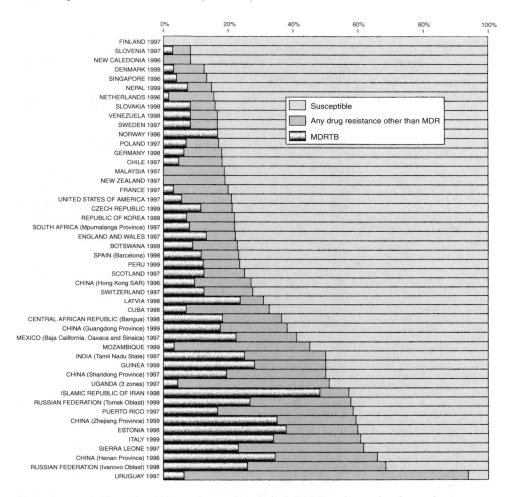

Figure 7.2. Prevalence of multidrug-resistant tuberculosis (MDRTB) and any other drug resistance among previously treated TB cases, 1996–1999 (source, with permission of the publisher: World Health Organization. (2000). Antituberculosis drug resistance in the world, report no. 2: Prevalence and trends. Geneva, Switzerland [WHO/CDS/TB/2000.278]).

1996–1999, and Figure 7.3 shows the prevalence for the same period for both new and retreatment cases. Figure 7.4 displays the global distribution of combined MDRTB prevalence for the same period.

A recent report provided the first comprehensive incidence estimates of the MDRTB burden for the 136 countries that constitute 97% of the total world population (Dye et al., 2002). Although the lower and upper bounds of the calculations differed by a factor of two, the number of incident MDRTB cases in 2000 was estimated at 273,000 (95% confidence

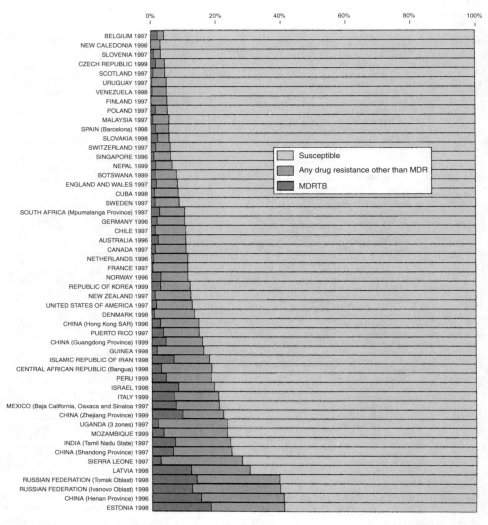

Figure 7.3. Prevalence of combined multidrug-resistant tuberculosis (MDRTB) and any other drug resistance, 1996–1999 (source, with permission of the publisher: World Health Organization. (2000). Antituberculosis drug resistance in the world, report no. 2: Prevalence and trends. Geneva, Switzerland [WHO/CDS/TB/2000.278]).

limits, 185,000 and 414,000), representing 3.2% of all incident TB cases. Nine countries (China, India, Pakistan, Philippines, Russia, Ethiopia, Nigeria, Sudan, and Afghanistan) were each estimated to have over 5,000 incident MDRTB cases in 2000; China and India each were estimated to have over 60,000 MDRTB cases. Given this unprecedented burden, the authors concluded that even with the favorable prices of second-line antituberculosis

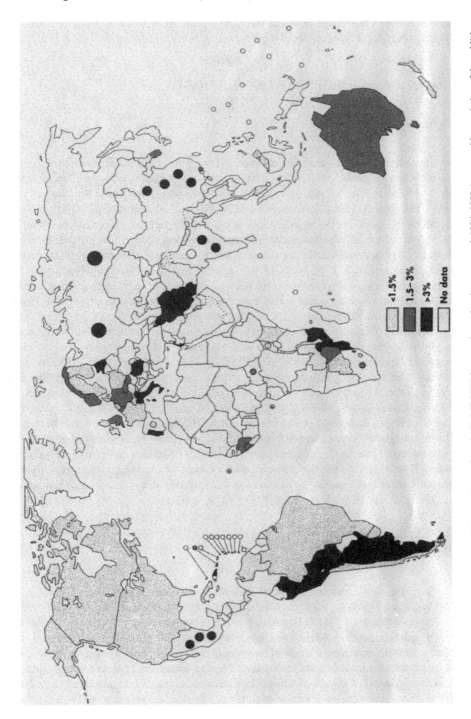

Figure 7.4. Prevalence of combined multidrug-resistant tuberculosis (MDRTB) in countries and regions surveyed, 1994–1999 (source, with permission of the publisher: World Health Organization. (2000). Antituberculosis drug resistance in the world, report no. 2: Prevalence and trends. Geneva, Switzerland [WHO/CDS/TB/2000.278]).

drugs offered through the WHO, it would likely cost more to treat the 3.2% of incident TB cases that were MDRTB than all other incident cases combined.

3. PRODUCTION AND PERPETUATION OF MDRTB

3.1. Mechanisms of Resistance

As mentioned at the outset of this chapter, MDRTB is a man-made phenomenon created primarily by inadequacies introduced by health care providers and, on a larger scale, TB control programs. Bluntly put, "you cannot cure multidrug-resistant TB as fast as you can create it" (Enarson, 2000). Patients with MDRTB must be "produced," and if persons with infectious MDRTB are not quickly identified and treated, they have the potential to transmit drug-resistant *M. tuberculosis* to others, thereby producing "new" MDRTB cases.

One way of producing MDRTB cases is through the use of repeated cycles of antituberculosis monotherapy. The problem of antituberculosis monotherapy arises from the existence of small numbers of resistant bacilli that develop through random, non-linked, spontaneous mutations. For patients with paucibacillary conditions resulting from exposure to drug-susceptible organisms (e.g., LTBI), the probability of the existence of these resistant variants is clinically irrelevant. In such a situation, treatment with a single bactericidal agent is sufficient and effective and will not result in the emergence of resistance. If, on the other hand, the patient has a large number of bacilli, as seen with extensive cavitary disease, harboring 10^9 or more tubercle bacilli, then there is a high probability that organisms resistant to a single agent are present. Since mutations conferring resistance to different drugs occur independently, the likelihood of simultaneous mutations conferring resistance to multiple drugs is equal to the product of the mutation rates for the individual drugs. In this respect, the anticipated probability of resistance to isoniazid and rifampin of a single tubercle bacillus is approximately 1 in 10^{14}. Even in the setting of cavitary pulmonary TB in which the bacillary burden may exceed 10^9 organisms, the probability of simultaneous mutations leading to resistance to multiple drugs is exceedingly small (Canetti, 1964; David, 1970; Mitchison, 1984). How, then, are such cases produced?

3.2. Clinical Errors

Errors in the clinical management of patients with either drug-susceptible or drug-resistant TB can lead to those patients developing MDRTB. Mahmoudi and Iseman (1993) described a case series of MDRTB patients referred to the National Jewish Center for Immunology and Respiratory Medicine from 1989 through 1990, identifying the common errors that led to the acquisition of antituberculosis drug resistance. Standards of practice were based on treatment guidelines promulgated by the American Thoracic Society (ATS), CDC, and the American College of Chest Physicians. Six common errors were identified: (1) addition of a single drug to a failing regimen (2) inadequate primary regimen, (3) failure to recognize initial or acquired resistance, (4) failure to recognize and deal with non-adherence, and (5) failure to provide directly observed therapy. Of the 35 cases reviewed, management errors were detected in 28, with an average nearly 4 errors per case. As a result of these treatment errors, the authors calculated that prolonged hospitalization, use of toxic second-line drugs, and high-risk resectional surgery, cost an average of $180,000 (in 1990 dollars) per patient. Another report described treatment errors by private practitioners, including chest physicians, and found that 50% of patients cared for outside the TB control program received treatment that deviated for CDC/ATS guidelines (Liu et al., 1998).

Failure to obtain or delays in obtaining the results of drug susceptibility tests (DST) may also lead to delays in the diagnosis of drug-resistant TB. Isolation and identification of *M. tuberculosis* by commonly used methods, such as Lowenstein–Jensen or Middlebrook 7H11 may require approximately 6–8 weeks, and DST of the isolates may require an additional 2–3 weeks. This extremely slow growth rate and the need for special laboratory containment facilities may complicate laboratory diagnosis. Although more rapid and reliable methods had been developed, many were not in widespread use in the early 1990s after the resurgence of TB had been recognized. In the first quarter of 1991, even after large outbreaks of MDRTB had occurred, only 60% of *M. tuberculosis* isolates had undergone DST (CDC, 1992a). Clearly, delays in the diagnosis of MDRTB, occasioned either by the unavailability or the failure to perform DST, prevent the timely and appropriate treatment of MDRTB and result in the clinical deterioration of patients, the development of additional drug resistance, and the continued transmission of MDR *M. tuberculosis* isolates.

3.3. Host Factors

Other host-related factors, apart from patient non-adherence, may contribute to the development of drug-resistant TB, particularly in the case of concurrent illnesses that impair drug absorption or require medications that interact with antituberculosis drugs. Malabsorption of antituberculosis agents has been described in patients with AIDS (Berning et al., 1992; Gordon et al., 1993; Patel et al., 1995; Peloquin et al., 1996; Sahai et al., 1997), and an association between HIV infection and primary rifampin monoresistance has been reported (Lutfey et al., 1996; Munsiff & Frieden, 1996; Nolan et al. 1995). Because its inclusion in treatment regimens greatly reduces the necessary duration of therapy, resistance to rifampin alone may seriously jeopardize the overall success of treatment. Ridzon et al. (1998) reported on a case-control study of risk factors for rifampin monoresistance, finding that HIV-infected cases were more likely than matched controls to have a history of diarrhea, prior rifabutin use, and antifungal therapy. In this group, rifampin monoresistance was associated with the use of rifabutin for the prevention or treatment of *M. avium* complex infection, which was consistent with previous reports and concern about its use on the emergence of rifampin resistance (Bishai et al., 1996; Reichman et al., 1994). In addition, drug–drug interactions between rifamycins and azole compounds have been described (Narang et al., 1994; Trapnell et al., 1996). Acquired rifamycin monoresistance has also been associated with widely spaced (once or twice weekly) intermittent rifamycin-containing regimens (CDC, 2002; Vernon et al., 1999).

3.4. Transmission and Outbreaks

The question of whether drug-resistant *M. tuberculosis* bacilli are less likely than drug-susceptible strains to produce infection and disease has persisted for decades. Although early studies using animal models suggested that drug-resistant bacilli were attenuated and less likely to produce disease (Cohn, 1970; Middlebrook & Cohn, 1953), other reports have demonstrated that transmission of drug-resistant *M. tuberculosis* occurs, even among immunocompetent persons (Kenyon et al., 1997; Ridzon et al., 1997a, 1997b). Another report found that the risk of infection among contacts of isoniazid- and strepto-mycin-resistant TB cases was no lower than that among contacts of drug-susceptible cases (Snider et al., 1985). A recent study reported limited transmission of MDR *M. tuberculosis* among patients in Los Angeles County, California (Nitta et al., 2002). In this report, the authors based their conclusions in part on the low number of skin test conversions among contacts of active cases; however, a large proportion of the contacts were foreign-born and likely were ineligible to meet the authors' definition of conversion. However, in a study assessing the relative "fitness," or the ability of *M. tuberculosis* isolates to survive and reproduce, Burgos et al. (2002) found that drug-resistant strains of *M. tuberculosis* were approximately half as likely as drug-susceptible strains to progress to active TB.

Whether or not drug-resistant *M. tuberculosis* strains are less transmissible than drug-susceptible bacilli, outbreaks of drug-resistant and MDRTB have occurred, demonstrating that MDRTB can result from direct transmission to persons without previous treatment for TB. Before the onset of the HIV epidemic, outbreaks of drug-resistant TB occurred largely in community settings. Steiner et al. (1970) reported a community outbreak of TB from a source case with isoniazid, streptomycin, and para-aminosalicylic acid resistance. All 23 members of the immediate household were found to be tuberculin reactors, including 6 with active disease (2 with bacteriologically proven resistant bacilli), and evidence of spread to the local community was indicated by a significant increase in the rate of tuber-culin reactors among non-household contacts of the source case. Another report described an outbreak of TB in a school and community in 1976 from a patient with an isolate resist-ant to isoniazid, streptomycin, and para-aminosalicylic acid. High rates of infection asso-ciated with exposure to the index case suggested that transmission of resistant organisms had occurred, and the subsequent appearance of bacteriologically proven isoniazid/streptomycin/para-aminosalicylic acid resistant TB in four school contacts of the index case confirmed that transmission of drug-resistant *M. tuberculosis* had occurred. Retrospective investigation revealed that the school outbreak was part of an ongoing com-munity outbreak dating back to at least 1964 (Reves et al., 1981).

Nothing brought the problem of the emergence of MDRTB to the attention of the pub-lic health community, and the public in general, more so than did a number of highly publicized outbreaks of MDRTB in the late 1980s and early 1990s. Over this period, multiple outbreaks of MDRTB occurred worldwide in institutional settings, such as hospitals, medical and dental clinics, substance abuse treatment centers, homeless shelters, and correctional facilities (Beck-Sague et al., 1992; Breathnach et al., 1998; CDC, 1985, 1991a, 1991b, 1996a; Cleveland et al., 1995; Coronado et al., 1993; Fischl et al., 1992a, 1992b; Frieden et al., 1996; Kenyon et al., 1997; Moro et al., 1998; Nardell et al., 1986; Pearson et al., 1992; Portugal et al., 1999; Reichler et al., 2000; Sacks et al., 1999;

Valway et al., 1994a, 1994b; Villarino et al., 1992). In large part, these outbreaks resulted from the convergence of highly susceptible HIV-infected persons and lapses in management and infection control practices, including delays in diagnosis, delays in obtaining drug susceptibility test results, and inadequate isolation of infectious cases.

In addition, several reports tracked the spread of MDR *M. tuberculosis* strains across the United States. In many situations, the resistant organism originated in New York City, shared a common ancestor and underwent clonal expansion by sequential acquisition of resistance-conferring mutations in several genes, most likely as a consequence of antibiotic selection of randomly occurring variants in concert with inadequately treated infections (Bifani et al., 1996). A particularly resistant outbreak strain, called strain W, was resistant to as many as eight antituberculosis drugs, and was tracked from New York City to several states and Puerto Rico (Agerton et al., 1999). An *M. tuberculosis* strain genotypically similar to strain W was also associated with a community outbreak of MDRTB in South Africa (van Rie et al., 1999). Transmission of strain W was also associated with a community outbreak and nosocomial transmission via a contaminated bronchoscope (Agerton et al., 1997).

3.5. Programmatic and Institutional Factors

TB control programs have two major aims (CDC, 1992b, 1992c). The first and highest priority is to detect persons with TB disease and treat them with effective antituberculosis drugs, which cure the vast majority of patients and stop the transmission of *M. tuberculosis* to other persons. If the patient does not take the proper drugs for the full treatment period, the disease may not be cured and relapse may occur. In the context of "producing" drug resistance, if medications are not taken correctly, selective multiplication may occur and lead to drug-resistant disease that can be transmitted to others. This is reflected by the higher proportion of drug-resistant disease in retreatment TB cases compared with new cases. The second major control intervention is to detect and treat persons with LTBI in order to prevent the development of disease. In cases of LTBI resulting from exposure to drug-susceptible *M. tuberculosis*, effective regimens exist to greatly diminish the probability that this will occur (CDC, 2000). On the other hand, persons with LTBI as a result of exposure to MDR *M. tuberculosis* have few clear cut options, and treatment, if undertaken, requires the use of empiric regimens whose efficacy have not been proven in controlled trials.

With an estimated one third of all humanity infected with *M. tuberculosis*, an estimated two million deaths a year resulting from TB, and the recognition of widespread antituberculosis drug resistance, the WHO identified critical programmatic inadequacies that contribute to the TB epidemic and the rise in drug-resistant cases (WHO, 1997). These include a reliance in many countries on special TB care facilities that fail to ensure directly observed treatment and that have not been accessible to large numbers of patients, use of inadequate treatment regimens and failure to use standardized regimens, and lack of an information management system for the rigorous evaluation of treatment outcomes. In response to these problems, the WHO developed a comprehensive TB control strategy, DOTS, consisting of five principal elements: (1) political commitment, (2) accurate laboratory-based case diagnosis, (3) directly observed treatment using standardized regimens, (4) an uninterrupted supply of antituberculosis drugs of high quality, and (5) a mechanism to monitor program activities and analyze treatment outcomes using a standardized reporting system (WHO, 1997). As of 2001, DOTS had been implemented in 148 countries (containing 55% of the world population), although many countries, such as Russia, are not universally covered (WHO, 2002), and at other sites purporting to employ DOTS programs, major deficiencies have been identified (Laserson et al., 2000).

But even sound programs using appropriate regimens for drug-susceptible TB cases may fare poorly when it comes to treating large numbers of cases at risk for drug-resistant disease. Use of a standard regimen of first-line antituberculosis drugs (isoniazid, rifampin, pyrazinamide, and ethambutol or streptomycin), generally employed in DOTS programs, is likely to have limited efficacy in these situations. In a prison setting in Azerbaijan, only 54% of patients had a successful treatment outcome, far short of the WHO target for cure rate of 85%, and mortality was high (11%). Resistance to two or more drugs, a sputum positive for acid-fast bacilli at the end of initial treatment, cavitary disease, and poor adherence were independently associated with treatment failure (Coninx et al., 1999). In a Siberian TB referral prison, among isolates from 164 patients examined, the rate of initial resistance to isoniazid and rifampin was 23%. In this setting, treatment failure was 35% despite implementation of a strict DOTS program and use of an expanded initial treatment regimen (Kimerling et al., 1999).

Given that the ability to perform DSTs is not widely available, especially in resource-poor settings, "standardized" antituberculosis regimens may in certain situations need to be preemptively structured to treat cases of TB with suspected drug resistance, particularly those with a high likelihood of rifampin resistance or MDR. Espinal et al. (2000) investigated the impact of MDRTB on the outcome of standard short-course chemotherapy in six countries or regions within countries (Dominican Republic, Hong Special Administrative Region [People's Republic of China], Italy, Ivanovo Oblast [Russia], the Republic of Korea, and Peru) with established DOTS programs. Treatment success was lower for retreatment (57%) than for new cases (83%). Overall, treatment failure (relative risk, 15.4; 95% confidence interval, 10.6–22.4) and mortality (relative risk, 3.73; 95% confidence interval, 2.13–6.53) were higher among new MDRTB cases than among new drug-susceptible cases. Even in settings using 100% direct observation, MDRTB cases (both new and retreatment) had a significantly higher failure rate than susceptible cases (10% vs. 0.7%). Treatment failure rates were also significantly higher among all cases with any rifampin or isoniazid resistance (other than MDRTB). The authors concluded that the standard DOTS regimen was inadequate for some patients with drug-resistant TB, and suggested modification of the strategy in some settings to identify drug-resistant cases sooner and to make use of second-line drugs. In response to the recognized inadequacy of standard DOTS regimens for many patients with drug-resistant TB, the WHO developed a new strategy, called "DOTS-Plus," which will be discussed in Section 7.2.

As in the case of TB caused by drug-susceptible *M. tuberculosis*, institutional factors may contribute to widespread transmission of drug-resistant TB, particularly in congregate settings lacking appropriate infection and environmental controls. In many cases, the lack of effective barriers to prevent transmission, such as negative pressure isolation rooms, contributed to the transmission of drug-resistant TB in nosocomial outbreaks (Edlin et al., 1992; Fischl et al., 1992b; Kenyon et al., 1997). In other outbreaks, institutional characteristics such as overcrowding and forced transfer or involuntary restriction of inmates also contributed to extensive *M. tuberculosis* transmission (Brewer & Heymann 1998; Valway et al., 1994a, 1994b).

Although no published reports have appeared, other high-risk situations and settings, where overcrowding occurs and a high prevalence of drug resistance exists, could potentially result in the widespread transmission of MDRTB. Numerous reports have demonstrated the widespread prevalence of infectious TB in refugee camps, along with the challenges of instituting sound TB control practices in such settings (Mastro & Coninx, 1988; Miles & Maat, 1984, 1987; Rieder, 1985; Shears, 1984; Spinaci, 1985). The epidemiology and factors contributing to the spread of TB among migrant farm workers in the United States (largely from high-prevalence countries with high levels of drug resistance) has also been demonstrated (CDC, 1986; Ciesielski et al., 1991; Hibbs et al., 1989; Jacobson et al., 1987).

A recent report illustrated the potential for *M. tuberculosis* transmission at medical waste processing plants (Johnson et al., 2000). The facility involved, in an area of low TB incidence (Washington State, US), accepted contaminated medical waste from a number of medical laboratories where it was shredded, blown, and compacted before sterilization. In this setting, three plant workers developed TB within a span of 5 months. All three workers had different *M. tuberculosis* strains demonstrated by DNA fingerprinting; one of the workers had MDRTB. Genotyping linked the MDRTB patient isolate to an MDR strain obtained from a laboratory that sent material to the plant for processing.

3.6. Substandard Antituberculosis Drugs

As mentioned, incomplete adherence to treatment and interruptions in drug supply can lead to the production of drug-resistant TB. Another factor, particularly relevant in areas of the world in which pharmaceutical manufacturing practices may lack consistent quality control or where improper storage may occur, involves the use of substandard antituberculosis drugs by TB control programs. Laserson and colleagues (2001) used a recently developed thin layer chromatography kit to assess the quality of isoniazid and rifampin in single and fixed-dose formulations in six countries (Colombia, Estonia, India, Latvia, Russia, and Vietnam). Of the 40 samples tested, 10% of all samples (including 13% of rifampin samples) contained less than 85% of stated content of drug. In this analysis, more fixed-dose than single-dose preparations were substandard. Although interpretation of the results was limited by the relatively small sample, the study demonstrated that thin layer chromatography was an effective and inexpensive method for the detection of substandard drugs that have a potential to induce drug-resistant TB. Similarly, in countries that allow over-the-counter purchase of rifampin for use in a variety of bacterial infections, increasing rates of rifampin monoresistance have been reported (Jarallah et al., 1994).

4. DIAGNOSIS

4.1. Risk Factors for MDRTB

Previous treatment for TB (particularly of extended duration), recent emigration from a geographic area with a high prevalence of antituberculosis drug resistance, and known exposure to a person with drug-resistant TB, are the principal predictors of drug resistance in a patient with TB (Barnes, 1987; Costello et al., 1980; Espinal et al., 2001a, 2001b; Frieden et al., 1993).

The clinical presentation of patients with MDRTB is similar to those of patients with drug-susceptible disease, although some of the descriptive studies to date involve subjects with HIV coinfection. One such study found dry cough to be more common and lymphadenopathy less common in MDRTB patients (Fischl et al., 1992a) than in patients with drug-susceptible TB. Another found that failure to defervesce while receiving a standard four-drug antituberculosis regimen was independently associated with MDRTB, and suggested that patients with prolonged fever who are receiving appropriate therapy may be a subgroup to target for broader empiric therapy (Salomon et al., 1995). Consistent with the propensity for TB to present as extrapulmonary disease in HIV-infected persons, these studies also demonstrated frequent extrapulmonary involvement in the patients studied. Other series, however, which include patients without HIV infection, have reported that large proportions of MDRTB cases present with cavitary lung lesions and smear-positive sputum (Goble et al., 1993; Iseman et al., 1990; Nitta et al., 2002).

4.2. Drug Susceptibility Tests

The performance of DST on *M. tuberculosis* isolates is essential to the identification and management of patients with MDRTB; unfortunately, the availability of such testing in many parts of the world is limited. The four DST standardized methods used throughout the world are the absolute concentration method, the resistance ratio method, the proportion method, and the BACTEC radiometric method (WHO, 1997).

The absolute concentration method was originally used to determine minimal inhibitory concentrations of isoniazid and streptomycin by adding a controlled inoculum of *M. tuberculosis* to the control and drug-containing media. Media containing sequential 2-fold dilutions of each drug are used, and resistance is indicated by the lowest concentration of the drug that will inhibit growth. This technique may be less reliable than others, because a satisfactory result can only be obtained if the inoculum size and the drug concentrations are standardized in each laboratory by reference to a "wildtype" culture (WHO, 1997).

The resistance ratio method is a variant of the absolute concentration method, and was introduced to prevent variation in minimal inhibitory concentrations of a given strain of *M. tuberculosis* when tested on different batches of drug-containing media (Canetti et al., 1969; Kent & Kubica, 1985). The resistance ratio is defined as the minimal inhibitory concentration of the test strain divided by that of the standard susceptible strain H37Rv in the same set of tests. A resistance ratio of two or less defines drug susceptibility, while eight or more is considered evidence of drug resistance. Although the quality of this method still depends on the standardization of the inoculum size, the critical concentration need not be determined because a susceptible control is provided by the standard strain (WHO, 1997).

The proportion method has gained acceptance in many countries throughout the world. With this method, the ratio between the number of colonies growing on drug-containing medium and the number of colonies growing on drug-free medium indicates the proportion of drug-resistant bacilli present in the bacterial population. High and low dilutions of the inoculum are placed on media so that isolated, countable colonies can be obtained. From these colony counts, the proportion of variants resistant to the drug concentration tested can be determined and expressed as a percentage of the total number of viable colony forming units in the population. Below and above a certain fraction, called the "critical proportion," a strain is classified as either susceptible or resistant, respectively (WHO, 1997). The principal advantages of this method are that standardization of the inoculum size is not crucial, and its validity has been correlated to bacteriological as well as clinical criteria (Laszlo et al., 1997; Mitchison & Nunn, 1986).

Given the importance of rapid identification of drug resistance in the management of patients with TB, the aforementioned methods are significantly limited from a clinical standpoint because of the time required to obtain test results. All are based on the use of conventional culture methods, and it may take over 2 months from the receipt of primary specimens before DST results are obtained. A fourth method, the BACTEC radiometric, was commercially developed in the 1980s for DST in liquid medium (Roberts et al., 1983), and results can be obtained as soon as 1 week following inoculation (Siddiqi, 1989). Now in use in many industrialized countries, it is a variant of the proportion method in which the production of 14C-labeled CO_2 (evidence of bacterial growth) in a standard *M. tuberculosis* inoculum in the presence of antimicrobials is compared to the labeled CO_2 produced by a 1/100 dilution of the original inoculum in the absence of antimicrobials. The principal disadvantages of the BACTEC method are that it requires appropriate laboratory infrastructure, including nuclear waste disposal, and it is more expensive than the nonradiometric proportion method (WHO, 1997).

4.3. New Methodologies for Rapid Detection of Drug Resistance

In areas of the world in which MDRTB is a significant public health problem, such as the Russian Federation, methods to rapidly detect drug resistance would greatly enhance TB control and treatment efforts. Given the importance of rifampin in the antituberculosis armamentarium, particularly in many of these same areas where isoniazid and streptomycin resistance is common, rapid detection of rifampin resistance alone would provide a significant alert for the need for treatment with second-line drugs. Rapid detection of rifampin resistance is technically feasible both by genotypic and phenotypic means (Schluger, 2001). A genotypic approach, called the line-probe assay, detects rifampin resistance-related mutations in the *rpoB* gene of *M. tuberculosis* and is currently available in Europe (Cooksey et al., 1997; Hirano et al., 1999; Marttila et al., 1999). These assays are currently not in use in the United States, and their cost in resource-limited settings may be prohibitive.

A potential phenotypic approach to the detection of drug resistance is the luciferase reporter gene assay, which involves transfecting *M. tuberculosis* from a clinical specimen with a luciferase-containing mycobacterial phage. If viable *M. tuberculosis* is present in the specimen, it will take up the phage and emit light. By inoculating the sample into antibiotic-containing medium, resistant bacilli will remain viable and continue to emit light (Jacobs et al., 1993). Although initial displays of this assay were impressive, its

development for clinical use has been slow. Field trials of this assay are currently underway in the United States and foreign settings (Schluger, 2001).

Another assay under development employs the use of molecular beacons, which are
molecules that emit light when a chemical reaction occurs (Leone et al., 1998). Recent
studies have demonstrated high sensitivity and specificity of this assay in detecting
M. tuberculosis as well as identifying mutations associated with drug resistance (Piatek
et al., 1998, 2000). Again, however, given the technical demands of the procedure, requiring
expensive and sophisticated laboratory equipment, may likely limit the adoption of this
technology to wealthy nations (Schluger, 2001).

5. TREATMENT

5.1. General Principles

In general, patients with TB with bacilli resistant to both isoniazid and rifampin have
a much worse prognosis than those patients who have drug-susceptible disease. Treatment
of TB resistant to any single first-line drug is accomplished by using other first-line drugs
to which the organism is susceptible, including isoniazid, rifampin, pyrazinamide, ethambutol, and streptomycin. If the organism is resistant to either isoniazid or streptomycin
alone, a 94–96% success rate has been reported, even with short course therapy (Hong
Kong Chest Service/British Medical Research Council, 1987). When the organism is
rifampin resistant, the outcome of therapy is less successful and second-line agents may be
recommended (Michison and Nunn, 1986).

Consultation with experts in the management of MDRTB is essential at the outset and
throughout the course of treatment. Initiation of treatment of patients with known MDRTB
requires a thorough and careful review of previous drug therapy, including the dates during which all agents were administered. Clearly, it is prudent to consider that drugs administered to a patient without direct observation might not have been ingested at all. Even
when in vitro sensitivities to previously used agents are demonstrated, these agents may not
prove to be as effective in a salvage regimen as the in vitro DST pattern predicts (Goble
et al., 1993). Second, the design of a retreatment regimen requires that meticulous laboratory
studies be performed to characterize the susceptibility of the specific strain. If current DST
results are not available, it is essential to review the results of those previously performed,
in addition to the treatment history. If resistance patterns in the record are inconsistent, this
may be the result of sampling of different populations of organisms in a patient with a large
bacillary load, or to different techniques of testing in different laboratories. In the design
of a retreatment regimen under these circumstances, the most conservative approach is to
assume that the worst combination of resistances found is correct, and proceed accordingly
(Harkin & Harris, 1996).

The selection of a regimen to treat a patient with MDRTB is critically important, and
complicated by the fact that the choice of secondary agents, with greater toxicity and less
efficacy, is limited. As is the case in the treatment of drug-susceptible TB, the use of multiple drugs is imperative to prevent the development of additional resistance. Given that

agents used in retreatment regimens are less effective, most experienced clinicians recommend a minimum of three or four drugs, and possibly as many as six or seven, including a parenteral agent (Goble et al., 1993; Iseman, 1993; Iseman & Madsen, 1989; Jancik et al., 1963; Somner and Brace, 1962). At minimum, three drugs should ideally meet two criteria: (1) the organism is known to be susceptible to the drugs and (2) the patient has never received the drugs (Harkin and Harris, 1996). If the patient has not received a quinolone for antituberculosis therapy in the past, an agent from this class of drug with demonstrated activity against *M. tuberculosis* may constitute a critical part of a salvage regimen, particularly when combined with a parenteral agent (American Thoracic Society/CDC, 1994; Iseman, 1993). In short, the development of a salvage regimen involves: (1) elimination of agents for which drug resistance has been documented, (2) avoidance of antituberculosis drugs that the patient has received in a failing regimen in the past, and (3) construction of a salvage regimen centered on the drugs that remain, with consideration of their potential toxicities (Harkin & Harris, 1996). The administration of all medications for the treatment of MDRTB should be directly observed, and given daily, with the exception of aminoglycoside agents. Ideally, the initiation of a salvage regimen for MDRTB should occur in the hospital to permit close observation of toxicity and intolerance, to perform peak and trough serum concentrations of medications (therapeutic drug monitoring [TDM]), and to allow for prompt adjustments in the regimen, as necessary (Iseman, 1993). For situations in which susceptibility of an *M. tuberculosis* isolate to a drug is reported as "intermediate," use of that drug in the treatment of MDRTB may be ill advised, particularly if the drug has been used previously or if its administration in a higher dose is likely to lead to toxicity.

5.2. Second-Line Antituberculosis Drugs, Toxicity, and Cross-Resistance

Isoniazid, rifampin, pyrazinamide, and ethambutol are considered first-line antituberculosis drugs because of their long history of use, efficacy, tolerance, and relatively low cost, and are the mainstay of treatment for TB today. Second-line agents, on the other hand, are not typically used in the treatment of drug-susceptible disease (although some have been used for such a purpose in the past), and generally have less effective antimycobacterial activity, are more toxic, and more costly to administer.

Parenteral antituberculosis drugs are streptomycin, amikacin, kanamycin, and capreomycin. Amikacin and kanamycin are structurally similar, and there is usually cross-resistance between them; however, cross-resistance between them and streptomycin is rare (Iseman, 1993). Capreomycin, a cyclic polypeptide, differs structurally and exhibits no uniform cross-resistance with the aminoglycosides (McClatchy et al., 1977). Amikacin, kanamycin, and streptomycin may be given intramuscularly, but are tolerated better intravenously if administration is required for an extended period of time. The principal adverse effects are nephrotoxicity and ototoxicity, and clinicians are many times in the position of choosing between continuing effective therapy with the possibility of permanent hearing loss, or risking less effective therapy in an attempt to preserve hearing (Johnson & Sepkowitz, 1995).

Fluoroquinolones, including ciprofloxacin, oflaxacin, and its L-isomer, levofloxacin, have shown considerable promise as antimycobacterial agents (Hong Kong Chest

Service/British Medical Research Council, 1992; Kahana & Spino, 1991; Kohno et al., 1992; Mohanty & Dhamgaye, 1993; Rastogi & Goh, 1991; Tsukamura et al., 1985). Ofloxacin was as effective as ethambutol in a 6-month, three-drug regimen (Kohno et al., 1992); however, the study did not include patients with MDRTB. Though limited, data on the use of fluoroquinolones in the treatment of MDRTB are encouraging; however, the emergence of fluoroquinolone resistance has been reported. In one study, ofloxacin was added to failing regimens in 19 patients with MDRTB. Five of these patients had sputum cultures convert to negative, despite what was essentially ofloxacin monotherapy; eleven patients had reductions in the numbers of bacilli in sputum, but all of these isolates had become ofloxacin-resistant (Tsukamura et al., 1985). In a more recent report from Turkey with MDRTB patients, the inclusion of ofloxacin in a retreatment regimen and its absence from a previous regimen were associated with a successful outcome (Tahouglu et al., 2001). Until controlled trials have been conducted that clearly delineate the role of fluoro-quinolones in the treatment of drug-susceptible and drug-resistant TB (and updated treatment guidelines are published), these agents should be reserved for use in multidrug salvage regimens for patients with known or suspected MDRTB (American Thoracic Society/CDC, 1994).

Aminosalicylic acid and ethionamide are poorly tolerated drugs, and treatment with these agents must be initiated slowly and proceeded cautiously. Gastrointestinal side effects are nearly universal. Because few patients can tolerate the doses of ethionamide necessary to achieve therapeutic serum concentrations, it should only be used when there are no alternatives (Iseman, 1993).

Cycloserine is another second-line antituberculosis drug, and is generally tolerated better with regard to gastrointestinal disturbance. It does, however, have significant central nervous system toxicity, and can precipitate focal or grand mal seizures with high serum concentrations. Psychotic disturbances and suicidal ideation have been reported with cycloserine, even in patients with appropriate serum concentrations. Pyridoxine is given with cycloserine with the intention of preventing neurologic toxicity, but its value has not been proved (Iseman, 1993).

Other oral medications that have been used for the treatment of MDRTB include thiacetazone, clofazamine, amoxicillin-clavulanate, macrolide antibiotics (clarithomycin and azithromycin), and other rifamycin agents (Iseman, 1993). Thiacetazone is not approved by the FDA, and has been associated with the development of erythema multiforme in HIV-infected patients (Nunn et al., 1991; Okwera et al., 1997). Clofazamine, an antileprosy drug, has in vitro but unproven clinical efficacy against *M. tuberculosis*, amoxicillin-clavulanate and macrolide agents have high minimal inhibitory concentrations for most strains of *M. tuberculosis* relative to achievable serum concentrations, and other rifamycins such as rifabutin often exhibit cross-resistance between it and rifampin (Frieden et al., 1996; Iseman, 1993). Table 7.1 displays the common adverse reactions to second-line antituberculosis agents used in a WHO-sponsored pilot project in Lima, Peru, as well as proposed adverse event management strategies.

As improvement in the results of bacteriologic tests of sputum is the principal marker of response, Iseman recommends that specimens be obtained weekly for smear and culture during the initial phase of treatment. Improvements in the chest radiograph may lag behind other changes, but decreased fever, cough, and sputum production, and increase in weight are indirect markers of clinical response. The optimal duration of treatment has not been

Table 7.1

Common Adverse Reactions Observed and Protocols for Management Strategies Proposed in a Pilot Project in Three Districts of Lima, Peru

Adverse reaction	Suspected agent(s)	Suggested management strategies	Comments
Seizures	Cs, H, O, L, Cx	(1) Initiate anticonvulsant therapy (e.g., phenytoin, valproic acid) (2) Increase pyridoxine to 300 mg daily (3) Lower dose of suspected agent. If this can be done without compromising regimen (4) Discontinue suspected agent if this can be done without compromising regimen	(1) Anticonvulsant is generally continued until multidrug-resistant tuberculosis (MDRTB) treatment completed or suspected agent discontinued (2) History of prior seizure disorder is not a contraindication to the use of agents listed here if patient's seizures are well-controlled and/or patient is receiving anticonvulsant therapy (3) Patients with history of prior seizures may be at increased risk for development of seizures during MDRTB therapy (4) Seizures not a permanent sequelae of MDRTB treatment
Peripheral neuropathy	Sm, Km, Amk, Cm, M Tha, Cs, E, O, L, Cx	(1) Increase pyridoxine to 300 mg daily (2) Change parenteral to Cm if patient has documented susceptibility to Cm (3) Begin exercise regimen, regions (4) Initiate therapy with tricyclic antidepressant drugs (5) Lower dose of suspected agent, if this can be done without compromising regimen (6) Discontinue suspected agent if this can be done without compromising regimen (7) Initiate therapy with neurontin	(1) Patients with comorbid disease (e.g. diabetes, HIV, alcoholism) may be more likely to develop peripheral neuropathy, but these conditions are not contraindications to the use of the agents listed here (2) Neuropathy is generally not reversible, although only a minority (approximately 10%) of patients require continued intervention to keep symptoms controlled once MDRTB treatment completed
Hearing loss	Sm, Km, Amk, Cm, Clr	(1) Change parenteral to Cm if patient has documented susceptibility to Cm (2) Lower does of suspected agent, if this can be done without compromising regimen	(1) If patients have received prior treatment with amino-glycosides, they may start therapy with hearing loss (2) Hearing loss is generally not reversible

(continued)

Table 7.1

(continued)

Adverse reaction	Suspected agent(s)	Suggested management strategies	Comments
		(3) Discontinue suspected agent if this can be done without compromising regimen	
Psychotic symptoms	Cs, O, L, Cx, H, Tha	(1) Initiate antipsychotic drugs (2) Hold suspected agent for short period of time (1–4 weeks) while psychotic symptoms brought under control (3) Lower dose of suspected agent, if this can be done without compromising regimen (4) Discontinue suspected agent if this can be done without compromising regimen	(1) Some patients will need to continue antipsychotic treatment throughout MDRTB therapy (2) Prior history of psychiatric disease is not a contraindication to the use of agents listed here but may increase the likelihood of development of psychotic symptoms (3) Psychotic symptoms generally reversible upon MDRTB treatment completion or discontinuation of offending agent
Depression	Socioeconomic circumstances, Cs, O, L, Cx, H, Tha	(1) Improve Socioeconomic conditions (2) Group or individual supportive counselling (3) Initiate anti-depressant drugs (4) Lower dose of suspected agent, if this can be done without compromising regimen (5) Discontinue suspected agent if this can be done without compromising regimen	(1) Importance of socioeconomic conditions should not be underestimated as contributing factor to depression (2) Depression and depressive symptoms may fluctuate during therapy (3) History of prior depression is not a contraindication to the use of the agents listed here, however, these patients may be at increased risk for developing depression during MDRTB treatment
Hypothyroidism	PAS, Tha, especially when given in combination	(1) Initiate thyroxine therapy (2) Substitute equally efficacious agent for Tha or PAS	(1) Completely reversible upon discontinuation of PAS or Tha
Nausea and vomiting	PAS, Tha, H, E, Cfz, PZ	(1) Rehydration (2) Initiate anti-emetic therapy (3) Lower dose of suspected agent, if this can be done without compromising regimen	(1) Nausea and vomiting ubiquitous in early weeks of therapy and usually abate with supportive therapy (2) Electrolytes should be monitored and repleted if vomiting severe

Table 7.1

(continued)

Adverse reaction	Suspected agent(s)	Suggested management strategies	Comments
		(4) Discontinue suspected agent if this can be done without compromising regimen	(3) Reversible upon discontinuation of suspected agent
Gastritis	PAS, Tha, H, E, Cfz, PZ	(1) Antacids (e.g., calcium carbonate, H$_2$-blockers, proton-pump isoniazidibitors) (2) Hold suspected agent(s) for short periods of time (e.g., 1–7 days) (3) Lower dose of suspected agent, if this can be done without compromising regimen (4) Discontinue suspected agent if this can be done without compromising regimen	(1) Severe gastritis, as manifest by hematemesis, melena or hematechezia and observed in this cohort (2) Dosing of antacids should be carefully timed so as to not interfere with the absorption of anti-TB drugs (3) Reversible upon discontinuation of suspected agent(s)
Hepatitis	PZ, H, R, Tha, O, L, Cx, E, PAS	(1) Stop therapy (2) Rule out other potential causes of hepatitis (3) Re-introduce drugs grouped serially while monitoring liver function, with most likely agent introduced last	(1) History of prior hepatitis should be carefully analyzed to determine most likely causative agent(s); these should be avoided in future regimens (2) Generally reversible upon discontinuation of suspected agent
Renal failure	Sm, Km, Amk, Cm	(1) Discontinue suspected agent (2) Consider using Cm if an aminoglycoside had been prior parenteral in regimen	(1) History of diabetes or renal disease is not a contraindication to the use of the agents listed here, although patients with these comorbidities may be at increased risk for developing renal failure (2) Renal impairment may be permanent
Optic neuritis	E	Stop E	(1) Not observed in this cohort of patients
Arthralgias	PZ, O, L, Cx	(1) Initiate therapy with non-steroidal antiinflammatory drugs (2) Initiate exercise regimen (3) Lower dose of suspected agent, if this can be done without compromising regimen	(1) Symptoms of arthralgia generally diminish over time, even without intervention (2) Uric acid levels may be elevated in some patients but are of little therapieutic relevance and anti-gout therapy (e.g., allopurinol,

(continued)

Table 7.1
(continued)

Adverse reaction	Suspected agent(s)	Suggested management strategies	Comments
		(4) Discontinue suspected agent if this can be done without compromising regimen	colchicine) is of no proven benefit in these patients

Key: Cs: Cycloserine; H: Isoniazid; Sm: Streptomycin; E: Ethambutol; Km: Kanamycin; Amk: Amikacin; Cm: Capreomycin; Clr: Clarithromycin; Tha: Thiacetazone; Cfz: Clofazimine; R: Rifampicin; Et: Ethionamide; PAS: Para-aminosalicyclic acid; O: Ofloxacin; L: Levofloxacin; Cx: Ciprofloxacin; PZ: Pyrazinamide.
Source, with permission of the publisher: World Health Organization. Scientific Panel of the Working Group on DOTS-Plus for MDRTB: (2000). Guidelines for establishing DOTS-Plus pilot projects for the management of multidrug-resistant tuberculosis. WHO. WHO/CDS/TB/2000.279.

clearly defined, though experience with large numbers of patients with MDRTB suggests that if chemotherapy is to achieve sputum conversion, it will do so within 4 months in most patients (Iseman, 1993). Susceptibility testing should be repeated on cultures that remain positive after 2–3 months of treatment to detect any additional evidence of drug resistance. Treatment with parenteral agents generally continues for 4–6 months in the absence of significant toxicity, and oral medications are administered for at least 18–24 months after the sputum culture has converted to negative. Though not rigorously documented, shorter duration of treatment has resulted in an increased risk of reactivation (Goble et al., 1993).

TDM should be considered for all patients with MDRTB. Close monitoring of anti-tuberculosis serum concentrations allows for the adjustment of drug doses to achieve the best peak serum to minimal inhibitory concentration, and may alert the clinician to the potential for toxicity before it occurs. Similarly, low serum concentrations of drug may be indicative of malabsorption, non-adherence, or a drug interaction (Seaworth, 2002).

5.3. Surgical Intervention

The most extensive experience with surgical intervention for MDRTB comes from Iseman and colleagues in Denver, Colorado (Iseman et al., 1990; Mahmoudi & Iseman, 1992). Surgical candidates were selected based on extensive drug resistance and poor response to medical therapy, and with disease sufficiently localized to permit resection of devitalized tissue (which may remain a focus for superinfection or relapse), while retaining sufficient respiratory capacity to predict recovery. The optimal timing of surgery is following 3–4 months of therapy and eradication of bacilli from the sputum, although patients who fail to convert their sputum to negative after such a period of intensive chemotherapy may still obtain benefit (Iseman et al., 1990; Treasure & Seaworth, 1995; Van Leuven et al., 1997). Surgical morbidity and mortality is infrequent, although complications such as bronchopleural fistula occur and may be devastating (Treasure & Seaworth, 1995). Of the

57 patients who underwent surgery in the Denver series, there was one postoperative death and six patients were left with persistent respiratory insufficiency; however, 49 of 50 patients remained smear and culture negative.

5.4. Novel Therapies

Although the fluoroquinolone agents have become a welcome addition to the antituberculosis armamentarium, particularly in the treatment of MDRTB, no new class of antituberculosis drug has been introduced since the development and release of rifampin in the early 1970s. Resistance to the fluoroquinolones is uncommon but has been reported and may occur rapidly (Sullivan et al., 1995). Newer compounds in this class, such as moxifloxacin and gatifloxacin, appear to be much more active against *M. tuberculosis* than any of the currently available agents (Fung-Tomc et al., 2000; Miyazaki et al., 1999). Rifabutin cross-resistance has been reported to occur in as many as 80% of patients with rifampin resistance (Frieden et al., 1996). Rifabutin is as effective as rifampin in the treatment of drug-susceptible TB, but data on its use in MDRTB is limited and controversial (Seaworth, 2002). Rifapentine, a rifamycin with a longer duration of activity, was approved for the treatment of TB in 1998, but has complete cross-resistance with rifampin and, therefore, is not of use in the treatment of MDRTB.

A recent study by Sacks et al. (2001) reviewed the use of inhaled aminoglycosides in the treatment of refractory drug-susceptible and drug-resistant TB. The potential advantage of such administration is the direct delivery of drug to pulmonary tissue and the avoidance of systemic toxicity. Among 12 patients with drug-resistant TB, 7 had conversion of the sputum smear to negative, and adverse events were limited to airway irritability.

Oxazolidinones, a novel class of antibacterial agents, are also of interest as antituberculosis drugs. Linezolid, a particular drug in this group, is approved for the treatment of resistant Gram-positive infections. Clinical studies in its use for the treatment of TB have not been done, but laboratory and murine data indicate some promise (Cynamon et al., 1999).

Another novel class is the nitroimidazopyrans, drugs related to nitroimidazoles that have been studied in the past as possible antituberculosis drugs. The most promising among these drugs is PA-824, which has a novel mechanism of action against *M. tuberculosis* and bactericidal capacity comparable with that of isoniazid (Stover et al., 2000). In addition, this drug appears to be active against nonreplicating organisms, suggesting that it might be a potent sterilizing agent capable of shortening treatment regimens significantly (O'Brien & Nunn, 2001).

Use of systemic gamma interferon for patients with nontuberculous mycobacterial disease has resulted in symptomatic and clinical improvement in some patients, and its mechanism of action may involve increased inhibition of mycobacterial growth by alveolar macrophages through enhanced production of reactive nitrogen species (Holland et al., 1994). Inhaled gamma interferon has also been studied in a small number of patients with MDRTB. Although sputum smears became negative in the five patients studied during the course of treatment, cultures remained positive, and all patients became sputum smear-positive again once treatment with interferon was discontinued (Condos et al., 1997).

5.5. Treatment Outcomes

Treatment outcomes have varied widely among patients with MDRTB, depending on the extent of pulmonary involvement and destruction, the number of antituberculosis drugs to which the patient remains susceptible, the treatment setting, and the patient's ability to tolerate and adhere to long-term treatment. Coinfection with the HIV, which will be discussed in the following section, has also been a critical determinant of treatment outcomes.

In a series involving 171 patients treated at the National Jewish Center from 1973 through 1983, 65% of the patients responded to chemotherapy, as indicated by negative sputum for at least three consecutive months (Goble et al., 1993). Twelve of the patients with responses subsequently had relapses, leaving an overall response rate of 56% over a mean period of 51 months. Of the 171 patients, 63 (37%) died, and 37 deaths were attributable to TB. In another series involving patients treated from 1983 through 1993, the median survival of HIV-seronegative patients with MDRTB was greater than 120 months (Park et al., 1996). In both of these series, however, most of the patients were referred to the tertiary centers after multiple treatment failures, and most had advanced disease.

Contrary to these reports, others have reported better treatment outcomes for patients with MDRTB. In a study of 25 HIV-seronegative patients in New York City treated in 1991 through 1994, 96% of patients had clinical responses, and 17 patients for whom data on microbiologic response were available had such a response (Telzak et al., 1995). The median follow-up for the patients who responded and who received appropriate therapy was 91 months. More recently, in a study of 158 patients with MDRTB treated at a tertiary referral center in Turkey, the overall success rate was 77%, which included cures and probable cures (Tahaoglu et al., 2001). The patients had previously received a mean of 5.7 antituberculosis drugs and had isolates that were resistant to a mean of 4.4 drugs. A successful outcome was independently associated with a younger age and the absence of previous treatment with ofloxacin.

6. HIV INFECTION AND MDRTB

6.1. Impact of HIV on the Epidemiology of MDRTB

In the 20 years since the first cases were recognized in 1981, the explosive spread of HIV/acquired immunodeficiency syndrome (AIDS) throughout the world has produced one of the most devastating pandemics of recorded history. As of 2001, The Joint United Nations Program on HIV/AIDS (UNAIDS) estimated that 20 million people have died of HIV/AIDS since 1981 and 40 million individuals worldwide are currently infected. Five million new infections occurred in 2001 alone (UNAIDS, 2002). Africa and Southeast Asia have been affected by HIV/AIDS most severely. An estimated 71% of persons with HIV worldwide live in Sub-Saharan Africa and 14% are in Southeast Asia; these subcontinental regions also account for the overwhelming majority of incident HIV infections and deaths (UNAIDS, 2002). Accordingly, the impact of HIV infection on TB has been greatest in these two regions because of the high prevalence of TB infection and disease in these areas, even before the HIV epidemic. Figure 7.5 displays the distribution of estimated global HIV/TB coinfection by country.

The major rise of TB in countries most affected by HIV results from the increased risk of progression from LTBI to active disease in coinfected persons, and the spread of HIV infection in populations where ongoing transmission of *M. tuberculosis* and latent TB infection are common. Figure 7.6 shows the relationship between the estimated incidence of TB and HIV prevalence in adults (age 15–49 years) from 18 African countries in 1999, demonstrating the linear rise in TB incidence as the prevalence of HIV infection in a population increases (WHO, 2001). Perhaps nowhere is the strong association of TB morbidity and mortality rates with the HIV epidemic more evident than in Botswana, a country that has had a strong NTP since 1975, and has strictly adhered to DOTS (Chaisson et al., 1999). Despite this, the incidence of TB more than doubled during the 1990s, from 202 cases per 100,000 population to 537 per 100,000 persons (Botswana Ministry of Health, 2000).

With regard to the transmission of drug-resistant *M. tuberculosis*, it is fortunate that the prevalence of MDRTB in Africa is relatively low. In the second round of the global survey of antituberculosis drug resistance, 7 of 56 countries or regions were in Sub-Saharan Africa (WHO, 2000). Compared with the global median rate of MDRTB of 1.0%, of these seven countries, only Mozambique was significantly higher, with 3.5% MDRTB. Three countries had values near the median, and the remaining three had less than 0.5% MDRTB. Although resistance to isoniazid was common, the relatively low prevalence of MDRTB in these countries has been attributed to the late introduction of rifampin and the unavailability of antituberculosis medications outside of NTPs (WHO, 2002). Even with the use of rifampin in short-course treatment regimens, the experience in Sub-Saharan Africa has shown that well-executed DOTS programs can prevent the growth in the number of MDRTB cases (Chaisson et al., 1999). In a nationwide survey in Botswana conducted in 1995 and 1996, MDRTB was found in less than 1% of new and 6% of retreatment cases (Kenyon et al., 1999).

In other areas of the world, where the prevalence of MDRTB is either known to be high or in which drug resistance surveys have not been performed, where the use of DOTS is limited, and where rifampin is available outside of national TB control programs, the potential impact of growing HIV prevalence on MDRTB remains a large source of concern. In the Russian Federation and among the republics of the former Soviet Union, increasing HIV incidence may have a devastating impact on an already serious TB and MDRTB epidemic (Kazionny et al., 2001). Data from China, where HIV incidence is increasing, show a worrisome prevalence of MDRTB, especially in areas where DOTS has not been implemented (WHO, 2000). Expansion of drug resistance surveillance is critically needed in the five countries with the greatest estimated incidence of TB worldwide (India, China, Indonesia, Pakistan, and Bangladesh), because the magnitude of the problem is not yet well known (WHO, 2000).

In the United States, the impact of HIV/AIDS on the epidemiology of MDRTB was well recognized in the late 1980s and early 1990s, when large institutional outbreaks of MDRTB occurred, as has been discussed. During these outbreaks, transmission of MDR *M. tuberculosis* occurred not only from patient to patient, but from patient to healthcare worker and prison staff as well. The epidemiologic evidence of institutional transmission was confirmed by DNA fingerprint data, which suggested that several of the outbreaks in

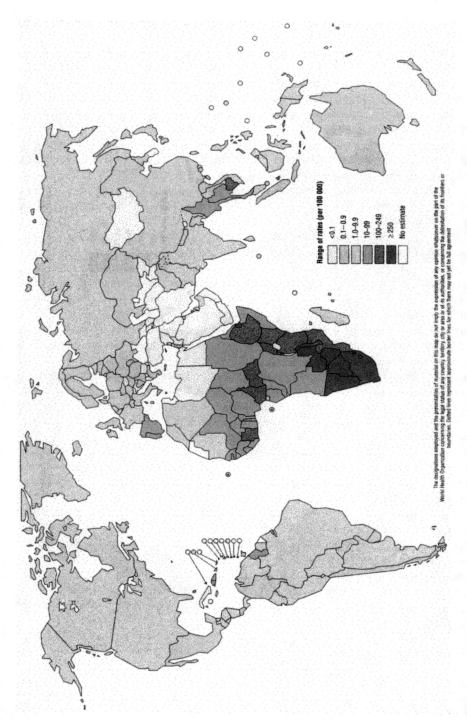

Figure 7.5. Estimated incidence rates of HIV-positive TB, 1999 (source, with permission of the publisher: World Health Organization. (2001). Global tuberculosis control, 2001. Geneva, Switzerland [WHO/CDS/TB/2001.287]).

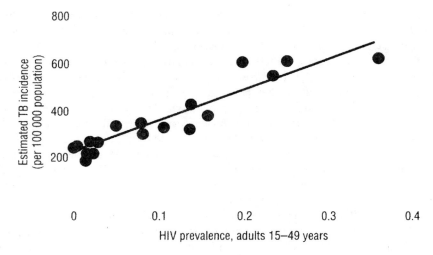

Figure 7.6. Relationship between estimated incidence of TB (all forms) and HIV prevalence in adults for 18 African countries in 1999 (HIV data supplied by UNAIDS) (source, with permission of the publisher: World Health Organization. (2001). Global tuberculosis control, 2001. Geneva, Switzerland [WHO/CDS/TB/2001.287]).

New York State were connected. In these outbreaks, a large proportion of the patients and staff involved were HIV-infected persons who became infected with highly resistant *M. tuberculosis*. More than 80% of the cases occurred in persons infected with HIV. Mortality in these outbreaks, as mentioned, was extraordinarily high, and in most of these outbreaks more than 70% of patients died, with a median survival ranging from 4 to 16 weeks (Beck-Sague et al., 1992; CDC, 1990, 1991a, 1992a; Dooley et al., 1992; Edlin et al., 1992; Fischl et al., 1992a, 1992b; Pearson et al., 1992; Valway et al., 1994a, 1994b; Villarino et al., 1992).

6.2. Impact on Diagnosis and Treatment

Whether HIV infection predisposes an individual to develop MDRTB has been debated. In a multicenter study performed in the United States of HIV-infected TB patients from 1992 to 1994, Gordin et al. (1996) found that HIV infection was a risk factor for drug resistance, independent of geographic location, history of prior therapy, age, and race. However, the patient population was not selected to reflect a sampling of all tuberculosis cases in the geographic areas included in the study, and may have reflected biases owing to characteristics of patients who used the participating facilities. In a later study, Telzak et al. (1999) found that a history of previous treatment for TB was the only predictor of MDRTB in a cohort of HIV-infected patients.

Similarly, the issue of whether HIV-infected patients with TB differ in their infectiousness compared with HIV-seronegative patients has also been investigated. Several studies investigating this issue, in both community and nosocomial settings, have produced conflicting results. In a study conducted at a tertiary referral hospital and its adjacent community in Kenya, Nunn et al. (1994) concluded that HIV-1 associated pulmonary TB was not more infectious than TB alone. In another study conducted in Miami/Dade County, Florida, contacts exposed to TB patients with AIDS or HIV infection were compared with contacts of HIV-negative TB patients for evidence of *M. tuberculosis* transmission. After an adjusted analysis, tuberculin positivity was 42% in contacts of HIV-negative TB patients compared with 29% and 31% in contacts of HIV-infected and AIDS TB patients, respectively. In this study, the authors concluded that TB patients with AIDS or HIV infection were less infectious and exposed fewer contacts than HIV-negative TB patients (Cauthen et al., 1996). To assess whether the relative infectiousness of patients with TB is enhanced by coinfection with HIV, Cruciani et al. (2001) performed a meta-analysis using data from six studies of 1,240 healthcare workers who had contact with TB patients, and from 11 studies of 10,714 household contacts of TB patients. In both settings, data suggested that TB patients with HIV infection were not intrinsically more infectious to their contacts than HIV-seronegative patients. In a subsequent correspondence, Pai et al. (2002) raised concerns about the meta-analysis, as its authors did not provide data on the quality of the studies included in the analysis, all of which were observational in nature and inherently more prone to bias.

Pulmonary disease is the most common presentation of TB in persons with HIV infection and is seen with or without extrapulmonary involvement (Theuer et al., 1990). Persons with early HIV infection present with the typical picture of cavitating upper lobe pulmonary TB. Symptoms include cough, chest pain, hemoptysis, fever, night sweats, and weight loss and are similar to those seen in persons with TB who do not have HIV infection. One report suggested that HIV-infected TB patients have smaller numbers of bacilli in sputum smears, and a smaller proportion have sputum smear-positive disease when compared with TB patients without HIV infection (Elliott et al., 1993).

Extrapulmonary disease is more common in persons with HIV infection. In one study in Africa, extrapulmonary TB (with or without pulmonary disease) was found in 60% of HIV-infected patients compared to 28% in those without HIV infection (Elliott et al., 1993). The occurrence of extrapulmonary TB and mycobacteremia increases with the level of immunosuppression (Havlir and Barnes, 1999). In many forms of extrapulmonary TB, symptoms are nonspecific, and extrapulmonary disease should be considered when a patient with HIV infection presents with fever of unknown origin. Since the majority of patients with extrapulmonary TB also have pulmonary involvement, a chest radiograph demonstrating pulmonary disease may be helpful in the diagnosis of extrapulmonary TB.

Several series have emphasized "atypical" radiographic presentations of TB among HIV-infected persons, with less frequent occurrence of cavitation and a higher frequency of adenopathy on chest radiographs than in HIV-uninfected adults (Batungwanayo et al., 1992; Mukadi et al., 1993). In a study of the effect of HIV disease stage on chest radiograph findings among patients with HIV-related pulmonary TB, Perlman et al. (1997) found that CD4+ lymphocyte counts of less than 200 per cubic millimeter were significantly associated with hilar and mediastinal adenopathy on chest radiograph, whereas CD4+ lymphocyte counts greater than 200 per cubic millimeter were more frequently associated with cavitation.

As the number of antiretroviral medications and use of highly active antiretroviral therapy (HAART) have proliferated, the complexity of treating HIV-related TB has concomitantly increased; however, for the treatment of MDRTB in HIV-infected persons on HAART, this complexity is ostensibly reduced because of rifampin resistance. In contrast, for patients on HAART with drug-susceptible TB, treatment is complicated by drug interactions between the rifamycins and both protease inhibitors (PIs) and non-nucleoside reverse transcriptase inhibitors (NNRTIs) (Burman et al., 1999; Burman & Jones, 2001; Small & Fujiwara, 2001). Guidelines have been issued with recommendations for concurrent treatment of HIV and TB (CDC, 1998b, 2000).

6.3. Impact on Treatment Outcomes

Patients with MDRTB have been shown to have worse clinical outcomes than patients with disease caused by susceptible isolates (Goble et al., 1993; Park et al., 1996). As mentioned, outbreaks of MDRTB, particularly those involving HIV-infected patients, have been associated with extraordinarily high mortality rates, often due to delays in the diagnosis and institution of appropriate therapy. Many of the patients died before the results of DST were known. In a study from Bellevue Hospital in New York City, 55% of a cohort of patients with MDRTB died, and the mortality was significantly greater for HIV-infected than for HIV-seronegative patients (72% vs. 20%) (Park et al., 1996). Institution of appropriate therapy was the factor most strongly associated with a favorable outcome. Other reports have supported the idea that rapid identification of risk factors for drug resistance, prompt institution of appropriate therapy tailored for drug-resistant disease (which employ empiric regimens using second-line antituberculosis drugs), and treatment within specialized MDRTB treatment programs can improve outcomes, even among HIV-infected persons (Salomon et al., 1995; Turett et al., 1995).

Given the copathogenesis of HIV and TB, improvements in the treatment of HIV disease with HAART will likely have a favorable impact on clinical outcomes in HIV-TB patients, benefits that may conceivably extend to patients with HIV-MDRTB. These advances, however, may be difficult to attain in many resource-poor settings, where the prevalence of HIV-TB is the greatest. In a report of patients with HIV-TB treated at a large urban U.S. hospital from 1991 through 2000, the 1-year survival rate for patients with HIV-TB was 58% in 1991, 81% in 1994, and 83% in 1997 (Leonard et al., 2002). The authors attributed the increase in survival to improved treatment of both HIV and TB, and to increased enrollment of patients in specialized HIV clinics. As the use of HAART expands into areas with a high prevalence of HIV-TB, it is likely that the concomitant use of standardized antituberculosis regimens will result in improved clinical outcomes and a significant reduction in mortality, as well as contribute to the prevention of MDRTB.

7. PREVENTION

7.1. Provider-Based

The best way to prevent MDRTB is to appropriately treat patients with drug-susceptible TB. Failure to do so can create enormous problems. Treatment of patients with MDRTB requires a minimum of 18–24 months and the use of less effective second line antituberculosis agents that are more costly and prone to produce serious adverse events. Cure of patients with MDRTB, when it can be accomplished, may often require risky surgical procedures, and may lead to major morbidity and mortality.

In the absence of primary exposure to drug-resistant bacilli, MDRTB occurs as the result of clinical mismanagement or patient non-adherence. The provider-based factors that may lead a patient with initially drug-susceptible disease to later develop MDRTB is described in Section 3.2. The principal common errors are: the addition of a single drug to a failing regimen, an inadequate primary regimen, failure to recognize initial or acquired resistance, failure to recognize and deal with non-adherence, and failure to provide directly observed therapy. Therefore, the first line of defense in the prevention of MDRTB falls on the shoulders of providers. Awareness and recognition of patients at risk for drug-resistant disease (previous treatment for TB, contact of a case of drug-resistant TB, being from an area with a high prevalence of drug-resistant TB) is critical, as delays in starting appropriate regimens and obtaining drug susceptibility test results can lead to continued transmission and the development of additional drug resistance. And as with any case of suspected TB, patients should be placed in respiratory isolation until the diagnosis of TB is excluded or when the patient is deemed noninfectious. In most situations, initial therapy should begin with four first line agents, including isoniazid, rifampin, pyrazinamide, and either ethambutol or streptomycin (CDC, 1993a). This regimen is effective even when the isolate is resistant to isoniazid (Hong Kong Chest Service/British Medical Research Council, 1987); however, if risk factors for drug resistance are present, an expanded initial regimen should be considered. If drug susceptibility test results indicate drug resistance, then the initial regimen should be altered as appropriate, as outlined in Section 5.1.

7.2. Institutional and Program-Based

If the first line of defense is the practicing physician, then the second is the laboratory (Bloch et al., 1996b; Tenover et al., 1993). Given the importance of drug susceptibility testing to the management of drug-resistant TB, laboratories need to be enabled by regulation to perform susceptibility testing on the initial isolates from every patient (CDC, 1993). Thus, even in the absence of a request for susceptibility testing from the provider, the laboratory should still proceed with such testing and report the results to both the provider and local health department.

The health department in many respects may serve as a safety net to back up the health care provider and is legally responsible for TB control (CDC, 1995). TB control programs can proactively prevent MDRTB by collecting information on patients with respect to initial regimen used, susceptibility testing, and drug resistance, and relay such information to providers so that effective interventions and corrective actions, if necessary, can be undertaken (Bloch et al., 1996a, 1996b; Sbarbaro 1996). Health departments, more so than private providers, are in a position to use directly observed therapy and other adherence promoting strategies to ensure completion of treatment, assuming that proper allocation of funding and resources for such measures is adequate (Bayer & Wilkinson, 1995; Reichman, 1991).

From an international perspective, in settings that may be relatively resource-limited, establishment of national TB control programs and implementation of the WHO DOTS strategy is essential to the prevention of MDRTB. During the early stages of a national TB control program, previously treated TB cases with drug resistance may represent up to half of all notified cases (WHO, 1997). The principal solution is to adopt the WHO recommended standard regimens of chemotherapy for new and retreatment cases, in order to stop the creation of more cases with drug resistance. Even if the proportion of MDRTB cases is high, program efforts must focus initially on the prevention of additional MDRTB cases (WHO, 1997).

As a result of information derived from the WHO/IUATLD Global project on antituberculosis drug resistance surveillance, it is clear that in some countries there exists a formidable MDRTB problem. Although appropriate treatment of drug-susceptible TB cases is crucial to the prevention of MDRTB, treatment of existing MDRTB cases is necessary to prevent further transmission of MDR bacilli and the creation of new MDRTB cases. The best manner with which to proceed in this pursuit has been the subject of debate. Providing reserve second line antituberculosis drugs to inefficient NTPs, which allow mistreatment and consequent MDRTB, might create an untreatable epidemic through additional misuse of reserve drugs. Ultimately, it was agreed that funds should be provided for these reserve drugs only to areas where there was a well-established successful DOTS-based program (WHO, 2000). In 2000, WHO developed guidelines for establishing pilot projects for the management of MDRTB, referred to as "DOT-Plus." DOTS-Plus for MDRTB is designed to manage MDRTB in areas where it has emerged and needs to be addressed in conjunction with the treatment of drug-susceptible TB cases. An effective DOTS-based TB control program must be in place before investing the considerable resources needed for the treatment of MDRTB, otherwise an inadequate program generates MDRTB cases faster than a DOTS-Plus program can treat them. In order for WHO to support potential pilot projects, such pilot projects require: (1) a review and approval by a coordinating expert body, known as the Green Light Committee, for the provision of second-line drugs; (2) continuous monitoring using standardized methods and indicators; and (3) periodic evaluation and prompt measures for adaptation or discontinuation of the pilot project depending on performance (WHO, 2000).

7.3. Treatment of Persons Exposed to MDRTB

Following the resurgence of TB in the 1980s and in the face of several large outbreaks of MDRTB, CDC issued guidelines for the management of persons exposed to MDRTB (CDC, 1992a). The approach to selecting drug regimens for the treatment of latent MDR *M. tuberculosis* infection hinges on two factors: (1) the likelihood of infection with MDR bacilli and (2) whether the exposed person has HIV infection, is at risk for HIV infection, or has other conditions known to substantially increase the risk of developing TB disease. One potential regimen is a combination of pyrazinamide and ethambutol at the recommended dose for the therapy of TB (pyrazinamide, daily oral dose 25–30 mg/kg; ethambutol, daily oral dose 15–25 mg/kg) (American Thoracic Society/CDC, 1986). Ethambutol at the 15 mg/kg dose is considered bacteriostatic, and in vitro studies show that ethambutol may be bactericidal at the 25 mg/kg dose (Crowle et al., 1985). If ethambutol is used at the higher dosage as part of a regimen to treat latent infection, the potential for higher rates of toxicity must be recognized and carefully monitored. The recommended duration of therapy is 6–12 months.

Another potential alternative regimen for treating latent MDR *M. tuberculosis* infection is pyrazinamide plus a fluoroquinolone. Gorzynski et al. (1989) reported that ofloxacin and ciprofloxacin had similar antimycobacterial potencies in vitro. Short-term administration of fluoroquinolones is generally well tolerated, but therapy of 6–12 months duration has not been fully studied. Arthropathy has been noted in experiments with immature animals, and rupture of hand, shoulder, and Achilles' tendons, requiring surgical repair, have been reported with levofloxacin and other fluoroquinolones (Physicians' Desk Reference, 2001). Therefore, fluoroquinolones should be used for the treatment of latent infection in children and pregnant patients only if the potential benefit justifies the potential side effects.

Intolerance to these regimens, however, has been reported. In a study of health care workers exposed to MDRTB (manifesting tuberculin skin test conversions), only 12.5% completed therapy with pyrazinamide and ofloxacin, and 43.8% experienced arthralgias. Fourteen of sixteen patients (87.5%) had reported some adverse effect, compared with 20.6% of another group on isoniazid treatment (Horn et al., 1995). Another report noted a high proportion of asymptomatic hepatitis with the use of pyrazinamide and ofloxacin for LTBI following exposure to MDRTB (Ridzon et al., 1997c). Two recent reports have also illustrated limited tolerability of levofloxacin and pyrazinamide for the treatment of presumed latent MDR *M. tuberculosis* infection (Lou et al., 2002; Papastavros et al., 2002). In these reports, treatment was discontinued for musculoskeletal, hepatic, central nervous system, gastrointestinal, and dermatological side effects; in the report by Lou et al., all 17 patients receiving levofloxacin and pyrazinamide had therapy discontinued due to adverse events.

To date, no controlled trials have been conducted to assess the efficacy of treatment for latent MDR *M. tuberculosis* infection; the decision to proceed with such treatment should involve the consultation of specialists in the treatment of MDRTB. In many situations, when adults and non-immunosuppressed persons with possible MDR *M. tuberculosis* infection are involved, a "watchful waiting" approach may be appropriate.

7.4. BCG and Vaccines

The ability by vaccination to prevent TB (and therefore, MDRTB) would have a profound effect on the global epidemiology of TB, as transmission models have indicated (Lietman & Blower, 2000). TB elimination probably cannot be achieved in the United States without the development of an effective vaccine (CDC, 1998a). The only vaccine in current use throughout the world, however, is BCG. BCG (the first live attenuated vaccine to be developed) is derived from an attenuated strain of *Mycobacterium bovis* originally produced by Calmette and Guerin at the Pasteur Institute in Lille, France, and first used in 1921 (CDC, 1996b; Grange et al., 1983). Both randomized placebo-controlled clinical trials and retrospective case-control and cohort studies have demonstrated a wide variation in vaccine efficacy, ranging from 80% to 0% (Anonymous, 1979; Rodriguez & Smith, 1990). Its use has been associated with a reduction of disseminated and meningeal TB in children. Although used extensively on a global basis, BCG vaccination is not routinely recommended in the United States, given its variable efficacy and tendency to produce a reactive tuberculin skin test in the absence of *M. tuberculosis* infection (CDC, 1996b).

Advances in molecular genetics, which have resulted in the establishment of the genomic sequence of *M. tuberculosis* H37 and identification of nearly 4,000 genes associated with activity of the bacterium, make it possible to generate a vast array of potential TB vaccine candidates (Cole et al., 1998; Young, 2000). Over the last few years, as many as 50–100 candidate vaccines have been developed to the stage of evaluation in animal models (Ginsberg, 2000). Vaccines conceivably could be used either before or after infection with *M. tuberculosis*. Pre-infection vaccines could be administered before infection with *M. tuberculosis*, and ideally would confer lifelong immunity to infection and disease. Post-infection vaccines would be given to persons already infected with *M. tuberculosis*, and would theoretically reduce the incident development of TB disease (CDC, 1998a). Three types of TB vaccines exist: (1) live attenuated vaccines, which are largely BCG-derived; (2) subunit vaccines, which are mycobacterial polypeptides and potentially lipid and carbohydrate antigens combined with adjuvants to augment antigenicity; and (3) naked DNA vaccines, which involve injection of DNA into host cells with the secondary expression of protective antigens (Ginsberg, 2000).

A major barrier to vaccine development, however, arises from insufficient knowledge about the roles of specific T-cell subsets, lymphokines, cytokines, and antibodies to *M. tuberculosis* in conferring and serving as surrogate markers of protection (Ginsberg, 2000). Currently, the only test available to determine protective immunity is assessment of the response to a virulent challenge in experimental animal models, mostly mice and guinea pigs (Young, 2000). Such an approach, given logistical constraints, not only severely limits the number of candidate vaccines that can be screened, but is additionally fraught with uncertainty over how vaccine efficacy in animal models relates to activity in humans.

8. SUMMARY

From a U.S. perspective, the problem of MDRTB has been greatly ameliorated through the use of standardized four-drug regimens in the initial phase of treatment, rapid DST, directly observed therapy, and improved infection control practices. The importation of MDRTB cases from countries with high levels of drug resistance, however, will continue to challenge TB control efforts in the United States. In other areas of the world, the rapid emergence of MDRTB represents an even greater challenge to such efforts, and will require the influx of significant resources and expertise to meet this challenge. Given that the best treatment of MDRTB is its prevention, the expansion of DOTS to prevent the production of MDRTB and the careful expansion of DOTS-Plus to treat existing cases and prevent further transmission of MDR *M. tuberculosis* are critical. In addition, as the HIV epidemic reaches areas in which the prevalence of TB and antituberculosis drug resistance are high, a concerted effort to treat these coexisting diseases will be essential to mitigate the convergence of factors that led to the large outbreaks of MDRTB that occurred in the United States in the early 1990s.

References

Agerton, T., Valway, S., Blinkhorn, R., Shilkret, K., Reves, R., Schluter, W., Gore, B., Pozsik, C., Plikaytis, B., Woodley, C., & Onorato, I. (1999). Spread of strain W, a highly drug-resistant strain of *Mycobacterium tuberculosis*, across the United States. *Clin Infect Dis, 29*, 85–92.

Agerton, T., Valway, S., Gore, B., Pozsik, C., Plikaytis, B., Woodley, C., & Onorato, I. (1997). Transmission of a highly drug-resistant strain (Strain W1) of Mycobacterium tuberculosis: Community outbreak and nosocomial transmission via a contaminated bronchoscope. *JAMA, 278*, 1073–1077.

Algerian Working Group/British Medical Research Council Cooperative Study. (1984). Controlled clinical trial comparing 6-month and a 12-month regimen in the treatment of pulmonary tuberculosis in the Algerian Sahara. *Am Rev Respir Dis, 129*, 921–928.

American Thoracic Society/CDC. (1986). Treatment of tuberculosis and tuberculosis infection in adults and children. *Am Rev Respir Dis, 134*, 355–363.

American Thoracic Society/CDC. (1994). Treatment of tuberculosis and tuberculosis infection in adults and children. *Am J Respir Crit Care Med, 149*, 1359–1374.

Anonymous. (1979). Trial of BCG vaccines in south India for tuberculosis prevention: First report. Tuberculosis Prevention Trial. *Bull World Health Organ, 57*, 819–827.

Barnes, P. (1987). The influence of epidemiologic factors on drug resistance rates in tuberculosis. *Am Rev Resp Dis, 136*, 325–328.

Batungwanayo, J., Taelman, H., Dhote, R., Bogaerts, J., Allen, S., & Van De Perre, P. (1992). Pulmonary tuberculosis in Kigali, Rwanda: Impact of human immunodeficiency virus infection on clinical and radiographic presentation. *Am Rev Respir Dis, 146*, 53–56.

Bayer, R., & Wilkinson, D. (1995). Directly observed therapy for tuberculosis: History of an idea. *Lancet, 345*, 1545–1548.

Beck-Sague, C., Dooley, S., Hutton, M., Otten, J., Breedon, A., Crawford, J., Pitchenik, A., Woodley, C., Cauthen, G., & Jarvis, W. (1992). Outbreak of multidrug resistant Mycobacterium tuberculosis infections in a hospital: Transmission to patients with HIV infection and staff. *JAMA, 268*, 1280–1286.

Ben-Dov, I., & Mason, G. (1987). Drug-resistant tuberculosis in a Southern California hospital: Trends from 1969 to 1984. *Am Rev Respir Dis, 135*, 1307.

Berning, S., Huitt, G., Iseman, M., & Peloquin, C. (1992). Malabsorption of antituberculosis drugs by a patient with AIDS. *N Engl J Med, 327*, 1817–1818.

Bifani, P., Plikaytis, B., Kapur, V., Stockbauer, K., Pan, X., Lutfey, M., Moghazeh, S., Eisner, W., Daniel, T., Kaplan, M., Crawford, J., Musser, J., & Kreiswirth, B. (1996). Origin and interstate spread of a New York City multidrug-resistant Mycobacterium tuberculosis clone family. *JAMA, 275*, 452–457.

Bishai, W., Graham, N., Harrington, S., Page, C., Moore-Rice, K., Hooper, N., & Chaisson, R. (1996). Rifampin-resistant tuberculosis in a patient receiving rifabutin prophylaxis. *N Engl J Med, 334*, 1573–1576.

Bloch, A., Cauthen, G., Onorato, I., Dansbury, K., Kelly, G., Driver, C., & Snider, D. (1994). Nationwide survey of drug-resistant tuberculosis in the United States. *JAMA* 271(9), 665–671.

Bloch, A., Onorato, I., Isle, W., Hadler, J., Hayden, C., & Snider, D. (1996a). Expanded tuberculosis surveillance in the United States: the need for epidemic intelligence. *Public Health Rep, 111*, 24–29.

Bloch, A., Simone, P., McCray, E., & Castro, K. (1996b). Preventing multidrug-resistant tuberculosis. *JAMA, 275*(6), 487–489.

Botswana Ministry of Health. (2000). Botswana National Tuberculosis Programme Report, 2000. Gabarone.

Breathnach, A., de Ruiter, A., Holdsworth, G., Bateman, N., O'Sullivan, D., Rees, P., Snashall, D., Milburn, H., Peters, B., Watson, J., Drobniewski, F., & French, G. (1998). An outbreak of multi-drug-resistant tuberculosis in a London teaching hospital. *J Hosp Infect, 39*, 111–117.

Brewer, T., & Heymann, S. (1998). Reducing the impact of tuberculosis transmission in institutions: Beyond infection control measures. *Int J Tuberc Lung Dis, 2*(9), S118–S123.

British Thoracic and Tuberculosis Association. (1975). Short-course chemotherapy in the treatment of tuberculosis. *Lancet, 1*, 119–121.

British Thoracic Association. (1982). A controlled trail of six months chemotherapy in pulmonary tuberculosis. Second report: Results during the 24 months after the end of chemotherapy. *Am Rev Respir Dis, 126*, 460–462.

Burgos, M., DeRiemer, K., Small, P., Hopewell, P., & Daley, C. (2002, May 17–22). Relative fitness of drug-resistant and drug-susceptible strains of Mycobacterium tuberculosis in San Francisco (abstract). American Thoracic Society International Conference, Atlanta, Georgia.

Burman, W., Gallicano, K., & Peloquin, C. (1999). Therapeutic implications of drug interactions in the treatment of human immunodeficiency virus-associated tuberculosis. *Clin Inf Dis, 28*, 419–430.

Burman, W., & Jones, B. (2001). Treatment of HIV-related tuberculosis in the era of effective anti-retroviral therapy. *Am J Resp Crit Care Med, 164*, 7–12.

Canetti, G. (1962). The eradication of tuberculosis: Theoretical problems and practical solutions. *Tubercle, 43*, 301–321.

Canetti, G. (1964). Host factors and chemotherapy of tuberculosis. In V. Barry (Ed.), *Chemotherapy of tuberculosis* (pp. 180–181). London: Butterworth.

Canetti, G. (1965). The J. Burns Amberson lecture: Present aspects of bacterial resistance in tuber-culosis. *Am Rev Resp Dis, 92*(5), 687–703.

Canetti, G., Fox, W., Khomenko, A., Mahler, H., Menon, N., Mitchison, D., Rist, N., & Smelev, N. (1969). Advances in techniques of testing mycobacterial drug sensitivity and the use of sensitiv-ity tests in tuberculosis control programmes. *Bull World Health Organ, 41*, 21–43.

Cauthen, G., Dooley, S., Onorato, I., Ihle, W., Burr, J., Bigler, W., Witte, J., & Castro, K. (1996). Transmission of *Mycobacterium tuberculosis* from tuberculosis patients with HIV infection or AIDS. *Am J Epidemiol, 144*, 69–77.

Cavalli-Sforza, L., & Lederberg, J. (1955). Isolation of pre-adaptive variants in bacteria by sib selec-tion. *Genetics, 41*, 367–381.

Cegielski, J., Chin, D., Espinal, M., Frieden, T., Rodriguez, R., Talbot, E., Weil, D., Zaleskis, R., & Raviglione, M. (2002). The global tuberculosis situation: Progress and problems in the 20th Century, prospects for the 21st Century. *Inf Dis Clin N Am, 16*(1), 1–58.

Centers for Disease Control and Prevention. (1983). Primary resistance to antituberculosis drugs—United States. *MMWR, 32*, 75.

Centers for Disease Control and Prevention. (1985). Drug resistant tuberculosis among the home-less—Boston. *MMWR, 34*, 429–431.

Centers for Disease Control and Prevention. (1986). Tuberculosis among migrant farm workers—Virginia. *MMWR, 35*, 467–469.

Centers for Disease Control and Prevention. (1990). Nosocomial transmission of multidrug resistant TB to healthcare workers and HIV-infected patients in an urban hospital—Florida. *MMWR, 39*, 718–722.

Centers for Disease Control and Prevention. (1991a). Nosocomial transmission of multidrug resist-ant tuberculosis among HIV-infected persons—Florida and New York, 1988–1991. *MMWR, 40*, 585–591.

Centers for Disease Control and Prevention. (1991b). Transmission of multidrug-resistant tubercu-losis from an HIV-positive client in a residential substance-abuse treatment facility—Michigan. *MMWR, 40*, 129–131.

Centers for Disease Control and Prevention. (1992a). Management of persons exposed to multidrug-resistant tuberculosis. *MMWR, 41*(RR-11).

Centers for Disease Control and Prevention. (1992b). National action plan to combat multidrug-resistant tuberculosis. *MMWR, 41*(RR-11), 1–45.

Centers for Disease Control and Prevention. (1992c). Prevention and control of tuberculosis in migrant farm worker. *MMWR, 41*(RR-10), 1–11.

Centers for Disease Control and Prevention. (1993). Tuberculosis control laws—United States, 1993: Recommendations of the Advisory Council for the Elimination of Tuberculosis (ACET). *MMWR, 42*(RR-15), 1–28.

Centers for Disease Control and Prevention. (1994). Expanded tuberculosis surveillance and tuberculosis morbidity—United States, 1993. *MMWR, 43*(20), 361–366.

Centers for Disease Control and Prevention. (1995). Essential components of a tuberculosis prevention and control program: Recommendations of the Advisory Council for the Elimination of Tuberculosis. *MMWR, 40*(RR-11), 1–16.

Centers for Disease Control and Prevention. (1996a). Prevention and control of tuberculosis in migrant farm workers. *MMWR, 41*(RR-10).

Centers for Disease Control and Prevention. (1996b). The role of BCG vaccine in the prevention and control of tuberculosis in the United States. *MMWR, 45*(RR-4).

Centers for Disease Control and Prevention. (1998a). Development of new vaccines for tuberculosis. *MMWR, 47*(RR-13), 1–6.

Centers for Disease Control and Prevention. (1998b). Prevention and treatment of tuberculosis among patients infected with human immunodeficiency virus: Principles of therapy and revised recommendations. *MMWR, 47*(RR-20), 1–58.

Centers for Disease Control and Prevention. (2000). Notice to readers: Updated guidelines for the use of rifabutin or rifampin for the treatment and prevention of tuberculosis among HIV-infected patients taking protease inhibitors or nonnucleoside reverse transcriptase inhibitors. *MMWR, 49,* 185–189.

Centers for Disease Control and Prevention. (2001, August). Reported Tuberculosis in the United States, 2000. Atlanta, GA: US Department of Health and Human Services, CDC.

Centers for Disease Control and Prevention. (2002). Acquired rifamycin resistance in persons with advanced HIV disease being treated for active tuberculosis with intermittent rifamycin-based regimens. *MMWR, 51,* 214–215.

Chaisson, R., Coberly, J., & DeCock, K. (1999). DOTS and drug resistance: A silver lining to a darkening cloud. *Int J Tuberc Lung Dis, 3,* 1–3.

Ciesielski, S., Seed, J., Esposito, P., & Hunter, N. (1991). The epidemiology of TB among North Carolina migrant farm workers. *JAMA, 265,* 1715–1719.

Cleveland, J., Kent, J., Gooch, B., Valway, S., Marianos, D., Butler, W., & Onorato, I. (1995). Multidrug-resistant *Mycobacterium tuberculosis* in an HIV dental clinic. *Infect Conrol Hosp Epidemiol, 16,* 7–11.

Cohn, D., Bustreo, F., & Raviglione, M. (1997). Drug-resistant tuberculosis: Review of the worldwide situation and WHO/IUATLD global surveillance project. *Clin Infect Dis, 24*(Suppl. 1), S121–130.

Cohn, M. (1970). Infectivity and pathogenicity of drug-resistant strains of tubercle bacilli studied by aerogenic infection of guinea pigs. *Am Rev Respir Dis, 102,* 97–100.

Cole, S. T., Brosch, R., Parkhill, J., Garnier, T., Churcher, C., Harris, D., Gordon, S. V., Eiglmeier, K., Gas, S., Barry, C. E., Tekaia, F., Badcock, K., Basham, D., Brown, D., Chillingworth, T., Connor, R., Davies, R., Devlin, K., Feltwell, T., Gentles, S., Hamlin, N., Holroyd, S., Hornsby, T., Agels, K., Krogh, A., McLean, J., Moule, S., Murphy, L., Oliver, K., Osborne, J., Quail, M. A., Rajandream, M. A., Rogers, J., Rutter, S., Seeger, K., Skelton, J., Squares, R., Squares, S., Suslston, J. E., Taylor, K., Whitehead, S., & Barrell, B. G. (1998). Deciphering the biology of *Mycobacterium tuberculosis* from the complete genomic sequence. *Nature, 393,* 537–544.

Condos, R., Rom, W., & Schluger, N. 1997. Treatment of multidrug-resistant pulmonary tuberculosis with interferon—via aerosol. *Lancet, 349*, 1513–1515.

Coninx, R., Mathieu, C., Debacker, M., Mirzoev, F., Ismaelov, A., de Haller, R., & Meddings, D. (1999). First-line tuberculosis therapy and drug-resistant *Mycobacterium tuberculosis* in prisons. *Lancet, 353*, 969–973.

Cooksey, R., Morlock, G., Glickman, S., & Crawford, J. (1997). Evaluation of a line probe assay kit for characterization of rpoB mutations in rifampin-resistant *Mycobacterium tuberculosis* isolates from New York City. *J Clin Microbiol, 35*, 1281–1283.

Coronado, V., Beck-Sague, C., Hutton, M., Davis, B., Nicholas, P., Villareal, C., Woodley, C., Kilburn, J., Crawford, J., Frieden, T., Sinkowitz, R., & Jarvis, W. (1993). Transmission of multidrug-resistant *Mycobacterium tuberculosis* among persons with human immunodeficiency virus infection in an urban hospital: Epidemiologic and restriction fragment length polymorphism analysis. *J Infec Dis, 168*, 1052–1055.

Costello, H., Caras, G., & Snider, D. (1980). Drug resistance among previously treated tuberculosis patients, a brief report. *Am Rev Resp Dis, 121*, 313–316.

Crofton, J., Chaulet, P., & Maher, D. (1997). Guidelines for the management of drug-resistant tuberculosis. WHO WHO/TB/96.210, 5–47.

Crofton, J., & Mitchison, D. (1948). Streptomycin resistance in pulmonary tuberculosis. *Brit Med J, 2*, 1009.

Crowle, A., Sbarbaro, J., Judson, F., & May, M. (1985). The effect of ethambutol on tubercle bacilli within cultured human macrophages. *Am Rev Respir Dis, 132*, 742–745.

Cruciani, M., Malena, M., Bosco, O., Gatti, G., & Serpelloni, G. (2001). The impact of human immunodeficiency virus type 1 on infectiousness of tuberculosis: A meta-analysis. *Clin Infect Dis, 33*, 1922–1930.

Cynamon, M., Klemens, S., Sharpe, C., & Chase, S. (1999). Activities of several novel oxazolidinones against *Mycobacterium tuberculosis* in a murine model. *Antimicrob Agents Chemother, 43*, 1189–1191.

David, H. (1970). Probability distribution of drug-resistant variants in unselected populations of *Mycobacterium tuberculosis*. *Appl Microbiol, 20*, 810–814.

Dickinson, J., & Mitchison, D. (1981). Experimental models to explain the high sterilizing activity of rifampin in the chemotherapy of tuberculosis. *Am Rev Resp Dis, 123*, 367–371.

Dooley, S., Jarvis, W., & Martone, W. (1992). Multidrug resistant tuberculosis (editorial). *Ann Intern Med, 117*, 257–258.

Doster, B., Caras, G., & Snider, D. (1976). A continuing survey of primary drug resistance in tuberculosis, 1961 to 1968. *Am Rev Respir Dis, 113*, 419.

Driver, C., Frieden, T., Bloch, A., & Onorato, I. (1994). Drug resistance among tuberculosis patients, New York City, 1991 and 1992. *Public Health Reports, 109*(5), 632–636.

Dye, C., Espinal, M., Watt, C., Mbiaga, C., & Williams, B. (2002). Worldwide incidence of multidrug-resistant tuberculosis. *J Inf Dis, 185*, 1197–1202.

Edlin, B., Tokars, J., Grieco, M., Crawford, J., Williams, J., Sordillo, E., Ong, K., Kilburn, J., Dooley, S., Castro, K., Jarvis, W., & Holmberg, S. (1992). An outbreak of multidrug resistant tuberculosis among hospitalized persons with the acquired immunodeficiency syndrome. *N Engl J Med, 326*, 1514–1521.

Elliott, A., Halwiindi, B., Hayes, R., Luo, N., Tembo, G., Machiels, L., Bern, C., Steenbergen, G., Pobee, J., & Nunn, P. (1993). The impact of human immunodeficiency virus on presentation and diagnosis of tuberculosis in a cohort study in Zambia. *J Trop Med Hyg, 96*, 1–11.

Enarson, D. (2000). Resistance to antituberculosis medication. Hard lessons to learn. *Arch Intern Med, 160*, 581–582.

Espinal, M., Kim, S., Suarez, P., Kam, K., Khomenko, A., Migliori, G. B., Baez, J., Kochi, A., Dye, C., & Raviglione, M. (2000). Standard short-course chemotherapy for drug-resistant tuberculosis: Treatment outcomes in six countries. *JAMA, 283*(19), 2537–2545.

Espinal, M. A., Laserson, K., Camacho, M., Fusheng, Z., Kim, S. J., Tlali, R. E., Smith, I., Suarez, P., Antunes, M. L., George, A. G., Martin-Casabona, N., Simelane, P., Weyer, K., Binkin, N., & Raviglione, M. C. (2001a). Determinants of drug-resistant tuberculosis: Analysis of 11 countries. *Int J Tuberc Lung Dis, 5*(10), 887–893.

Espinal, M., Laszlo, A., Simonsen, L., Boulahbal, F., Kim, S., Reniero, A., Hoffner, S., Rieder, H., Binkin, N., Dye, C., Williams, R., & Raviglione, M. (2001b). Global trends in resistance to anti-tuberculosis drugs. *N Engl J Med, 344,* 1294–1303.

Fischl, M., Daikos, G., Uttamchandani, R., Poblete, R., Moreno, J., Reyes, R., Boota, A., Thompson, L., Cleary, T., & Oldham, S. (1992a). Clinical presentation and outcome of patients with HIV infection and tuberculosis caused by multiple-drug resistant bacilli. *Ann Intern Med, 117,* 184–190.

Fischl, M., Uttamchandani, R., Daikos, G., Poblete, R., Moreno, J., Reyes, R., Boota, A., Thompson, L., Cleary, T., & Lai, S. (1992b). An outbreak of tuberculosis caused by multiple-drug resistant tubercle bacilli among patients with HIV infection. *Ann Intern Med, 117,* 177–183.

Frieden, T. R., Sherman, L. F., Maw, K. L., Fujiwara, P. I., Crawford, J. T., Nivin, B., Sharp, V., Hwelett, D., Jr., Brudney, K., Alland, D., & Kreiswroth, B. N. (1996). A multi-institutional outbreak of highly drug-resistant tuberculosis: Epidemiology and clinical outcomes. *JAMA, 276,* 1229–1235.

Frieden, T., Sterling, T., Pablos-Mendez, A., Kilburn, J., Cauthen, G., & Dooley, S. (1993). The emergence of drug-resistant tuberculosis in New York City. *N Engl J Med, 328*(8), 521–526.

Fung-Tomc, J., Minassian, B., Kolek, B., Washo, T., Huczko, E., & Bonner, D. (2000). In vitro antibacterial spectrum of a new broad-spectrum 8-methoxy fluoroquinolone, gatifloxacin. *J Antimicrob Chemother, 45,* 437–446.

Ginsberg, A. (2000). A proposed national strategy for tuberculosis vaccine development. *Clin Infect Dis, 30*(Suppl 3), S233–S242.

Goble, M., Iseman, M., Madsen, L., Waite, D., Ackerson, L., & Horsburgh, C. (1993). Treatment of 171 patients with pulmonary tuberculosis resistant to isoniazid and rifampin. *N Engl J Med, 328,* 527–532.

Gordin, F., Nelson, E., Matts, J., Cohn, D., Ernst, J., Benator, D., Besch, C., Crane, L., Sampson, J., Bragg, P., El-Sadr, W., and the Terry Beirn Community Programs for Clinical research on AIDS. (1996). The impact of human immunodeficiency virus infection on drug-resistant tuberculosis. *Am J Respir Crit Care Med, 154,* 1478–1483.

Gordon S. M., Horsburgh, C. R., Jr., Peloquin, C. A., Havlik, J. A., Jr., Metchock, B., Heifits, L., McGowan, J. E., Jr., & Thompson, S. E. (1993). Low serum levels of oral antimycobacterial agents in patients with disseminated *Mycobacterium avium* complex disease. *J Infect Dis, 168,* 1559–1562.

Gorzynski, E., Gutman, S., & Allen, W. (1989). Comparative antimycobacterial activities of difloxacin, temafloxacin, enoxacin, perfloxacin, reference fluoroquinolones, and a new macrolide, clarithromycin. *Antimicrob Agents Chemother, 33,* 591–592.

Grange, J., Gibson, J., Osborn, T., Collins, C., & Yates, M. (1983). What is BCG? *Tubercle, 64,* 129–139.

Harkin, T., & Harris, H. (1996). Treatment of multidrug-resistant tuberculosis. In W. Rom & S. Garay (Eds.), *Tuberculosis* (pp. 843–850). Boston: Little, Brown and Company.

Havlir, D., & Barnes, P. 1999. Tuberculosis in patients with human immunodeficiency virus infection. *N Engl J Med, 340,* 367–373.

Hibbs, J., Xeager, S., & Cochran, J. (1989). Tuberculosis among migrant farm workers. *JAMA, 262,* 1775.

Hirano, K., Abe, C., & Takahashi, M. (1999). Mutations in the rpoB gene of rifampin-resistant *Mycobacterium tuberculosis* strains isolated mostly in Asian countries and their rapid detection by line probe assay. *J Clin Microbiol, 37,* 2663–2666.

Holland, S., Eisenstein, E., Kuhns, D., Turner, M., Fleisher, T., Strober, W., & Gallin, J. (1994). Treatment of refractory disseminated nontuberculous mycobacteria infection with gamma interferon. *N Engl J Med, 330*, 1348–1355.

Hong Kong Chest Service/British Medical Research Council. (1987). Five year follow-up of a controlled trial of five 6 month regimes of chemotherapy for pulmonary tuberculosis. *Am Rev Respir Dis, 136*, 1339–1342.

Hong Kong Chest Service/British Medical Research Council. (1992). A controlled study of rifabutin and an uncontrolled study of ofloxacin in the retreatment of patients with pulmonary tuberculosis resistant to isoniazid, streptomycin, and rifampicin. *Tuberc Lung Dis, 73*, 59–67.

Horn, D., Hewlett, D., Alfalia, C., Pella, P., Franchini, D., Peterson, S., & Opal, S. (1995). Limited tolerance of ofloxacin and pyrazinamide prophylaxis in health care workers following exposure to rifampin-isoniazid-streptomycin-ethambutol-resistant tuberculosis. *Infect Dis Clin Prac, 4*, 219–225.

Howard, W., Maresh, F., Mueller, E., Yanitelli, S., & Woodruff, G. (1949). The role of pulmonary cavitation in the development of bacterial resistance to streptomycin. *Am Rev Tuberc, 59*, 391.

Howlett, H., O'Connor, J., Sadusk, J., Swift, J., & Beardsley, F. (1949). Sensitivity of tubercle bacilli to streptomycin: The influence of various factors upon the emergence of resistant strains. *Am Rev Tuberc, 59*, 402.

Iseman, M. (1993). Treatment of multidrug-resistant tuberculosis. *N Engl J Med, 329*, 784–791.

Iseman, M., & Madsen, L. (1989). Drug-resistant tuberculosis. *Clin Chest Med, 10*, 341–353.

Iseman, M., Madsen, L., Goble, M., & Pomerantz, M. (1990). Surgical intervention in the treatment of pulmonary disease caused by drug-resistant *Mycobacterium tuberculosis*. *Am Rev Resp Dis, 141*, 623–625.

Jacobs, W., Barletta, R., Udani, R., Chan, J., Kalkut, G., Sosne, G., Kieser, T., Sarkis, G., Hatfull, G., & Bloom, B. (1993). Rapid assessment of drug susceptibilities of *Mycobacterium tuberculosis* by means of luciferase reporter phages. *Science, 260*, 819–822.

Jacobson, M., Mercer, M., Miller, L., & Simpson, T. (1987). Tuberculosis risk among migrant farm workers on the Delmarva peninsula. *Am J Public Health, 77*, 29–32.

Jancik, E., Zelenka, M., Tousek, J., & Makova, M. (1963). Chemotherapy for patients with cultures resistant to streptomycin, isoniazid, and PAS. *Tubercle, 44*, 443–445.

Jarallah, J., Elias, K., Hajjaj, A., Bukhar, M., Shareef, A., & Al-Shammari, S. (1994). High rate of rifampicin resistance of *Mycobacterium tuberculosis* in the Taif region of Saudi Arabia. *Tubercle, 73*, 113–115.

Johnson, K., Braden, C., Cairns, L., Field, K., Colombel, A., Yang, Z., Woodley, C., Morlock, G., Weber, A., Boudreau, A., Bell, T., Onorato, I., Valway, S., & Stehr-Green, P. (2000). Transmission of *Mycobacterium tuberculosis* from medical waste. *JAMA, 284*(13), 1683–1688.

Johnson, L., & Sepkowitz, K. (1995). Treatment of multi-drug-resistant tuberculosis. In L. Lutwick (Ed.), *Tuberculosis* (pp. 316–330). London: Chapman and Hall Medical.

Kahana, L., & Spino, M. (1991). Ciprofloxacin in patients with mycobacterial infections: Experience in 15 patients. *DICP Ann Pharmacother, 25*, 919–924.

Kazionny, B., Wells, C., Kluge, H., Gusseynova, N., & Milotilov, V. (2001). Implications of the growing HIV-1 epidemic for tuberculosis control in Russia. *Lancet, 358*, 1513–1514.

Kent, J. (1993). The epidemiology of multidrug-resistant tuberculosis in the United States. *Med Clin N Am, 77*(6), 1391–1409.

Kent, P., & Kubica, G. (1985). *Public health mycobacteriology. A guide for the level III laboratory* (pp. 159–184). Atlanta, Georgia: U.S. Department of Health and Human Services. Centers for Disease Control.

Kenyon, T., Mwasekaga, M., Huebner, R., et al. (1999). Low levels of drug resistance amidst rapidly increasing tuberculosis and human immunodeficiency virus coepidemics in Botswana. *Int J Tuberc Lung Dis, 3*, 4–11.

Kenyon, T., Ridzon, R., Luskin-Hawk, R., Schultz, C., Paul, W., Valway, S., Onorato, I., & Castro, K. (1997). A nosocomial outbreak of multidrug-resistant tuberculosis. *Ann Intern Med, 127*(1), 32–36.

Kimerling, M., Kluge, H., Vezhnina, N., Iacovazzi, T., Demeulenaere, T., Portaels, F., & Matthys, F. (1999). Inadequacy of the current WHO re-treatment regimen in a central Siberian prison: Treatment failure and MDR-TB. *Int J Tuberc Lung Dis, 3*, 451–453.

Kohno, S., Koga, H., Kaku, M., Maesaki, S., & Hara, K. (1992). Prospective comparative study of ofloxacin or ethambutol for the treatment of pulmonary tuberculosis. *Chest, 102*, 1815–1818.

Laserson, K., Kenyon, A., Kenyon, T., Layloff, T., & Binkin, N. (2001). Substandard tuberculosis drugs on the global market and their simple detection. *Int J Tuberc Lung Dis, 5*(5), 448–454.

Laserson, K., Osorio, L., Sheppard, J., Hernandez, H., Benitez, A., Brim, S., Woodley, C., Hazbon, M., Villegas, M., Castano, M., Henriquez, N., Rodriguez, E., Metchock, B., & Binkin, N. (2000). Clinical and programmatic mismanagement rather than community outbreak as the cause of chronic, drug-resistant tuberculosis in Buenaventura, Colombia, (1998). *Int J Tuberc Lung Dis, 4*(7), 673–683.

Laszlo, A., Rahman, M., Ravilglione, M., Bustreo, F., WHO/IUATLD Network of Supranational Laboratories. (1997). Quality assurance programme for drug susceptibility testing of Mycobacterium tuberculosis in the WHO/IUATLD Supranational Laboratory Network: First round of proficiency testing. *Int J Tuberc Lung Dis, 1*, 231–238.

Lederberg, J., & Lederberg, E. (1952). Replica plating and indirect selection of bacterial variants. *J Bact, 63*(3), 399–406.

Lietman, T., & Blower, S. (2000). Potential impact of tuberculosis vaccines as epidemic control agents. *Clin Infect Dis, 30*(Suppl 3), S316–322.

Leonard, M., Larsen, N., Drechsler, H., Blumber, H., Lennox, J., Arrellano, M., Filip, J., & Horsburgh, C. (2002). Increased survival of persons with tuberculosis and human immunodeficiency virus infection, 1991–2000. *Clin Infect Dis, 34*, 1002–1007.

Leone, G., van Schijndel, H., van Gemen, B., Kramer, F., & Schoen, C. (1998). Molecular beacon probes combined with amplification by NASBA enable homologous, real-time detection of RNA. *Nucleic Acids Res, 26*, 2150–2155.

Liu, A., Shilkret, K., & Finelli, L. (1998). Initial drug regimens for the treatment of tuberculosis: Evaluation of physician prescribing practices in New Jersey, 1994–1995. *Chest, 113*, 1446–1451.

Lou, H., Shullo, M., & McKaveney, T. (2002). Limited tolerability of levofloxacin and pyrazinamide for multidrug-resistant tuberculosis prophylaxis in a solid organ transplant population. *Pharmacotherapy 22*, 701–704.

Lutfey, M., Della-Latta, P., Kapur, V., & Palumbo, L. (1996). Independent origin of mono-resistant Mycobacterium tuberculosis in patients with AIDS. *Am J Resp Crit Care Med, 153*, 837–840.

McClatchy, L., Kane, S., Davidson, P., & Moulding, T. (1977). Cross-resistance in *M. tuberculosis* to kanamycin, capreomycin and viomycin. *Tubercle, 58*, 29–34.

Mahmoudi, A., & Iseman, M. (1993). Pitfalls in the care of patients with tuberculosis. *JAMA, 270*(1), 65–68.

Mahmoudi, A., & Iseman, M. (1992). Surgical intervention in the treatment of drug-resistant tuberculosis: Update and extended follow-up. *Am Rev Respir Dis, 145*, A816.

Marttila, H., Soini, H., Vyshnevskaya, E., Vyshnevskiy, B., Otten, T., Vasilyef, A., & Viljanen, M. (1999). Line probe assay in the rapid detection rifampin-resistant *Mycobacterium tuberculosis* directly from clinical specimens. *Scand J Infect Dis, 31*, 269–273.

Mastro, T., & Coninx, R. (1988). The management of tuberculosis in refugees along the Thai-Kampuchean border. *Tubercle, 69*, 95–103.

Middlebrook, G. (1952). Sterilization of tubercle bacilli by isonicotinic acid hydrazide and the incidence of variants resistant to the drug in vitro. *Am Rev Tuberc, 65*, 765–767.

Middlebrook, G. (1954). Isoniazid-resistance and catalase activity of the tubercle bacilli: A preliminary report. *Am Rev Tuberc, 69*, 471–472.

Middlebrook, G., & Cohn, M. (1953). Some observations on the pathogenicity of isoniazid-resistant variants of tubercle bacilli. *Science, 118*, 297–299.

Miles, S., & Maat, R. (1984). A successful supervised outpatient short-course tuberculosis treatment program in an open refugee camp on the Thai-Cambodian border. *Am Rev Respir Dis, 130*, 827–830.

Miles, S., & Maat, R. (1987). Follow-up on tuberculosis treatment in a Cambodian refugee camp (letter). *Am Rev Respir Dis, 135*, 512.

Mitchison, D. (1950). Development of streptomycin resistant strains of tubercle bacilli in pulmonary tuberculosis. *Thorax, 4*, 144.

Mitchison, D. (1965). Chemotherapy of tuberculosis: A bacteriologist's viewpoint. *Brit Med J, 1*, 1333–1340.

Mitchison, D. (1984). Drug resistance in mycobacteria. *Br Med Bull, 40*, 84–90.

Mitchison, D., & Nunn, A. (1986). Influence of initial drug resistance on the response to short-course chemotherapy of pulmonary tuberculosis. *Am Rev Respir Dis, 133*, 423–430.

Miyazaki, E., Miyazaki, M., Chen, J., Chaisson, R., & Bishai, W. (1999). Moxifloxacin (BAY12–8039), a new 8-methoxyquinolone, is active in a mouse model of tuberculosis. *Antimicrob Agents Chemother, 43*, 85–89.

Mohanty, K., & Dhamgaye, T. (1993). Controlled trial of ciprofloxacin in short-term chemotherapy for pulmonary tuberculosis. *Chest, 104*, 1194–1198.

Moore, M., Onorato, I., McCray, E., & Castro, K. (1997). Trends in drug-resistant tuberculosis in the United States, 1993–1996. *JAMA, 278*, 833–837.

Moro, M., Gori, A., Errante, I., Infuso, A., Franzetti, F., Sodano, L., Iemoli, E., and the Italian Multidrug-Resistant Tuberculosis Outbreak Study Group. (1998). An outbreak of multidrug-resistant tuberculosis involving HIV-infected patients of two hospitals in Milan, Italy. *AIDS, 12*, 1095–1102.

Mukadi, Y., Perriens, J., St. Louis, M., Brown, C., Prignot, J., Willame, J., Pouthier, F., Kaboto, M., Ryder, R., & Portaels, F. (1993). Spectrum of immunodeficiency in HIV-1-infected patients with pulmonary tuberculosis in Zaire. *Lancet, 342*, 143–146.

Munsiff, S., & Frieden, T. (1996). Mono-refampin resistant tuberculosis, New York City, 1993–1994 (Abstract No. C118). In Abstracts of the 36th Interscience Conference on Antimicrobial Agents and Chemotherapy (New Orleans, LA, p. 55). American Society for Microbiology, Washington, DC.

Narang, P., Trapnell, C., Schoenfelder, J., Lavelle, J., & Bianchine, J. (1994). Fluconazole and enhanced effect of rifabutin prophylaxis. *N Engl J Med, 330*, 1316.

Nardell, E., McInnes, B., Thomas, B., & Weidhaas, S. (1986). Exogenous reinfection with tuberculosis in a shelter for the homeless. *N Engl J Med, 315*, 1570–1575.

Nitta, A., Knowles, L., Kim, J., Lehnkering, E., Borenstein, L., Davidson, P., Harvey, S., & DeKoning, M. (2002). Limited transmission of multidrug-resistant tuberculosis despite a high proportion of infectious cases in Los Angeles County, California. *Am Rev Resp Crit Care Med, 165*, 812–817.

Nolan, C., Williams, D., Cave, M., Eisenach, K., El-Hajj, H., Hooton, T., Thompson, R., & Goldberg, S. (1995). Evolution of rifampin resistance in human immunodeficiency virus-associated tuberculosis. *Am J Resp Crit Care Med, 152*, 1067–1071.

Nunn, P., Kibuga, D., Gathua, S., Brindle, R., Imalingat, A., Wasunna, K., Lucas, S., Gilks, C., Omwega, M., & Were, J. (1991). Cutaneous hypersensitivity reactions due to thiacetazone in HIV-1 seropositive patients treated for tuberculosis. *Lancet, 337*, 627–630.

Nunn, P., Mungai, M., Nyamwaya, J., Gicheha, C., Brindle, R., Dunn, D., Githui, W., Were, J., & McAdam, K. (1994). The effect of human immunodeficiency virus type-1 on the infectiousness of tuberculosis. *Tuberc Lung Dis, 75*, 25–32.

O'Brien, R., & Nunn, P. (2001). The need for new drugs against tuberculosis: Obstacles, opportunities, and next steps. *Am J Respir Crit Care Med, 162*, 1055–1058.

Okwera, A., Johnson, J., Vjecha, M., Wolski, K., Whalen, C., Hom, D., Huebner, R., Mugerwa, R., &
    Ellner, J. (1997). Risk factors for adverse drug reactions during thiacetazone treatment of pulmonary
    tuberculosis in human immunodeficiency virus infected adults. *Int J Tuberc Lung Dis, 1*, 441–445.
Pablos-Mendez, A., Raviglione, M., Laszlo, A., Binkin, N., Rieder, H., Bustreo, F., Cohn, D.,
    Lambregts-van Weezenbeek, C., Kim, S., Chaulet, P., & Nunn, P. (1998). Global surveillance for
    antituberculosis-drug resistance, 1994–1997. *N Engl J Med, 338*, 1641–1649.
Pai, M., McCulloch, M., & Colford, J. (2002). Meta-analysis of the impact of HIV on the infec-
    tiousness of tuberculosis: Methodological concerns (letter). *Clin Infect Dis, 34*, 1285–1287.
Papastavros, T., Dolovich, L., Holbrook, A., Whitehead, L., & Loeb, M. (2002). Adverse events asso-
    ciated with pyrazinamide and levofloxacin in the treatment of latent multidrug-resistant tubercu-
    losis. *Can Med Assoc J, 167*, 131–136.
Park, M., Davis, A., Schluger, N., Cohen, H., & Rom, W. (1996). Outcome of MDR-TB patients,
    1983–1993: Prolonged survival with appropriate therapy. *Am J Resp Crit Care Med, 153*,
    317–324.
Patel, K. B., Belmonte, R., & Crowe, H. M. (1995). Drug malabsorption and resistance in HIV-
    infected patients. *N Engl J Med, 332*, 326–337.
Pearson, M., Jereb, J., Frieden, T., Crawford, J., Davis, B., Dooley, S., & Jarvis, W. (1992).
    Nosocomial transmission of multidrug resistant *Mycobacterium tuberculosis*. A risk to patients
    and healthcare workers. *Ann Intern Med, 117*, 191–196.
Peloquin, C., Nitta, A., Burman, W., Brudney, K., Miranda-Massari, J., McGuiness, M., Berning, S., &
    Gerena, G. (1996). Low antituberculosis drug concentrations in patients with AIDS. *Ann
    Pharmacother, 30*, 919–925.
Perlman, D., El-Sadr, W., Nelson, E., Matts, J., Telzak, E., Salomon, N., Chirgwin, K., Hafner, R., for
    the Terry Beirn Community Programs for Clinical Research on AIDS (CPCRA) and the AIDS
    Clinical Trial Group (ACTG). (1997). Variation of chest radiographic patterns in pulmonary tuber-
    culosis by degree of human immunodeficiency virus-related immunosuppression. *Clin Inf Dis, 25*,
    242–246.
Physicians' Desk Reference Electronic Library. (2001). Medical Economics Company, Inc.
    http://www.pdrel.com/
Piatek, A., Telenti, A., Murray, M., El-Hajj, H., Jacobs, W., Kramer, F., & Alland, D. (2000).
    Genotypic analysis of *Mycobacterium tuberculosis* in two distinct populations using molecular
    beacons: implications for rapid susceptibility testing. *Antimicob Agents Chemother, 44*, 103–110.
Piatek, A., Tyagi, S., Pol, A., Telenti, A., Miller, L., Kramer, F., & Alland, D. (1998). Molecular bea-
    con sequence analysis for detecting drug resistance in *Mycobacterium tuberculosis*. *Nat
    Biotechnol, 16*, 359–363.
Portugal, I., Covas, M. J., Brum, L., Viveiros, M., Ferrinho, P., Moniz-Pereira, J., & David, H. (1999).
    Outbreak of multidrug-resistant tuberculosis in Lisbon: Detection by restriction fragment length
    polymorphism analysis. *Int J Tuberc Lung Dis, 3*, 207–213.
Pyle, M. (1947). Relative numbers of resistant tubercle bacilli in patients before and during treatment
    with streptomycin. *Proc Staff Meet Mayo Clin, 22*, 465–488.
Rastogi, N., & Goh, K. (1991). In vitro activity of the new difluorinated quinolone sparfloxacin (AT-
    4140) against *Mycobacterium tuberculosis* compared with activities of ofloxacin and
    ciprofloxacin. *Antimicrob Agents Chemother, 35*, 1933–1936.
Reichler, M., Valway, S., & Onorato, I. (2000). Transmission in the United States Virgin Islands and
    Florida of a multidrug-resistant *Mycobacterium tuberculosis* strain acquired in Puerto Rico. *Clin
    Infect Dis, 30*, 617–618.
Reichman, L. (1991). The U-shaped curve of concern. *Am Rev Respir Dis, 144*, 741–742.
Reichman, L., McDonald, R., & Mangura, B. (1994). Rifabutin prophylaxis against *Mycobacterium
    avium* complex infection. *N Engl J Med, 330*, 437–438.

Reves, R., Blakey, D., Snider, D., & Farer, L. (1981). Transmission of multiple drug-resistant tuberculosis: Report of a school and community outbreak. *Am J Epidemiol, 113*, 423–435.

Ridzon, R., Kent, J., Valway, S., Weismuller, P., Maxwell, R., Elcock, M., Meador, J., Royce, S., Shefer, A., Smith, P., Woodley, C., & Onorato, I. (1997a). Outbreak of drug-resistant tuberculosis with second generation transmission in a high school in California. *J Pediatr* 131(6), 863–868.

Ridzon, R., Kenyon, T., Luskin-Hawk, R., Schultz, C., Valway, S., & Onorato, I. (1997b). Nosocomial transmission of human immunodeficiency virus and subsequent transmission of multidrug-resistant tuberculosis in a healthcare worker. *Infect Control Hosp Epidemiol, 18*, 422–423.

Ridzon, R., Meador, J., Maxwell, R., Higgins, K., Weismuller, P., & Onorato, I. (1997c). Asymptomatic hepatitis in persons who received alternative preventive therapy with pyrazinamide and ofloxacin. *Clin Infec Dis, 24*, 1264–1265.

Ridzon, R., Whitney, C., McKenna, M., Taylor, J., Ashkar, S., Nitta, A., Harvey, S., Valway, S., Woodley, C., Cooksey, R., & Onorato, I. (1998). Risk factors for rifampin mono-resistant tuberculosis. *Am Rev Respir Crit Care Med, 157*, 1881–1884.

Rieder, H. (1985). Tuberculosis in an Indochinese refugee camp: Epidemiology, management and therapeutic results. *Tubercle, 66*, 179–186.

Roberts, G., Goodman, N., Heifits, L., Larsh, H., Lindner, T., McClatchy, J., McGinnis, M., Siddiqi, S., & Wright, P. (1983). Evaluation of the BACTEC radiometric method for recovery of mycobacteria and drug susceptibility testing of *Mycobacterium tuberculosis* from acid-fast smear-positive specimens. *J Clin Microbiol, 18*, 689–696.

Rodriguez, L., & Smith, P. (1990). Tuberculosis in developing countries and methods for its control. *Trans R Soc Trop Med Hyg, 84*, 739–744.

Rouse, D., Li, Z., & Morris, S. (1995). Characterization of the katG and inhA genes of isoniazid-resistant clinical isolates of *Mycobacterium tuberculosis*. *Antimicrob Agents Chemother, 39*, 2472–2477.

Sacks, L., Pendle, S., Orlovic, D., Andre, M., Popara, M., Moore, G., Thonell, L., & Hurwitz, S. (2001). Adjunctive salvage therapy with inhaled aminoglycosides for patients with persistent smear-positive pulmonary tuberculosis. *Clin Infect Dis, 32*, 44–49.

Sacks, L., Pendle, S., Orlovic, D., Blumberg, L., & Constantinou, C. (1999). A comparison of outbreak- and nonoutbreak-related multidrug-resistant tuberculosis among human immunodeficiency virus-infected patients in a South African Hospital. *Clin Infect Dis, 29*, 96–101.

Sahai, J., Gallicano, K., Swick, L., Tailor, S., Garber, G., Seguin, I., Oliveras, S., Walker, S., Rachlis, A., & Cameron, D. (1997). Reduced plasma concentrations of antituberculosis drugs in patients with HIV infection. *Ann Intern Med, 127*, 289–293.

Salomon, N., Perlman, D., Friedmann, P., Buchstein, S., Kreiswirth, B., & Mildvan, D. (1995). Predictors and outcome of multidrug-resistant tuberculosis. *Clin Inf Dis, 21*, 1245–1252.

Sbarbaro, J. (1996). Tuberculosis control is indeed an exercise in vigilance. *Public Health Rep, 111*, 30–31.

Schluger, N. (2001). Changing approaches to the diagnosis of tuberculosis. *Am J Respir Crit Care Med, 164*, 2020–2024.

Seaworth, B. (2002). Multidrug-resistant tuberculosis. *Infect Dis Clin N Am, 16*, 73–105.

Shears, P. (1984). Tuberculosis control in Somali refugee camps. *Tubercle, 65*, 111–116.

Siddiqi, S. (1989). *Bactec TB System. Product and Procedure Manual*. Towson, MD, USA: Becton Dickinson.

Small, P., & Fujiwara, P. (2001). Management of tuberculosis in the United States. *N Engl J Med, 345*, 189–200.

Snider, D., Cauthen, G., Farer, L., Kelly, G., Kilburn, J., Good, R., & Dooley, S. (1991). Drug-resistant tuberculosis. *Am Rev Resp Dis, 144*, 732.

Snider, D., Graczyk, J., Bek, E., & Rogowski, J. (1984). Supervised six-months treatment of newly diagnosed pulmonary tuberculosis using isoniazid, rifampin, pyrazinamide with and without streptomycin. *Am Rev Respir Dis, 130*, 1091–1094.

Snider, D., Kelly, G., Cauthen, G., Thompson, N., & Kilburn, J. (1985). Infection and disease among contacts of tuberculosis cases with drug-resistant and drug-susceptible bacilli. *Am Rev Resp Dis, 132*, 125–132.

Somner, A., & Brace, A. (1962). Ethionamide, pyrazinamide, and cycloserine used successfully in the treatment of chronic pulmonary tuberculosis. *Tubercle, 43*, 345–360.

Spinaci, S. (1985, November 19–21). Tuberculosis problems among Afghan refugees in N.W.F.P. (Pakistan). *Workshop on the Afghan Refuge Health Programme*, Islamabad.

Steiner, M., Chaves, A., Lyons, H., Steiner, P., & Portugaleza, C. (1970). Primary drug-resistant tuberculosis: Report of an outbreak. *N Engl J Med, 283*, 1353–1358.

Stottmeier, K. (1976). Emergence of rifampin-resistant *Mycobacterium tuberculosis* in Massachusetts. *J Infect Dis, 133*, 88.

Stover, C., Warrener, P., VanDevanter, D., Sherman, D., Arain, T., Langhorne, M., Anderson, S., Towell, J., Yaun, Y., McMurray, D., Kresiwirth, B., Barry, C., & Baker, W. (2000). A small-molecule nitroimidazopyran drug candidate for the treatment of tuberculosis. *Nature, 405*, 962–966.

Sullivan, E., Kreiswirth, B., Palumbo, L., Kapur, V., Musser, J., Ebrahimzadeh, A., & Frieden, T. (1995). Emergence of fluoroquinolone-resistant tuberculosis in New York City. *Lancet, 345*, 1148–1150.

Tahaoglu, K., Torun, T., Sevim, T., Atac, G., Kir, A., Karasulu, L., Ozmen, I., & Kapakli, N. (2001). The treatment of multidrug-resistant tuberculosis in Turkey. *N Engl J Med, 345*, 170–174.

Telenti, A., Imboden, P., Marchesi, F., Lowrie, D., Cole, S., Colston, M., Matter, L., Schopfer, K., & Bodmer, T. (1993). Detection of rifampin-resistance mutations in *Mycobacterium tuberculosis*. *Lancet, 341*, 647–650.

Telzak, E., Chirgwin, K., Nelson, E., Matts, J., Sepkowitz, K., Benson, C., Perlman, D., El-Sadr, W., for the Terry Beirn Community Programs for Clinical Research on AIDS (CPCRA) and the AIDS Clinical trial Group (ACTG), National institutes of Health. (1999). Predictors for multidrug-resistant tuberculosis among HIV-infected patients and responses to specific drug regimens. *Int J Tuberc Lung Dis, 3*, 337–343.

Telzak, E., Sepkowitz, K., Alpert, P., Mannheimer, S., Medard, F., El-Sadr, W., Blum, S., Gagliardi, A., Salomon, N., & Turett, G. (1995). Multidrug-resistant tuberculosis in patients without HIV infection. *N Engl J Med, 333*, 907–911.

Tenover, F. C., Crawford, J. T., Huebner, R. E., Geiter, L. J., Horsburgh, C. R. J., & Good, R. C. (1993). The resurgence of tuberculosis: Is your laboratory ready? *J Clin Microbiol, 31*, 767–770.

Theuer, C., Hopewell, P., Elias, D., Schecter, G., Rutherford, G., & Chaisson, R. (1990). Human immunodeficiency virus infection in tuberculosis patients. *J Infect Dis, 162*, 8–12.

Trapnell, C., Narrowing, P., Li, R., & Lavelle, J. (1996). Increased plasma rifabutin levels with concomitant fluconazole therapy in HIV-infected patients. *Ann Intern Med, 124*, 573–576.

Treasure, R., & Seaworth, B. (1995). Current role of surgery in *Mycobacterium tuberculosis*. *Ann Thorac Surg, 59*, 1405–1407.

Tsukamura, M., Nakamura, E., Yoshii, S., & Amano, H. (1985). Therapeutic effect of a new antibacterial substance ofloxacin (DL8280) on pulmonary tuberculosis. *Am Rev Respir Dis, 131*, 352–356.

Turett, G., Telzak, E., Torian, L., Blum, S., Alland, D., Weisfuse, I., & Fazal, B. (1995). Improved outcomes for patients with multidrug-resistant tuberculosis. *Clin Infect Dis, 21*, 1238–1244.

UNAIDS. (2002). Report on the global HIV/AIDS epidemic, Geneva, Switzerland, UNAIDS, UNAIDS/02.26E.

Valway, S., Greifinger, R., Papania, M., Kilburn, J., Woodley, C., DiFernando, G., & Dooley, S. (1994a). Multidrug-resistant tuberculosis in the New York State prison system, 1990–1991. *J Infect Dis, 170*, 151–156.

Valway, S., Richards, S., Kovacovich, J., Greifinger, R., Crawford, J., & Dooley, S. (1994b). Outbreak of multidrug-resistant tuberculosis in a New York State prison. *Am J Epidemiol, 140,* 113–122.

Van Leuven, M., De Groot, M., Shean, K., Von Oppell, U., & Willcox, P. (1997). Pulmonary resection as an adjunct in the treatment of multiple drug-resistant tuberculosis. *Ann Thorac Surg, 63,* 1363–1368.

Van Rie, A., Warren, R., Beyers, N., Gie, R., Classen, C., Richardson, M., Sampson, S., Victor, T., & van Helden, P. (1999). Transmission of a multidrug-resistant *Mycobacterium tuberculosis* strain resembling "strain W" among noninstitutionalized, human immunodeficiency virus-seronegative patients. *J Inf Dis, 180,* 1609–1615.

Vernon, A., Burman, W., Benator, D., Khan, A., Bozeman, L., Tuberculosis Trials Consortium. (1999). Acquired rifamycin monoresistance in patients with HIV-related tuberculosis treated with once-weekly rifapentine and isoniazid. *Lancet, 353,* 1843–1847.

Villarino, M., Geiter, L., & Simone, P. (1992). The multidrug resistant tuberculosis challenge to public health efforts to control tuberculosis. *Public Health Rep, 107,* 616–625.

Wehrli, W. (1988). Rifampin: Mechanisms of action and resistance. *Rev Infect Dis, 5,* 407–411.

World Health Organization. (1997). Anti-tuberculosis drug resistance in the world: The WHO/IUATLD global project on anti-tuberculosis drug resistance surveillance, 1994–1997. Geneva, Switzerland, WHO/TB/97.229, 1–229.

World Health Organization. (2000a). Anti-tuberculosis drug resistance in the world, report no. 2: Prevalence and trends. Geneva, Switzerland, WHO/CDS/TB/2000.278.

World Health Organization. (2000b). Scientific Panel of the Working Group on DOTS-Plus for MDRTB. Guidelines for establishing DOTS-Plus pilot projects for the management of multidrug-resistant tuberculosis. *WHO,* WHO/CDS/TB/2000.279, 5–95.

World Health Organization. (2001). Global tuberculosis control, 2001. Geneva, Switzerland. WHO/CDS/TB/2001.287.

World Health Organization. (2002). WHO report 2002: Global tuberculosis control. Geneva, Switzerland. WHO/CDS/TB/2002.295.

Yeager, R., Monroe, W., & Dessau, F. (1952). Pyrazinamide in the treatment of pulmonary tuberculosis. *Am Rev Tuberc, 65,* 523–546.

Young, D. (2000). Current tuberculosis vaccine development. *Clin Infect Dis, 30*(Suppl. 3), S254–S256.

Zhang, Y., Heym, B., Allen, B., Young, D., & Cole, S. (1992). The catalase-peroxidase gene and isoniazid resistance of *Mycobacterium tuberculosis. Nature, 358,* 591–593.

8

Controlling Antibiotic Resistance: Strategies Based on the Mutant Selection Window

Karl Drlica and Xilin Zhao

1. INTRODUCTION

Antimicrobial resistance has become an important factor in the reemergence of microbial pathogens, particularly in hospital settings. Among the more publicized examples are staphylococci that are resistant to all common antibiotics except vancomycin (Holder & Neely, 1998; Murray, 1997). Even vancomycin may soon be rendered ineffective, since prolonged exposure selects for isolates with reduced susceptibility (Hiramatsu et al., 1997; Tenover et al., 1998). Moreover, vancomycin-resistance genes can move into staphylococci from enterococci, at least in laboratory settings (Noble et al., 1992). Thus we can expect untreatable staphylococcal infections to be increasingly common. Other types of infection are also beginning to exhibit resistance. For example, *Streptococcus pneumoniae*, a common cause of community-acquired pneumonia, is losing its susceptibility to penicillin (Ball, 1999; Doern, 2001), and multidrug-resistant tuberculosis is spreading through the Russian prison system (Coninx et al., 1999). In most cases increasing resistance is attributed to misuse and overuse of antibiotics, two practices that are difficult to change (Levy, 2001; Pechere, 2001; Sbarbaro, 2001; Zinner et al., 2001b). Hope is often placed on the development of new agents; however, the same factors will also erode new agents, if and when they become available.

In the present chapter we argue that eliminating misuse will fail to correct the resistance problem fully because traditional dosing strategies keep us only one mutational step ahead of the pathogens. These strategies allow antimicrobial concentrations to fall inside a concentration range that enriches the mutant fraction of pathogen populations. If host defense systems fail to remove resistant mutants faster than they are enriched, the mutant fraction will gradually increase. To restrict the development of resistance, it may be necessary to change the paradigm used to establish dosing regimens. One approach would be to shift our goal from efficacious treatment of the presenting infection to explicitly avoiding the development of resistance. This strategy focuses on blocking the growth of mutants rather than susceptible cells.

Reemergence of Established Pathogens in the 21st Century
Edited by Fong and Drlica, Kluwer Academic/Plenum Publishers, New York, 2003

2. THE RESISTANCE PROBLEM

A microbiological perspective of antimicrobial resistance can be obtained from surveillance studies. In one of the many examples, a teaching hospital in the United States recently reported that 36% of the Gram-positive and 25% of the Gram-negative organisms associated with infection from trauma and general surgery were resistant to at least one agent (Sawyer et al., 2001). Since patient care is more expensive for resistant than susceptible infections (Carmeli et al., 1999), one of the consequences of resistance is increased cost. In 1995 the cost of resistance was estimated to be about $4 billion per year in the United States (Boyce, 2001). Table 8.1 shows that the problem is neither restricted to the United States nor limited to just a few pathogens.

Table 8.1
Examples of Reduced Susceptibility to Antibacterial Agents

Pathogen species	Antibacterial agent	Geographic location	Percentage resistant[a]	Reference
Campylobacter sp.				
	Fluoroquinolone	Denmark	20 (1999)	Engberg et al. (2001)[b]
		Italy	35 (1998)	Engberg et al. (2001)[b]
		Spain	70 (1998)	Engberg et al. (2001)[b]
		Thailand	83 (1995)	Engberg et al. (2001)[b]
		United States	20 (1995)	Engberg et al. (2001)[b]
E. faecium				
	Ampicillin	Israel	67 (1996)	Marcus et al. (1997)[b]
	Gentamycin	Argentina	33 (1996–1998)	Bantar et al. (2000)
		Israel	66 (1996)	Marcus et al. (1997)[b]
	Streptomycin	Argentina	37 (1996–1998)	Bantar et al. (2000)
	Vancomycin	Israel	50 (1996)	Marcus et al. (1997)[b]
		United Kingdom	24 (1998)	Reacher et al. (2000)
E. coli				
	Ampicillin	Europe	45 (1997)	Jones et al. (1999)
		Korea	79 (1997)	Chong et al. (1998)
		Taiwan	76 (1998)	Ho et al. (1999)
	Fluoroquinolone	Beijing	50–60 (1997–1998)	Wang et al. (2001)
		Greece	4–13 (1997)	Vatopoulos et al. (1999)
		Hong Kong	16 (1997)	Ling et al. (2001)[b]
		Korea	24 (1997)	Chong et al. (1998)
		Venezuela	21 (1997–1998)	Guzman-Blanco et al. (2000)
	Tetracycline	Europe	51 (1997)	Jones et al. (1999)
		Korea	69 (1997)	Chong et al. (1998)
H. pylori				
	Clarithromycin	Belgium	11 (1995–1997)	(Glupczynski, 1998)[b]
		Spain	12 (1995–1997)	(Glupczynski, 1998)[b]
		United States	13 (1995–1997)	(Glupczynski, 1998)[b]
H. influenzae				
	Ampicillin	France	28 (1997–1998)	Sahm et al. (2000)
		Spain	32 (1997–1998)	Sahm et al. (2000)
	Azithromycin	Spain	10 (1996–1997)	Garcia-Rodriguez et al. (1999)

Table 8.1

(*continued*)

Pathogen species	Antibacterial agent	Geographic location	Percentage resistant[a]	Reference
	Clarithromycin	Spain	37 (1996–1997)	Garcia-Rodriguez et al. (1999)
	Ciprofloxacin	Spain	2 (1996–1997)	Garcia-Rodriguez et al. (1999)
	Cefactor	Spain	7 (1996–1997)	Garcia-Rodriguez et al. (1999)
K. pneumoniae				
	Amikacin	Croatia	61 (1990–1995)	Barsic et al. (1997)
		Hong Kong	16 (1997)	Ling et al. (2001)[b]
		Taiwan	8 (1998)	Ho et al. (1999)
	Ceftazidime	Croatia	68 (1990–1995)	Barsic et al. (1997)
		Hong Kong	17 (1997)	Ling et al. (2001)[b]
	Ciprofloxacin	Croatia	25 (1990–1995)	Barsic et al. (1997)
	Gentamycin	Croatia	81 (1990–1995)	Barsic et al. (1997)
		Korea	27 (1997)	Chong et al. (1998)
		Taiwan	14 (1998)	Ho et al. (1999)
M. tuberculosis				
	Isoniazid	United States	8 (1996)	Moore et al. (1997)[b]
	Ofloxacin	Spain	6 (1998?)	Casal et al. (2000)
	Rifampin	United States	2 (1996)	Moore et al. (1997)[b]
N. gonorrhoeae				
	Ciprofloxacin	India	6 (1999)	Ray et al. (2000)[b]
		Japan	62 (1993–1997)	Tanaka et al. (2000)
	Penicillin	Japan	24 (1986)	Bal (1999)
		Philippines	71 (1994)	Bal (1999)
		Thailand	18 (1995)	Bal (1999)
		United States	11 (1991)	Gorwitz et al. (1993)[b]
	Tetracycline	India	6 (1999)	Ray et al. (2000)[b]
		United States	6 (1991)	Gorwitz et al. (1993)[b]
P. aeruginosa				
	Amikacin	Croatia	49 (1990–1995)	Barsic et al. (1997)
		Europe	9 (1997)	Jones et al. (1999)
		Latin America	16 (1997)	Diekema et al. (1999)
		Taiwan	13 (1998)	Ho et al. (1999)
	Ciprofloxacin	Croatia	66 (1990–1995)	Barsic et al. (1997)
		Europe	23 (1997)	Jones et al. (1999)
		Latin America	26 (1997)	Diekema et al. (1999)
		Taiwan	13 (1998)	Ho et al. (1999)
		United States	12 (1997)	Diekema et al. (1999)
Salmonella enterica ser. *typhimurium*				
	Ampicillin	Barcelona	80 (1994)	Gallardo et al. (1999)[b]
	Chloramphenicol	Barcelona	80 (1994)	Gallardo et al. (1999)[b]
	Tetracycline	Barcelona	90 (1994)	Gallardo et al. (1999)[b]
Shigella sp.				
	Ampicillin	Bangladesh	90 (1987)	Bennish et al. (1992)[b]
		Greece	46 (1991–1995)	Maraki et al. (1998)
		Latin America	40–98 (1998)	Guzman-Blanco et al. (2000)
	Nalidixic acid	Bangladesh	60 (1990)	Bennish et al. (1992)[b]
	Tetracycline	Greece	48 (1991–1995)	Maraki et al. (1998)
		Latin America	75 (1998)	Guzman-Blanco et al. (2000)

(*continued*)

Table 8.1
(continued)

Pathogen species	Antibacterial agent	Geographic location	Percentage resistant[a]	Reference
S. aureus				
	Methicillin	Argentina	58 (1996–1998)	Bantar et al. (2000)
		Europe	22 (1997)	Jones et al. (1999)
		United Kingdom	21 (1996)	Johnson (1998)[b]
Staphylococci, coagulase negative				
	Methicillin	United States	60 (1989)	Thornsberry (1995)[b]
		Argentina	56 (1996–1998)	Bantar et al. (2000)
S. pneumoniae				
	Penicillin	France	25 (1993)	Baquero (1996)[b]
		Japan	10 (1997–1998)	Sahm et al. (2000)
		Spain	25 (1997–1998)	Sahm et al. (2000)
		France	34 (1997–1998)	Sahm et al. (2000)
		Alaska	13 (1998)	Rudolph et al. (2000)[b]
		London	12 (1994–1995)	Johnson (1998)[b]
		USA	16 (1997)	Doern et al. (1998)
		Canada	8 (1997)	Doern et al. (1998)
		Hungary	35 (1988–1999)	Marton (1992)[b]
		Spain	37 (1996–1997)	Baquero et al. (1999)
		Taiwan	13 (1996–1997)	Fung et al. (2000)
	Cefuroximine	Spain	46 (1996–1997)	Baquero et al. (1999)
		Japan	37 (1997–1998)	Sahm et al. (2000)
		France	55 (1997–1998)	Sahm et al. (2000)
		USA	19 (1997)	Doern et al. (1998)
	Aminopenicillins	Spain	24 (1996–1997)	Baquero et al. (1999)
	Cefotaximine	Spain	13 (1996–1997)	Baquero et al. (1999)
		USA	4 (1997)	Doern et al. (1998)
	Azithromycin	Taiwan	74 (1996–1997)	Fung et al. (2000)
		Japan	66 (1997–1998)	Sahm et al. (2000)
		China	72 (1997–1998)	Sahm et al. (2000)
		Spain	37 (1997–1998)	Sahm et al. (2000)
		France	57 (1997–1998)	Sahm et al. (2000)
		Italy	23 (1997–1998)	Sahm et al. (2000)
V. cholerae				
	Nalidixic acid	India	98 (1994)	Garg et al. (2001)[b]
	Ciprofloxacin	India	39 (1999)	Garg et al. (2001)[b]

[a] Percentage resistant excludes intermediate susceptibility, which may exceed the percentage considered resistant by breakpoints. The data in the table are listed without distinction among types of patients, types of tissues infected, or local origin (nosocomial or community-acquired). Numbers in parenthesis indicate year of determination.
[b] Indicates time course reported.

Before considering the scope of the resistance problem, it is useful to define terms. In the broadest sense, resistance to an antimicrobial agent means that a particular microorganism is able to reproduce in the presence of the agent under specified conditions. Resistance is usually associated with a specific, heritable alteration (exceptions include induction of protective genes such as those encoding β-lactamases [Hanson & Sanders, 1999; Phillips & Shannon, 1993]). Heritability would seem to make resistance an absolute term, since changes in DNA primary structure are unequivocal. However, in some cases resistance genes are not fully protective. Consequently, the term "resistant" must be qualified to take into account the antimicrobial concentration.

Among the more widely used measures of concentration are susceptibility breakpoints. These antimicrobial concentrations are empirically derived thresholds that indicate whether a favorable clinical outcome is likely. If the minimal inhibitory concentration (MIC) observed with a pathogen from a patient sample exceeds the breakpoint, the outcome is likely to be unfavorable; that isolate is considered resistant. Conversely, an isolate is considered to be susceptible if the MIC for a particular compound is below the breakpoint, even though the microbial cells may carry many mutations that reduce susceptibility.

In general, organisms considered resistant by microbiological standards increase the frequency of treatment failure, relapse, and mortality (examples are observed with *Mycobacterium tuberculosis* [O'Brien, 1994; Portaels et al., 1999], *S. pneumoniae* [Moran, 2001], *Staphylococcus aureus* [Rello et al., 1994], *Pseudomonas aeruginosa* [Carmeli et al., 1999; Olson et al., 1985], and *Neisseria gonorrhoeae* [Rahman et al., 2001]). For a given patient, however, treatment may be successful even though the infection is caused by a pathogen deemed to be resistant by breakpoint criteria (Jacobs et al., 1996). As a result, arguments arise concerning whether breakpoints are set so low that some patients are denied a treatment that would have a reasonable probability for cure. But if breakpoints are set too high, some of the "susceptible" strains may have mutations that compromise treatment. For example, cases have been described in which nalidixic acid-resistant mutants of *Salmonella enterica* ser. *typhi* were considered to be susceptible to the more potent quinolone ofloxacin, even though the bacteria contained a resistance mutation in *gyrA*, a gene encoding a quinolone target (Wain et al., 1997). These "susceptible" infections responded poorly to ofloxacin treatment (the median fever-clearance time was nearly twice as long), and treatment failure among patients with nalidixic acid-resistant isolates was 10 times higher than among those with nalidixic acid-susceptible strains.

Continued use of antimicrobial agents against bacterial populations that have already been enriched for first-step mutants could facilitate the selection of second- and third-step mutants (Li et al., 2002; Urban et al., 2001), thereby shortening the lifespan of an entire class of antimicrobial. This principle raises an important question: should breakpoints be set to maximize the number of patients cured or to minimize the selection of resistant mutants? The answer may lie in how rapidly resistance is increasing.

Estimating the prevalence of resistance and its rate of increase is not straightforward. One reason is that samples are often not collected when patients are treated successfully (MacGowan et al., 1998; Wise & Andrews, 1998; Zinner et al., 2001a). Consequently, resistance, when expressed as a fraction of the isolates tested, may overestimate the actual value (underestimation is discussed in a subsequent section). The overestimation problem can be bypassed by assuming a similar, unreported fraction for longitudinal surveys conducted in the same geographical region. Such studies show that once the prevalence of resistance begins to increase noticeably, it can advance from below 5% to above 20% within a few years (Figure 8.1). The fraction of resistant isolates can reach 90% (Figure 8.1a); however, it often hovers around the 20–30% mark (Baquero, 1996; Johnson, 1998), perhaps because physicians switch to other agents when they notice the failures. The speed at which resistance is developing, coupled with our inability to rapidly identify new classes of antimicrobial agent, suggest that conservation of existing compounds is required.

(a)

(b)

(c)

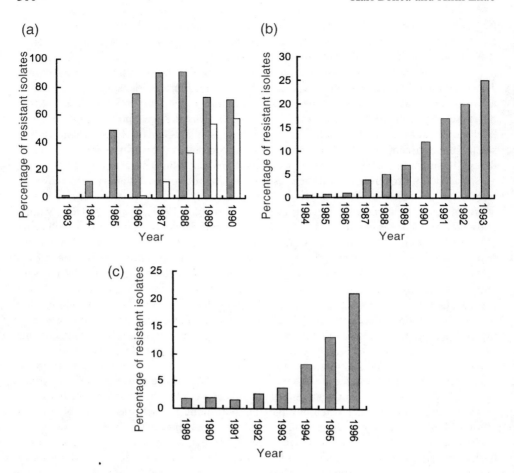

Figure 8.1. Rate of resistance development. Results of multiyear antibiotic surveillance are shown for several diseases and antibacterial agents. (a) Ampicillin (solid bars) and nalidixic acid (open bars) resistance of *S. dysenteriae* in Bangladesh (figure taken from Bennish et al., 1992). (b) Penicillin resistance of *S. pneumoniae* in France (redrawn from Baquero, 1996). (c) Methicillin resistance of *S. aureus* in Great Britain (Johnson, 1998). The panels have been prepared with permission of the publishers of the original papers.

Increasing resistance has been attributed to several factors. One is the high consumption of antimicrobial agents. For example, during the 1970s erythromycin consumption in Japan reached 170 tons per year and macrolide resistance among group A streptococci got as high as 80% (Low, 2001). In Canada, the number of prescriptions for fluoroquinolones increased from 0.8 per 100 persons per year in 1988 to 5.5 in 1997; fluoroquinolone resistance among strains of *S. pneumoniae* climbed from 0 in 1993 to 1.7% in 1997 and 1998 (among adults, the number reached 2.9%; Chen et al., 1999). Indeed, the correlation between consumption and resistance can be quite high (Baquero et al., 1991). Supporting the consumption hypothesis is the observation that decreases in consumption sometimes correlate with decreases in resistance (Austin et al., 1999; Nowak, 1994). In a subsequent section we discuss this phenomenon in terms of antibiotic cycling. A second factor involved in increasing resistance is the number of persons having weakened immune systems. Over 36 million persons are currently infected with the human immunodeficiency virus (Piot et al., 2001), and millions of others have had their immune systems compromized by aging, autoimmune diseases, and chemotherapy. A third factor is dissemination through global travel. Examples include penicillin-resistant pneumococcus that spread from Spain to several other countries (Gasc et al., 1995; Kristinsson et al., 1992; Munoz et al., 1991; Reichmann et al., 1995; Soares et al., 1993) and resistant typhoid fever that is associated with travel from undeveloped to developed countries (Ackers et al., 2000). None of the "resistance factors" can be changed easily: efforts to slow consumption have been disappointing (Harrison & Svec, 1998; McGowan & Gerding, 1996), and it is unlikely that aging populations, AIDS, and global travel will soon stop increasing. Thus the prevalence of resistance will continue to rise unless drastic changes are made.

Below we consider how resistance can develop even when antimicrobial concentrations are considered appropriate by traditional standards. The key idea is that a concentration range, the mutant selection window, exists in which resistant mutants are selected (Zhao & Drlica, 2001, 2002). Therapies designed only to provide a favorable patient outcome often place antimicrobial concentrations in the window. Thus repeated cycles of pathogen outgrowth followed by selective pressure gradually enrich bacterial populations for resistant mutants. It may be possible to severely restrict the development of genetic resistance by keeping antimicrobial concentrations out of the selection window.

3. MUTANT SELECTION WINDOW

The mutant selection window hypothesis evolved from the suggestion of Baquero (Baquero, 1990; Baquero & Negri, 1997) that a dangerous concentration range exists in which mutants are most frequently selected. We were later able to experimentally define the boundaries of the range when we noticed that the recovery of mycobacterial mutants from agar plates displays a characteristic response to fluoroquinolone concentration. Increasing concentration initially causes the recovery of colonies to drop sharply as the growth of wild-type cells is inhibited. Then a distinct plateau is observed, and finally a second sharp decline in mutant recovery occurs (Figure 8.2). The plateau arises from the outgrowth of resistant mutants (Dong et al., 1999; Zhou et al., 2000). The second sharp decline occurs when concentrations are reached that block the growth of all single-step mutants (Sindelar et al., 2000). Thus mutants are selectively enriched at fluoroquinolone concentrations between the two sharp drops in colony recovery.

The lower boundary of the window is the lowest concentration that blocks the growth of the majority of drug-susceptible cells. This concentration can be approximated by the MIC for half the cells in the population ($MIC_{(50)}$; note that this definition of MIC is much less stringent than that specified by the National Committee for Clinical Laboratory Standards, NCCLS). The upper boundary of the window is the drug concentration that blocks the growth of the most resistant, single-step mutant. Above this boundary, cell growth requires the presence of two or more resistance mutations. Since two concurrent mutations are expected to arise rarely (Iseman, 1994; Ng et al., 1996; Pan et al., 1996; Zhao et al., 1997; Zhao & Drlica, 2001), few mutants will be selectively amplified

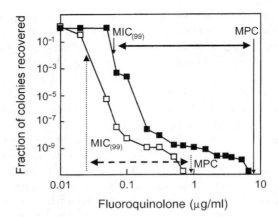

Figure 8.2. Mutant selection window when one drug target is present. Wild-type cells of *Mycobacterium bovis* BCG were applied to agar plates containing the indicated concentrations of fluoroquinolone. After incubation, colonies were recovered and retested for growth at each concentration. The fraction of resistant colonies, relative to input cells, was then determined. Symbols and abbreviations: open squares, PD161148, a C-8-methoxy fluoroquinolone; solid squares, PD160793, a C-8-H fluoroquinolone otherwise identical to PD161148; double-headed arrows, mutant selection windows; $MIC_{(99)}$, minimal drug concentration that blocks colony formation by 99%; MPC, minimal drug concentration that blocks colony formation when more than 10^{10} cells are applied to agar plates. The figure, which was adapted from Dong et al. (1999), is reproduced with permission of the publisher.

when drug concentrations exceed the upper boundary. For example, with fluoroquinolones the mutation frequency for resistance due to target mutations can be less than 10^{-7} (Zhou et al., 2000); consequently, more than 10^{14} bacteria would be required to find a cell with two concurrent fluoroquinolone-resistant target mutations. In clinical cases, bacterial populations may reach 10^{10} cells within an infected individual (Bingen et al., 1990; Fagon et al., 1990; Feldman, 1976; Low, 2001; Mitchison, 1984; Wimberley et al., 1979), but 10^{14} is unlikely. Thus resistance is expected to develop rarely when drug concentrations are above the upper boundary of the mutant selection window. This expectation led to the upper boundary being designated as the mutant prevention concentration (MPC; Dong et al., 1999). MPC is approximated experimentally as the lowest concentration that allows no colony growth when more than 10^{10} cells are applied to drug-containing agar plates.

The window changes slightly when antibacterial agents have more than one intracellular target. For example, DNA gyrase and DNA topoisomerase IV are both targets of the fluoroquinolones in pathogens other than *M. tuberculosis* (Cole et al., 1998), *Helicobacter pylori* (Tomb et al., 1997), and *Treponema pallidum* (Fraser et al., 1998). Generally one of the two targets is more sensitive than the other (with *Escherichia coli*, gyrase activity is inhibited at lower concentrations of fluoroquinolone than is topoisomerase IV activity). The presence of two targets means that concentrations high enough to attack both targets will require two mutations for growth. If the two targets have similar drug sensitivities, the plateau in the mutant selection curve will be short, constituting little more than an inflection point (filled squares, Figure 8.3; also see Dong et al., 1999; Li et al., 2002). As expected, a good correlation exists between concentrations that inhibit growth of the least susceptible first-step mutant and MPC (Li et al., 2002; Sindelar et al., 2000).

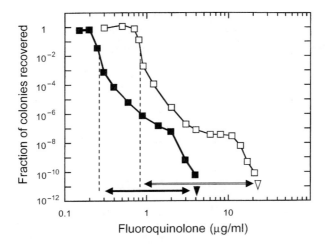

Figure 8.3. Mutant selection window when two drug targets are present. Wild-type cells of *S. aureus* were applied to agar plates containing the indicated concentrations of fluoroquinolone. After incubation, colonies were recovered and retested for growth at each concentration. The fraction of resistant colonies, relative to input cells, was then determined. Symbols: open squares, norfloxacin; filled squares, ciprofloxacin; dashed lines, $MIC_{(99)}$; triangles, MPC; double-headed arrows, mutant selection windows. The figure was modified from Zhao and Drlica (2002) with permission of the publisher.

We emphasize that although MPC was initially defined with respect to susceptible populations, the idea applies to any step in the process of gradual accumulation of mutations. In a broad sense MPC correlates with the MIC of the most resistant, next-step mutant. A relevant example may involve the development of fluoroquinolone resistance, since administration of low doses is likely to enrich efflux mutants. The reduced intracellular drug concentration in these mutants may then raise the MIC of target mutants and thereby raise MPC.

The concentration boundaries of the selection window (MIC and MPC) place no restriction on the types of mutant selected. Among those expected are uptake, efflux, degradation, and drug target mutants. Fluoroquinolone treatment of mycobacteria serves as an example: more than 20 different gyrase alleles have been recovered, and nontarget mutants can be so abundant at low drug concentrations that gyrase mutants are difficult to detect (Zhou et al., 2000).

The most resistant mutant need not be available in pure culture to determine the upper boundary of the window (MPC), since the boundary is estimated using a large population of susceptible cells (see Figures 8.2 and 8.3). Likewise, the mechanism of resistance need not be known to use the selection window idea for restricting the development of resistance. However, the mechanism of resistance is likely to influence the height of the window. In Table 8.2 the size of the selection window is estimated for a variety of agents (for convenience, the lower boundary of the window is taken to be the drug concentration that blocks growth of 99% of the cells, $MIC_{(99)}$; and the upper boundary is the concentration that prevents colony growth when 10^{10} cells are applied to agar plates, MPC). When the window opening is represented by the ratio of MPC to $MIC_{(99)}$, some compounds, such as rifampicin, have very wide windows. For such agents the protective effects of mutations cannot be easily overcome by high concentrations of drug. Other compounds have narrower windows.

Table 8.2
Mutant Selection Window Parameters[a]

Organism (hr)	Compound	MIC$_{(99)}$ (μg/ml)	MPC (μg/ml)	MPC/MIC$_{(99)}$	C$_{max}$ (μg/ml)	C$_{max}$/MPC	t$_{1/2}$
E. coli							
	Tobramycin	1.2	25	21	52.2	2.1	1.8
	Chloramphenicol	1.9	12	6.3	26	2.2	6.5
	Rifampin	7	>4,000	>570	9.5	<0.002	2
	Penicillin G	2.4	300	125	512	1.7	0.9
	Norfloxacin	0.045	1.6	36	1.3	0.81	5.1
S. aureus							
	Tobramycin	0.27	20	74	52.2	2.6	1.8
	Chloramphenicol	1.9	40	21	26	0.65	6.5
	Rifampin	0.003	480	160,000	9.5	0.02	2
	Penicillin G	0.015	1	67	512	512	0.9
	Vancomycin	0.65	40	62	39	1	6.5
	Norfloxacin	0.85	22	26	1.3	0.06	5.1
	Ciprofloxacin	0.3	4	13	6	1.5	3.9
	PD135042[b]	0.076	0.45	6	na[c]	na	na
	Ofloxacin	0.28	4.5	16	4.5	1.0	4.6
	Levofloxacin	0.18	2.5	14	5.2	2.1	7.4
	Moxifloxacin	0.05	0.6	12	2.5	4.2	13
	Bay y3114[d]	0.05	1.7	34	na	na	na
M. tuberculosis							
	Rifampin	0.02	>80	>4000	9.5	<0.12	2
	Streptomycin	0.2	>320	>1600	34	<0.11	4
	Isoniazid	0.06	20	330	7.6	0.38	2.5
	Capreomycin	2.0	160	800	33	0.2	3
	Kanamycin	1.5	>800	>530	21	<0.03	2.3
	Cycloserine	14	70	5	35	0.5	22
	Ciprofloxacin	0.15	8.0	53	4.4	0.56	3.9
	Levofloxacin[e]	0.15	7.5	50	5.7	0.76	8
	Moxifloxacin	0.037	2.5	67	4.5	1.8	13
	Gatifloxacin	0.03	1.5	50	3.7	2.4	8
	Sparfloxacin	0.075	2.5	33	1.4	0.56	16

[a] Data taken from Dong et al. (2000) and Zhao and Drlica (2002).
[b] PD135042 has the same structure as ciprofloxacin except that the former contains a C-8 methoxy group.
[c] Not available.
[d] Bay y3114 has the same structure as moxifloxacin but lacks the C-8 methoxy group.
[e] Experimental data obtained from Y. Dong, unpublished observations.

The mutant selection window can be depicted with pharmacokinetic profiles in which serum or tissue drug concentration is expressed as a function of time after drug administration (Figure 8.4). This representation has led to a pharmacodynamic test of the selection window idea: A. Firsov, S. Zinner, and associates (unpublished data) adjusted an in vitro pharmacodynamic model (Firsov et al., 2001) using *S. aureus* such that fluoroquinolone concentrations were (1) always above MPC; (2) between MIC and MPC; or (3) below MIC. Only concentrations between MIC and MPC, that is, in the window, selected mutants.

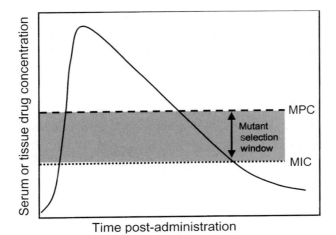

Time post-administration

Figure 8.4. Pharmocokinetic representation of mutant selection window. Stylized representation of serum drug concentrations obtained following administration of fluoroquinolones to human volunteers. $MIC_{(99)}$ and MPC were determined from data of the type shown in Figures 8.3 and 8.4. Double-headed arrow indicates mutant selection window.

4. DEVELOPMENT OF RESISTANCE

Antimicrobials are usually administered to produce tissue concentrations above the MIC, the minimal concentration that prevents pathogen growth. Blocking the growth of susceptible bacteria then enables host defense systems to reduce the pathogen population enough that bacterial outgrowth and disease symptoms do not occur after treatment is stopped. Bactericidal agents probably directly reduce pathogen numbers. However, hundreds, and perhaps even thousands of resistant cells can be present prior to administration of antibiotic, since mutation frequencies are often on the order of 10^{-6} to 10^{-8} while, as pointed out above, bacterial infections can contain 10^{10} organisms. Doses of antimicrobial that simply exceed the MIC allow growth of the mutant portion of the population. Patients with weakened defense systems are expected to be particularly vulnerable to enrichment of resistant mutants. That could make nursing homes, oncology departments, and intensive care units of hospitals sources of resistant strains.

When episodes of infection are brief, the enrichment of mutants in an individual patient may not be easily detected. Nevertheless, the passage of a pathogen through many individual, treated patients is expected to gradually increase the mutant fraction of the population. Thus an antimicrobial agent may cure 99.9% of the cases, but when millions are considered, the development of resistance is an inevitable consequence of MIC-based dosing strategies.

Consideration of the mutant selection window allows us to divide the development of antimicrobial resistance into two categories. In one, resistance arises in a single step—a mutation reduces susceptibility so much that no tolerable concentration of drug can block growth, that is, the upper boundary of the window (MPC) is above the maximum tolerable drug concentration. With this type of resistance, individual organisms in a bacterial population are either very susceptible or highly resistant (Murray, 1997). Well-known examples involve resistance determinants carried by mobile genetic elements such as plasmids and integrons (Carattoli, 2001; Navarro et al., 2001; Oppegaard et al., 2001; Salyers & Amabile-Cuevas, 1997). They enter a population horizontally, often after having achieved high-level resistance elsewhere, sometimes in another species or even another genus (see Chapter 6). The all-or-none category also includes many chromosomal resistance mutations. For example, most antituberculosis agents, as well as many compounds used against *E. coli* and *S. aureus*, have values of MPC that exceed maximal serum concentrations (Table 8.2). Preventing the enrichment of mutants in this category requires a strategy of multidrug, combination therapy designed so that the concentration of no single agent is above its MIC while the concentrations of the other agents are below their MICs (discussed in a subsequent section).

The second pattern of resistance requires the presence of more than one mutation for a cell to be considered resistant. With this pattern, resistant populations develop stepwise through the gradual accumulation of mutations that individually reduce susceptibility by low-to-moderate increments. When individual cells are tested, some are found to have intermediate levels of susceptibility. An example of this pattern is the development of penicillin resistance in *S. pneumoniae* (Barry, 1999; Jacobs, 1999; Tomasz, 1999). Treatment failure due to penicillin resistance was initially so uncommon that low-dose therapy was often used, but that approach caused an increase in the carriage of resistant isolates (Guillemot et al., 1998). After the mutants spread to fresh hosts, curing infection required higher doses of penicillin, new derivatives having greater potency, or new derivatives having different penicillin-binding protein targets (Goldstein & Garau, 1997). That led to selective enrichment of mutants having even lower susceptibility. These gradual, stepwise challenges with β-lactams, coupled with dissemination and plasmid-borne factors, have made penicillin ineffective against a third of the *S. pneumoniae* isolates in some countries (Table 8.1).

Fluoroquinolone resistance also develops in a stepwise manner, as illustrated by treatment of cholera in India. The use of a marginally effective quinolone, nalidixic acid, selected mutants of *V. cholerae* (Garg et al., 2001). Those mutants remained susceptible to the more potent quinolone ciprofloxacin, but within a few years resistance also developed against ciprofloxacin (Garg et al., 2001). A similar situation is likely to occur with *S. pneumoniae*. Clinical isolates already contain a variety of target and nontarget resistance mutations (Bast et al., 2000; Blondeau et al., 2001; Jones et al., 2000; Pestova et al., 2000; Urban et al., 2001) due to the use of ciprofloxacin and levofloxacin. More potent compounds, such as moxifloxacin, gatifloxacin, and gemifloxacin, have been identified, but they readily select resistant mutants if strains already contain a mutation (Li et al., 2002; Urban et al., 2001). With laboratory challenge of *S. pneumoniae* up to 7 mutations have been observed (Urban et al., 2001). Thus, developing new compounds of the same class may prolong the lifespan of the class, but that does not solve the resistance problem initiated by the older compounds.

Loss of susceptibility is expected to occur more readily with agents whose concentrations remain inside the window for long periods of time (Baquero & Negri, 1997; Zhao & Drlica, 2001). That may help explain why long-term, low-dose use of β-lactams selectively enriches penicillin-resistant *S. pneumoniae* that persist after treatment (Guillemot et al., 1998).

Stepwise loss of susceptibility is also expected to occur more readily when a bacterial population contains a diverse array of resistant mutants that are associated with many different levels of susceptibility. As pointed out above, many different fluoroquinolone-resistance mutations have been found in the gyrase genes (Drlica & Zhao, 1997; Nakamura, 1997; Zhou et al., 2000). But more insidious are the nontarget resistance mutants. They are so abundant at low quinolone concentration that few target mutants can be detected (Li et al., 2002; Zhou et al., 2000), and they are associated with increased frequency for subsequent resistance mutations (Takiff et al., 1996). Thus the use of low drug concentrations that enrich nontarget mutants may *accelerate* the selection process.

Dosing to place fluoroquinolone concentrations high in the selection window should reduce the development of resistance from factors other than target mutations, since nontarget mutations are usually selected only at low drug concentrations (Zhou et al., 2000). A clinical study reported by Schentag and associates (Thomas et al., 1998) can be interpreted within this framework. They determined (1) the pharmacokinetics of ciprofloxacin for patients hospitalized with pneumonia caused by *P. aeruginosa*; (2) the MIC for each infecting strain; and (3) whether treatment failure was associated with bacterial resistance. Low values of the pharmacodynamic parameter AUC/MIC, which correspond to dosing in the lower portion of the window, invariably resulted in resistance and treatment failure (AUC is the area under the time–concentration curve measured after administration of the antimicrobial). Higher values that placed concentrations near the middle of the window (AUC/MIC >100) were associated with only 25% resistance and failure (in these experiments the maximal concentration reached 5 times MIC [Thomas et al., 1998] or about 50% MPC [J. Blondeau, personal communication]). We predict that when mutants recovered from this type of study are examined, nontarget mutants will predominate among the low AUC/MIC cases while gyrase (target) mutants will be found in the high ones. Consistent with these ideas, low AUC/MIC conditions select predominantly efflux mutants in a rat pseudomonal pneumonia model (Join-Lambert et al., 2001).

The ideas developed above indicate that the use of low antimicrobial concentrations or weak agents will selectively enrich resistant mutants faster than more stringent conditions. Hospital benchmarking studies are beginning to support this concept. During the 1990s some hospitals in the United States switched from ciprofloxacin to the less potent fluoroquinolones ofloxacin and levofloxacin for treatment of infections caused by *P. aeruginosa*. The switch increased the prevalence of fluoroquinolone-resistant *P. aeruginosa* and expenditures for antimicrobials (Bhavnani et al., 1999; Rifenburg et al., 1999). A similar conclusion can be drawn from a single-hospital study (Peterson et al., 1998).

5. RESTRICTING RESISTANCE: MONODRUG THERAPY

5.1. Drug Concentrations above MPC

According to the selection window hypothesis, antimicrobial concentrations at the site of infection should be kept outside the window to avoid selective enrichment of resistant mutants. Since concentrations below the window are unlikely to be effective even against susceptible cells, restricting resistance generally means that concentrations should be kept above the upper boundary, above the MPC. In this sense, the MPC serves as a threshold for limiting the development of resistance.

The limited data in Table 8.2 show that for many compounds serum concentrations fail to exceed MPC. For agents whose serum concentrations do exceed MPC, only chloramphenicol with *E. coli*, moxifloxacin, levofloxacin, and penicillin G with *S. aureus*, and gatifloxacin or moxifloxacin with *M. tuberculosis* have a long enough dosing interval (>7 hr) to be easily administered (for details see Zhao & Drlica, 2002). For penicillin G and chloramphenicol, high-level resistance often enters a bacterial population horizontally (Tenover & McGowan, 1998), further reducing the number of drug–pathogen combinations for which concentations can exceed MPC with monotherapy. Although a more extensive survey may identify more compounds that might be suitable for dosing above the MPC, we expect the number to be small because the agents currently available were developed for dosing above MIC rather than above MPC.

The conclusions drawn above are based primarily on plasma pharmacokinetics. When tissue concentrations at the site of infection become better defined, some of the detailed statements may require modification. However, the general features of the selection window should remain unchanged. The current challenge is to design a clinical test of the selection window hypothesis. Two compounds, moxifloxacin and levofloxacin, may be appropriate for a test with *S. pneumoniae*. At recommended doses, serum concentrations of moxifloxacin exceed a provisional MPC while those of levofloxacin do not (Blondeau et al., 2001; Li et al., 2002); consequently, a prediction is that resistance will develop less often in medical centers using moxifloxacin than in those using levofloxacin. For such a trial it is important that resistance develop often enough to be detected. Recent case studies suggest that detecting resistance with levofloxacin may not be difficult (Davidson et al., 2002; Fishman et al., 1999; Kays et al., 2002; Urban et al., 2001; Weiss et al., 2001).

5.2. Dual Targetting and Closing the Mutant Selection Window

Hooper (Ng et al., 1996) and Fisher (Pan et al., 1996) pointed out that an antimicrobial agent that inhibits two different targets with equal efficacy would require a cell to acquire two concurrent mutations for growth. Only rarely would resistant mutants be recovered; within the context of the selection window hypothesis, the window would be closed (MIC = MPC). Since many bacterial species have two intracellular targets for the fluoroquinolones (DNA gyrase and DNA topoisomerase IV), these agents have been investigated for dual targetting. Several of the new compounds (moxifloxacin, gatifloxacin, gemifloxacin, and clinafloxacin) approach the dual target situation with *S. pneumoniae* as judged (1) by very low mutation frequencies (Pan & Fisher, 1998); (2) in one case by recovery of both *gyrA* and *parC* resistance mutations from the same bacterial population (Pan & Fisher, 1998); and (3) by a diminished plateau (inflection point) in plots of mutant recovery versus fluoroquinolone concentration (Li et al., 2002). Dual targetting compounds offer many of the advantages of combination therapy without the problems associated with pharmacokinetic mismatches (discussed below).

Another way to close the window is to seek compounds that exhibit a small difference between MIC and MPC without explicitly considering the targets. An example of how this might be accomplished is seen in a comparison of fluoroquinolones with respect to two

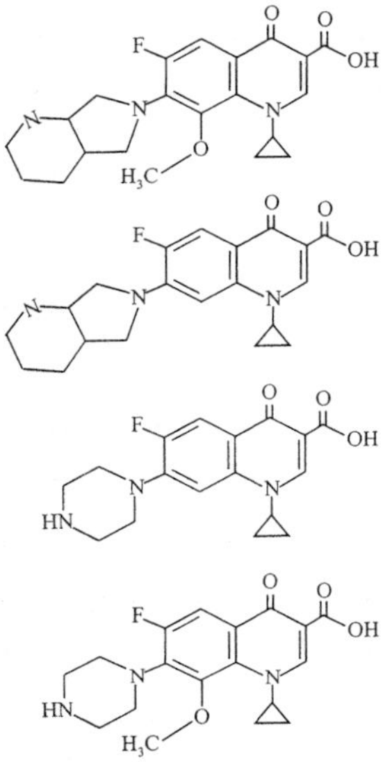

	MPC (μg/ml)	MIC$_{(99)}$ (μg/ml)	MPC/MIC$_{(99)}$
(a)	0.6	0.05	12
(b)	1.7	0.05	34
(c)	4	0.3	13
(d)	0.45	0.08	6

Figure 8.5. Effect of fluoroquinolone structure on the mutant selection window. MIC$_{(99)}$ and MPC were determined experimentally with *S. aureus* for (a) moxifloxacin, (b) Bay y3114, (c) ciprofloxacin, and (d) PD135042. The ratio of MPC to MIC$_{(99)}$ was then calculated. Data taken from Zhao and Drlica (2002) with permission of the publisher.

structural features that affect the window opening (Figure 8.5). One is the moiety at the C-8 position: the value of MPC/MIC$_{(99)}$ is lower for moxifloxacin than for its C-8 hydrogen cognate, Bay y3114. The other feature is the size of the C-7 ring system (ciprofloxacin has a lower value of MPC/MIC$_{(99)}$ than Bay y3114, a compound that has a larger C-7 group). These two features can be combined by adding a C-8 methoxy group to ciprofloxacin. The resulting compound, PD135042, has the lowest MPC to MIC$_{(99)}$ ratio of the quinolones tested. Once a compound is found that lacks a mutant selection window, few mutants will be selected regardless of how the compound is administered.

5.3. Numerical Considerations

As mentioned above, the MPC is estimated experimentally as the drug concentration that allows no mutant growth when more than 10^{10} cells are applied to agar plates. For most bacterial species 10^{-10} is several orders of magnitude below the frequency at which the least susceptible, first-step mutant is expected to be present. Moreover, 10^{10} cells generally exceed the number of bacterial cells present in an infection. In principle, antimicrobial agents can be compared for the ability to restrict the development of resistance by determining the length of time that available concentrations in relevant tissues is above MPC. Inaccuracies are introduced by uncertainties in determining relevant pharmacokinetics. For example, many compounds bind to proteins and are therefore expected to be only partially available for antimicrobial activity.

MPC determination may sometimes require adjustment of the number of cells tested, particularly if the pathogen load is very high, mutation frequency is high, or if the number of patients is large (the probability of a mutant being present is related to the number of bacteria per patient times the number of patients). The number of patients also bears on whether it is necessary to maintain drug concentrations above MPC for infections that contain few bacterial cells.

5.4. Standard Pharmacodynamic Approach

The MPC-based strategy differs conceptually from other pharmacodynamic approaches that have been advocated for restricting the development of resistance (Craig, 2001a; Drusano, 2000; Schentag, 1999). MPC establishes a concentration threshold that must be exceeded throughout therapy unless a compound is exceptionally lethal (discussed in a subsequent section). In contrast, monodrug strategies based on time above MIC, AUC/MIC, or C_{max}/MIC allow concentrations to be in the mutant selection window. The latter reflect the cumulative attack of susceptible cells, and they correlate with patient outcome (Preston et al., 1998). When measured with patients, these parameters bypass uncertainties associated with estimating available drug concentration at the site of infection.

When the endpoint is the restriction of resistance rather than patient cure, raising the AUC/MIC is expected to move the drug concentration higher in the selection window. Then fewer of the low- and moderate-level resistant mutants are likely to be selected. But at the recommended C_{max}/MIC of 10 or 12 (Craig, 1998, 2001b), the time that the drug concentration exceeds MPC may or may not be a long enough portion of the dosing period to restrict selection of the least susceptible, single-step mutants. For example, with the fluoroquinolone levofloxacin and the pathogen *S. pneumoniae*, doses of 500 and 750 mg generate C_{max}/MIC ratios of 5.7 and 8.6, respectively. For this compound the serum concentration barely exceeds MPC (Figure 8.6a). Even if higher serum concentrations are extrapolated from existing data, at C_{max}/MIC = 12 the projected serum concentration would exceed MPC for only 5 hr each day (1 g administered once daily can generate a value of C_{max}/MIC of 11.8 [Chien et al., 1998]; for this illustration we use a conservative, provisional value of MPC, which we estimate to be about twice the MPC [Blondeau et al., 2001]). During the remainder of the time the concentration would be inside the mutant selection window. Moxifloxacin is a more potent compound, but even at C_{max}/MIC = 18 the plasma drug concentration is expected to exceed the provisional MPC for only 15 hr (Figure 8.6b).

If C_{max}/MIC and AUC/MIC are raised to high enough levels, drug concentration will exceed MPC throughout therapy. At that point the empirical pharmacodynamic parameters should converge with the selection window concept. If a compound is particularly effective at killing *resistant* mutants, MPC may overestimate the concentration needed to restrict the enrichment of mutants (MPC is a bacteriostatic parameter). On the other hand, the standard pharmcodynamic parameters tend to underestimate mutant restriction if care is not taken to assure that the test population is large enough to have subpopulations that contain the most resistant, first-step mutant. That was unlikely to have been the case in a widely cited work (Blaser et al., 1987); whether a followup animal study (Drusano et al.,

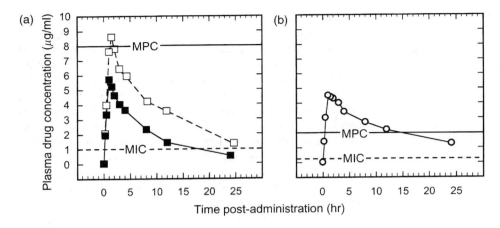

Figure 8.6. Relationship of MPC and pharmacokinetic profile for fluoroquinolones with *S. pneumoniae*. Serum concentrations of (a) levofloxacin and (b) moxifloxacin were determined at various times after administration of 500 mg levofloxacin (filled squares), 750 mg levofloxacin (open squares), or 400 mg moxifloxacin (open circles) to human volunteers (Chien et al., 1997, 1998). Values for MIC and MPC were estimated with clinical isolates of *S. pneumoniae* as reported in Blondeau et al. (2001). Provisional data for MPC, which may overestimate MPC by 2-fold due to inoculum effects, are used in the figure.

1993) blocked the outgrowth of mutants other than low-level, efflux mutants was not established (such mutants are readily recovered; Join-Lambert et al., 2001). Such considerations are important because the treatment of millions of patients makes underestimation undesirable with respect to mutant selection.

6. RESTRICTING RESISTANCE: COMBINATION THERAPY

Combination therapy was introduced to avoid treatment failure due to the development of resistance. Conceptually, a combination treatment regimen containing two or more drugs of different classes should require at least two distinct resistance mutations for the pathogen to grow. The simultaneous occurrence of two such mutations is expected only in bacterial populations of much greater size than is normally present within any individual patient; consequently, combination therapy with two distinct antibiotic types provides a way to reduce mutant selection using moderate concentrations of compounds that may individually have very high MPCs. Consideration of the mutant selection window reveals an additional issue: if times exist during therapy when the concentration of one compound is above MIC, but below MPC, while that of the other is below MIC, resistant mutants will be selectively enriched. This phenomenon, which we call pharmacokinetic mismatch, is discussed after a brief overview of combination therapy.

Animal studies demonstrate that combination therapy reduces the frequency of resistance (Michea-Hamzehpour et al., 1986). The best human examples of combination therapy are found with tuberculosis. The standard agents used for treating patients with this disease cannot be dosed at concentrations that exceed the respective MPCs of these drugs

(Table 8.2), and so resistance readily arises during monotherapy (British Medical Research Council, 1950; East African Hospitals & British Medical Research Council, 1960; Moulding et al., 1995). Multidrug therapies are used routinely to reduce the number of treatment failures (the frequency can be as low as 0.01%; Mitchison & Nunn, 1986). Drug resistance still develops among tuberculosis patients, but it is generally attributed to the failure of patients to comply fully with therapy regimens (Mason & Nitta, 1997; Second East African/British Medical Research Council Study, 1974). In effect, sporadic episodes of noncompliance allow periods of bacterial population expansion to punctuate therapy that is sometimes equivalent to monotherapy. To improve patient compliance, a major effort has been placed on "directly observed therapy" (DOT). That significantly lowers the incidence of treatment failure (Balasubramanian et al., 2000; Roosihermiatie et al., 2000; Weis et al., 1994). However, noncompliance still arises and contributes to treatment failure (noncompliance with DOT can be as high as 18%; Burman et al., 1997).

The potential importance of pharmacokinetic mismatch is illustrated by a small clinical trial involving HIV-1-positive, pulmonary tuberculosis patients (Vernon et al., 1999). About 60 patients were first treated for 2 months with a standard four-drug regimen that consisted of isoniazid, rifampin, pyrazinamide, and ethambutol. The patients were then divided into two groups for an additional four months of therapy. One group was given a once-weekly treatment of isoniazid and rifapentine, a long-acting derivative of rifampin (the half-life of rifapentine is 8 times that of rifampin). In this regimen, the total serum concentration of rifapentine was above MIC while isoniazid was below MIC for nearly 6 days each week (Figure 8.7a)—for most of the treatment period, rifapentine acted as a monodrug therapy. Under such circumstances, rifapentine/rifampin resistance is expected to develop. Relapses occurred with five patients, of whom four developed resistance.

The second group of patients received a twice-weekly, isoniazid–rifampin regimen. In this protocol the total rifampin concentration in the serum dropped below the MIC roughly 17 hr after drug administration, and the isoniazid concentration dropped below MIC about 8 hr later (Figure 8.7b). The lack of effective antibiotic for several days after each dose probably allowed growth of *M. tuberculosis*. As with the first protocol, relapse occurred in about 10% of the cases. Since rifampin concentration dropped below its MIC before isoniazid concentration, no case of rifampicin resistance was expected, and none of the three relapse cases produced rifampin-resistant bacilli.

Although the number of cases in the tuberculosis trial was small and uncertainties exist concerning the relevant tissue concentration of the agents, the trial does call attention to what may happen when mismatches in antibiotic pharmacokinetics exist. The solution to the mismatch problem is conceptually straightforward: formulate and administer combination therapies such that pharmacokinetic profiles, normalized to MIC, superimpose. Treatment failure due to other factors, such as lack of patient compliance with therapy regimens, would still occur. However, few new multidrug-resistant strains should be enriched as long as the equivalent of monotherapy is avoided.

To examine the idea that mutant enrichment is severely restricted when the concentrations of two compounds both exceed MIC, we determined rifampin and tobramycin combinations that prevent colony formation by *S. aureus* when more than 10^{10} cells are applied to drug-containing agar (these conditions allow us to estimate a combination MPC). Combinations of rifampin and tobramycin that are above the combination MPC and

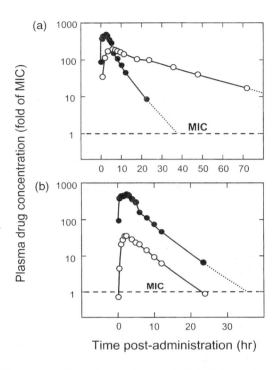

Figure 8.7. Pharmacokinetic comparison of two anti-tuberculosis dual-drug regimens. Pharmacokinetic profiles of isoniazid, rifampin, and rifapentine were normalized to their respective MICs to generate the plots. (a) Isoniazid (900 mg) + rifapentine (600 mg) twice weekly. (b) Isoniazid (900 mg) + rifampin (600 mg) once weekly. Symbols: isoniazid, filled circles; rifampin/rifapentine, open circles. Figure taken from Drlica (2001) with the permission of the publisher.

also within achievable serum concentrations are shown by the shaded portion of Figure 8.8. The mutant selection window extends from the data points down to the dashed lines in Figure 8.8. Below the dashed lines the concentration of neither compound is above its $MIC_{(99)}$. The minimal concentration for restricting resistance is 2 and 4 times the $MIC_{(99)}$ for rifampin and tobramycin, respectively (arrow, Figure 8.8). Thus each agent in the combination must by itself block bacterial growth.

The next step is to relate the in vitro determinations to pharmacokinetics. The time required for rifampin to drop from its C_{max} to twice the $MIC_{(99)}$ is more than 22 hr (11 times $t_{1/2}$); more than 13 hr (7 times $t_{1/2}$) is needed for tobramycin concentration to fall from C_{max} to 4 times its $MIC_{(99)}$ (see Table 8.2 for values of $t_{1/2}$). If we assume that the total serum drug concentration represents the effective concentration at the site of infection, twice daily dosing would maintain concentrations above the combination MPC. Thus, combination therapy, after experimental determination of appropriate doses, provides a way to administer antimicrobial agents outside the mutant selection window with compounds whose concentrations during monotherapy exceed MPC only briefly, if at all. Now it is necessary to adjust concentrations to reflect those that are available at the site of

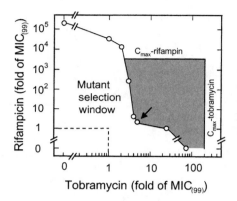

Figure 8.8. Combination treatment of *S. aureus* by rifampin and tobramycin. *S. aureus* cells, in excess of 10^{10} colony-forming units, were applied to agar plates containing the indicated concentrations of rifampin and tobramycin (expressed as multiples of $MIC_{(99)}$). Combinations that prevented colony growth (MPC) are shown as open circles. C_{max}-rifampin and C_{max}-tobramycin indicate maximal serum concentrations of rifampin and tobramycin, respectively. Shaded area indicates achievable serum drug concentration combinations that exceed MPC. Dashed lines approximate the lower boundary of the selection window. Figure taken from Zhao and Drlica (2002) with permission of the publisher.

infection. Uncertainties in the effects of drug binding to protein and in patient-to-patient variation make such determinations difficult. However, the general strategy of using an experimental determination of combination MPC to define dosing intervals should help restrict the development of resistance for most antibacterial agents.

The combination MPC/pharmacokinetic overlap approach described above differs conceptually from the use of AUC/MIC to restrict mutant enrichment during combination treatment because the latter places no restriction on periods equivalent to monotherapy. It has been suggested that maintaining a combined value of AUC/MIC above 100 for ciprofloxacin treatment of *P. aeruginosa* would reduce the rate at which resistance develops (Thomas et al., 1998). That is the case; however, failure still occurs in more than 3% of the cases (27/779) when combination therapy is implemented (Fish et al., 1995; Thomas et al., 1998). While 3% may be an acceptable risk for an individual patient, it could make compounds difficult to preserve when administered to large numbers of persons.

7. IMPORTANCE OF LETHAL ACTION

Many very successful antibiotics are bacteriostatic agents. Indeed, application of the selection window hypothesis to restrict mutant enrichment is based on bacteriostatic activity. Lethal action by an antimicrobial agent should help host defenses eliminate susceptible pathogens, thereby shortening treatment times. That will then reduce costs, toxic side effects, and the chance that new resistance will develop. Removal of susceptible cells should also increase the probability that host defense systems will eliminate resistant mutants. That action, plus direct killing of mutants by the antimicrobials, should reduce the time that drug concentrations must exceed MPC. Those times now need to be estimated with pharmacodynamic models.

An added feature of highly lethal agents, observed with compounds for which resistance is recessive, is a lower frequency for selection of resistant mutants. The lower frequency occurs because a recessive resistance mutation is not phenotypically expressed until the resistant, mutant protein has replaced the sensitive, wild-type one. Until that time, the mutants will be killed. An example is seen when DNA gyrase is the principal target of quinolones (Hane & Wood, 1969). When topoisomerase IV is the main target, resistance is codominant (Khodursky & Cozzarelli, 1998), which means that resistance would be expressed soon after the mutation occurred. Such dominance considerations may contribute to the frequency for obtaining target mutants of *S. pneumoniae* being 1,000 times higher for fluoroquinolones that target topoisomerase IV than for those whose primary target is gyrase (Fukuda et al., 2001; Li et al., 2002).

Enhanced killing of resistant mutants should also contribute to the ability of a compound to control a larger bacterial population. For example, if the mutation frequency for resistance is about 10^{-8}, then a population of 10^9 cells would contain on average 10 mutants. A compound that kills more than 99% of the mutant cells during an overnight treatment would reduce the number of mutants present from 10 to fewer than 1, assuming that the mutants cannot grow in the presence of such concentrations of the agent. In contrast, a compound that kills 99% of the susceptible cells, but not mutants, would allow all 10 mutants to persist and perhaps reproduce. That would enrich the mutant fraction of the population by at least 100-fold. Thus, simply improving lethality against susceptible microbes may not actually suppress the development of resistance if the mutants are allowed to reproduce, as might be the case in immunocompromised hosts. Indeed, it may actually speed the enrichment process by killing susceptible cells.

The ability to kill resistant mutants has been part of the characterization of fluoroquinolones. For example, C-8-methoxy derivatives avidly kill resistant mutants, and they are better able to suppress the development of resistance in vitro than older C-8-H derivatives (Dong et al., 1998; Li et al., 2002; Lu et al., 2001; Zhao et al., 1997). Direct attack of mutants at high drug concentrations may help explain why large, infrequent doses of fluoroquinolone are less likely to selectively enrich resistant mutants than multiple, moderate doses over the same time period (Marchbanks et al., 1993).

8. CROSS-RESISTANCE

Cross-resistance among compounds can cause a marginally active derivative to render other members of the class ineffective when it selectively enriches resistant mutants. Occasionally resistance mutations have subtle effects. For example, resistance to an older compound can have little effect on susceptibility to a new derivative yet profoundly raise the frequency at which the newer compound selects subsequent mutations. Such a case was observed with the fluoroquinolone ciprofloxacin. In the late 1980s and early 1990s ciprofloxacin was used against methicillin-resistant *S. aureus* (MRSA; Acar & Goldstein, 1997). Resistance was readily selected, as expected for a compound whose pharmocokinetic profile falls inside the selection window for long periods of time (Figure 8.9). Dissemination within health care institutions aggravated the situation, and now some hospitals report that more than 90% of the MRSA strains are fluoroquinolone resistant

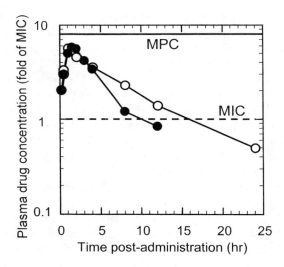

Figure 8.9. Relationship of MPC and pharmacokinetic profile for ciprofloxacin with *S. aureus* and levofloxacin with *S. pneumoniae*. Pharmacokinetic profiles for ciprofloxacin (filled circles; mean steady-state concentration after 750 mg twice daily oral dose; Shah et al., 1994) and levofloxacin (open circles; mean steady-state concentration after 500 mg once daily oral dose; Chien et al., 1997) are shown after normalization to MIC of *S. aureus* (X. Zhao et al., unpublised data) and *S. pneumoniae* (Dalhoff, 1999) respectively. MPC was taken from Blondeau et al. (2001) for *S. pneumoniae* and from unpubished observations (X. Zhao et al.) for *S. aureus*. Figure taken from Tillotson et al. (2001) with permission of the publisher.

(Acar & Goldstein, 1997; Schmitz et al., 1999). New fluoroquinolones, such as garenoxacin (BMS-284756), have been developed that are active enough for some ciprofloxacin-resistant MRSA to be considered susceptible (Jones et al., 2001). However, the MPC for garenoxacin with ciprofloxacin-resistant strains of *S. aureus* is so high that MPC cannot be exceeded for long, if at all, by serum levels (X. Zhao et al., unpublished observations). Thus the new fluoroquinolones are expected to readily select resistant mutants having even lower susceptibilities. Had ciprofloxacin not been used with MRSA, a fluoroquinolone might soon be available that would have been an effective alternative for these strains.

The same phenomenon may apply to fluoroquinolone treatment of streptococcal pneumonia (Tillotson et al., 2001). In the late 1990s the fluoroquinolone levofloxacin was widely used, usually with good patient outcome (Fogarty et al., 2001). However, the pharmacodynamics of levofloxacin with *S. pneumoniae* are similar to those for ciprofloxacin with MRSA (Figure 8.9); consequently, resistance is expected to increase (between 1997–1998 and 1998–1999 samplings, the prevalence of levofloxacin-resistant *S. pneumoniae* increased from 0.1 to 0.6% [Sahm et al., 2001]; the following year a value of 0.5% was recorded [Selman et al., 2000]; indicating that the 0.6% number is probably reliable). A local study from Indianapolis revealed that in 1999–2000 about 1.7% of the isolates collected were levofloxacin resistant (Kays & Denys, 2001); in Hong Kong, where resistance is beginning to disseminate, the nonsusceptible isolates had reached 13% by 2000 (Ho et al., 2001a). At the same time, case reports of treatment failure being associated with levofloxacin therapy began to appear (Davidson et al., 2002; Empey et al., 2001; Fishman et al., 1999; Ho et al., 2001b; Urban et al., 2001). The levofloxacin-resistance mutations are

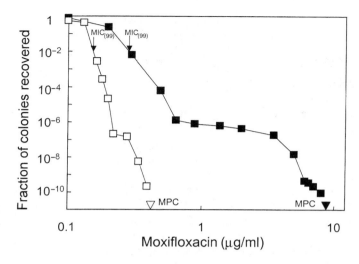

Figure 8.10. Recovery of second-step resistant mutants of *S. pneumoniae*. Cells were applied to fluoroquinolone-containing agar, and the fraction of cells recovered as mutants was determined. Filled symbols represent data obtained with a ParC (topoisomerase IV) variant. Open symbols represent data obtained for wild-type cells included as a reference. $MIC_{(99)}$ and MPC are indicated. The figure was adapted from data in Li et al. (2002) with permission of the publisher.

expected to have a profound effect on the ability of newer compounds, such as moxifloxacin, gatifloxacin, and gemifloxacin, to control *S. pneumoniae*. One reason is that the MPC for the mutants is above available serum concentrations (with susceptible cells the MPC is below maximal concentrations, at least for moxifloxacin [Blondeau et al., 2001; Li et al., 2002]). Another reason is that the mutation frequency is orders of magnitude higher with first-step, levofloxacin-resistant mutants than with wild-type cells (Figure 8.10). Thus even though the new derivatives prefer a different intracellular target than levofloxacin or ciprofloxacin and may cure disease caused by first-step mutants, resistance to the newer compounds is expected to develop more quickly due to the use of the older derivatives.

9. SURVEILLANCE OF RESISTANCE

Surveillance studies measure the fraction of clinical isolates that are considered to be resistant; consequently, they reveal when antibiotic use strategies have allowed resistant mutants to develop within pathogen populations. Such studies are important, since with the exception of tuberculosis, resistance tends to arise too infrequently with individual patients to be readily noticeable until it is widespread. At the local level, surveillance studies improve empirical therapies by alerting physicians to outbreaks of resistant organisms. The studies also help identify failed strategies or compounds. For example, even a small sampling from the surveillance literature suggests that the utility of many antimicrobials is being lost (Table 8.1; Figure 8.1).

The prevalence of resistant isolates is generally based on determination of MIC followed by comparison with breakpoints that relate to clinical outcome. If several mutations are required to lower susceptibility enough to cross a breakpoint, surveillance studies will be insensitive to the accumulation of mutant strains until susceptibility is close to the breakpoint. A lack of sensitivity also arises from the nature of pathogen samples taken from individual patients. Those samples often represent only the majority members of the infecting population—subpopulations tend to be excluded during sample preparation. Thus patients can harbor many undetected mutant cells. The use of breakpoints, coupled with the inability of standard MIC determination to reveal small subpopulations, causes the gradual process of mutant accumulation to be seen as an all-or-none phenomenon. Resistance can appear to develop suddenly (Figure 8.1), even though it may actually develop gradually (other factors, such as rapid dissemination of resistant strains, can cause an increase in resistance to actually be rapid).

One consequence of the all-or-none property is that treatment failure is rarely attributed to the development of resistance during therapy. Until the resistance threshold is reached, therapy will generally be successful. If the threshold is quickly crossed, most of the resistance-dependent treatment failures will appear to have arisen because the pathogen had lost susceptibility before, rather than during the round of infection being examined. The practice of using breakpoints obscures the enriching effect of dosing within the mutant selection window, and it may provide a false sense of security when the prevalence of resistance is low. Thus surveillance studies can reveal the failure of treatment strategies, but they are not designed to accurately reflect success.

10. REVERSING RESISTANCE AND ANTIBIOTIC CYCLING

Several situations have been described in which rapid increases in resistance have elicited a reduction in antibiotic consumption. One occurred in Iceland following the introduction of penicillin-resistant pneumococci from Spain. Restrictions were placed on overall antibiotic use, especially on macrolide and trimethoprim-sulfamethoxazole consumption for childhood infections caused by *S. pneumoniae* (Kristinsson et al., 1995), and the fraction of resistant isolates declined in a predictable way (Austin et al., 1999). Another community-based study occurred in Finland where restrictions were imposed in the early 1990s because erythromycin resistance among group A streptococci had risen from 5 to 13% between 1988–1989 and 1990. By 1995 the frequency of macrolide resistance had dropped to 8.6% (Seppala et al., 1997). Reduction of macrolide use in Japan also correlated with a marked decrease in resistance (Low, 2001), and several rollbacks of resistance have been reported for hospital settings (Quale et al., 1996; Rahal et al., 1998; Rice et al., 1996). Although none of these examples contained controls to rule out a decrease in resistance unrelated to consumption (Phillips, 2001), they have provided hope that a drastic lowering of antibiotic use might halt, if not reverse, the development of antibiotic resistance.

If resistance could be reversed, then it might be possible to use antibiotic rotation or cycling to extend the lifespan of antibiotics (Gruson et al., 2000; John & Rice, 2000; Kollef et al., 1997; McGowan & Gerding, 1996). In principle, selective pressure would be removed long enough for the presumably more fit, wild-type cells to overgrow the mutants. Then the agent could be used again. For this scheme to work, resistance needs to impair fitness. Examples can be found in which this is the case, at least when measured as growth in vitro (Bagel et al., 1999; Gillespie et al., 2002; Olson et al., 1985). However, reversibility of resistance is not likely to be a general occurrence, partially because loss of fitness tends to be corrected by the acquisition of additional mutations, often without loss of resistance (Bagel et al., 1999; Bjorkman et al., 2000). It has been argued that reversion of an evolved, resistant strain to susceptibility would be difficult (Andersson & Levin, 1999; Schrag et al., 1997). Even plasmids that are initially a burden to their bacterial host can evolve with the host such that the presence of the plasmid eventually becomes beneficial in the absence of drug (Lenski et al., 1994). These findings, plus the possibility that some resistance alleles cause little or no disadvantage in growth rate, suggest that reversal of resistance may be the exception rather than the rule.

Cases in which resistance has been partially reversed can exhibit a rapid return to resistance after readministration of the agent (Gerding, 2000; Gerding et al., 1991). This is the expected result when years of therapy at concentrations inside the selection window have allowed the enrichment of multiple resistance alleles, many of which are lost slowly when the selective pressure is removed. Among the problem strains that are likely to be enriched by repeated antimicrobial treatment are those that contain mutator mutations. These strains, which exhibit a mutation frequency of up to 10^{-3}–10^{-4} (Metzger & Wills, 2000; Miller, 1996), can be highly enriched by selective pressure (Mao et al., 1997). In one study up to 36% of cystic fibrosis patients were colonized by mutator strains (Oliver et al., 2000). Mutators are likely to persist and proliferate during antibiotic cycling, which will keep mutation rates high. Then the net result of cycling could be selection of multidrug-resistant mutants.

Even if the bacteria themselves do not revert to susceptibility, strategies that lengthen the time that an antibiotic concentration exceeds MPC could lower the prevalence of resistance. For example, if patients entering an intensive care unit are infected with a susceptible strain of *P. aeruginosa* and if those strains develop resistance inside the unit, raising the concentration or potency of the antibiotic to restrict the development of new resistance would gradually lower the overall prevalence as new patients replaced the old ones.

11. CONCLUDING REMARKS

Resistant mutants are generated by nucleotide sequence changes, either spontaneously or through horizontal transfer. It is difficult to prevent those changes. However, in individual patients the mutant fraction of susceptible populations is often small enough, usually on the order of one in 10^6–10^8 cells, to be removed by host defense systems if antimicrobial treatment eliminates wild-type cells. But repeated cycles of selective pressure within the mutant selection window, coupled with population expansion, gradually erode the usefulness of any agent when millions of patients are considered (50 million prescriptions are written annually in the United States [Bell, 2001]; in 2001 the number for fluoroquinolones was above 31 million [G. Tillotson, personal communication]). The repeated cycles can occur within a single host, as when tuberculosis patients take antimicrobials sporadically, or the cycles can be spread over many hosts, as seen with streptococcal pneumonia (when many hosts are involved, population expansion occurs in each fresh or recurrent host prior to administration of antibiotic). Misuse and overuse of antimicrobials speed the selection process (Low, 2001; Monroe & Polk, 2000).

We can interfere with mutant selection by administering antimicrobials so that relevant tissue concentrations are high enough to directly attack mutants. For monodrug therapies, such concentrations would be above the mutant selection window (above MPC). With combination therapies, a crucial factor is the adjustment of pharmacokinetics to avoid creating periods of monotherapy within the mutant selection window. For both situations, halting the development of resistance requires dosing at higher levels than are usually required to cure infection.

Selection window strategies differ conceptually from standard, empirical pharmacodynamic efforts. The latter focus on achieving a successful outcome with individual patients, and no effort is made to avoid dosing within the selection window. Since it may be difficult to examine enough patients to be assured that a given drug concentration prevents the outgrowth of the least susceptible mutant, empirical pharmacodynamics will tend to underestimate the necessary concentration. The selection window idea probably overestimates how long the drug concentration must be kept above the MPC, since the ability of a compound to kill resistant mutants is not taken into account. The two approaches will tend to converge as the stringency of the pharmacodynamic endpoint is increased and as MPC and pharmacokinetic measurements are refined.

MPC can be measured in vitro for various pathogen–antimicrobial combinations, and the suitability of a given agent for single or combination therapy can be estimated (Zhao & Drlica, 2002). Resistance that enters a population horizontally requires special consideration for two reasons. First, the level of protection conferred by the resistance genes is usually so high that MPC (and sometimes MIC) is above achievable tissue concentrations that are safe. Thus, combination therapy with two effective agents of different classes is often required even though the fraction of resistant cells may be small. Second, the frequency at which resistance enters the bacterial population horizontally may be higher than spontaneous mutation frequency. If so, combination therapies may require three or more agents to make it unlikely for a large bacterial population to contain a multiple mutant that is resistant to all of the agents. It is important to note that phenotypic resistance, exemplified by induction of β-lactamases, currently falls outside the scope of the mutant selection window hypothesis. However, mutational resistance to β-lactamase inhibitors and mutationally constitutive depression of β-lactamase gene expression should behave according to the hypothesis.

As mentioned above, clinical tests for restriction of resistance are difficult to carry out because the low frequency at which resistance arises requires examination of large numbers of patients. Surrogate tests, such as coupling MPC with pharmacokinetics, are imprecise because drug concentrations at the site of infection are often not known and because factors such as drug binding to host proteins may markedly reduce effectiveness (Craig & Suh, 1978). Moreover, patient-to-patient variation can be considerable (Marchant, 1981; Sweeney, 1983; Vesell, 1991). Thus many aspects of the mutant selection window hypothesis require additional refinement and testing.

Even when the window becomes precisely defined clinically, using the information to restrict mutant enrichment will be difficult. A substantial problem can be expected at the prescriber level because immediate, individual health often takes precedence over public health concerns—using drug concentrations that fall within the mutant selection window is often of less concern than is the risk of toxic side-effects. This is partly because the frequency at which resistance arises is low. Even with difficult diseases such as tuberculosis, the chance of a successful outcome is better than 94% when combination drug regimens are carefully followed (Roosihermiatie et al., 2000). For most other infections the odds are probably better, even with single-drug therapy. Thus for most prescribers resistance is an intellectual, rather than an experiential phenomenon. Another factor is the false sense of security provided by surveillance studies. They reveal failures, but continued low prevalence of resistance does not exclude mutant accumulation and the gradual increase in MIC and MPC.

In conclusion, trying to stay only one step ahead of the pathogens may be a flaw in the traditional use of antimicrobials because it allows gradual, stepwise enrichment of mutant bacteria. In cases where clinical resistance arises from the gradual accumulation of several resistance mutations, staying two or more steps ahead may be necessary to severely restrict the emergence of resistance. The mutant selection window hypothesis suggests several ways to have antimicrobial agents directly attack resistant mutants so that susceptible cells must acquire at least two mutations for growth during therapy. Whether being two mutational steps ahead of the pathogens is enough remains to be seen. To minimize problems arising from dosing errors, new compounds need to have such a narrow selection window that even extensive misuse barely enriches mutants.

ACKNOWLEDGMENTS

We thank M. Gennaro, S. Kayman, D. Low, E. Rubinstein, F. Schmitz, G. Tillotson, C. Urban, and S. Zinner for critical comments on the manuscript. The authors' work has been supported by NIH grant AI35257 and grants from Bayer AG, Bristol-Myers-Squibb, and Mylan Pharmaceutical Co.

References

Acar, J., & Goldstein, F. (1997). Trends in bacterial resistance to fluoroquinolones. *Clin Infect Dis, 24*, S67–S73.

Ackers, M., Puhr, N., Tauxe, R., & Mintz, E. (2000). Laboratory-based surveillance of *Salmonella* serotype *typhi* infections in the United States. *JAMA, 283*, 2668–2673.

Andersson, D., & Levin, B. (1999). The biological cost of antibiotic resistance. *Curr Opin Microbiol, 2*, 489–493.

Austin, D., Kristinsson, K., & Anderson, R. (1999). The relationship between the volume of antimicrobial consumption in human communities and the frequency of resistance. *Proc Natl Acad Sci USA, 96*, 1152–1156.

Bagel, S., Hullen, V., Wiedemann, B., & Heisig, P. (1999). Impact of *gyrA* and *parC* mutations on quinolone resistance, doubling time, and supercoiling degree of *Escherichia coli. Antimicrob Agents Chemother, 43*, 868–875.

Bal, C. (1999). Increasing antimicrobial resistance in STDs and the need for surveillance: *Neisseria gonorrhoeae* as a model. *FEMS Immunol Med Microbiol, 24*, 447–453.

Balasubramanian, V., Oommen, K., & Samuel, R. (2000). DOT or not: Direct observation of anti-tuberculosis treatment and patient outcomes, Kerala State, India. *Int J Tuberc Lung Dis, 4*, 409–413.

Ball, P. (1999). Therapy for pneumococcal infection at the millennium: Doubts and certainties. *Am J Med, 107*(1A), 77S–85S.

Bantar, C., Famiglietti, A., Goldberg, M., Antimicrobial Committee, & National Surveillance Program. (2000). Three-year surveillance study of nosocomial bacterial resistance in Argentina. *Int J Inf Dis, 4*, 85–90.

Baquero, F. (1990). Resistance to quinolones in Gram-negative microorganisms: Mechanisms and prevention. *Eur Urol, 17*(Suppl. 1), 3–12.

Baquero, F. (1996). Trends in antibiotic resistance of respiratory pathogens: An analysis and commentary on a collaborative surveillance study. *J Antimicrob Chemother, 38*(Suppl. A), 117–132.

Baquero, F., Garcia-Rodriguez, J., deLomas, J., Aguilar, L., & Spanish Surveillance Group. (1999). Antimicrobial resistance of 1,113 *Streptococcus pneumoniae* isolates from patients with respiratory tract infections in Spain: Results of a 1-year (1996–97) multicenter surveillance study. *Antimicrob Agents Chemother, 43*, 357–359.

Baquero, F., Martinez-Beltran, J., & Loza, E. (1991). A review of antibiotic resistance patterns of *Streptococcus pneumoniae* in Europe. *J Antimicrob Chemother, 28*(Suppl. C), 31–38.

Baquero, F., & Negri, M. C. (1997). Strategies to minimize the development of antibiotic resistance. *J Chemother, 9*(Suppl. 3), 29–37.

Barry, A. (1999). Antimicrobial resistance among clinical isolates of *Streptococcus pneumoniae* in North America. *Am J Med, 107*, 28S–33S.

Barsic, B., Beus, I., Marton, E., Himbele, J., Kuzmanovic, N., Bejuk, D., Boras, A., & Klinar, I. (1997). Antibiotic resistance among Gram-negative nosocomial pathogens in the intensive care unit: Results of 6-year body-site monitoring. *Clin Therapeut, 19*, 691–700.

Bast, D., Low, D., Duncan, C., Kilburn, L., Mandell, L., Davidson, R., & deAzavedo, J. (2000). Fluoroquinolone resistance in clinical isolates of *Streptococcus pneumoniae*: Contributions of type II topoisomerase mutations and efflux on levels of resistance. *Antimicrob Agents Chemother, 44*, 3049–3054.

Bell, D. (2001). Promoting appropriate antimicrobial drug use: Perspective from the Centers for Disease Control and Prevention. *Clin Inf Dis, 33*(Suppl. 3), S245–S250.

Bennish, M., Salam, M. A., Hossain, M. A., Myaux, J., Khan, E. H., Chakraborty, J., Henry, F., & Ronsmans, C. (1992). Antimicrobial resistance of Shigella isolates in Bangladesh, 1983–1990: Increasing frequency of strains multiply resistant to ampicillin, trimethoprim-sulfamethoxazole, and nalidixic acid. *Clin Infect Dis, 14*, 1055–1060.

Bhavnani, S., Forrest, A., Collins, D., Paladino, J., & Schentag, J. (1999). Association between fluoroquinolone expenditures and ciprofloxacin susceptibility of *Pseudomonas aeruginosa* among U.S. hospitals. *39th ICAAC*, San Francisco.

Bingen, E., Lambert-Zechovsky, N., Mariani-Kurkdjian, P., Doit, C., Aujard, Y., Fournerie, F., & Mathieu, H. (1990). Bacterial counts in cerebrospinal fluid of children with meningitis. *Eur J Clin Microbiol Infect Dis, 9*, 278–281.

Bjorkman, J., Nagaev, I., Berg, O., Hughes, D., & Andersson, D. (2000). Effects of environment on compensatory mutations to ameliorate costs of antibiotic resistance. *Science, 287*, 1479–1482.

Blaser, J., Stone, B., Groner, M., & Zinner, S. (1987). Comparative study with enoxacin and netilmicin in a pharmacodynamic model to determine importance of ratio of antibiotic peak concentration to MIC for bactericidal activity and emergence of resistance. *Antimicrob Agents Chemother, 31*, 1054–1060.

Blondeau, J., Zhao, X., Hansen, G., & Drlica, K. (2001). Mutant prevention concentrations (MPC) for fluoroquinolones with clinical isolates of *Streptococcus pneumoniae*. *Antimicrob Agents Chemother, 45*, 433–438.

Boyce, J. (2001). Consequences of inaction: Importance of infection control practices. *Clin Inf Dis, 33*(Suppl. 3), S133–S137.

British Medical Research Council. (1950). Treatment of pulmonary tuberculosis with streptomycin and para-amino-salicylic acid. *Br Med J, 2*, 1073–1085.

Burman, W. J., Rietmeijer, C. A., & Sbarbaro, J. A. (1997). Noncompliance with directly observed therapy for tuberculosis: Epidemiology and effect on the outcome of treatment. *Chest, 111*, 1168–1173.

Carattoli, A. (2001). Importance of integrons in the diffusion of resistance. *Vet Res, 32*, 243–259.

Carmeli, Y., Troillet, N., Karchmer, A., & Samore, M. (1999). Health and economic outcomes of antibiotic resistance in *Pseudomonas aeruginosa*. *Arch Intern Med, 159*, 1127–1132.

Casal, M., Ruiz, P., Herreras, A., & Spanish Study Group of *M. tuberculosis* Resistance. (2000). Study of the in vitro susceptibility of *M. tuberculosis* to ofloxacin in Spain. *Int J Tuberc Lung Dis, 4*, 588–591.

Chen, D. K., McGeer, A., deAzavedo, J. C., & Low, D. E. (1999). Decreased susceptibility of *Streptococcus pneumoniae* to fluoroquinolones in Canada. *N Engl J Med, 341*, 233–239.

Chien, S.-C., Wong, F., Fowler, C., Callery-D'Amico, S., Williams, R., Nayak, R., & Chow, A. (1998). Double-blind evaluation of the safety and pharmacokinetics of multiple oral once-daily 750 milligram and 1-gram doses of levofloxacin in healthy volunteers. *Antimicrob Agents Chemother, 42*, 885–888.

Chien, S.-H., McRogge, Gisclon, L., Curtin, C., Wong, F., Natarajan, J., Williams, R., Fowler, C., Cheung, W., & Chow, A. (1997). Pharmacokinetic profile of levofloxacin following once-daily 500 mg oral or intravenous doses. *Antimicrob Agents Chemother, 41*, 2256–2260.

Chong, Y., Lee, K., Park, Y., Jeon, D., Lee, M., Kim, M., Chang, C., Kim, E., Lee, N., & Kim, H. (1998). Korean nationwide surveillance of antimicrobial resistance of bacteria in 1997. *Yonsei Med J, 39*, 569–577.

Cole, S. T., Brosch, R., Parkhill, J., Garnier, T., Churcher, C., Harris, D., Gordon, S., Eiglmeier, K., Gas, S., & Barry, C. E. (1998). Deciphering the biology of *Mycobacterium tuberculosis* from the complete genome sequence. *Nature, 393*, 537–544.

Coninx, R., Mathieu, C., Debacker, M., Mirzoev, F., Ismaelov, A., DeHaller, R., & Meddings, D. R. (1999). First-line tuberculosis therapy and drug-resistant *Mycobacterium tuberculosis* in prisons. *The Lancet, 353*, 969–973.

Craig, W. (1998). Pharmacokinetic/pharmacodynamic parameters: Rationale for antibacterial dosing of mice and men. *Clin Infect Dis, 26*, 1–12.

Craig, W. (2001a). Does the dose matter? *Clin Inf Dis, 33*, S233–S237.

Craig, W. (2001b). Introduction. *Respir Med, 95*, S2–S4.

Craig, W., & Suh, B. (1978). Theory and practical impact of binding of antimicrobials to serum proteins and tissue. *Scand J Inf Dis, 14*(Suppl.), 92–99.

Dalhoff, A. (1999). In vitro activity of quinolones. *Exp Opin Invest Drugs, 8*, 123–137.

Davidson, R., Cavalcanti, R., Brunton, J., Bast, D. J., deAzavedo, J. C., Kibsey, P., Fleming, C., & Low, D. E. (2002). Resistance to levofloxacin and failure of treatment of pneumococcal pneumonia. *N Engl J Med, 346*, 747–750.

Diekema, D., Pfaller, M., Jones, R., Doern, G., Winokur, P., Gales, A., Sader, H., Kugler, K., Beach, M., & SENTRY Participants Group. (1999). Survey of bloodstream infections due to Gram-negative bacilli: Frequency of occurrence and antimicrobial susceptibility of isolates collected in the United States, Canada, and Latin America for the SENTRY antimicrobial surveillance program, 1997. *Clin Inf Dis, 29*, 595–607.

Doern, G. (2001). Antimicrobial use and the emergence of antimicrobial resistance with *Streptococcus pneumoniae* in the United States. *Clin Inf Dis, 33*(Suppl. 3), S187–S192.

Doern, G., Pfaller, M., Kugler, K., Freeman, J., & Jones, R. (1998). Prevalence of antimicrobial resistance among respiratory tract isolates of *Streptococcus pneumoniae* in North America: 1997 results from the SENTRY antimicrobial surveillance program. *Clin Inf Dis, 27*, 764–770.

Dong, Y., Xu, C., Zhao, X., Domagala, J., & Drlica, K. (1998). Fluoroquinolone action against mycobacteria: Effects of C8 substituents on bacterial growth, survival, and resistance. *Antimicrob Agents Chemother, 42*, 2978–2984.

Dong, Y., Zhao, X., Domagala, J., & Drlica, K. (1999). Effect of fluoroquinolone concentration on selection of resistant mutants of *Mycobacterium bovis* BCG and *Staphylococcus aureus*. *Antimicrob Agents Chemother, 43*, 1756–1758.

Dong, Y., Zhao, X., Kreiswirth, B., & Drlica, K. (2000). Mutant prevention concentration as a measure of antibiotic potency: Studies with clinical isolates of *Mycobacterium tuberculosis*. *Antimicrob Agents Chemother, 44*, 2581–2584.

Drlica, K. (2001). A strategy for fighting antibiotic resistance. *ASM News, 67*, 27–33.

Drlica, K., & Zhao, X. (1997). DNA gyrase, topoisomerase IV, and the 4-quinolones. *Microbiol Mol Rev, 61*, 377–392.

Drusano, G. (2000). Fluoroquinolone pharmacodynamics: Prospective determination of relationships between exposure and outcome. *J Chemother, 12SB*, 21–26.

Drusano, G. L., Johnson, D., Rosen, M., & Standiford, H. (1993). Pharmacodynamics of a fluoroquinolone antimicrobial agent in a neutropenic rat model of *Pseudomonas* sepsis. *Antimicrob Agents Chemother, 37*, 483–490.

East African Hospitals, & British Medical Research Council. (1960). Comparative trial of isoniazid alone in low and high dosage and isoniazid plus PAS in the treatment of acute pulmonary tuberculosis in East Africa. *Tubercle, 40*, 83–102.

Empey, P., Jennings, H., Thornton, A., Rapp, R., & Evans, M. (2001). Levofloxacin failure in a patient with pneumococcal pneumonia. *Ann Pharmacother, 35*, 687–690.

Engberg, J., Aarestrup, F., Taylor, D., Gerner-Smidt, P., & Nachamkin, I. (2001). Quinolone and macrolide resistance in *Campylobacter jejuni* and *C. coli*: Resistance mechanisms and trends in human isolates. *Emerging Inf Dis, 7*, 24–34.

Fagon, J., Chastre, J., Trouillet, J., Domart, Y., Dombret, M., Bornet, M., & Gibert, C. (1990). Characterization of distal bronchial microflora during acute exacerbation of chronic bronchitis. *Am Rev Respir Dis, 142*, 1004–1008.

Feldman, W. (1976). Concentrations of bacteria in cerebrospinal fluid of patients with bacterial meningitis. *J Pediatr, 88*, 549–552.

Firsov, A., Lubenko, I., Portnoy, Y., Zinner, S., & Vostrov, S. (2001). Relationships of the area under the curve/MIC ratio to different integral endpoints of the antimicrobial effect: Gemifloxacin pharmacodynamics in an in vitro dynamic model. *Antimicrob Agents Chemother, 45*, 927–931.

Fish, D., Piscitelli, S., & Danziger, L. (1995). Development of resistance during antimicrobial therapy: A review of antibiotic classes and patient characteristics in 173 studies. *Pharmacotherapy, 15*, 279–291.

Fishman, N. O., Suh, B., Weigel, L. M., Lorber, B., Gelone, S., Truant, A. L., & Gootz, T. D. (1999). Three levofloxacin treatment failures of pneumococcal respiratory tract infections. *39th ICAAC*, San Francisco.

Fogarty, C., Greenberg, R., Dunbar, L., Player, R., Marrie, T., Kojak, C., Morgan, N., & Williams, R. (2001). Effectiveness of levofloxacin for adult community-acquired pneumonia caused by macrolide-resistant *Streptococcus pneumoniae*: Integrated results from four open-label, multicenter, phase III clinical trials. *Clin Therap, 23*, 425–439.

Fraser, C., Norris, S., Weinstock, G., White, O., Sutton, G., Dodson, R., Gwinn, M., Hickey, E., Clayton, R., & Ketchum, K. (1998). Complete genome sequence of *Treponema pallidum*, the syphilis spirochete. *Science, 281*, 375–388.

Fukuda, H., Kishi, R., Takei, M., & Hosaka, M. (2001). Contributions of the 8-methoxy group of gatifloxacin to resistance selectivity, target preference, and antibacterial activity against *Streptococcus pneumoniae*. *Antimicrob Agents Chemother, 45*, 1649–1653.

Fung, C., Hu, B., Lee, S., Liu, P., Jang, T., Leu, H., Kuo, B., Yen, M., Liu, C., & Liu, Y. (2000). Antimicrobial resistance of *Streptococcus pneumoniae* isolated in Taiwan: An island-wide surveillance study between 1996 and 1997. *J Antimicrob Chemother, 45*, 49–55.

Gallardo, F., Ruiz, J., Marco, F., Towner, K., & Vila, J. (1999). Increase in incidence of resistance to ampicillin, chloramphenicol, and trimethoprim in clinical isolates of *Salmonella* serotype Typhimurium with investigation of molecular epidemiology and mechanisms of resistance. *J Med Microbiol, 48*, 367–374.

Garcia-Rodriguez, J., Baquero, F., Lomas, J. G. D., Aguilar, L., & Spanish Surveillance Group. (1999). Antimicrobial susceptibility of 1,422 *Haemophilus influenzae* isolates from respiratory tract infections in Spain. Results of a 1-year (1996–97) multicenter surveillance study. *Infection, 27*, 265–267.

Garg, P., Sinha, S., Chakraborty, R., Bhattacharya, S., & Ramamurthy, T. (2001). Emergence of fluoroquinolone-resistant strains of *Vibrio cholerae* 01 biotype E1 Tor among hospitalized patients with cholera in Calcutta, India. *Antimicrob Agents Chemother, 45*, 1605–1606.

Gasc, A., Geslin, P., & Sicard, A. (1995). Relatedness of penicilllin-resistant *Streptococcus pneumoniae* serogroup 9 strains from France and Spain. *Microbiol, 141*, 623–627.

Gerding, D. (2000). Antimicrobial cycling: Lessons learned from the aminoglycoside experience. *Infect Control Hosp Epidemiol, 21*, S12–S17.

Gerding, D., Larson, T., Hughes, R., Weiler, M., Shanholtzer, C., & Peterson, L. (1991). Aminoglycoside resistance and aminoglycoside usage: Ten years of experience in one hospital. *Antimicrob Agents Chemother, 35*, 1284–1290.

Gillespie, S. H., Voelker, L. L., & Dickens, A. (2002). Evolutionary barriers to quinolone resistance in *Streptococcus pneumoniae*. *Microb Drug Resist, 8*, 79–84.

Glupczynski, Y. (1998). Antimicrobial resistance in *Helicobacter pylori*: A global overview. *Acta Gastroenter Belg, 61*, 357–366.

Goldstein, F., & Garau, J. (1997). Thirty years of penicillin-resistant *S. pneumoniae*: Myth or reality? *Lancet, 350*, 233–234.

Gorwitz, R., Nakashima, A., Moran, J., & Knapp, J. (1993). Sentinel surveillance for antimicrobial resistance in *Neisseria gonorrhoeae*—United States, 1988–1991. *MMWR, 42*, 29–39.

Gruson, D., Hilbert, G., Vargas, F., Valentino, R., Bebear, C., Allery, A., Bebear, C., Gbikpi-Benissan, G., & Cardinaud, J. (2000). Rotation and restricted use of antibiotics in a medical intensive care unit. *Am J Crit Care Med, 162*, 837–843.

Guillemot, D., Carbon, C., Balkau, B., Geslin, P., Lecoeur, H., Vauzelle-Kervroedan, F., Bouvenot, G., & Eschwege, E. (1998). Low dosage and long treatment duration of β-lactam. *JAMA, 279*, 365–370.

Guzman-Blanco, M., Casellas, J., & Sader, H. (2000). Bacterial resistance to antimicrobial agents in Latin America. *Inf Dis Clin North Am, 14*, 67–81.

Hane, M. W., & Wood, T. H. (1969). *Escherichia coli* K-12 mutants resistant to nalidixic acid: Genetic mapping and dominance studies. *J Bacteriol, 99*, 238–241.

Hanson, N., & Sanders, C. (1999). Regulation of inducible AmpC β-lactamase expression in Enterobacteriaceae. *Curr Pharm Des, 5*, 881–894.

Harrison, J., & Svec, T. (1998). The beginning of the end of the antibiotic era? Part II. Proposed solutions to antibiotic abuse. *Quintessence Int, 29*, 223–229.

Hiramatsu, K., Aritaka, N., Hanaki, H., Kawasaki, S., Hosoda, Y., Hori, S., Fukuchi, Y., & Kobayashi, I. (1997). Dissemination in Japanese hospitals of strains of *Staphylococcus aureus* heterogeneously resistant to vancomycin. *Lancet, 350*, 1670–1673.

Ho, M., McDonald, C., Lauderdale, T., Yeh, L., Chen, P., & Shiau, Y. (1999). Surveillance of antibiotic resistance in Taiwan, 1998. *J Microbiol Immunol Infect, 32*, 239–249.

Ho, P., Yung, R., Tsang, D., Que, T., Ho, M., Seto, W., Ng, T., Yam, W., & Ng, W. (2001a). Increasing resistance of *Streptococcus pneumoniae* to fluoroquinolones: Results of a Hong Kong multicentre study in 2000. *J Antimicrob Chemother, 48*, 659–665.

Ho, P. L., Tse, W. S., Tsang, K., Kwok, T., Ng, T., Cheng, V., & Chan, R. (2001b). Risk factors for acquisition of levofloxacin-resistant *Streptococcus pneumoniae*: A case–control study. *Clin Inf Dis, 32*, 701–707.

Holder, I., & Neely, A. (1998). Fear of MRSA—potential for future disaster. *Burns, 24*, 99–103.

Iseman, M. (1994). Evolution of drug-resistant tuberculosis: A tale of two species. *Proc Natl Acad Sci USA, 91*, 2428–2429.

Jacobs, M. (1999). Drug-resistant *Streptococcus pneumoniae*: Rational antibiotic choices. *Am J Med, 106*, 19S–25S.

Jacobs, R., Kaplan, S., Schutze, G., Dajani, A., Leggiadro, R., Rim, C., & Puri, S. (1996). Relationship of MICs to efficacy of cefotaxime in treatment of *Streptococcus pneumoniae* infections. *Antimicrob Agents Chemother, 40*, 895–898.

John, J., & Rice, L. (2000). The microbial genetics of antibiotic cycling. *Infect Control Hosp Epidemiol, 21*(Suppl.), S22–S31.

Johnson, A. P. (1998). Antibiotic resistance among clinically important Gram-positive bacteria in the UK. *J Hosp Infect, 40*, 17–26.

Join-Lambert, O., Michéa-Hamzehpour, M., Köhler, T., Chau, F., Faurisson, F., Dautrey, S., Vissuzaine, C., Carbon, C., & Pechére, J.-C. (2001). Differential selection of multidrug efflux mutants by trovafloxacin and ciprofloxacin in an experimental model of *Pseudomonas aerugiosa* acute pneumonia in rats. *Antimicrob Agents Chemother, 45*, 571–576.

Jones, M., Schmitz, F., Fluit, A., Acar, J., Gupta, R., Verhoef, J., & SENTRY Participants Group. (1999). Frequency of occurrence and antimicrobial susceptibility of bacterial pathogens associated with skin and soft tissue infections during 1997 from an international surveillance program. *Eur J Clin Microbiol, 18*, 403–408.

Jones, M. E., Sahm, D. F., Martin, N., Scheuring, S., Heisig, P., Thornsberry, C., Köhrer, K., & Schmitz, F.-J. (2000). Prevalence of *gyrA*, *gyrB*, *parC*, and *parE* mutations in clinical isolates of *Streptococcus pneumoniae* with decreased susceptibilities to different fluoroquinolones and originating from worldwide surveillance studies during the 1997–1998 respiratory season. *Antimicrob Agents Chemother, 44*, 462–466.

Jones, R., Pfaller, M., Stilwell, M., & SENTRY Antimicrobial Surveillance Program Participants Group. (2001). Activity and spectrum of BMS 284756, a new des-F (6) quinolone, tested against strains of ciprofloxacin-resistant Gram-positive cocci. *Diagn Microbiol Inf Dis, 39*, 133–135.

Kays, M., & Denys, G. (2001). Fluoroquinolone susceptibility, resistance, and pharmacodynamics versus clinical isolates of *Streptococcus pneumoniae* from Indiana. *Diagn Microbiol Infect Dis, 40*, 193–198.

Kays, M., Smith, D., Wack, M., & Denys, G. (2002). Levofloxacin treatment failure in a patient with fluoroquinolone-resistant *Streptococcus pneumoniae*. *Pharmacotherapy, 22*, 395–399.

Khodursky, A., & Cozzarelli, N. (1998). The mechanism of inhibition of topoisomerase IV by quinolone antibacterials. *J Biol Chem, 273*, 27668–27677.

Kollef, M. H., Vlasnik, J., Sharpless, L., Pasque, C., Murphy, D., & Fraser, V. (1997). Scheduled change of antibiotic classes: A strategy to decrease the incidence of ventilator-associated pneumonia. *Am J Respir Crit Care Med, 156*, 1040–1048.

Kristinsson, K., Hjalmarsdottir, M., & Steingrimsson, O. (1992). Increasing penicillin resistance in penumococci in Iceland. *The Lancet, 339*, 1606–1607.

Kristinsson, K. G., Hjalmarsdottir, M. A., & Gudnason, T. (1995). Epidemiology of penicillin resistant pneumococci in Iceland—hope for the future? *35th ICAAC*, San Francisco.

Lenski, R., Simpson, S., & Nguyen, T. (1994). Genetic analysis of a plasmid-encoded, host genotype-specific enhancement of bacterial fitness. *J Bacteriol, 176*, 3140–3147.

Levy, S. (2001). Antibiotic resistance: Consequences of inaction. *Clin Inf Dis, 33*(Suppl. 3), S124–S129.

Li, X., Zhao, X., & Drlica, K. (2002). Selection of *Streptococcus pneumoniae* mutants having reduced susceptibility to levofloxacin and moxifloxacin. *Antimicrob Agents Chemother, 46*, 522–524.

Ling, T., Liu, E., & Cheng, A. (2001). A 13-year study of antimicrobial susceptibility of common Gram-negative bacteria isolated from the bloodstream in a teaching hospital. *Chemotherapy, 47*, 29–38.

Low, D. (2001). Antimicrobial drug use and resistance among respiratory pathogens in the community. *Clin Inf Dis, 33*(Suppl. 3), S206–S213.

Lu, T., Zhao, X., Li, X., Drlica-Wagner, A., Wang, J.-Y., Domagala, J., & Drlica, K. (2001). Enhancement of fluoroquinolone activity by C-8 halogen and methoxy moieties: Action against a gyrase resistance mutant of *Mycobacterium smegmatis* and a gyrase-topoisomerase IV double mutant of *Staphylococcus aureus*. *Antimicrob Agents Chemother, 45*, 2703–2709.

MacGowan, A., Bowker, K., Bennett, P., & Lovering, A. (1998). Surveillance of antimicrobial resistance. *Lancet, 352*, 1783.

Mao, E. F., Lane, L., Lee, J., & Miller, J. H. (1997). Proliferation of mutators in a cell population. *J Bacteriol, 179*, 417–422.

Maraki, S., Georgiladakis, A., Christidou, A., Scoulica, E., & Tselentis, Y. (1998). Antimicrobial susceptibilities and beta-lactamase production of *Shigella* isolates in Crete, Greece, during the period 1991–1995. *APMIS, 106*, 879–883.

Marchant, B. (1981). Pharmacokinetic factors influencing variability in human drug response. *Scand J Rheumatol Suppl, 39*, 5–14.

Marchbanks, C. R., McKiel, J. R., Gilbert, D. H., Robillard, N. J., Painter, B., Zinner, S., & Dudley, M. N. (1993). Dose ranging and fractionation of intravenous ciprofloxacin against *Pseudomonas aeruginosa* and *Staphylococcus aureus* in an in vitro model of infection. *Antimicrob Agents Chemother, 37*, 1756–1763.

Marcus, N., Peled, N., & Yagupsky, P. (1997). Rapid increase in the prevalence of antimicrobial drug resistance among enterococcal blood isolates in southern Israel. *Eur J Clin Microbiol Infect Dis, 16*, 913–915.

Marton, A. (1992). Pneumococcal antimicrobial resistance; the problem in Hungary. *Clin Inf Dis, 15*, 106–111.

Mason, G. R., & Nitta, A. (1997). Emergence of MDR TB during standard therapy in AIDS. *Am J Respir Crit Care Med, 155*, A221.

McGowan, J. E., & Gerding, D. N. (1996). Does antibiotic restriction prevent resistance? *New Horiz, 4*, 370–376.

Metzger, D., & Wills, C. (2000). Evidence for the adaptive evolution of mutation rates. *Cell, 101*, 581–584.

Michea-Hamzehpour, M., Pechere, J., Marchou, B., & Auckenthaler, R. (1986). Combination therapy: A way to limit emergence of resistance. *Am J Med, 80*, 138–142.

Miller, J. (1996). Spontaneous mutators in bacteria: Insights into pathways of mutagenesis and repair. *Annu Rev Microbiol, 50*, 625–643.

Mitchison, D. A. (1984). Drug resistance in mycobacteria. *Brit Med Bull, 40*, 84–90.

Mitchison, D. A., & Nunn, A. J. (1986). Influence of initial drug resistance on the response to short-course chemotherapy on pulmonary tuberculosis. *Am Rev Respir Dis, 133*, 423–430.

Monroe, S., & Polk, R. (2000). Antimicrobial use and bacterial resistance. *Curr Opin Microbiol, 3*, 496–501.

Moore, M., Onorato, I., McCray, E., & Castro, K. (1997). Trends in drug-resistant tuberculosis in the United States, 1993–1996. *JAMA, 278*, 833–837.

Moran, G. (2001). New directions in antiinfective therapy for community-acquired pneumonia in the emergency department. *Pharmacotherapy, 21*, 95S–99S.

Moulding, T., Dutt, A., & Reichman, L. B. (1995). Fixed-dose combinations of antituberculous medications to prevent drug resistance. *Ann Intern Med, 122*, 951–954.

Munoz, R., Coffey, T., Daniels, M., Dowson, C., Laible, G., Casal, J., Hakenbeck, R., Jacobs, M., Musser, J., & Spratt, B. (1991). Intercontinental spread of a multiresistant clone of serotype 23F *Streptococcus pneumoniae. J Inf Dis, 164*, 302–306.

Murray, B. E. (1997). Antibiotic resistance. *Adv Int Med, 42*, 339–367.

Nakamura, S. (1997). Mechanisms of quinolone resistance. *J Infect Chemother, 3*, 128–138.

Navarro, F., Perz-Trallero, E., Marimon, J., Aliaga, R., Gomariz, M., & Mirelis, B. (2001). CMY-2-producing *Salmonella enterica, Klebsiella pneumoniae, Klebsiella oxytoca, Proteus mirabilis,* and *Escherichia coli* strains isolated in Spain (October 1999–December 2000). *J Antimicrob Chemother, 48*, 383–389.

Ng, E. Y., Trucksis, M., & Hooper, D. C. (1996). Quinolone resistance mutations in topoisomerase IV: relationship to the *flqA* locus and genetic evidence that topoisomerase IV is the primary target and DNA gyrase is the secondary target of fluoroquinolones in *Staphylococcus aureus. Antimicrob Agents Chemother, 40*, 1881–1888.

Noble, W., Virani, Z., & Cree, R. (1992). Co-transfer of vancomycin and other resistance genes from *Enterococcus faecalis* NCTC 12201 to *Staphylococcus aureus. FEMS Microbiol Lett, 93*, 195–198.

Nowak, R. (1994). Hungary sees an improvement in penicillin resistance. *Science, 264*, 364.

O'Brien, R. (1994). Drug-resistant tuberculosis: Etiology, management, and prevention. *Semin Respir Infect, 9*, 104–112.

Oliver, A., Canton, R., Campo, P., Baquero, F., & Blazquez, J. (2000). High frequency of hyper-mutable *Pseudomonas aeruginosa* in cystic fibrosis lung infection. *Science, 288*, 1251–1253.

Olson, B., Weinstein, B., Nathan, C., Chamberlin, W., & Kabins, S. (1985). Occult aminoglycoside resistance in *Pseudomonas aeruginosa*: Epidemiology and implications for therapy and control. *J Inf Dis, 152*, 769–774.

Oppegaard, H., Steinum, T., & Wasteson, Y. (2001). Horizontal transfer of a multi-drug resistance plasmid between coliform bacteria of human and bovine origin in a farm environment. *App Environ Microbiol, 67*, 3732–3734.

Pan, X., & Fisher, L. M. (1998). DNA gyrase and topoisomerase IV are dual targets of clinafloxacin action in *Streptococcus pneumoniae. Antimicrob Agents Chemother, 42*, 2810–2816.

Pan, X.-S., Ambler, J., Mehtar, S., & Fisher, L. M. (1996). Involvement of topoisomerase IV and DNA gyrase as ciprofloxacin targets in *Streptococcus pneumoniae. Antimicrob Agents Chemother, 40*, 2321–2326.

Pechere, J.-C. (2001). Patients' interviews and misuse of antibiotics. *Clin Inf Dis, 33*(Suppl. 3), S170–S173.

Pestova, E., Millichap, J., Noskin, G., & Peterson, L. (2000). Intracellular targets of moxifloxacin: A comparison with other fluoroquinolones. *J Antimicrob Chemother, 45*, 583–590.

Peterson, L., Postelnick, M., Pozdol, T., Reisberg, B., & Noskin, G. (1998). Management of fluoroquinolone resistance in *Pseudomonas aeruginosa*—outcome of monitored use in a referral hospital. *Int J Antimicrob Agents, 10*, 207–214.

Phillips, I. (2001). Prudent use of antibiotics: Are our expectations justified? *Clin Inf Dis, 33*(Suppl. 3), S130–S132.

Phillips, I., & Shannon, K. (1993). Importance of beta-lactamase induction. *Eur J Clin Microbiol Infect Dis, 12*, S19–S26.

Piot, P., Bartos, M., Ghys, P., Walker, N., & Schwartlander, B. (2001). The global impact of HIV/AIDS. *Nature, 410*, 968–973.

Portaels, F., Rigouts, L., & Bastian, I. (1999). Addressing multidrug-resistant tuberculosis in penitentiary hospitals and in the general population of the former Soviet Union. *Int J Tuberc Lung Dis, 3*, 582–588.

Preston, S., Drusano, G., Berman, A., Fowler, C., Chow, A., Dornseif, B., Reichi, V., Natarajan, J., & Corrado, M. (1998). Pharmacodyamics of levofloxacin: A new paradigm for early clinical trials. *JAMA, 279*, 125–129.

Quale, J., Landman, D., Saurina, G., Atwood, E., DiTore, V., & Patel, K. (1996). Manipulation of a hospital antimicrobial formulary to control an outbreak of vancomycin-resistant enterococci. *Clin Inf Dis, 23*, 1020–1025.

Rahal, J., Urban, C., Horn, D., Freeman, K., Segal-Maurer, S., Maurer, J., Mariano, N., Marks, S., Burns, J., & Dominick, D. (1998). Class restriction of cephalosporin use to control total cephalosporin resistance in nosocomial *Klebsiella. JAMA, 280*, 1233–1237.

Rahman, M., Alam, A., Nessa, K., Nahar, S., Dutta, D., Yasmin, L., Monira, S., Sultan, Z., Khan, S., & Albert, M. (2001). Treatment failure with the use of ciprofloxacin for gonorrhea corelates with the prevalence of fluoroquinolone-resistant *Neisseria gonorrhoeae* strains in Bangladesh. *Clin Inf Dis, 32*, 884–889.

Ray, K., Bala, M., Kumar, J., & Misra, R. (2000). Trend of antimicrobial resistance in *Neisseria gonorrhoeae* at New Delhi, India. *Int J STD AIDS, 11*, 115–118.

Reacher, M., Shah, A., Livermore, D., Wale, M., Graham, C., Johnson, A., Heine, H., Monnickendam, M., Barker, K., & James, D. (2000). Bacteraemia and antibiotic resistance of its pathogens reported in England and Wales between 1990 and 1998: Trend analysis. *Brit Med J, 320*, 213–216.

Reichmann, P., Varon, E., Gunther, E., Reinerts, R., Luttiken, R., Marton, A., Geslin, P., Wagner, J., & Hakenbeck, R. (1995). Penicillin-resistant *Streptococcus pneumoniae* in Germany: Genetic relationship to clones from other European countries. *J Med Microbiol, 43*, 377–385.

Rello, J., Torres, A., Ricart, M., Valles, J., Gonzalez, J., Artigas, A., & Rodriguez, R. (1994). Ventilator-associated pneumonia by *Staphylococcus aureus*. Comparison of methicillin-resistant and methicillin-sensitive episodes. *Am J Crit Care Med, 150*, 1545–1549.

Rice, L., Eckstein, E., DeVente, J., & Shlaes, D. (1996). Ceftazidime-resistant *Klebsiella pneumoniae* isolates recovered at the Cleveland Department of Veterans Affairs Medical Center. *Clin Inf Dis, 23*, 118–124.

Rifenburg, R., Paladino, J., Bhavnani, S., DenHaese, D., & Schentag, J. (1999). Influence of fluoroquinolone purchasing patterns on antimicrobial expenditures and *Pseudomonas aeruginosa* susceptibiltity. *Am J Health-Syst Pharmacy, 56*, 2217–2223.

Roosihermiatie, B., Nashiyama, M., & Nakae, K. (2000). The comparison of tuberculosis treatments: A short course therapy and the directly observed short course teratment (DOTS), East Java Province, Indonesia. *Southeast Asian J Trop Med Public Health, 31*, 85–88.

Rudolph, K., Parkinson, A., Reasonover, A., Bulkow, L., Parks, D., & Butler, J. (2000). Serotype distribution and antimicrobial resistance patterns of invasive isolates of *Streptococcus pneumoniae*: Alaska, 1991–1998. *J Infect Dis, 182*, 490–496.

Sahm, D., Jones, M., Hickey, M., Diakun, D., Mani, S., & Thornsberry, C. (2000). Resistance surveillance of *Streptococcus pneumoniae, Haemophilus influenzae*, and *Moraxella catarrhalis* isolated from Asia and Europe, 1997–1998. *J Antimicrob Chemother, 45*, 457–466.

Sahm, D., Karlowsky, J., Kelly, L., Critchley, I., Jones, M., Thornsberry, C., Mauriz, Y., & Kahn, J. (2001). Need for annual surveillance of antimicrobial resistance in *Streptococcus pneumoniae* in the United States: 2-year longitudinal analysis. *Antimicrob Agents Chemother, 45*, 1037–1042.

Salyers, A., & Amabile-Cuevas, C. (1997). Why are antibiotic resistance genes so resistant to elimination. *Antimicrob Agents Chemother, 41*, 2321–2325.

Sawyer, R., Raymond, D., Pelletier, S., Crabtree, T., Gleason, T., & Pruett, T. (2001). Implications of 2,457 consecutive surgical infections entering year 2000. *Ann Surg, 233*, 867–874.

Sbarbaro, J. (2001). Can we influence prescribing patterns? *Clin Inf Dis, 33*(Suppl. 3), S240–S244.

Schentag, J. (1999). Antimicrobial action and pharmacokinetics/pharmacodynamics: The use of AUIC to improve efficacy and avoid resistance. *J Chemother, 11*, 426–439.

Schmitz, F.-J., Fluit, A., Brisse, S., Verhoef, J., Koher, K., & Milatovic, D. (1999). Molecular epidemiology of quinolone resistance and comparative in vitro activities of new quinolones against European *Staphylococcus aureus* isolates. *FEMS Immunol Med Microbiol, 26*, 281–287.

Schrag, S., Perrot, V., & Levin, B. (1997). Adaptation to the fitness costs of antibiotic resistance in *Escherichia coli. Proc R Soc Lond B, 264*, 1287–1291.

Second East African/British Medical Research Council Study. (1974). Controlled clinical trial of four short-course (6-month) regimens of chemotherapy for treatment of pulmonary tuberculosis. *Lancet, 2*, 1100–1106.

Selman, L. J., Mayfield, D. C., Thornsberry, C., Mauriz, Y., & Sahm, D. F. (2000). Changes in single- and multiple-drug resistance among *Streptococcus pneumoniae* over three years (1997–2000). *40th ICAAC*, Toronto.

Seppala, H., Klaukka, T., Vuopio-Varkila, J., Maotiala, A., Helenius, H., & Lager, K. (1997). The effect of changes in the consumption of macrolide antibiotics on erythromycin resistance in group A streptococci in Finland. *N Engl J Med, 337*, 441–446.

Shah, A., Lettieri, J., Kaiser, L., Echols, R., & Heller, A. (1994). Comparative pharmacokinetics and safety of ciprofloxacin 400 mg iv thrice daily versus 750 mg PO twice daily. *J Antimicrob Chemother, 33*, 795–801.

Sindelar, G., Zhao, X., Liew, A., Dong, Y., Zhou, J., Domagala, J., & Drlica, K. (2000). Mutant prevention concentration as a measure of fluoroquinolone potency against mycobacteria. *Antimicrob Agents Chemother, 44*, 3337–3343.

Soares, S., Kristinsson, K., Musser, J., & Tomasz, A. (1993). Evidence for the introduction of a multiresistant clone of serotype 6B *Streptococcus pneumoniae* from Spain to Iceland in the late 1980s. *J Inf Dis, 168*, 158–163.

Sweeney, G. D. (1983). Variability in the human drug response. *Thromb Res Suppl, 4*, 3–15.

Takiff, H. E., Cimino, M., Musso, M. C., Weisbrod, T., Martinez, R., Delgado, M. B., Salazar, L., Bloom, B. R., & Jacobs, W. R. (1996). Efflux pump of the proton antiporter family confers low-level fluoroquinolone resistance in *Mycobacterium smegmatis. Proc Natl Acad Sci USA, 93*, 362–366.

Tanaka, M., Nakayama, H., Haraoka, M., Saika, T., Kobayashi, I., & Naito, S. (2000). Susceptibilities of *Neisseria gonorrhoeae* isolates containing amino acid substitutions in *gyrA*, with or without substitutions in *parC*, to newer fluoroquinolones and other antibiotics. *Antimicrob Agents Chemother, 44*, 192–195.

Tenover, F., Lancaster, M., Hill, B., Steward, C., Stocker, S., Hancock, G., O'Hara, C., Clark, N., & Hiramatsu, K. (1998). Characterization of staphylococci with reduced susceptibilities to vancomycin and other glycopeptides. *J Clin Microbiol, 36*, 1020–1027.

Tenover, F., & McGowan, J. E. (1998). The epidemiology of bacterial resistance to antimicrobial agents. In A. S. Evans & P. S. Brachman (Eds.), *The epidemiology of bacterial resistance to antimicrobial agents* (pp. 83–93). New York: Plenum Medical Book Company.

Thomas, J., Forrest, A., Bhavnani, S., Hyatt, J., Cheng, A., Ballow, C., & Schentag, J. (1998). Pharmacodynamic evaluation of factors associated with the development of bacterial resistance in acutely ill patients during therapy. *Antimicrob Agents Chemother, 42*, 521–527.

Thornsberry, C. (1995). Trends in antimicrobial resistance among today's bacterial pathogens. *Pharmacotherapy, 15*, 3S–8S.

Tillotson, G., Zhao, X., & Drlica, K. (2001). Fluoroquinolones as pneumococcal therapy: Closing the barn door before the horse escapes. *Lancet Inf Dis, 1*, 145–146.

Tomasz, A. (1999). New faces of an old pathogen: Emergence and spread of multi-drug resistant *Streptococcus pneumoniae. Am J Med, 107*(1A), 55S–62S.

Tomb, J., White, O., Kerlavage, A., Clayton, R., Sutton, G., Fleischmann, R., Ketchum, K., Klenk, H., Gill, S., & Dougherty, B. (1997). The complete genome sequence of the gastric pathogen *Helicobacter pylori. Nature, 388*, 539–547.

Urban, C., Rahman, N., Zhao, X., Mariano, N., Segal-Maurer, S., Drlica, K., & Rahal, J. (2001). Fluoroquinolone-resistant *Streptococcus pneumoniae* associated with levofloxacin therapy. *J Inf Dis, 184*, 794–798.

Vatopoulos, A., Kalapothaki, V., Network, G., & Legakis, N. (1999). Bacterial resistance to ciprofloxacin in Greece: Results from the national electronic surveillance system. *Emerging Inf Dis, 5*, 471–475.

Vernon, A., Burman, W., Benator, D., Khan, A., & Bozeman, L. (1999). Acquired rifamycin monoresistance in patients with HIV-related tuberculosis treated with once-weekly rifapentine and isoniazid. *The Lancet, 353*, 1843–1847.

Vesell, E. (1991). Genetic and environmental factors causing variation in drug response. *Mutat Res, 247*, 241–257.

Wain, J., Hoa, N., Chinh, N., Vinh, H., Everett, M., Diep, T., Day, N., Solomon, T., White, N., & Piddock, L. (1997). Quinolone-resistant *Salmonella typhi* in Vietnam: Molecular basis of resistance and clinical response to treatment. *Clin Inf Dis, 25*, 1404–1410.

Wang, H., Dzink-Fox, J., Chen, M., & Levy, S. (2001). Genetic characterization of highly fluoroquinolone-resistant clinical *Escherichia coli* strains from China: Role of *acrR* mutations. *Antimicrob Agents Chemother, 45*, 1515–1521.

Weis, S., Slocum, P., Blais, F., King, B., Nunn, M., Matney, G., Gomez, E., & Foresman, B. (1994). The effect of directly observed therapy on the rates of drug resistance and relapse in tuberculosis. *N Engl J Med, 330*, 1179–1184.

Weiss, K., Restieri, C., Gauthier, R., Laverdiere, M., McGeer, A., Davidson, R., Kilburn, L., Bast, D., deAzavedo, J., & Low, D. E. (2001). A nosocomial outbreak of fluoroquinolone-resistant *Streptococcus pneumoniae. Clin Infect Dis, 33*, 517–522.

Wimberley, N., Faling, L., & Bartlett, J. (1979). A fiberoptic bronchoscopy technique to obtain uncontaminated lower airway secretions for bacterial culture. *Am Rev Respir Dis, 119*, 337–343.

Wise, R., & Andrews, J. M. (1998). Local surveillance of antimicrobial resistance. *Lancet, 352*, 657–658.

Zhao, X., & Drlica, K. (2001). Restricting the selection of antibiotic-resistant mutants: A general strategy derived from fluoroquinolone studies. *Clin Infect Dis, 33*(Suppl. 3), S147–S156.

Zhao, X., & Drlica, K. (2002). Restricting the selection of antibiotic-resistant mutants: Measurement and potential uses of the mutant selection window. *J Inf Dis, 185*, 561–565.

Zhao, X., Xu, C., Domagala, J., & Drlica, K. (1997). DNA topoisomerase targets of the fluoroquinolones: A strategy for avoiding bacterial resistance. *Proc Natl Acad Sci USA, 94*, 13991–13996.

Zhou, J.-F., Dong, Y., Zhao, X., Lee, S., Amin, A., Ramaswamy, S., Domagala, J., Musser, J. M., & Drlica, K. (2000). Selection of antibiotic resistance: Allelic diversity among fluoroquinolone-resistant mutations. *J Inf Dis, 182*, 517–525.

Zinner, S., Wise, R., & Moellering, R. (2001a). General discussion. *Clin Inf Dis, 33*(Suppl. 3), S251–S260.

Zinner, S., Wise, R., & Moellering, R. (2001b). Maximizing antimicrobial efficacy, minimizing antimicrobial resistance; a paradigm for the new millenium. *Clin Inf Dis, 33*(Suppl. 3), S107.

Section III

Resistant Parasitic Infections

9

Drug-Resistant Malaria

Mona R. Loutfy and Kevin C. Kain

1. INTRODUCTION

Malaria is one of the most important causes of global morbidity and mortality. Since the areas of the world that suffer the greatest burden of disease, have the least developed systems of health, reporting the quoted figures for annual deaths and clinical cases are best estimates (Phillips, 2001; Snow et al., 1999). The World Health Organization (WHO) estimates that malaria is responsible for 300–500 million cases of clinical disease and 1.5–2.7 million deaths each year, most of which are children under 5 years of age in sub-Saharan Africa. These may be underestimates due to gross underreporting and failure to appreciate gaps in the burden of disease including cerebral malaria with resulting neurological sequelae, severe anemia, hypoglycemia, respiratory distress and malaria-associated complications of pregnancy, which may double commonly accepted malaria fatality rates (Murphy & Breman, 2001). Malaria represents a significant public health problem for approximately 2.4 billion people residing in over 90 countries (Phillips, 2001) and for the estimated 70 million travellers who visit malaria-endemic regions each year (Breman & Campbell, 1988; Murphy & Breman, 2001; Phillips, 2001; Schwartlander, 1997; Sturchler, 1989; WHO, 1997). The burden of malaria falls most heavily on sub-Saharan Africa, where >90% of these deaths occur and ~5% of children die from the disease before reaching 5 years of age (Phillips, 2001). A child is estimated to die from malaria every 12 s; virtually all these deaths are due to *Plasmodium falciparum*. In addition to the health impacts, the economic burden of malaria is enormous with up to US$12 billion in lost productivity attributed each year in Africa to malaria (Gallup & Sachs, 2001).

Although most malaria-associated mortality is due to *P. falciparum*, *Plasmodium vivax* malaria results in ~80 million cases annually with considerable morbidity, particularly in countries outside of Africa. Repeated attacks and relapses from *P. vivax* contribute to deleterious effects on personal health, growth, development, and health economics (Mendis et al., 2001; White, 2000). *P. vivax* infection has recently been linked to adverse outcomes in pregnancy (Nosten et al., 1999).

Reemergence of Established Pathogens in the 21st Century
Edited by Fong and Drlica, Kluwer Academic/Plenum Publishers, New York, 2003

Malaria incidence has increased in the last two decades and several factors are contributed to this distressing trend. Since malaria is transmitted by the Anopheles mosquito, a major strategy of control is to attack the vector with insecticides. However, extended use of insecticides has led to the emergence of insecticide-resistant vectors (Phillips, 2001). In addition, the cost of such control programs has forced their reduction or total abandonment in many malaria-endemic regions (Phillips, 2001). New mosquito breeding sites have also been created by environmental changes including road building, deforestation, mining, irrigation projects, and new agricultural practices (Campbell, 1997; Phillips, 2001).

Rises in population density in malaria-endemic areas, combined with migration from rural to more populated urban areas, have led to higher rates of transmission. This migration has resulted in increased exposure of individuals with little or no immunity to higher rates of infection (Breman & Campbell, 1988; Phillips, 2001). Finally, drug resistance has contributed significantly to the escalating rates of malaria-associated morbidity and mortality (Trape, 2001). As a safe and inexpensive drug, chloroquine has been the mainstay of malaria control and treatment for decades. Chloroquine resistance has now become an established problem in South America, Asia, and Africa; however, because of a lack of affordable alternatives, chloroquine remains widely used in many endemic regions in particular sub-Saharan Africa. In Southeast Asia and elsewhere, increasing reliance on second and third line agents has led to the emergence of resistance to these alternative drugs including sulfadoxine/pyrimethamine (SP), mefloquine, halofantrine, and quinine. The future prospect for new antimalarials is relatively bleak given that few major pharmaceutical companies have demonstrated any sustained interest in developing new antimalarial drugs. Nonetheless, much progress has been made in understanding the mechanisms of drug action and drug-resistance, in predicting treatment failures, in the use of drug combinations to combat resistance, and in the area of vaccine development. In this chapter, these topics along with a review of the epidemiology of drug resistant falciparum and vivax malaria will be summarized.

2. DRUG-RESISTANT FALCIPARUM MALARIA

2.1. Epidemiology and Worldwide Distribution

With the possible exception of artemisinin derivatives, resistance to all antimalarials has been reported but has developed at dramatically different rates (White, 1992, 1996, 1998). Cinchona bark was used to treat intermittent fevers in South America and was introduced into Europe in the 17th century by Jesuit priests returning from Peru. Quinine was isolated from this "Jesuit bark" by the French chemists Caventou and Pelletier in 1820. Despite over 350 years of use, quinine remains an effective antimalarial agent throughout most of the world. Quinine resistance was first described in 1908 in Brazil and confirmed in human volunteers in Brazil and Southeast Asia in the 1960s. However unlike most antimalarials and for reasons that are not entirely clear, quinine resistance has not rapidly progressed. Since the 1980s quinine cure rates have declined particularly in Southeast Asia and quinine is now combined with other agents such as tetracyclines, SP, or clindamycin to maintain efficacy. Combination quinine therapy continues to provide cure rates of

85–90% even against multidrug-resistant (MDR) falciparum malaria in Southeast Asia (White, 1998). However, common adverse effects of cinchonism (headache, tinnitis, deafness, dysphoria) limit adherence with quinine-containing drug regimens.

Chloroquine was originally synthesized by a team of German chemists in the mid-1930s and after the World War II, rapidly became the drug of choice for the prevention and treatment of malaria. It is well tolerated and inexpensive, at around US$0.08 per treatment and in 1994 was said to be the second or third most widely consumed drug in the world after aspirin and paracetamol (Foster, 1994). Chloroquine had a relatively long and effective period of deployment; however the first reports of resistance appeared in the late 1950s from South America and the Thai–Cambodian border and more significant reports in 1961 (Wernsdorfer & Payne, 1991). Initially spreading through South America and Southeast Asia, chloroquine resistant-*P. falciparum* malaria reached East Africa in late 1970s and crossed the entire continent by 1985 (Bjorkman & Phillips-Howard, 1990). Data from Africa indicates that chloroquine-resistance has had a major but often underestimated impact on public health. In Senegal and other sentinel sites in West Africa, the emergence of chloroquine-resistance has been associated with a 2–6-fold increase in malaria-associated mortality and hospital admissions for severe disease in children (Trape, 2001; Trape et al., 1998). Nonetheless, primarily because of the lack of affordable alternatives and since partial immunity enhances the effect of the drug, chloroquine is still widely used in much of sub-Saharan Africa. Currently, falciparum malaria resistant to chloroquine are reported throughout the sub-tropics and tropics with the exception of Central America (above the Panama canal), Caribbean (Haiti and Dominican Republic) or Northern Africa, and Middle East (Figure 9.1).

In the face of escalating chloroquine resistance, antifolate drug combinations such as SP became drugs of choice in many malaria-endemic areas. The extensive use of SP has led to the selection of drug-resistance, which is now common and widespread throughout Asia, parts of sub-Saharan Africa, and South America (Cowman, 1995; Nzila et al., 2000a, 2000b; Peterson et al., 1990). The mechanism of resistance is single point mutations in enzymes involved in the folate biosynthetic pathway, which may rapidly develop resulting in drug resistance (Phillips, 2001). Resistance to the combination of SP took only 5 years to develop in Thailand and only 3 years to develop in Africa (Peterson et al., 1990; Warhurst, 1999). Data from the East Africa Network for Monitoring Antimalarial Treatment (EANMAT; Monica Parise, CDC, personal communication) report RII/RIII resistance rates to SP that range from 0% to 22% in West Africa and 0% to 72% in East Africa, suggesting that in many locations in Africa, SP can no longer be relied upon to provide an effective cure. Rates of SP resistance are very high in the Amazon basin and Southeast Asia but there is little data on SP efficacy elsewhere is Asia. SP is now being combined with artemisinin derivatives in an effort to delay the development and spread of drug resistance and to reduce malaria transmission (von Seidlein et al., 2000).

Mefloquine is a quinoline methanol compound with good activity against chloroquine-resistant *P. falciparum* and has been widely used in Southeast Asia and South America. Resistance to mefloquine was recognized even before the drug was brought into routine use in Southeast Asia and Africa but resistance levels have remained low in most malaria-endemic areas except the eastern and western borders of Thailand. Mefloquine was initially combined with SP in an effort to prevent resistance but this failed largely because isolates were already SP resistant in Southeast Asia at the time of deployment.

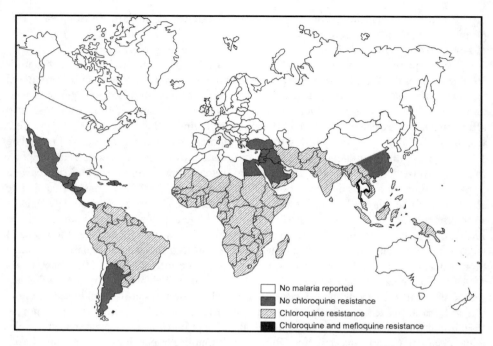

Figure 9.1. Map showing malaria-endemic zones worldwide. *Note*. This map is meant as a visual aid only. This figure was adapted from the CDC, CATMAT, and the WHO with permission from the publishers. The reader is referred to Centers for Disease Control and Prevention (CDC, 2002), CATMAT (2003), WHO (2002), www.cdc.gov (See *Health information for international travel 2001–2002*), and www.who.int/ith/ (See *International travel and health*) for country specific malaria risk.

Mefloquine was then used alone at a dose of 15 mg/kg until high failure rates led to a dose increase to 25 mg/kg. This proved to be only a stopgap measure and rates of mefloquine treatment failure at this higher dose approach 50% in regions of Thailand, particularly on the Thai–Myanmar and Thai–Cambodian borders (Nosten et al., 1991; ter Kuile et al., 1992; White, 1998). Although mefloquine resistance has been described in South America and Africa, it has not been an operational problem to date (Brasseur et al., 1990; Raccurt et al., 1991). Surveillance of Peace Corp volunteers in sub-Saharan Africa over a 6 year period identified only five cases likely due to mefloquine-resistant falciparum malaria; and most individuals who developed malaria reported noncompliance with mefloquine (Lobel et al., 1998).

2.2. Mechanisms of Action and Resistance

2.2.1. Chloroquine

Chloroquine, like other aminoquinoline antimalarials, has its primary effect on the mature stages of the asexual life cycle of the parasite (Cowman, 1995). The mature parasite rapidly degrades hemoglobin, taken in from the cytoplasm of the infected erythrocyte.

This occurs in a lysosome-like organelle termed the food vacuole in which hemoglobin is broken down to amino acids releasing large amounts of hematin. Hematin is toxic to the parasite and is sequestered as a crystalline-like structure called hemozoin, which is a non-toxic, insoluble polymer of heme units linked by the central ferric ion of one unit to the carboxylic side group of the next heme group (Slater et al., 1991). Chloroquine is thought to accumulate to high levels in the food vacuole where it binds with hematin, interfering with polymerization and detoxification and thereby destroying the parasite (Chou et al., 1980; Chou & Fitch, 1980, 1981; Fitch et al., 1983; Pagola et al., 2000; Sullivan et al., 1996; Wellems & Plowe, 2001).

The precise molecular mechanism of resistance to chloroquine remains uncertain; however, significant advances have been made in our understanding in the past decade. Chloroquine-resistant parasites survive by effectively preventing accumulation of chloroquine in the digestive vacuole. How this is achieved remains to be elucidated but may involve increased efflux or decreased import of the drug across the cytoplasm or vacuolar membrane combined with changes in the vacuolar pH (Warhurst, 1999; Wellems & Plowe, 2001). There has been a focused effort to identify the genetic basis of resistance to chloroquine. Three genes have been implicated in the process: the "multidrug resistance" gene (*pfmdr1*) on chromosome 5 (Foote et al., 1990; Wilson et al., 1989), which encodes Pgh1; a determinant, *cg2*, identified via a genetic cross (Su et al., 1997); and, most recently *pfcrt* (chloroquine resistance transporter gene) (Fidock et al., 2000), which is closely linked to *cg2* on chromosome 7.

Pgh1 was initially implicated following observations that verapamil and other agents that inhibit P-glycoprotein-mediated multidrug resistance in mammalian tumour cells, partly reversed chloroquine resistance in malarial parasites in vitro (reviewed in White, 1998). Foote et al. (1990), studying laboratory-cultured *P. falciparum* isolates, identified two *pfmdr1* alleles linked with chloroquine resistance; one characterized by an Asn → Tyr mutation at amino acid 86 (N86Y), and the other by mutations S1034C, N1042D, and D1246Y. Most field studies have investigated the N86Y allele, which was associated with chloroquine resistance in some studies but not in others (Awad-El-Kariem et al., 1992; Babiker et al., 2001; Basco et al., 1995; Foote et al., 1990; Haruki et al., 1994; Pillai et al., 2001; Wellems et al., 1990). Recent transfection studies have demonstrated that mutations in *pfmdr1* can decrease chloroquine resistance from high to moderate levels in vitro (Reed et al., 2000). Therefore mutations in *pfmdr1* are not required for chloroquine resistance but may play a role in modulating the level of resistance (Reed et al., 2000).

Using a genetic cross between chloroquine-sensitive and resistant isolates of *P. falciparum*, Wellem and colleagues mapped the chloroquine-resistance determinant to a 36-kb region of chromosome 7 that did not contain the *pfmdr1* gene (Su et al., 1997; Wellems et al., 1990, 1991). Initial work identified complex polymorphisms in a candidate gene in this region, *cg2*, with chloroquine-resistance in vitro (Su et al., 1997). Although *cg2* was originally believed to be a principal determinant of resistance, it was not consistently associated with resistance in field studies (Durand et al., 1999; Pillai et al., 2001; Su et al., 1997) and *cg2* resistant alleles were unable to confer resistance in transfection-based studies (Fidock et al., 2000). Further analysis eventually demonstrated an association between chloroquine resistance and mutations in a new candidate gene, *pfcrt* (chloroquine resistance transporter) (Fidock et al., 2000). *pfcrt* encodes PfCRT, a transmembrane protein that localizes to the digestive vacuole and as such might play a role in regulating digestive vacuole pH and/or drug flux across this membrane. Eight point mutations in *pfcrt* were associated with chloroquine resistance in vitro in *P. falciparum* lines from Africa, South America, and Southeast Asia. One mutation, the substitution of Thr → Lys at position 76 (K76T), was present in all resistant isolates and absent from all sensitive lines tested in vitro. The most definitive evidence for a key role for pfcrt in chloroquine resistance came from genetic-transformation experiments in which mutant forms of *pfcrt* were able to confer chloroquine resistance to different chloroquine-sensitive clones in vitro. PfCRT mutations were also associated with increased acidification of digestive vacuoles potentially resulting in altered chloroquine uptake or binding to hematin.

A number of field studies have examined the predictive role of mutations in *pfcrt* in chloroquine treatment outcome and the use of K76T as a molecular surveillance marker for in vivo chloroquine resistance (Babiker et al., 2001; Djimde et al., 2001; Pillai et al., 2001; Wellems & Plowe, 2001). In studies in Mali, in which 86% of patients who presented with malaria responded fully to therapy with chloroquine, the baseline prevalence of the *pfcrt* K76T mutation was 41% (Djimde et al., 2001). The presence of K76T mutation was strongly associated with chloroquine resistance (odds ratio 18.8; 95% CI 6.5–58.3), however the positive predictive value of T76 in predicting treatment outcome was only 30%. Similarly, Pillai et al. (2001) and others (Babiker et al., 2001; Dorsey et al., 2001; Mayor et al., 2001) found that although the *pfcrt* K76T mutation was perfectly associated with in vivo chloroquine treatment failure, the mutation was also present in in vivo sensitive isolates which limited its utility as a molecular marker to predict clinical outcome or for the molecular surveillance of in vivo chloroquine resistance. Collectively these studies support a key role for *pfcrt* mutations in conferring chloroquine resistance but highlight the important observation that many individuals infected with parasites possessing the T76 mutation will clear infections following standard chloroquine therapy. Treatment outcome is clearly influenced by additional host, and perhaps parasite factors, including variable degrees of underlying innate and acquired immunity (premunition), variations in drug absorption, distribution, and metabolism, and possibly the presence of additional mutations in or compensatory changes in expression of other parasite genes that may influence the level of resistance and ultimately the treatment outcome (Babiker et al., 2001; Reed et al., 2000). The use of T76 as a molecular marker of resistance will be most worthwhile in the areas of the world where chloroquine resistance is declining or still uncommon.

2.2.2. Antifolates

Antifolate drugs include proguanil, chlorproguanil, and pyrimethamine and the sulfa drugs dapsone, sulphalene, and sulfadoxine. Proguanil and chlorproguanil are metabolized to generate the active metabolites cycloguanil and chlorcycloguanil, respectively, that together with pyrimethamine bind to and inhibit the plasmodial enzyme dihydrofolate reductase (DHFR). The sulpha drugs compete with *p*-aminobenzoic acid and inhibit the malarial enzyme dihydropteroate synthase (DHPS). DHFR and DHPS are enzymes in the folate biosynthetic pathway essential for DNA synthesis. Antifolate drug resistance is mediated by the development of point mutations in DHFR and DHPS that rapidly developed when these agents were used alone for therapy (Foote & Cowman, 1994; Urdaneta et al., 1999). In an effort to relay resistance, antifolate combinations such as SP known as Fansidar™ (Hoffmann-La Roche Inc., Nutley, NJ), were developed that demonstrated synergistic and sequential inhibition of folate biosynthesis. SP has been widely used and has replaced chloroquine in a number of countries in sub-Saharan Africa (Warhurst, 1999). However, extensive use has resulted in the emergence of SP resistance related to point mutations in the *dhps* and *dhfr* genes (Brooks et al., 1994; Plowe et al., 1997). For DHFR inhibitors the initial mutation is generally at position 108, with S108N conferring pyrimethamine resistance and S108T combined with A16V conferring cycloguanil but not pyrimethamine resistance (Cortese & Plowe, 1998; Foote et al., 1990; Peterson et al., 1991). Additional mutations at positions 51, 59, and 164 of DHFR mediate escalating levels of resistance to both drugs in vitro (Foote and Cowman, 1994). Similarly, initial mutation in DHPS is usually A437G and additional mutations at positions 436, 540, and 613 confer increasing levels of suphadoxine resistance in vitro (Foote & Cowman, 1994; Phillips, 2001; Warhurst, 1999).

Recently a number of field studies have attempted to determine whether *dhps* and *dhfr* genotypes can be used to predict treatment outcome. Basco et al. (2000) evaluated the in vivo response to SP of 75 adults in Cameroon. In that study triple *dhfr* mutations were associated with in vivo resistance to SP; the *dhps* genotype had no measurable influence on outcome. In a study in two locations in Kenya (one epidemic and one holoendemic), the relationship of genotype to outcome with SP was more complex. In an epidemic area of study, mutations in both *dhfr* and *dhps* were predictive of outcome; in the holoendemic area, ≥2 mutations in *dhfr* and ≥1 mutation in *dhps* were predictive of treatment failure (Omar et al., 2001).

2.2.3. Mefloquine

Mefloquine's mechanism of action, like chloroquine, is likely mediated via inhibition of heme polymerization and detoxification. The precise mechanism of drug resistance to mefloquine although unknown, appears to be distinct from chloroquine. In regions where there is decreased susceptibility to both drugs, chloroquine and mefloquine resistance are inversely correlated and mefloquine resistance is reversed in vitro by penfluridol but not verapamil; whereas verapamil will reverse chloroquine resistance in vitro but not pen-fluridol. Several studies have suggested a link between mefloquine resistance and alter-ations in *pfmdr1* (Cowman, 1995; Peel et al., 1993; Wilson et al., 1993). In vitro selection studies and in vivo data linked decreased susceptibility to mefloquine and halofantrine to increased mRNA expression and/or gene amplification of *pfmdr1* (Cowman, 1995; Price et al., 1999; Wilson et al., 1993). On the other hand, other studies have failed to detect consistent gene amplification of *pfmdr1* in mefloquine-resistant isolates suggesting that additional mechanisms can mediate the mefloquine-resistant phenotype (Chaiyaroj et al., 1999). By genetically crossing HB3 and 3D7 strains of *P. falciparum*, Duraisingh et al. (2000) found complete allelic association between the HB3-like *pfmdr1* allele and increased sensitivity to the combination of mefloquine and artemisinin. The most direct evidence to date implicating *pfmdr1* in mefloquine resistance comes from genetic transfection experiments in which the introduction of the D10 *pfmdr1* allele (S1034, N1042, D1246) into the mefloquine sensitive line 7G8, conferred mefloquine and halofantrine resistance in vitro. Conversely, introduction of the 7G8 *pfmdr1* allele (C1034, D1042, Y1246) into the quinine sensitive D10 line conferred quinine resistance (Reed et al., 2000).

Of particular concern is the development of cross-resistance between antimalarials. Mefloquine is structurally related to quinine and halofantrine, and Peel et al. (1993) suggested that mefloquine resistance might drive halofantrine and quinine resistance. The development of halofantrine resistance has paralleled that of mefloquine resistance in Southeast Thailand and cross-resistance is supported by the above transformation studies. There is less data linking quinine and mefloquine resistance and the transformation studies would appear to contradict cross-resistance at least as mediated by *pfmdr1* (Reed et al., 2000; Wongsrichanalai et al., 1992).

2.2.4. Atovaquone/Proguanil

A fixed dose combination of atovaquone and proguanil hydrochloride is now available in adult and pediatric formulations (Malarone™, Glaxo Wellcome, Inc., Research Triangle Park, NC). Atovaquone acts by inhibition of parasite mitochondrial electron transport at the level of the cytochrome bc_1 complex and collapses mitochondrial membrane potential (Fry & Pudney, 1992; Pudney et al., 1999; Srivastava et al., 1997, 1999). The plasmodial electron transport system is a 1000-fold more sensitive to atovaquone than the mammalian electron transport system, which likely explains the selective action and limited side effects of this drug (Pudney et al., 1999). Proguanil is metabolized to cycloguanil, which acts by inhibiting DHFR impeding the synthesis of folate, which is required for parasite DNA synthesis. However, it appears that the mechanism of synergy of proguanil with atovaquone is via its biguanide mode of action rather than through its cycloguanil metabolite (Srivastava et al., 1999). In a mouse model, proguanil alone had no effect on mitochondrial membrane potential or electron transport, but significantly enhanced the ability of atovaquone to collapse mitochondrial membrane potential when used in combination (Srivastava et al., 1999). This might explain why proguanil displays synergistic activity with atovaquone even in the presence of documented proguanil resistance (Looareesuwan et al., 1996) or in patient populations who are deficient in cytochrome P450 enzymes required for the conversion of proguanil to cycloguanil (Helsby et al., 1990).

Used as a sole therapeutic agent atovaquone has high recrudescent rates (~33%). In vitro and in vivo drug resistance to atovaquone appears to be associated with mutations in the *cytochrome b* gene (Korsinczky et al., 2000; Srivastava et al., 1999). In vitro and in vivo atovaquone resistant isolates possess single or double amino acid mutations in the putative atovaquone-binding site of cytochrome bc_1 complex. Mutations such as Y268S confer a decrease of almost 100,000-fold in susceptibility to atovaquone. Other mutations including M133I and M133I plus G280D confer lesser degrees of in vitro resistance, 25-fold to ~900-fold increases in inhibitory concentration 50 (IC_{50}), respectively. Similarly, proguanil used alone for treatment in Southeast Asia is associated with very high failure rates (~94%) and as discussed above, resistance involves point mutations in the *dhfr* gene (Foote & Cowman, 1994). However, the combination of atovaquone and proguanil (AP) is effective against strains that are resistant to a variety of other antimalarial drugs and that possess DHFR, DHPS, and Pgh1 mutations (Gay et al., 1997). To date there are little data characterizing isolates that display true in vivo or in vitro resistance to the combination drug.

2.3. Management

Only falciparum malaria infections unequivocally acquired in chloroquine-sensitive areas (e.g., those from North Africa, Central America north of the Panama Canal, Haiti, Dominican Republic, or the Middle East) should be treated with chloroquine. *P. falciparum* malaria acquired elsewhere should be assumed to be chloroquine-resistant and the choice of therapy is generally between AP (Malarone™), mefloquine (Larium™), and quinine combined with doxycycline, SP (not for infections acquired in Southeast Asia or the Amazon basin), or less optimally, clindamycin. For MDR malaria, three drug combinations have been shown to be effective: an artemisinin derivative plus mefloquine, atovoquone plus proguanil, and artemether plus lumefantrine (Riamet™, Coartem™) (Labbe et al., 2001).

2.3.1. Sulfadoxine–pyrimethamine

Chloroquine-resistant falciparum malaria in Africa and parts of Asia may still respond to single-dose therapy with SP (Fansidar™). SP should not be used for therapy of falciparum malaria acquired in South America and Southeast Asia due to high rates of resistance. Furthermore, escalating resistance to Fansidar™ in parts of sub-Saharan Africa is limiting its use as sole or standby therapy for falciparum malaria, particularly for nonimmune individuals and travellers.

2.3.2. Mefloquine

Mefloquine alone (15 mg/kg) has low cure rates in regions of Thailand but it remains efficacious in much of Africa and South America (>90% efficacy) (Kain, 1996). When studied in 94 Brazilian patients with falciparum malaria, mefloquine (1,000 mg single dose) had a reported cure rate of 99% (95% Confidence Interval, CI 94.2–99.7%) (Cerutti et al., 1999). Higher doses of mefloquine (25 mg/kg as a divided dose) remain efficacious in Southeast Asia except on the Thai–Myanmar and Thai–Cambodian borders. However, high-dose mefloquine is poorly tolerated with significant side effects including nausea, vomiting, and gastrointestinal discomfort.

2.3.3. Halofantrine

Although effective against chloroquine-resistant malaria, halofantrine's cardiotoxicity has limited its use as a therapeutic agent. A recent in vitro electrophysiologic study confirmed that halofantrine prolonged the QT interval by blocking the delayed rectifier potassium channel in animal myocytes. Therefore halofantrine, like quinidine and class III antiarrhythmics, is able to prolong repolarization, and high plasma levels should be avoided. There is little if any indication to use halofantrine as a first line antimalarial. Halofantrine should not be used concurrently with mefloquine and other drugs known to affect cardiac conduction, nor in anyone with congenital or acquired conduction cardiac abnormalities. Continuous cardiac monitoring is recommended during its use (Wesche et al., 2000; WHO, 2000).

2.3.4. Atovaquone plus Proguanil

The combination of AP has been shown to be highly efficacious in the treatment of falciparum malaria in clinical trials and has successfully cured MDR falciparum malaria after failure of other antimalarial regimens. In 10 open-label clinical trials, treatment of uncomplicated falciparum malaria with 1,000 mg atovoquone and 400 mg proguanil hydrochloride once daily for three days achieved cure in 514 of 521 (99%) evaluated patients (Kremser et al., 1999). In several of these trials, AP was compared to other antimalarial drugs and cure rates with AP were found to be significantly higher than with chloroquine, mefloquine, amodiaquine, or a combination of chloroquine and SP. AP therapy has been demonstrated to be effective in semi-immune populations in Africa and also in Thai patients with little or no immunity and in nonimmune travellers returning to France. AP is well tolerated with few reported treatment-limiting adverse events. Interestingly, a recent study revealed that AP may significantly reduce the infectivity of *P. falciparum*-infected individuals compared to chloroquine, suggesting that AP may inhibit infectivity of gametocytes to mosquitoes (Enosse et al., 2000).

2.3.5. Artemisinin Derivatives

The artemisinin derivatives are the most rapidly acting of all antimalarial drugs. These drugs are not currently registered or available in many Western countries, but they have been used extensively for the treatment of drug-resistant falciparum malaria in China, Southeast Asia, and more recently in Africa. Five compounds have been used: the parent, artemisinin, and four more active derivatives (two water soluble hemisuccinates, artesunate, and artelinate, and two oil-soluble ethers, artemether, and arteether), which are metabolized to a biologically active metabolite, dihydroartemisinin (White, 1996, 1998). When used alone, the artemisinin derivatives need to be given for at least 5–7 days in order to prevent recurrent infections. However, artemisinins are preferably used in combination with other antimalarial agents including mefloquine, SP, doxycycline, or lumefantrine (benflumetol), in order to increase cure rates, shorten the duration of therapy, and lower gametocyte carriage and therefore transmission rates (McIntosh and Olliaro, 2000; White et al., 1999). A well-studied and highly efficacious regimen for treating uncomplicated MDR falciparum malaria in Southeast Asia, is 3 days of oral artesunate (4 mg/kg/day for 3 days) plus mefloquine (25 mg/kg given as a divided dose 8–24 hr apart). Efficacy rates of 94% in adults were reported in 63-day follow-up studies in Thailand (Looareesuwan et al., 1997; Na-Bangchang et al., 1999). A double blind, randomized trial studied the efficacy of artesunate plus SP for uncomplicated falciparum malaria in 600 Gambian children (von Seidlein et al., 2000). Treatment failure rates at day 14 were 3.1% in the one-dose SP alone group, 3.7% in the one-dose SP plus artesunate group and 1.6% in the one-dose SP plus 3-dose artesunate group ($p = 0.048$). Combination therapy with artemisinin derivatives should delay the emergence of resistance since the artemisinin derivative effectively and rapidly eliminates most of the parasite biomass, leaving only a small residual number of parasites to be eradicated by the second agent. This reduces the selective pressure for the development of resistance and reduces the number of gametocytes and therefore transmission of drug-resistant parasites. However, some controversy exists regarding the potential neurotoxicity of these drugs, particularly the lipid-soluble derivatives (Genovese et al., 1998; van Vugt et al., 2000; White, 2000). In animal studies using lipid soluble derivatives at elevated doses, brainstem nuclei damage was consistently observed (Genovese et al., 1998). However, in large clinical trials involving >7,000 patients who underwent detailed neurologic evaluations, no evidence of CNS dysfunction following treatment with artemisinin derivatives was identified (White, 2000). In recent studies, rectal suppositories of artemisinin derivatives have proved as effective as parental administration providing a useful treatment strategy for the treatment of severe malaria in rural locations (Sabchareon et al., 1998; White, 2000). In a number of large comparative trials of patients with severe falciparum malaria, treatment with artemisinin derivatives accelerated parasite clearance but slightly prolonged recovery from coma, and did not reduce mortality significantly in comparison with quinine. These results indicate that artemisinins are an acceptable and well-tolerated alternative to quinine in severe malaria but that they do not appear to improve outcome (Hien et al., 1996; van Hensbroek et al., 1996).

3. DRUG-RESISTANT VIVAX MALARIA

3.1. Epidemiology

The global impact of *P. vivax* malaria is often overshadowed by the lethality of *P. falciparum* malaria. Although rarely fatal, *P. vivax* is nonetheless a serious public health problem with a profound impact on quality of life and economic productivity. It is the second most common cause of malaria worldwide and the annual rates of *P. vivax* cases range from 75 to 90 million (Nomura et al., 2001). Chloroquine has been the treatment of choice for eliminating the blood stages of *P. vivax* for over 40 years, but resistance has been an increasing problem since it was first recognised in Oceania in 1989 (Rieckmann et al., 1989). Despite similar exposure of *P. vivax* and *P. falciparum* malaria to chloroquine over the last 50 years, the emergence of chloroquine resistance in *P. vivax* occurred three decades after that in *P. falciparum* (Harinasuta et al., 1965; Young & Moore, 1961). Chloroquine-resistant *P. vivax* was first reported in Papua New Guinea in 1989 (Rieckmann et al., 1989) and Indonesia in 1991 (Baird et al., 1991; Schwartz et al., 1991). The recognized geographic distribution of chloroquine-resistant *P. vivax* has since extended to India (Dua et al., 1996; Garg et al., 1995; Singh, 2000), Myanmar (Marlar-Than et al., 1995; Myat-Phone-Kyaw, et al., 1993), and in the western hemisphere to Guyana (Phillips et al., 1996), Colombia (Soto et al., 2001), and Brazil (Alecrim et al., 1999; Garavelli & Corti, 1992).

Field trials in Papua New Guinea and Papua (formerly Irian Jaya) revealed recrudescent rates of 22% for *P. vivax*-infected patients after treatment with standard courses of chloroquine (Murphy et al., 1993). Baird et al. (1995, 1996) found even higher failure rates in the same area with 28-day cumulative failure rates of 64%. Chloroquine resistance was also identified in 14% of infections acquired off the coast of northwestern Sumatra (Baird et al., 1996), and in up to 52% of infections in West Kalimantan and North Sulawesi (Fryauff et al., 1995, 1998). Chloroquine monotherapy can no longer be relied upon for prophylaxis or treatment of blood stage vivax malaria acquired in New Guinea, Oceania, and much of Indonesia.

Relapse of *P. vivax* malaria after standard courses of primaquine (15 mg base/day for 14 days) is also commonly reported from Papua New Guinea, Papua, Thailand and other parts of Southeast Asia and Oceania (failure rates approximately 35%), and less commonly from India and Colombia. Smoak et al. (1997) reported high relapse rates in American soldiers deployed to Somalia. Of 60 *P. vivax*-infected soldiers treated with standard doses of chloroquine and primaquine (15 mg base/day for 14 days), 26 relapsed for a failure rate of 43%. Eight soldiers had a second relapse following another course of chloroquine plus primaquine therapy including three who completed a high-dose regimen (30 mg base/day × 14 days).

3.2. Mechanism of Resistance

The delay in emergence of chloroquine resistance in *P. vivax* compared to *P. falciparum* combined with the different recurrence profile of chloroquine-resistant *P. vivax*, suggests that the mechanism of resistance differs between these two species. Nomura et al. (2001) assessed whether mutations in *pfcrt* associated with chloroquine-resistance in *P. falciparum*, were also associated with chloroquine resistance in other malaria species. To identify *pfcrt* orthologues in *P. vivax, Plasmodium knowlesi, Plasmodium berghei*, and *Dictyostelium discoideum*, codon-adjusted primers were used to amplify the corresponding genes from each species. Striking conservation in the amino acid sequence and structure was found between the homologues and PfCRT protein. However, the authors found no codon mutations in the *P. vivax* orthologue, *pvcg10*, associated with chloroquine-resistance in three resistant monkey adapted *P. vivax* isolates nor five chloroquine-resistant *P. vivax* patient isolates from Papua New Guinea. The authors concluded that the molecular mechanisms that confer chloroquine resistance in *P. vivax* differ from those found in *P. falciparum*.

3.3. Management

Few studies have examined alternative drugs for the treatment of vivax malaria. Quinine was found to be effective but was often required in higher doses or combined with doxycycline to cure strains from Papua New Guinea (Murphy et al., 1993). Based on the observation that primaquine has blood stage antimalarial activity against *P. vivax*, Baird et al. (1995) examined the efficacy of halofantrine versus chloroquine plus high-dose primaquine for the treatment of chloroquine-resistant *P. vivax* in Irian Jaya. Halofantrine was found to be highly efficacious with a 28-day cure rate of 94%. Standard doses of chloroquine (25 mg/kg) combined with high doses of primaquine, either 2.5 mg/kg over 48 hr or 10 mg/kg over 28 days, had 28-day cure rates of 85% compared with 22% for chloroquine alone. In Thailand, four treatment regimens were assessed in *P. vivax*-infected patients from the Thailand–Myanmar border: (1) Fansidar alone (3 tablets); (2) Fansidar (3 tablets) and then primaquine (30 mg base/day for 14 days); (3) primaquine (30 mg base/day for 14 days); and (4) artesunate (200 mg once a day for 3 days) and then primaquine (30 mg base/day for 14 days) (Wilairatana et al., 1999). The 28-day cure rates were 40%, 100%, 100%, and 100% for regimens 1, 2, 3, and 4, respectively. Artesunate plus primaquine cleared the parasitemia faster than the other regimens. Fansidar™ alone was found to be ineffective for the treatment of *P. vivax*. Other potential treatment options include mefloquine (15 mg/kg), AP plus primaquine, and artemether plus lumefantrine.

The timing of recurrent *P. vivax* parasitemia can be informative in distinguishing recrudescence (treatment failure) from relapse. If the recurrence occurs within 28 days of supervised treatment, then *P. vivax* is most likely resistant to chloroquine (Baird et al., 1997). If the recurrence occurs more than 28 days after treatment, then relapse is unlikely (Baird et al., 1997).

Patients who relapse following a standard course of primaquine should receive two times the standard dose (30 mg base/day for 14 days) or a total dose of 6 mg/kg of primaquine to prevent further relapse (Kain, 1996).

4. MALARIA PREVENTION

4.1. Malarial Control

The WHO suggests that there are three essential elements of malaria control and prevention (WHO, 1995). The first element is the selective application of vector control by the reduction of the numbers of vector mosquitoes either by eliminating or reducing mosquito breeding sites; destroying larval, pupal, and adult mosquitoes; and reducing human–mosquito contact. The second element consists of early diagnosis and effective prompt treatment of malarial disease, which also reduces a source of parasites for infection of mosquitoes as well as reducing morbidity and mortality. The third element is early detection or forecasting of epidemics and rapid application of control measures.

Chemicals are the mainstay of mosquito control and multiple products are used. Dichlorodiphenyltrichloroethane (DDT), an organochlorine, is the predominant product used. The rationale for its use for indoor spraying is that it remains active on the sprayed surface for weeks or even months and kills or at least repels the female mosquito (WHO, 1995). The problem of DDT resistance has been reported and has increased with time and use, from two species of mosquito being resistant to DDT in 1946 to 55 or more species being resistant to one or more insecticides 50 years later (Bruce-Chwatt, 1993; WHO, 1995). DDT has likely contributed to saving hundreds of thousands of lives, but because of the over-emphasized neurotoxicity, 120 countries are currently negotiating a treaty to ban the production and use of DDT by 2007 (Phillips, 2001).

Protection of the individual from mosquitoes can be achieved through a number of personal protection methods including mosquito repellents, protective clothing, insect screens, improvement of the design and construction of dwellings, and bed nets. One of the most encouraging recent developments in malaria control has been the finding that impregnation of bed nets and curtains with insecticides can significantly reduce malaria-associated morbidity and mortality (Langeler et al., 1997). Choi et al. (1995) concluded that studies in Asia and Africa in different epidemiological situations found that insecticide-impregnated bed nets reduce the incidence of clinical attacks by ~50%. A trial in Gambia showed that insecticide-impregnated bed nets using permethrin reduced overall mortality by >50% (Alonso et al., 1991). Further trials in other countries after the success in Gambia did not show such a beneficial effect on mortality rates, but nonetheless, there was a reduction in overall child mortality of 17–33% (Snow et al., 1996). The long-term impact of bed net programs is a matter of debate (Trape & Rogier, 1996). The reduced level

of exposure through bed net intervention may have an adverse effect on the natural acquisition of immunity, and there are concerns that any beneficial outcome may be transitory
in areas of high transmission (Trape & Rogier, 1996).

4.2. Chemoprophylaxis

Antimalarial drugs are selected based on individual risk assessment (as discussed
below) and drug-resistance patterns (Figure 9.1, Table 9.1). In addition, the reader is
referred to detailed on-line sources of country specific malaria risk and additional data on
drug doses and adverse events (www.cdc.gov See *Health information for international
travel 2001–2002*; www.who.int/ith/ See *International travel and health*).

The use of antimalarial drugs and their potential adverse effects must be weighed
against the risk of acquiring malaria. Estimating a traveller's risk is based on a detailed
travel itinerary and specific risk behaviors of the traveller. The risk of acquiring malaria
will vary according to the geographic area visited (e.g., Africa vs. Southeast Asia), the

Table 9.1

Malaria Chemoprophylactic Regimens for At Risk Individuals[a]
According to Zones of Drug-Resistance

Zone	Drug(s) of choice[b]	Alternatives
No chloroquine resistance	Chloroquine	Mefloquine, doxycycline, or atovaquone/proguanil (AP)
Chloroquine resistance	Mefloquine or AP or Doxycycline	1st choice: primaquine[c] 2nd choice: chloroquine plus proguanil[d]
Chloroquine & Mefloquine resistance	Doxycycline	

Adult doses	
Chloroquine phosphate	300 mg (base) weekly
Mefloquine	250 mg (salt in the USA; base elsewhere) weekly
AP	One tablet daily (250 mg/100 mg)
Doxycycline	100 mg daily
Primaquine	30 mg (base) daily[c]
Proguanil	200 mg daily

[a] Protection from mosquito bites (insecticide-treated bed nets, N,N-diethyl-m-toluamide now called
N,N-diethyl-3-methylbenzamide, (DEET)-based insect repellents, etc.) is the first line of defence
against malaria for *all* travellers. In the Americas and Southeast Asia, chemoprophylaxis is recommended *only* for travellers who will be exposed outdoors during evening or night time in rural areas.
[b] Chloroquine and mefloquine are to be taken once weekly, beginning one week before entering the
malarial area, during the stay and for 4 weeks after leaving. Doxycycline and proguanil are taken
daily, starting 1 day before entering malarial areas, during the stay and for 4 weeks after departure.
AP and primaquine are taken once daily, starting one day before entering the malarial area, during
the stay and may be discontinued 7 days after leaving the endemic area.
[c] Contraindicated in G6PD (glucose-6-phosphate dehydrogenase) deficiency and during pregnancy.
Not presently licensed for this use. Must perform a G6PD level before prescribing.
[d] Chloroquine plus proguanil is less efficacious than mefloquine, doxycycline, or AP in these areas.

travel destination within different geographic areas (e.g., urban vs. rural travel), type of accommodation (camping vs. well-screened or air conditioned), duration of stay (1 week business travel vs. 3 month overland trek), time of travel (high or low transmission season), elevation of destination (transmission is rare above 2000 meters), and efficacy of and compliance with preventive measures used (e.g., treated bed nets, chemoprophylactic drugs).

It is important to note that most travellers to low risk areas such as urban areas and tourist resorts of Southeast Asia do not require antimalarial drugs since the risk of infection is minimal. Travellers should be informed that personal protection measures and antimalarials will markedly decrease the risk of contracting malaria. However, *these interventions do not guarantee complete protection. The most important factors that determine outcome are early diagnosis and appropriate therapy. Travellers and health-care providers alike must consider and urgently rule out malaria in any febrile illness that occurs during or after travel to a malaria-endemic area.*

4.2.1. Areas with Chloroquine-Sensitive P. falciparum *Malaria*

Chloroquine should only be used as chemoprophylaxis for at-risk individuals travelling to areas, which are unequivocally chloroquine-sensitive (e.g., North Africa, Central America north of the Panama Canal, Haiti, Dominican Republic, or the Middle East) (Kain et al., 2001). Figure 9.1 and Table 9.1 summarize the drug-resistant malaria areas.

4.2.2. Areas with Chloroquine-Resistant P. falciparum *Malaria*

The choice of chemoprophylaxis agent for most travellers at risk of chloroquine-resistant falciparum malaria has traditionally been between mefloquine, doxycycline, or, less optimally, chloroquine plus proguanil. The advantages and disadvantages of these agents have recently been reviewed (Kain, 1999; Kain et al., 2001; Schlagenhauf, 1999). Mefloquine and doxycycline are both highly efficacious (protective efficacy >90%) against chloroquine-resistant malaria. Mefloquine-resistant malaria exists on the Thai–Myanmar and Thai–Cambodian border areas; doxycycline is the agent of choice for at risk travellers to these areas. A number of failures and several deaths have been reported in travellers to Africa taking chloroquine/proguanil combinations and this regimen is no longer recommended.

Malarone™, the combination of AP is a new option for malaria prophylaxis in chloroquine-resistant areas (Shapiro et al., 1999). Volunteer challenge studies have established that AP has causal prophylactic activity (i.e., activity against the liver stage parasite) (Berman et al., 2001). As a causal chemoprophylactic agent, travellers would need to take AP daily during periods of exposure and for only 1 week after departure from malaria-endemic areas. This avoids the requirement to complete 4 weeks of prophylaxis following exposure (a common reason for nonadherence) and makes this agent particularly attractive for travellers with short or repeated exposures in high-risk areas.

Three double-blind, randomized, placebo-controlled chemoprophylaxis trials have been conducted in semi-immune residents in Kenya, Zambia, and Gabon (Lell et al., 1998; Shanks et al., 1998; Sukwa et al., 1999). The overall efficacy for preventing malaria in these trials was 98% (95% CI, 91.9–99.9%). The most commonly reported adverse events attributed to the study drug were headache, abdominal pain, dyspepsia, and diarrhea. However, of note, all adverse events occurred with similar frequency in subjects treated with placebo or AP and there were no serious adverse events.

Studies among nonimmune travellers have recently been completed. In randomized, double-blind studies, ~2,000 nonimmune subjects travelling to a malaria-endemic area received either AP, daily for 1–2 days before travel until 7 days after travel, mefloquine, or chloroquine/proguanil, from 1 to 3 weeks before travel until 4 weeks after travel (Hogh et al., 2000, Overbosch et al., 2001). No confirmed diagnosis of malaria occurred with either AP or mefloquine but 3 documented cases of falciparum malaria occurred in travellers using chloroquine/proguanil. All drugs were well tolerated but AP was significantly better tolerated than either mefloquine or chloroquine/proguanil in these studies. Drug-related discontinuation rates for AP versus mefloquine were 1.2% versus 5% ($p = 0.001$) and for AP versus chloroquine/proguanil were 0.2% versus 2% ($p = 0.015$). In a comparative trial of AP versus doxycycline in 175 Australian military participants, AP was significantly better tolerated with a lower rate of gastrointestinal (29% vs. 53%) adverse events (Edstein et al., 2001). Taken together, the studies to date indicate that AP is a well tolerated and efficacious chemoprophylactic regimen for *P. falciparum*. Additional data are required to establish the efficacy against non-falciparum malaria but these trials are underway. Preliminary data from a randomized-controlled trial in nonimmune transmigrants in Papua, indicate a protective efficacy of 84% (95% CI, 45–95%) against *P. vivax* and 96% (95% CI, 71–99%) against *P. falciparum* (Baird, personal communication).

Primaquine is an 8-aminoquinoline that has activity against both blood and tissue (liver) stages of malaria and therefore can eliminate infections that are developing in the liver (causal prophylaxis). Randomized-controlled trials of primaquine as a prophylactic agent (0.5 mg/kg base/day; adult dose 30 mg base/day) in nonimmune adults who were not G6PD-deficient, have demonstrated a protective efficacy of 85–95% against both *P. falciparum* and *P. vivax* infections (Fryauff et al., 1995; Shanks et al., 2001; Soto et al., 1998, 1999). However, primaquine it is not currently licensed for this indication. Like AP, travellers would be required to take primaquine only during periods of exposure and for 1 week after departure from malaria-endemic areas. Primaquine is generally well tolerated but may cause nausea and abdominal pain, which can be decreased by taking the drug with food (CATMAT, 2000). More importantly, primaquine may cause oxidant-induced hemolytic anemia with methemogloginemia, particularly in individuals with G6PD deficiency and is therefore contraindicated in those individuals and during pregnancy. If the risk of *P. vivax* infection is thought to be particularly high (e.g., long term ex-patriots, soldiers, etc.), consideration may be given to the use of primaquine ("terminal" prophylaxis) to eliminate latent hepatic parasites; this is given at the conclusion of the standard post-travel chemoprophylaxis regimen.

5. FUTURE DIRECTION

5.1. New Agents

5.1.1. Lumefantrine plus Artemether

Although few pharmaceutical companies are currently developing new antimalarials, a couple of promising agents have been studied in phase I through III trials. Lumefantrine (formerly benflumetol) is a new drug developed in China with a mode of action similar to quinoline antimalarials. It has a slow onset of action and has been formulated in combination with artemether; which has a rapid onset of action but is associated with recurrent infections unless used for extended periods as monotherapy. This combination (Raimet™/Coartem™, formerly CGP 56697) should permit rapid onset of action and high cure rates with short course therapy. Initially a four-dose regimen given over 3 days of oral artemether plus lumefantrine were compared to artesunate plus mefloquine in Thai adults and Gambian children. In Thailand, parasite clearance and defervescence times were similar between the treatment arms but side-effects were significantly less in the CGP 56697 treatment group. The efficacy of CGP 56697 at 63 days was 81% versus 94% for artesunate–mefloquine. When CGP 56697 was compared to halofantrine in a double-blinded trial, CGP 56697 was superior with respect to parasite clearance time (32 vs. 48 hr, $p < 0.001$) and parasite reduction at 24 hr (99.7% vs. 89.6%, $p < 0.001$) (van Agtmael et al., 1999). However, the 28-day cure rate was 82% for CGP 56697 and 100% for halofantrine. In another randomized trial of CGP 56697 compared to mefloquine in Thai adults, the 28-day cure rate with CGP 56697 was 69.3% compared to 82.4% for mefloquine ($p < 0.001$) (Looareesuwan et al., 1999). Similar results were found in a randomized controlled trial of CGP 56697 versus SP (von Seidlein et al., 1998). These studies indicate that higher doses will likely be required to improve the cure rate. A number of studies have now examined six-dose schedules. Six-dose regimens gave adjusted 28-day cure rates of 96.9% and 99.12% compared with 83.3% for the four-dose regimen (van Vugt et al., 1999). The six-dose regimen was recently compared to artesunate plus mefloquine against MDR falciparum malaria in a randomized trial in Thailand. The 28-day cure rates for artemether–lumefantrine were 95.5% (95% CI, 91.7–97.9%) versus 100% (95% CI, 94.5–100%) for artesunate–mefloquine (Lefevre et al., 2001). Collectively these studies indicate that combination lumefantrine–artemether is an efficacious and well-tolerated regimen for MDR malaria.

5.2.2. Tafenaquine

Another promising new antimalarial agent is tafenoquine, a long-acting primaquine analogue (elimination half-life of 14–28 days vs. 4–6 hr for primaquine) (Brueckner et al., 1998, Shanks et al., 2001). Tafenoquine has activity against liver, blood, and transmission stages of malaria. In vitro and in vivo animal models have shown that tafenoquine is more potent and less toxic than primaquine. A phase I clinical study demonstrated that tafenoquine was well tolerated, with gastrointestinal disturbances as possible side effects especially at higher drug doses (Brueckner et al., 1998). In a human challenge model, a single oral dose administered 1 day prior to challenge, successfully protected 3 of 4 subjects. The 4th subject developed parasitemia on day 31 (vs. development of parasitemia on day 10 for the 2 placebo recipients). Phase III studies are completed or ongoing in Kenya, Thailand, Gabon, Bougainville, Irian Jaya, and Ghana (Brueckner et al., 1998; Shanks et al., 2001; Walsh et al., 1999). Early reports from these trials indicate that weekly dosage of tafenoquine (200 or 400 mg base) is protective against P. falciparum (efficacy >90%). A loading dosage of tafenaquine alone (200 mg base for 3 days) provided 100% protection for up to 10 weeks (Lell et al., 2000). Tafenoquine also has potential as a transmission-blocking agent. In the trials to date, tafenoquine was well tolerated when given to adults with normal G6PD activity. However, significant hemolysis can occur in G6PD-deficient subjects and testing is essential before use (Brueckner et al., 1998; Shanks et al., 1999, 2001).

6. CONCLUSION

Drug-resistant malaria is a major public health problem worldwide, however substantial progress has been made in the last decade in elucidating the underlying mechanisms of drug action and resistance. This knowledge should facilitate the rationale design of new effective and well-tolerated antimalarial drugs. Combination therapies, particularly regimens that include the rapid-acting artemisinin derivatives, are important new strategies to prevent drug resistance, increase treatment efficacy, and lower transmission rates in malaria-endemic areas (White et al., 1996). This strategy combined with other cost-effective interventions such as the implementation of insecticide impregnated bed nets, should substantially reduce malaria-associated morbidity and mortality in the short term, a fundamental objective of the Roll Back Malaria initiative of the WHO. Finally, the sequencing of the *Plasmodium* and human genomes should contribute substantially to our understanding of the pathophysiology of severe and fatal malaria and permit the identification of novel therapeutic strategies and new plasmodial targets for drug and vaccine development (Carucci, 2001; Fletcher, 1998; Hoffman et al., 1997, 1998; Riley, 1995).

References

Alecrim, M. G., Alecrim, W., & Macedo, V. (1999). *Plasmodium vivax* resistance to chloroquine (R2) and mefloquine (R3) in Brazilian Amazon region. *Rev Soc Bras Med Trop, 32*, 67–68.

Alonso, P. L., Lindsay, S. W., Armstrong, J. R., Conteh, M., Hill, A. G., David, P. H., Fegan, G., de Francisco, A., Hall, A. J., & Shenton, F. C. (1991). The effect of insecticide-treated bed nets on mortality of Gambian children. *Lancet, 337*, 1499–1502.

Awad-el-Kariem, F. M., Miles, M. A., & Warhurst, D. C. (1992). Chloroquine-resistant *Plasmodium falciparum* isolates from the Sudan lack two mutations in the *pfmdr1* gene thought to be associated with chloroquine resistance. *Trans R Soc Trop Med Hyg, 86*, 587–589.

Babiker, H. A., Pringle, S. J., Abdel-Muhsin, A., Mackinnon, M., Hunt, P., & Walliker, D. (2001). High-level chloroquine resistance in Sudanese isolates of *Plasmodium falciparum* is associated with mutations in the chloroquine resistance transporter gene *pfcrt* and the multidrug resistance gene *pfmdr1*. *J Infect Dis, 183*, 1535–1538.

Baird, J. K., Basri, H., Jones, T. R., Purnomo, Bangs, M. J., & Ritonga, A. (1991). Resistance to antimalarials by *Plasmodium falciparum* in Arso PIR, Irian Jaya, Indonesia. *Amer J Trop Med Hyg, 44*, 640–644.

Baird, J. K., Basri, H., Purnomo, Bangs, M. J., Subianto, B., Patchen, L. C., & Hoffman, S. L. (1991). Resistance to chloroquine by *Plasmodium vivax* in Irian Jaya, Indonesia. *Amer J Trop Med Hyg, 44*, 547–552.

Baird, J. K., Basri, H., Subianto, B., Fryauff, D. J., McElroy, P. D., Leksana, B., Richie, T. L., Masbar, S., Wignall, F. S., & Hoffman, S. L. (1995). Treatment of chloroquine-resistant *Plasmodium vivax* with chloroquine and primaquine or halofantrine. *J Infect Dis, 171*, 1678–1682.

Baird, J. K., Leksana, B., Masbar, S., Fryauff, D. J., Sutanihardja, M. A., Suradi, Wignall, F. S., & Hoffman, S. L. (1997). Diagnosis of resistance to chloroquine by *Plasmodium vivax*: Timing of recurrence and whole blood chloroquine levels. *Amer J Trop Med Hyg, 56*, 621–626.

Baird, J. K., Sustriayu, Nalim, M. F., Basri, H., Masbar, S., Leksana, B., Tjitra, E., Dewi, R. M., Khairani, M., & Wignall, F. S. (1996). Survey of resistance to chloroquine by *Plasmodium vivax* in Indonesia. *Trans R Soc Trop Med Hyg, 90*, 409–411.

Baird, J. K., Wiady, I., Fryauff, D. J., Sutanihardja, M. A., Leksana, B., Widjaya, H., Kysdarmanto, & Subianto, B. (1997). In vivo resistance to chloroquine by *Plasmodium vivax* and *Plasmodium falciparum* at Nabire, Irian Jaya, Indonesia. *Amer J Trop Med Hyg, 56*, 627–631.

Basco, L. K., Le Bras, J., Rhoades, Z., & Wilson, C. M. (1995). Analysis of pfmdr1 and drug susceptibility in fresh isolates of *Plasmodium falciparum* from subsaharan Africa. *Mol Biochem Parasitol, 74*, 157–166.

Basco, L. K., Tahar, R., Keundjian, A., & Ringwald, P. (2000). Sequence variations in the genes encoding dihydropteroate synthase and dihydrofolate reductase and clinical response to sulfadoxine–pyrimethamine in patients with acute uncomplicated falciparum malaria. *J Infect Dis, 182*, 624–628.

Berman, J. D., Nielson, R., Chulay, J. D., Dowler, M., Kain, K. C., Kester, K. E., Williams, J., Whelen, A. C., & Shmuklarsky, M. J. (2001). Causal prophylactic efficacy of atovaquone–progunail (Malarone) in a human challenge model. *Trans Roy Soc Trop Med Hyg, 95*, 429–432.

Bjorkman, A., & Phillips-Howard, P. A. (1990). The epidemiology of drug-resistant malaria. *Trans R Soc Trop Med Hyg, 84*, 177–180.

Brasseur, P., Kouamouo, J., Moyou, R. S., & Druilhe, P. (1990). Emergence of mefloquine-resistant malaria in Africa without drug pressure. *Lancet, 336*, 59.

Breman, J. G., & Campbell, C. C. (1988). Combating severe malaria in African children. *Bull World Health Organ, 66*, 611–620.

Brooks, D. R., Wang, P., Read, M., Watkins, W. M., Sims, P. F., & Hyde, J. E. (1994). Sequence variation of the hydroxymethyldihydropterin pyrophosphokinase: Dihydropteroate synthase gene in lines of the human malaria parasite, *Plasmodium falciparum*, with differing resistance to sulfadoxine. *Eur J Biochem, 224*, 397–405.

Bruce-Chwatt, L. (1993). In H. M. Gillies and D. A. Warrall (Eds.), *Essential malariology*. London, United Kingdom: Edward Arnold.

Brueckner, R. P., Coster, T., Wesche, D. L., Shmuklarsky, M., & Schuster, B. G. (1998). Prophylaxis of *Plasmodium falciparum* infection in a human challenge model with WR 238605, a new 8-aminoquinoline antimalarial. *Antimicrob Agents Chemother, 42*, 1293–1294.

Brueckner, R. P., Lasseter, K. C., Lin, E. T., & Schuster, B. G. (1998). First-time-in-humans safety and pharmacokinetics of WR 238605, a new antimalarial. *Amer J Trop Med Hyg, 58*, 645–649.

Campbell, C. C. (1997). Malaria: An emerging and re-emerging global plague. *FEMS Immunol Med Microbiol, 18*, 325–331.

Carucci, D. J. (2001). Genomic tools for gene and protein discovery in malaria: Toward new vaccines. *Vaccine, 19*, 2315–2318.

Centers for Disease Control and Prevention (2001). Health information for international travel 2001–2002. Atlanta, GA: DHHS.

Cerutti, Jr., C., Durlacher, R. R., de Alencar, F. E., Segurado, A. A., & Pang, L. W. (1999). In vivo efficacy of mefloquine for the treatment of falciparum malaria in Brazil. *J Infect Dis, 180*, 2077–2080.

Chaiyaroj, S. C., Buranakiti A., Angkasekwinai, P., Looressuwan, S., & Cowman, A. F. (1999). Analysis of mefloquine resistance and amplification of *pfmdr1* in multidrug-resistant *Plasmodium falciparum* isolates from Thailand. *Amer J Trop Med Hyg, 61*, 78078–78083.

Choi, H. W., Breman, J. G., Teutsch, S. M., Liu, S., Hightower, A. W., & Sexton, J. D. (1995). The effectiveness of insecticide-impregnated bed nets in reducing cases of malaria infection: A meta-analysis of published results. *Amer J Trop Med Hyg, 52*, 377–382.

Chou, A. C., Chevli, R., & Fitch, C. D. (1980). Ferriprotoporphyrin IX fulfills the criteria for identification as the chloroquine receptor of malaria parasites. *Biochemistry, 19*, 1543–1549.

Chou, A. C., & Fitch, C. D. (1980). Hemolysis of mouse erythrocytes by ferriprotoporphyrin IX and
chloroquine. Chemotherapeutic implications. *J Clin Invest, 66(4)*, 856–858.

Chou, A. C., & Fitch, C. D. (1981). Mechanism of hemolysis induced by ferriprotoporphyrin IX.
J Clin Invest, 68, 672–677.

Committee to advise on tropical medicine and travel (CATMAT). (2000). Canadian recommendations for the prevention and treatment of malaria among international travellers. Ottawa, ON:
Laboratory Centre for Disease Control, Health Canada.

Cortese, J. F., & Plowe, C. V. (1998). Antifolate resistance due to new and known *Plasmodium
falciparum* dihydrofolate reductase mutations expressed in yeast. *Mol Biochem Parasitol, 94*,
205–214.

Cowman, A. F. (1995). Mechanisms of drug resistance in malaria. *Aust N Z J Med, 25(6)*, 837–844.

Djimde, A., Doumbo, O. K., Cortese, J. F., Kayentao, K., Doumbo, S., Diourte, Y., Dicko, A., Su, X. Z.,
Nomura, T., Fidock, D. A., Wellems, T. E., Plowe, C. V., & Coulibaly, D. (2001). A molecular
marker for chloroquine-resistant falciparum malaria. *N Engl J Med, 344*, 257–263.

Dorsey, G., Kamya, M. R., Singh, A., & Rosenthal, P. J. (2001). Polymorphisms in the *Plasmodium
falciparum pfcrt* and *pfmdr-1* genes and clinical response to chloroquine in Kampala, Uganda.
J Infect Dis, 183, 1417–1420.

Dua, V. K., Kar, P. K., & Sharma, V. P. (1996). Chloroquine resistant *Plasmodium vivax* malaria in
India. *Trop Med Int Health, 1*, 816–819.

Duraisingh, M. T., Roper, C., Walliker, D., & Warhurst, D. C. (2000). Increased sensitivity to the
antimalarials mefloquine and artemisinin is conferred by mutations in the *pfmdr1* gene of
Plasmodium falciparum. *Mol Microbiol, 36*, 955–961.

Durand, R., Gabbett, E., Di Piazza, J. P., Delabre, J. F., & Le Bras, J. (1999). Analysis of kappa and
omega repeats of the cg2 gene and chloroquine susceptibility in isolates of *Plasmodium falciparum* from sub-Saharan Africa. *Mol Biochem Parasitol, 101*, 185–197.

Edstein, M. D., Walsh, D. S., Eamsila, C., Sasiprapha, T., Nasveld, P. E., Kitchener, S., &
Rieckmann, K. H. (2001). Malaria prophylaxis/radical cure: Recent experiences of the Australian
Defence Force. *Med Trop (Mars), 61*, 56–58.

Enosse, S., Butcher, G. A., Margos, G., Mendoza, J., Sinden, R. E., & Hogh, B. (2000). The mosquito transmission of malaria: The effect of atovaquone–proguanil (Malarone™) and chloroquine.
Trans R Soc Trop Med Hyg, 94, 77–82.

Fidock, D. A., Nomura, T., Talley, A. K., Cooper, R. A., Dzekunov, S. M., Ferdig, M. T., Ursos, L. M.,
Sidhu, A. B., Naude, B., Deitsch, K. W., Su, X. Z., Wootton, J. C., Roepe, P. D., & Wellems, T. E.
(2000). Mutations in the *P. falciparum* digestive vacuole transmembrane protein PfCRT and evidence for their role in chloroquine resistance. *Mol Cell, 6*, 861–871.

Fitch, C. D., Chevli, R., Kanjananggulpan, P., Dutta, P., Chevli, K., & Chou, A. C. (1983).
Intracellular ferriprotoporphyrin IX is a lytic agent. *Blood, 62*, 1165–1168.

Fletcher, C. (1998). The *Plasmodium falciparum* genome project. *Parasitol Today, 14*, 342–344.

Foote, S. J., & Cowman, A. F. (1994). The mode of action and the mechanism of resistance to
antimalarial drugs. *Acta Trop, 56*, 157–171.

Foote, S. J., Kyle, D. E., Martin, R. K., Oduola, A. M., Forsyth, K., Kemp, D. J., & Cowman, A. F.
(1990). Several alleles of the multidrug-resistance gene are closely linked to chloroquine resistance in *Plasmodium falciparum*. *Nature, 345*, 255–258.

Foster, S. (1994). Economic prospects for a new antimalarial drug. *Trans R Soc Trop Med Hyg,
88*(Suppl. 1), S55–S56.

Fry, M., & Pudney, M. (1992). Site of action of the antimalarial hydroxynaphthoquinone, 2-[trans-4-
(4'-chlorophenyl)cyclohexyl]-3-hydroxy-1,4-naphthoquinone (566C80). *Biochem Pharmacol, 43*,
1545–1553.

Fryauff, D. J., Baird, J. K., Basri, H., Sumawinata, I., Purnomo, Richie, T. L., Ohrt, C. K., Mouzin, E., Church, C. J., & Richards, A. L. (1995). Randomised placebo-controlled trial of primaquine for prophylaxis of falciparum and vivax malaria. *Lancet, 346,* 1190–1193.

Fryauff, D. J., Tuti, S., Mardi, A., Masbar, S., Patipelohi, R., Leksana, B., Kain, K. C., Richie, T. L., & Baird, J. K. (1998). Chloroquine-resistant *Plasmodium vivax* in transmigrant settlements of West Kalimantan. *Amer J Trop Med Hyg, 59,* 513–518.

Gallup, J. L., & Sachs, J. D. (2001). The economic burden of malaria. *Amer J Trop Med Hyg, 64*(Suppl. 1–2), 85–96.

Garavelli, P. L., & Corti, E. (1992). Chloroquine resistance in *Plasmodium vivax*: The first case in Brazil. *Trans R Soc Trop Med Hyg, 86,* 128.

Garg, M., Gopinathan, N., Bodhe, P., & Kshirsagar, N. A. (1995). Vivax malaria resistant to chloro- quine: Case reports from Bombay. *Trans R Soc Trop Med Hyg, 89,* 656–657.

Gay, F., Bustos, D., & Traore, B. (1997). In vitro response of *Plasmodium falciparum* to atovaquone and correlation with other antimalarials: Comparison between African and Asian strains. *Amer J Trop Med Hyg, 56,* 315–317.

Genovese, R. F., Newman, D. B., Li, Q., Peggin, J. O., & Brewer, T. G. (1998). Dose-dependent brain- stem neuropathology following repeated arteether administration in rats. *Brain Res Bull, 45,* 199–202.

Harinasuta, T., Suntharasamai, P., & Viravan, C. (1965). Chloroquine-resistant falciparum malaria in Thailand. *Lancet, 2,* 657–660.

Haruki, K., Bray, P. G., Ward, S. A., Hommel, M., & Ritchie, G. Y. (1994). Chloroquine resistance of *Plasmodium falciparum*: Further evidence for a lack of association with mutations of the pfmdr1 gene. *Trans R Soc Trop Med Hyg, 88,* 694.

Helsby, N. A., Ward, S. A., Edwards, G., Howells, R. E., & Breckenridge, A. M. (1990). The phar- macokinetics and activation of proguanil in man: Consequences of variability in drug metabolism. *Br J Clin Pharmacol, 30,* 593–598.

Heppner, D. G., & Ballou, W. R. (1998). Malaria in 1998: Advances in diagnosis, drug and vaccine development. *Curr Opinion Inf Dis, 11,* 519–530.

Hien, T. T., Day, N. P. J., & Phu, N. H. (1996). A controlled trial of artemether or quinine in Vietnamese adults with severe malaria. *N Engl J Med, 335,* 76–83.

Hoffman, S. L., Bancroft, W. H., Gottlieb, M., James, S. L., Burroughs, E. C., Stephenson, J. R., & Morgan, M. J. (1997). Funding for malaria genome sequencing. *Nature, 387,* 647.

Hoffman, S. L., Rogers, W. O., Carucci, D. J., & Venter, J. C. (1998). From genomics to vaccines: Malaria as a model system. *Nat Med, 4,* 1351–1353.

Hogh, B., Clarke, P. D., Camus, D., Nothdurft, H. D., Overbosch, D., Gunther, M., Joubert, I., Kain, K. C., Shaw, D., Roskell, N. S., Chulay, J. D., & Malarone International Study Team. (2000). Atovaquone–proguanil versus chloroquine–proguanil for malaria prophylaxis in non-immune travellers: A randomised, double-blind study. Malarone International Study Team. *Lancet, 356,* 1888–1894.

Kain, K. C. (1996). Chemotherapy of drug-resistant malaria. *Can J Infect Dis, 7,* 25–33.

Kain, K. C. (1999). Prophylactic drugs for malaria: Why do we need another one? *J Travel Med, 6,* S2–S7.

Kain, K. C., Shanks, G. D., & Keystone, J. S. (2001). Malaria chemoprophylaxis in the age of drug resistance. i. currently recommended drug regimens. *Clin Infect Dis, 33,* 226–234.

Korsinczky, M., Chen, N., Kotecka, B., Saul, A., Rieckmann, K., & Cheng, Q. (2000). Mutations in *Plasmodium falciparum* cytochrome b that are associated with atovaquone resistance are located at a putative drug-binding site. *Antimicrob Agents Chemother, 44,* 2100–2108.

Kremser, P. G., Looareesuwan, S., & Chulay, J. D. (1999). Atovaquone and proguanil hydrochloride for treatment of malaria. *J Travel Med, 6*(Suppl. 1), S18–S20.

Labbe, A. C., Loutfy, M. R., & Kain, K. C. (2001). Recent Advances in the Prophylaxis and Treatment of Malaria. *Curr Infect Dis Rep, 3,* 68–76.

Langeler, C., Smith, T. A., & Schemmenberg, J. A. (1997). Focus on the effects of bed nets on malaria morbidity and mortality. *Parasitol Today, 87,* 235–238.

Lefevre, G., Looareesuwan, S., Treeprasertsuk, S., Krudsood, S., Silachamroon, U., Gathmann, I., Mull, R., & Bakshi, R. (2001). A clinical and pharmacokinetic trial of six doses of artemether–lumefantrine for multidrug-resistant *Plasmodium falciparum* malaria in Thailand. *Amer J Trop Med Hyg, 64,* 247–256.

Lell, B., Faucher, J. F., & Missinou, M. A. (2000). Malaria chemoprophylaxis with tafenoquine: A randomized study. *Lancet, 355,* 2041–2045.

Lell, B., Luckner, D., Ndjave, M., Scott, T., & Kremsner, P. G. (1998). Randomised placebo-controlled study of atovaquone plus proguanil for malaria prophylaxis in children. *Lancet, 351,* 709–713.

Lobel, H., Varma, J., Miani, M., Green, M., Todd, G., Grady, K., & Barber, A. (1998). Monitoring for mefloquine-resistant *Plasmodium falciparum* in Africa: Implications for travellers' health. *Amer J Trop Med Hyg, 59,* 129–132.

Looareesuwan, S., Viravan, C., Webster, H. K., Kyle, D. E., Hutchinson, D. B., & Canfield, C. J. (1996). Clinical studies of atovaquone, alone or in combination with other antimalarial drugs, for treatment of acute uncomplicated malaria in Thailand. *Amer J Trop Med Hyg, 54,* 62–66.

Looareesuwan, S., Wilairatana, P., Chokejindachai, W., Chalermrut, K., Wernsdorfer, W., Gemperli, B., Gathmann, I., & Royce, C. (1999). A randomized, double-blind, comparative trial of a new oral combination of artemether and benflumetol (CGP 56697) with mefloquine in the treatment of acute *Plasmodium falciparum* malaria in Thailand. *Amer J Trop Med Hyg, 60,* 238–243.

Looareesuwan, S., Wilairatana, P., Viravan, C., Vanijanonta, S., Pitisuttithum, P., & Kyle, D. E. (1997). Open randomized trial of oral artemether alone and a sequential combination with mefloquine for acute uncomplicated falciparum malaria. *Amer J Trop Med Hyg, 56,* 613–617.

Marlar-Than, Myat-Phone-Kyaw, Aye-Yu-Soe, Khaing-Khaing-Gyi, Ma-Sabai, & Myint-Oo. (1995). Development of resistance to chloroquine by *Plasmodium vivax* in Myanmar. *Trans R Soc Trop Med Hyg, 89,* 307–308.

Mayor, A. G., Gomez-Olive, X., Aponte, J. J., Casimiro, S., Mabunda, S., Dgedge, M., Barreto, A., & Alonso, P. L. (2001). Prevalence of the K76T mutation in the putative *Plasmodium falciparum* chloroquine resistance transporter (*pfcrt*) gene and its relation to chloroquine resistance in Mozambique. *J Infect Dis, 183,* 1413–1416.

McIntosh, H. M., & Olliaro, P. (2000). Artemisinin derivatives for treating uncomplicated malaria. *Cochrane Database Syst Rev, 2,* CD000256.

Mendis, K., Sina, B. J., Marchesini, P., & Carter, R. (2001). The neglected burden of *Plasmodium vivax* malaria. *Amer J Trop Med Hyg, 64*(Suppl. 1–2), 97–106.

Murphy, G. S., Basri, H., Purnomo, Andersen, E. M., Bangs, M. J., Mount, D. L., Gorden, J., Lal, A. A., Purwokusumo, A. R., & Harjosuwarno, S. (1993). Vivax malaria resistant to treatment and prophylaxis with chloroquine. *Lancet, 341,* 96–100.

Murphy, S., & Breman, J. (2001). Gaps in the childhood malaria burden in Africa: Cerebral malaria, neurological sequelae, anemia, respiratory distress, hypoglycemia, & complications of pregnancy. *Amer J Trop Med Hyg, 64*(Suppl. 1), 57–67.

Myat-Phone-Kyaw, Myint-Oo, Myint-Lwin, Thaw-Zin, Kyin-Hla-Aye, & Nwe-Nwe-Yin. (1993). Emergence of chloroquine-resistant *Plasmodium vivax* in Myanmar (Burma). *Trans R Soc Trop Med Hyg, 87,* 687.

Na-Bangchang, K., Tippanangkosol, P., Ubalee, R., Chaovanakawee, S., Saenglertsilapachai, S., & Karbwang, J. (1999). Comparative clinical trial of four regimens of dihydroartemisinin–mefloquine in multidrug-resistant falciparum malaria. *Tropical Med Int Health, 4,* 602–610.

Nomura, T., Carlton, J. M., Baird, J. K., del Portillo, H. A., Fryauff, D. J., Rathore, D., Fidock, D. A., Su, X., Collins, W. E., McCutchan, T. F., Wootton, J. C., & Wellems, T. E. (2001). Evidence for different mechanisms of chloroquine resistance in two *Plasmodium* species that cause human malaria. *J Infect Dis, 183,* 1653–1661.

Nosten, F., McGready, R., Simpson, J. A., Thwai, K. L., Balkan, S., Cho, T., Hkirijaroen, L., Looareesuwan, S., & White, N. J. (1999). Effects of *Plasmodium vivax* malaria in pregnancy. *Lancet, 354*, 546–549.

Nosten, F., ter Kuile, F., Chongsuphajaisiddhi, T., Luxemburger, C., Webster, H. K., Edstein, M., Phaipun, L., Thew, K. L., & White, N. J. (1991). Mefloquine-resistant falciparum malaria on the Thai–Burmese border. *Lancet, 337*, 1140–1143.

Nzila, A. M., Nduati, E., Mberu, E. K., Hopkins Sibley, C., Monks, S. A., Winstanley, P. A., & Watkins, W. M. (2000a). Molecular evidence of greater selective pressure for drug resistance exerted by the long-acting antifolate pyrimethamine/sulfadoxine compared with the shorter-acting chlorproguanil/dapsone on Kenyan *Plasmodium falciparum. J Infect Dis, 181*, 2023–2028.

Nzila, A. M., Mberu, E. K., Sulo, J., Dayo, H., Winstanley, P. A., Sibley, C. H., & Watkins, W. M. (2000b). Towards an understanding of the mechanism of pyrimethamine–sulfadoxine resistance in *Plasmodium falciparum*: Genotyping of dihydrofolate reductase and dihydropteroate synthase of Kenyan parasites. *Antimicrob Agents Chemother, 44*, 991–996.

Omar, S. A., Adagu, I. S., & Warhurst, D. C. (2001). Can pretreatment screening for *dhps* and *dhfr* point mutations in *Plasmodium falciparum* infections be used to predict sulfadoxine–pyrimethamine treatment failure? *Trans R Soc Trop Med Hyg, 95*, 315–319.

Overbosch, D., Schilthuis, H., Bienzle, U., Behrens, R. H., Kain, K. C., Clarke, P. D., Toovey, S., Knobloch, J., Nothdurft, H. D., Shaw, D., Roskell, N. S., & Chulay, J. D. (2001). Atovaquone–proguanil versus mefloquine for malaria prophylaxis in nonimmune travellers: Results from a randomized, double-blind study. *Clin Infect Dis, 33*, 1015–1021.

Pagola, S., Stephens, P. W., Bohle, D. S., Kosar, A. D., & Madsen, S. K. (2000). The structure of malaria pigment beta-haematin. *Nature, 404*, 307–310.

Peel, S. A., Merritt, S. C., Handy, J., & Baric, R. S. (1993). Derivation of highly mefloquine-resistant lines from *Plasmodium falciparum* in vitro. *Amer J Trop Med Hyg, 48*, 385–397.

Peterson, D. S., Di Santi, S. M., Povoa, M., Calvosa, V. S., Do Rosario, V. E., & Wellems, T. E. (1991). Prevalence of the dihydrofolate reductase Asn-108 mutation as the basis for pyrimethamine-resistant falciparum malaria in the Brazilian Amazon. *Amer J Trop Med Hyg, 45*, 492–497.

Peterson, D. S., Milhous, W. K., & Wellems, T. E. (1990). Molecular basis of differential resistance to cycloguanil and pyrimethamine in *Plasmodium falciparum* malaria. *Proc Natl Acad Sci USA, 87*, 3018–3022.

Phillips, E. J., Keystone, J. S., & Kain, K. C. (1996). Failure of combined chloroquine and high-dose primaquine therapy for *Plasmodium vivax* malaria acquired in Guyana, South America. *Clin Infect Dis, 23*, 1171–1173.

Phillips, R. S. (2001). Current status of malaria and potential for control. *Clin Microbiol Rev, 14*, 208–226.

Pillai, D. R., Labbe, A. C., Vanisaveth, V., Hongvangthong, B., Pomphida, S., Inkathone, S., Zhong, K., & Kain, K. C. (2001). *Plasmodium falciparum* malaria in Laos: Chloroquine treatment outcome and predictive value of molecular markers. *J Infect Dis, 183*, 789–795.

Plowe, C. V., Cortese, J. F., Djimde, A., Nwanyanwu, O. C., Watkins, W. M., Winstanley, P. A., Estrada-Franco, J. G., Mollinedo, R. E., Avila, J. C., Cespedes, J. L., Carter, D., & Doumbo, O. K. (1997). Mutations in *Plasmodium falciparum* dihydrofolate reductase and dihydropteroate synthase and epidemiologic patterns of pyrimethamine–sulfadoxine use and resistance. *J Infect Dis, 176*, 1590–1596.

Price, R. N., Cassar, C., Brockman, A., Duraisingh, M., van Van Vugt, M., White, N. J., Nosten, F., & Krishna, S. (1999). The *pfmdr1* gene is associated with a multidrug-resistant phenotype in *Plasmodium falciparum* from the western border of Thailand. *Antimicrob Agents Chemother, 43*, 2943–2949.

Pudney, M., Gutteridge, W., & Zeman, A. (1999). Atovaquone and proguanil hydrochloride: A review of nonclinical studies. *J Travel Med, 6*, S8–S12.

Raccurt, C. P., Dumestre-Toulet, V., Abraham, E., Le Bras, M., Brachet-Liermain, A., & Ripert, C. (1991). Failure of falciparum malaria prophylaxis by mefloquine in travellers from West Africa. *Amer J Trop Med Hyg, 45*, 319–324.

Reed, M. B., Saliba, K. J., Caruana, S. R., Kirk, K., & Cowman, A. F. (2000). Pgh1 modulates sensitivity and resistance to multiple antimalarials in *Plasmodium falciparum. Nature, 403*, 906–909.

Riley, E. (1995). Malaria vaccine trials: SPf66 and all that. *Curr Opin Immunol, 7*, 612–616.

Rieckmann, K. H., Davis, D. R., & Hutton, D. C. (1989). *Plasmodium vivax* resistance to chloroquine? *Lancet, 2*, 1183–1184.

Sabcharoen, A., Attanath, P., Chanthavanich, P., Phanuaksook, P., Prarinyanupharb, V., Poonpanich, Y., Mookmanee, D., Teja-Isavadharm, P., Heppner, D. G., Brewer, T. G., & Chongsuphajaisiddhi, T. (1998). Comparative clinical trial of artesunate suppositories and oral artesunate in combination with mefloquine in the treatment of acute falciparum malaria. *Amer J Trop Med Hyg, 58*, 11–16.

Schlagenhauf, P. (1999). Mefloquine for malaria chemoprophylaxis 1992–1998: A review. *J Travel Med, 6*, 122–133.

Schwartlander, B. (1997). Global burden of disease. *Lancet, 350*, 141–142.

Schwartz, I. K., Lackritz, E. M., & Patchen, L. C. (1991). Chloroquine-resistant *Plasmodium vivax* from Indonesia. *N Engl J Med, 324*, 927.

Shanks, G. D. (1999). Possible options for malaria chemoprophylaxis on the horizon. *J Travel Med, 6*, S31–S32.

Shanks, G. D., Gordon, D. M., Klotz, F. W., Aleman, G. M., Oloo, A. J., Sadie, D., & Scott, T. R. (1998). Efficacy and safety of atovaquone/proguanil as suppressive prophylaxis for *Plasmodium falciparum* malaria. *Clin Infect Dis, 27*, 494–499.

Shanks, G. D., Kain, K. C., & Keystone, J. S. (2001). Malaria chemoprophylaxis in the age of drug resistance. ii. Drugs that may be available in the future. *Clin Infect Dis, 33*, 381–385.

Shanks, G. D., Kremser, P. G., & Sukwa, T. Y. (1999). Atovaquone and proguanil hydrochloride for prophylaxis of malaria. *J Travel Med, 6*, S21–S27.

Shapiro, T. A., Ranasinha, C. D., Kumar, N., & Barditch-Crovo, P. (1999). Prophylactic activity of atovaquone against *Plasmodium falciparum* in humans. *Amer J Trop Med Hyg, 60*, 831–836.

Singh, R. K. (2000). Emergence of chloroquine-resistant vivax malaria in south Bihar (India). *Trans R Soc Trop Med Hyg, 94*, 327.

Slater, A. F., Swiggard, W. J., Orton, B. R., Flitter, W. D., Goldberg, D. E., Cerami, A., & Henderson, G. B. (1991). An iron–carboxylate bond links the heme units of malaria pigment. *Proc Natl Acad Sci USA, 88*, 325–329.

Smoak, B. L., DeFraites, R. F., Magill, A. J., Kain, K. C., & Wellde, B. T. (1997). *Plasmodium vivax* infections in U.S. Army troops: Failure of primaquine to prevent relapse in studies from Somalia. *Amer J Trop Med Hyg, 56*, 231–234.

Snow, R. W., Craig, M. H., Deichmann, U., & le Sueur, D. (1999). A preliminary continental risk map for malaria mortality among African children. *Parasitol Today, 15*, 99–104.

Snow, R. W., Molyneux, C. S., Warn, P. A., Omumbo, J., Nevill, C. G., Gupta, S., & Marsh, K. (1996). Infant parasite rates and immunoglobulin M seroprevalence as a measure of exposure to *Plasmodium falciparum* during a randomized controlled trial of insecticide-treated bed nets on the Kenyan coast. *Amer J Trop Med Hyg, 55*, 144–149.

Soto, J., Toledo, J., Rodriquez, M., Sanchez, J., Herrera, R., Padilla, J., & Berman, J. (1998). Primaquine prophylaxis against malaria in nonimmune Colombian soldiers: Efficacy and toxicity. A randomized, double-blind, placebo-controlled trial. *Ann Intern Med, 129*, 241–244.

Soto, J., Toledo, J., Rodriquez, M., Sanchez, J., Herrera, R., Padilla, J., & Berman, J. (1999). Double-blind, randomized, placebo-controlled assessment of chloroquine/primaquine prophylaxis for malaria in nonimmune Colombian soldiers. *Clin Infect Dis, 29*, 199–201.

Soto, J., Toledo, J., Gutierrez, P., Luzz, M., Llinas, N., Cedeno, N., Dunne, M., & Berman, J. (2001). *Plasmodium vivax* clinically resistant to chloroquine in Colombia. *Amer J Trop Med Hyg, 65*, 90–93.

Srivastava, I. K., Morrisey, J. M., Darrouzet, E., Daldal, F., & Vaidya, A. B. (1999). Resistance mutations reveal the atovaquone-binding domain of cytochrome *b* in malaria parasites. *Mol Microbiol, 33*, 704–711.

Srivastava, I. K., Rottenberg, H., & Vaidya, A. B. (1997). Atovaquone, a broad spectrum antiparasitic drug, collapses mitochondrial membrane potential in a malarial parasite. *J Biol Chem, 272*, 3961–3966.

Srivastava, I. K., & Vaidya, A. B. (1999). A mechanism for the synergistic antimalarial action of atovaquone and proguanil. *Antimicrob Agents Chemother, 43*, 1334–1339.

Sturchler, D. (1989). How much malaria is there worldwide? *Parasitol Today, 5*, 39–40.

Su, X., Kirkman, L. A., Fujioka, H., & Wellems, T. E. (1997). Complex polymorphisms in an approximately 330 kDa protein are linked to chloroquine-resistant *P. falciparum* in Southeast Asia and Africa. *Cell, 91*, 593–603.

Sukwa, T. Y., Mulenga, M., Chisdaka, N., Roskell, N. S., & Scott, T. R. (1999). A randomized, double-blind, placebo-controlled field trial to determine the efficacy and safety of Malarone (atovaquone/proguanil) for the prophylaxis of malaria in Zambia. *Amer J Trop Med Hyg, 60*, 521–525.

Sullivan, D. J., Jr., Gluzman, I. Y., Russell, D. G., & Goldberg, D. E. (1996). On the molecular mechanism of chloroquine's antimalarial action. *Proc Natl Acad Sci USA, 93*, 11865–11870.

ter Kuile, F., Nosten, F., & Thieren, M. (1992). High dose mefloquine in the treatment of multidrug-resistant falciparum malaria. *J Infect Dis, 166*, 1393–1400.

Trape, J. F. (2001). The public health impact of chloroquine resistance in Africa. *Amer J Trop Med Hyg, 64*(Suppl. 1), 12–17.

Trape, J. F., Pison, G., Preziosi, M. P., Enel, C., Desgrees du Lou, A., Delaunay, V., Samb, B., Lagarde, E., Molez, J. F., & Simondon, F. (1998). Impact of chloroquine resistance on malaria mortality. *C R Acad Sci III, 321*, 689–697.

Trape, J. F., & Rogier, C. (1996). Combating malaria morbidity and mortality by reducing transmission. *Parsitol Today, 12*, 236–240.

Urdaneta, L., Plowe, C., Goldman, I., & Lal, A. A. (1999). Point mutations in dihydrofolate reductase and dihydropteroate synthase genes of *Plasmodium falciparum* isolates from Venezuela. *Amer J Trop Med Hyg, 61*, 457–462.

van Agtmael, M., Bouchaud, O., Malvy, D., Delmont, J., Danis, M., Barette, S., Gras, C., Bernard, J., Touze, J. E., Gathmann, I., & Mull, R. (1999). The comparative efficacy and tolerability of CGP 56697 (artemether + lumefantrine) versus halofantrine in the treatment of uncomplicated falciparum malaria in travellers returning from the Tropics to The Netherlands and France. *Int J Antimicrob Agents, 12*, 159–169.

van Hensbroek, M. B., Onyiorah, E., & Jaffar, S. (1996). A controlled trial of artemether or quinine in children with cerebral malaria. *N Engl J Med, 335*, 69–75.

van Vugt, M., Angus, B. J., Price, R. N., Mann, C., Simpson, J. A., Poletto, C., Htoo, S. E., Looareesuwan, S., White, N. J., & Nosten, F. (2000). A case-controlled auditory evaluation of patients treated with artemisinin derivatives for multidrug-resistant *Plasmodium falciparum* malaria. *Amer J Trop Med Hyg, 6*, 65–69.

van Vugt, M. V., Wilairatana, P., Gemperli, B., Gathmann, I., Phaipun, L., Brockman, A., Luxemburger, C., White, N. J., Nosten, F., & Looareesuwan, S. (1999). Efficacy of six doses of artemether–lumefantrine (benflumetol) in multidrug-resistant *Plasmodium falciparum* malaria. *Amer J Trop Med Hyg, 60*, 936–942.

von Seidlein, L., Bojang, K., Jones, P., Jaffar, S., Pinder, M., Obaro, S., Doherty, T., Haywood, M., Snounou, G., Gemperli, B., Gathmann, I., Royce, C., McAdam, K., & Greenwood, B. (1998). A randomized, controlled trial of artemether/benflumetol, a new antimalarial, & pyrimethamine/sulfadoxine in the treatment of uncomplicated falciparum malaria in African children. *Amer J Trop Med Hyg, 58*, 638–644.

von Seidlein, L., Milligan, P., Pinder, M., Bojang, K., Anyalebechi, C., Gosling, R., Coleman, R., Ude, J. I., Sadiq, A., Duraisingh, M., Warhurst, D., Alloueche, A., Targett, G., McAdam, K.,

Greenwood, B., Walraven, G., Olliaro, P., & Doherty, T. (2000). Efficacy of artesunate plus pyrimethamine–sulfadoxine for uncomplicated malaria in Gambian children: A double-blind randomized, controlled trial. *Lancet, 355*, 352–357.

Walsh, D. S., Looareesuwan, S., Wilairatana, P., Heppner, D. G. Jr., Tang, D. B., Brewer, T. G., Chokejindachai, W., Viriyavejakul, P., Kyle, D. E., Milhous, W. K., Schuster, B. G., Horton, J., Braitman, D. J., & Brueckner, R. P. (1999). Randomized dose-ranging study of the safety and efficacy of WR 238605 (tafenoquine) in the prevention of relapse of *Plasmodium vivax* malaria in Thailand. *J Infect Dis, 180*, 1282–1287.

Warhurst, D. C. (1999). Drug resistance in *Plasmodium falciparum* malaria. *Infection, 27* (Suppl. 2), S55–S58.

Wellems, T. E., Panton, L. J., Gluzman, I. Y., do Rosario, V. E., Gwadz, R. W., Walker-Jonah, A., & Krogstad, D. J. (1990). Chloroquine resistance not linked to *mdr*-like genes in a *Plasmodium falciparum* cross. *Nature, 345*, 253–255.

Wellems, T. E., & Plowe, C. V. (2001). Chloroquine-resistant malaria. *J Infect Dis, 184*, 770–776.

Wellems, T. E., Walker-Jonah, A., & Panton, L. J. (1991). Genetic mapping of the chloroquine-resistance locus on *Plasmodium falciparum* chromosome 7. *Proc Natl Acad Sci USA, 88*, 3382–3386.

Wernsdorfer, W. H., & Payne, D. (1991). The dynamics of drug resistance in *Plasmodium falciparum*. *Pharmacol Ther, 50*, 95–121.

Wesche, D. L., Schuster, B. G., Wang, W. X., & Woosley, R. L. (2000). Mechanism of cardiotoxicity of halofantrine [In Process Citation]. *Clin Pharmacol Ther, 67*, 521–529.

White, N. J. (1992). Antimalarial drug resistance: The pace quickens. *J Antimicrob Chemother, 30*, 571–585.

White, N. J. (1996). The treatment of malaria. *N Engl J Med, 335*, 800–806.

White, N. J. (1998). Drug resistance in malaria. *British Med Bull, 54*, 703–715.

White, N. J. (2000). Neurological dysfunction following malaria: Disease-or-drug related, *Clin Infect Dis, 30*, 836.

White, N. J., Nosten, F., & Looareesuwan, S. (1999). Averting a malaria disaster. *Lancet, 353*, 1965–1967.

White, N. J., & Olliaro, P. L. (1996). Strategies for the prevention of antimalarial drug resistance: Rationale for combination chemotherapy for malaria. *Parasitol Today, 12*, 399–401.

Wilairatana, P., Silachamroon, U., Krudsood, S., Singhasivanon, P., Treeprasertsuk, S., Bussaratid, V., Phumratanaprapin, W., Srivilirit, S., & Looareesuwan, S. (1999). Efficacy of primaquine regimens for primaquine-resistant *Plasmodium vivax* malaria in Thailand. *Amer J Trop Med Hyg, 61*, 973–977.

Wilson, C. M., Serrano, A. E., Wasley, A., Bogenschutz, M. P., Shankar, A. H., & Wirth, D. F. (1989). Amplification of a gene related to mammalian *mdr* genes in drug-resistant *Plasmodium falciparum*. *Science, 244*, 1184–1186.

Wilson, C. M., Volkman, S. K., Thaithong, S., Martin, R. K., Kyle, D. E., Milhous, W. K., & Wirth, D. F. (1993). Amplification of pfmdr 1 associated with mefloquine and halofantrine resistance in *Plasmodium falciparum* from Thailand. *Mol Biochem Parasitol, 57*, 151–160.

Wongsrichanalai, C., Webster, H. K., Wimonwattrawatee, T., Sookto, P., Chuanak, N., Thimasarn, K., & Wernsdorfer, W. H. (1992). Emergence of multidrug-resistant *Plasmodium falciparum* in Thailand: In vitro tracking. *Amer J Trop Med Hyg, 47*, 112–116.

World Health Organization, 1995, Vector control for malaria and other mosquito-borne diseases. *World Health Organ Tech Rep Ser, 857*, 1–97.

World Health Organization. (1997). World malaria situation in 1994. Part I. Population at risk. *Wkly Epidemiol Rec, 72*, 269–274.

World Health Organization. (2000). WHO Expert Committee on Malaria. *World Health Organ Tech Rep Ser, 892*, i–v, 1–74.

Young, M. D., & Moore, D. V. (1961). Chloroquine resistance in *Plasmodium falciparum*. *Amer J Trop Med Hyg, 10*, 317–320.

Index

Index